Springer
Specialist
Surgery
Series

*Other titles in this series include:*

Transplantation Surgery, edited by Hakim & Danovitch, 2001
Neurosurgery: Principles and Practice, edited by Moore & Newell, 2004

John W. L. Fielding and Michael T. Hallissey

# Upper Gastrointestinal Surgery

Series Editor: John Lumley

With 156 Illustrations

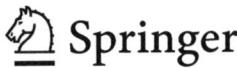

John W. L. Fielding
Department of Surgery
The Queen Elizabeth Hospital
Birmingham, UK

Michael T. Hallissey
Department of Surgery
The Queen Elizabeth Hospital
Birmingham, UK

British Library Cataloguing in Publication Data
Upper gastrointestinal surgery – (Springer specialist surgery series)
  1. Digestive organs – Surgery
  I. Fielding, J. W. L. (John William Lewis) II. Hallissey, Michael T.
  617.4′3

Library of Congress Cataloging-in-Publication Data
Upper gastrointestinal surgery/[edited by] John W. L. Fielding and Michael T. Hallissey.
    p.cm. – (Springer specialist surgery series)
    Includes bibliographical references and index.

  1. Digestive organs – Surgery.   2. Gastrointestinal system – Surgery.   3. Liver – Surgery.
  4. Upper Gastrointestinal Surgery.   I. Fielding, J. W. L.   II. Hallissey, Michael T.   III. Series.
  [DNLM:   1. Digestive System Surgical Procedures.   2. Biliary Tract Diseases – surgery.
  3. Gastrointestinal Diseases – surgery.   4. Liver Diseases – surgery. WI 900 H529 2004]
RD540.5.H47 2004
617.4′3–dc22                              2004042555

Apart from any fair dealing for the purposes of research or private study, or criticism or review, as permitted under the Copyright, Designs and Patents Act 1988, this publication may only be reproduced, stored or transmitted, in any form or by any means, with the prior permission in writing of the publishers, or in the case of reprographic reproduction in accordance with the terms of licences issued by the Copyright Licensing Agency. Enquiries concerning reproduction outside those terms should be sent to the publishers.

ISBN 978-1-84996-888-1           e-ISBN 978-1-84628-066-5
Springer-Verlag is part of Springer Science+Business Media
Springeronline.com

© Springer-Verlag London Limited 2005
Softcover reprint of the hardcover 1st edition 2005

The use of registered names, trademarks, etc. in this publication does not imply, even in the absence of a specific statement, that such names are exempt from the relevant laws and regulations and therefore free for general use.

Product liability: The publisher can give no guarantee for information about drug dosage and application thereof contained in this book. In every individual case the respective user must check its accuracy by consulting other pharmaceutical literature.

28/3830-543210 Printed on acid-free paper

# Foreword

Surgical practice and training are undergoing a worldwide revolution, with increased super-specialisation, at the expense of the generalist, giving rise to much heated debate. The pathway towards specialisation has been accompanied by an increase in interdisciplinary care, with the development of the multidisciplinary team approach. This has included expansion of diagnostic imaging, and of medical, chemotherapy and radio therapeutic regimes. The introduction of minimally invasive techniques and image guidance, have increased surgical precision and refinement, while in other areas interventional radiology has become the treatment of choice.

Training and assessment have followed these trends, but often in a disorganised fashion, without due concern for curricular development and adequate integration of basic and advanced educational requirements.

Regardless of these arguments, all surgeons working in a field require appropriate skills and the best available information to deliver optimal care; the *Springer Specialist Surgical Series* addresses these needs.

This volume considers the upper gastrointestinal tract, from the oesophagus to the small bowel. The liver, biliary tree and pancreas make up a separate volume, but the spleen, that orphan of the upper abdomen, is expertly covered, providing the reader with an added bonus.

The editors have skilfully chosen topics that provide a comprehensive cover of the field, while emphasizing the growing edges and future direction of their speciality. They have brought together a unique group of authors, each a recognized expert in the field. The resultant text is compelling and essential reading for all those involved in the management of disease of the upper alimentary tract, whatever their discipline.

# Contents

**Foreword**
*by Professor John Lumley* .................................................. v

**Contributors** .................................................. ix

1. The Anatomy and Physiology of the Oesophagus
   *Peter J. Lamb and S. Michael Griffin* .................................. 1

2. The Anatomy and Physiology of the Stomach
   *Ian R. Daniels and William H. Allum* .................................. 17

3. The Anatomy and Physiology of the Small Bowel
   *David Gourevitch* .................................................. 39

4. The Anatomy and Physiology of the Diaphragm
   *George R. Harrison* .................................................. 45

5. The Spleen
   *Hugo W. Tilanus* .................................................. 59

6. Benign Disease of the Oesophagus
   *Stephen E.A. Attwood and Christopher J. Lewis* .................. 69

7. Benign Diseases of the Stomach
   *Robert C. Mason* .................................................. 91

8. Benign Disease of the Small Bowel
   *Ling S. Wong, Emmanuel A. Agaba and Michael R.B. Keighley* .... 101

9. Benign Disease of the Diaphragm
   *Juliet E. King and Pala B. Rajesh* .................................. 117

10. Benign Diseases of the Spleen
    *Refaat B. Kamel* .................................................. 127

11. Epithelial Neoplasms of the Oesophagus
    *Derek Alderson and Jonathan H. Vickers* .................. 155

12. Epithelial Neoplasms of the Stomach
    *Peter McCulloch* .................................................. 167

13. Cancer at the Gastro-oesophageal Junction (Epidemiology)
    Gill M. Lawrence .......................................... 181

14. Neoplasms of the Small Bowel
    Aviram Nissan and Martin S. Karpeh ........................ 193

15. Stromal Upper GI Tract Neoplasms
    Stephan T. Samel and Stefan Post ........................... 207

16. Neoplasms of the Spleen
    Mark G. Coleman and Michael R. Thompson ................... 221

17. Lymphomas
    Mark Deakin, A. Murray Brunt, Mark Stephens and
    Richard C. Chasty ......................................... 231

18. Pathology of the Oesophagus and Stomach
    Sukhvinder S. Ghataura and David C. Rowlands .............. 241

19. Premalignant Lesions of the Oesophagus: Identification
    to Management
    Andrew Latchford and Janusz A.Z. Jankowski ................ 259

20. High Risk Lesions in the Stomach
    Marc C. Winslet and S. Frances Hughes ..................... 271

21. Upper GI Endoscopy
    Michael T. Hallissey ...................................... 279

22. Imaging in GI Surgery
    Julie F. C. Olliff and Peter J. Guest ..................... 287

23. High Risk Lesions in the Oesophagus and Nuclear Medicine
    Andrew Phillip Chilton and Janusz A. Z. Jankowski ......... 307

24. Surgical Resection for Oesophageal Cancer: Role of Extended
    Lymphadenectomy
    Hubert J. Stein, Jörg Theisen and Jörg-Rüdiger Siewert .... 317

25. Surgical Resection of the Stomach with Lymph Node Dissection
    Mitsuru Sasako, Takeo Fukagawa, Hitoshi Katai and Takeshi Sano  335

26. Chemotherapy of Upper GI Neoplasms: Proven/Unproven
    Niall C. Tebbutt and David Cunningham ..................... 349

27. Radiotherapy in Upper GI Tract Neoplasms
    M. Suhail Anwar, Ju Ian Geh and David Spooner ............. 359

Index ........................................................ 369

# Contributors

Emmanuel A. Agaba MB BS, FRCS
Department of Surgery
Walsgrave Hospital
University Hospitals Coventry and
Warwickshire NHS Trust
Coventry
UK

Derek Alderson MB BS, MD, FRCS
Division of Surgery
University Department of Surgery
Bristol Royal Infirmary
Bristol
UK

William H. Allum BSc, MD, FRCS
Department of Surgery
Royal Marsden Hospital NHS Trust
Sutton
Surrey
UK

M. Suhail Anwar BSc, MBBS, MRCP,
FRCR
Department of Oncology
Cancer Centre
Queen Elizabeth Hospital
Birmingham
UK

Stephen E. A. Attwood MD, MB BCh,
FRCSI, FRCS
Regional Laparoscopic Unit
Northumbria Healthcare Trust
North Tyneside
Northumberland
UK

A. Murray Brunt MB BS, MRCP, FRCR
Department of Oncology
University Hospital of North Staffordshire
Stoke-on-Trent
UK

Richard C. Chasty MB BS, MD, FRCP,
MRCPath
Department of Haematology
University Hospital of North Staffordshire
Stoke-on-Trent
UK

Andrew Phillip Chilton MRCP
Department of Gastroenterology
Kettering General Hospital
Kettering
Northamptonshire
UK

Mark G. Coleman MD, FRCS
The Colorectal Unit
Derriford Hospital
Plymouth
UK

David Cunningham MD, FRCP
Department of Medicine
The Royal Marsden Hospital
Sutton, Surrey
UK

Ian R. Daniels MB, FRCS
Department of Surgery
Pelican Centre
North Hampshire Hospital
Basingstoke
Hampshire, UK

Mark Deakin ChM, FRCS, FRCSE
Department of Surgery
University Hospital of North Staffordshire
Stoke on Trent
UK

John W. L. Fielding MD, FRCS
Department of Surgery
Queen Elizabeth Hospital
Birmingham
UK

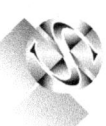

## CONTRIBUTORS

Takeo Fukagawa MD, PhD
Department of Surgical Oncology
National Cancer Centre Hospital
Tokyo
Japan

Ju Ian Geh MB BS, MRCP, FRCR
Department of Oncology
Cancer Centre
Queen Elizabeth Hospital
Birmingham, UK

Sukhvinder S. Ghataura MB ChB, FRCS
Department of Pathology
Medical School
University Hospital
Birmingham, UK

David Gourevitch MBChB, MD, FRCP
Department of Surgery
Upper GI Surgical Unit
Queen Elizabeth Hospital
Birmingham
UK

S. Michael Griffin MB BS, MD, FRCS
Northern Oesophago-Gastric Unit
Royal Victoria Infirmary
Newcastle upon Tyne
UK

Peter J. Guest MRCP, FRCR
Department of Imaging
University Hospital Birmingham
Queen Elizabeth Hospital
Birmingham
UK

Michael T. Hallissey MD, FRCS
Queen Elizabeth Medical Centre
Department of Surgery
Queen Elizabeth Hospital
Birmingham
UK

George R. Harrison BSc, MB BS, FFARCS
Department of Pain Management
Selly Oak Hospital
Birmingham
UK

S. Frances Hughes MS, FRCS
Department of Surgery
Royal London and St Bartholomew's
Hospital
London, UK

Janusz A. Z. Jankowski FRCP, PhD, MD,
MRCP, MB ChB
University Department of Cancer Studies
and Molecular Medicine
Leicester Medical School
Leicester Royal Infirmary
Leicester
UK

Refaat B. Kamel MD, FICS, FACS
Department of General Surgery
Faculty of Medicine
Ain-Shams University
International College of Surgeons
Cairo
Egypt

Martin S. Karpeh MD
The State University of New York
Division of Surgical Oncology
Health Sciences Center
Stony Brook, NY
USA

Hitoshi Katai MD, PhD
Department of Surgical Oncology
National Cancer Centre Hospital
Tokyo
Japan

Michael R.B. Keighley MB BS, MS, FRCS
Department of Surgery
University of Birmingham
Queen Elizabeth Hospital
Birmingham
UK

Juliet E. King BM, FRCS
Department of Thoracic Surgery
Birmingham Heartlands Hospital
Birmingham
UK

Peter J. Lamb MB BS, FRCS
Northern Oesophago-Gastric Cancer Unit
Royal Victoria Infirmary
Newcastle upon Tyne
UK

Andrew Latchford MB BS, BSc, MRCP
Department of Gastroenterology
St Mark's Hospital
Harrow
Middlesex
UK

# CONTRIBUTORS

Gill M. Lawrence PhD
West Midlands Cancer Intelligence Unit
The University of Birmingham
Birmingham

Christopher J. Lewis MB BCh, MRCS
Department of Upper GI Surgery
Hope Hospital
Salford
UK

Robert C. Mason BSc, MB ChB, MD, FRCS
Department of Surgery
St Thomas' Hospital
London
UK

Peter McCulloch MB ChB, MD, FRCS
Academic Unit of Surgery
University Hospital Aintree
University of Liverpool
Liverpool, UK

Aviram Nissan MD
Gastric and Mixed Tumor Service
Department of Surgery
Memoral Sloan-Kettering Cancer Center
New York, NY
USA

Julie F.C. Olliff MRCP, FRCR
Department of Imaging
University Hospital Birmingham
Queen Elizabeth Hospital
Birmingham
UK

Stefan Post MD
Surgery Clinic
University Hospital
Mannheim
Germany

Pala B. Rajesh MB BS, FRCS, FETCS
Regional Department of Thoracic Surgery
Birmingham Heartlands Hospital
Birmingham
UK

David C. Rowlands FRCPath
Department of Histopathology
The Medical School
University of Birmingham
Queen Elizabeth Medical Centre
Birmingham
UK

Stephan T. Samel MD
Group Practice Dres. Schiller / Samel
Göttingen
Germany

Takeshi Sano MD, PhD
Department of Surgical Oncology
National Cancer Centre Hospital
Tokyo
Japan

Mitsuru Sasako MD, PhD
Department of Surgical Oncology
National Cancer Center Hospital
Tokyo
Japan

Jörg-Rüdiger Siewert MD, FACS, FRCS
Chiurg. Klinik und Poliklinik
Klinikum rechts der Isar der TU München
München
Germany

David Spooner MB ChB, BSc, FRCP, MRCP, FRCR
Department of Oncology
Cancer Centre
Queen Elizabeth Hospital
Birmingham
UK

Hubert J. Stein MD
Chirurgische Klinik und Poliklinik
Klinikum rechts der Isar der TU München
München
Germany

Mark Stephens MB BCh, MRCPath
Department of Histopathology
Central Pathology Laboratory
Stoke-on-Trent
UK

Niall C. Tebbutt BM BCh, PhD, MRCP, FRACP
Department of Oncology
Austin Hospital
Heidelberg, Victoria
Australia

Jörg Theisen MD
Chirurgische Klinik und Poliklinik
Klinikum rechts der Isar der TU München
München
Germany

## CONTRIBUTORS

Michael R. Thompson MD, FRCS
Department of Surgery
Queen Alexandra Hospital
Portsmouth

Hugo W. Tilanus MD, PhD
Department of Gastrointestinal Surgery and Transplantation
Erasmus Medical Centre
Rotterdam
Netherlands

Jonathan H. Vickers MD ChB, BSc
Department of Surgery
Weston General Hospital
Weston Super Mare
North Somerset
UK

Marc C. Winslet MS, FRCS
Department of Surgery
Royal Free & University College Medical School
The Royal Free Hospital
London
UK

Ling S. Wong MD, FRCS
Department of Surgery
Walsgrave Hospital
University Hospitals Coventry and Warwickshire NHS Trust
Coventry
UK

# 1

# The Anatomy and Physiology of the Oesophagus

Peter J. Lamb and S. Michael Griffin

## Aims

- To develop an understanding of the surgical anatomy of the oesophagus.
- To establish the normal physiology and control of swallowing.
- To determine the structure and function of the antireflux barrier.
- To evaluate the effect of surgery on the function of the oesophagus.

## Introduction

The oesophagus is a muscular tube connecting the pharynx to the stomach and measuring 25–30 cm in the adult. Its primary function is as a conduit for the passage of swallowed food and fluid, which it propels by antegrade peristaltic contraction. It also serves to prevent the reflux of gastric contents whilst allowing regurgitation, vomiting and belching to take place. It is aided in these functions by the upper and lower oesophageal sphincters sited at its proximal and distal ends. Any impairment of oesophageal function can lead to the debilitating symptoms of dysphagia, gastro-oesophageal reflux or oesophageal pain.

The apparently simple basic structure of the oesophagus belies both its physiological importance and the dangers associated with surgical intervention. As a consequence of its location deep within the thorax and abdomen, a close anatomical relationship to major structures throughout its course and a marginal blood supply, the surgical exposure, resection and reconstruction of the oesophagus are complex. Despite advances in perioperative care, oesophagectomy is still associated with the highest mortality of any routinely performed elective surgical procedure [1].

In order to understand the pathophysiology of oesophageal disease and the rationale for its medical and surgical management a basic knowledge of oesophageal anatomy and physiology is essential. The embryological development of the oesophagus, its anatomical structure and relationships, the physiology of its major functions and the effect that surgery has on them will all be considered in this chapter.

## Embryology

The embryonic development of the oesophagus like that of all major organ systems takes place between the fourth and eighth weeks of gestation as the three germ layers differentiate into specific tissues. During the fourth week, as the embryo folds, part of the dorsal yolk sac is incorporated into the developing head as the foregut (Figure 1.1a). This ultimately develops into not only the oesophagus, stomach and duodenum but also the pharynx, lower respiratory system, liver, pancreas and biliary tree.

Early in the fourth week the laryngotracheal diverticulum develops in the midline of the ventral wall of the foregut. This extends caudally and becomes separated from the foregut by growth of the tracheo-oesophageal folds, which fuse to form the tracheo-oesophageal septum (Figure 1.1b and c). This creates the laryngotracheal tube (ultimately the larynx, trachea, bronchi and lungs) and dorsally the oesophagus [2]. Failure of this separation can occur due to a shortage of proliferating endothelial cells in the tracheo-oesophageal folds. This results in a tracheo-oesophageal fistula, which is commonly associated with oesophageal atresia. Complete failure to close the tracheo-oesophageal septum is much less common and results in a laryngo-oesophageal cleft. Normally the oesophagus lengthens rapidly as a result of cranial body growth (with descent of the heart and lungs) to reach its final relative length by the seventh week. During elongation the lumen is temporarily obliterated by proliferation of endodermal cells and failure to recanalise results in oesophageal atresia.

Oesophageal atresia is present in approximately 1 in 3000 live births. In 85% of cases there is proximal oesophageal atresia with a fistula between the distal oesophagus and the respiratory tract, usually the trachea. Less common combinations are oesophageal atresia without a fistula (10%), a fistula without atresia (2%) and a fistula between the upper oesophagus and trachea (1%). Because of the embryonic time period during which these failures take place 50% of oesophageal malformations are associated with major defects in other organ systems. In 25% these are cardiovascular, most commonly a patent ductus arteriosus, although musculoskeletal and other gastrointestinal defects, classically an imperforate anus, are also seen.

The artery of the foregut is the coeliac axis and whilst this supplies the distal oesophagus, more proximally it takes branches directly from the developing aorta. During the developmental sequence described, the epithelium and glands of the oesophagus are derived from endoderm. The striated skeletal muscle of the proximal third of the oesophagus is derived from mesenchyme in the caudal branchial arches whilst the smooth muscle of the more distal oesophagus develops from surrounding splanchnic mesenchyme. Even in the fetus the oesophagus is of vital functional importance, allowing swallowed amniotic fluid to pass to the intestines for absorption and placental transfer to maternal blood.

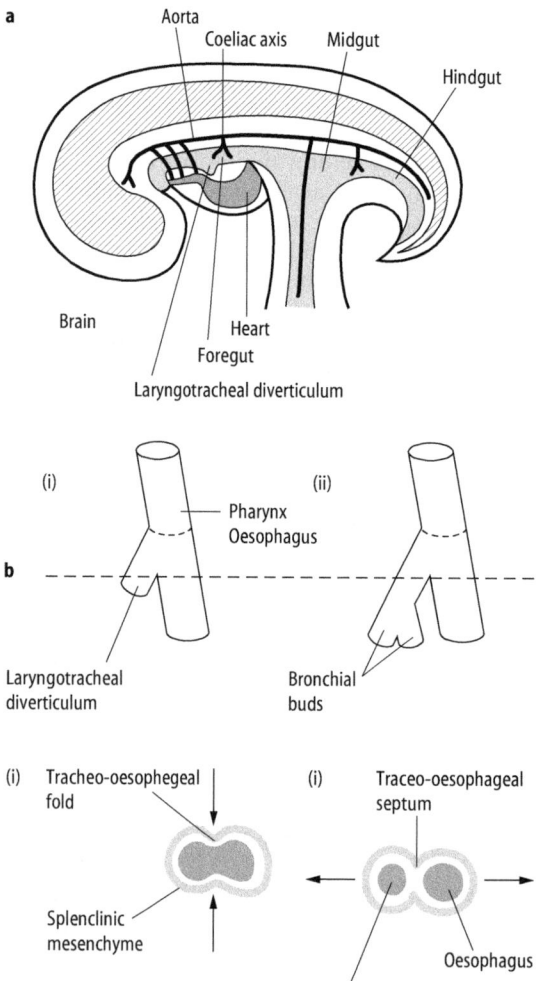

**Figure 1.1. a–c** The embryological development of the oesophagus. **a** Sagittal section of a 4-week-old embryo. **b–c** The development of the tracheo-oesophageal septum and separation of the oesophagus and laryngotracheal tube.

# Adult Oesophageal Anatomy

The oesophagus is a muscular tube protected at its ends by the upper and lower oesophageal

# THE ANATOMY AND PHYSIOLOGY OF THE OESOPHAGUS

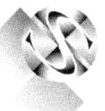

sphincters. It commences as a continuation of the pharynx at the lower border of the cricopharyngeus muscle, at the level of the sixth cervical vertebra (C6). The surface marking for this point is the lower border of the cricoid cartilage. It enters the chest at the level of the suprasternal notch and descends through the superior and posterior mediastinum along the front of the vertebral column. It passes though the oesophageal hiatus in the diaphragm at the level of the tenth thoracic vertebra to end at the gastro-oesophageal junction. The surface marking for this point is the left seventh costal cartilage. The oesophagus measures 25–30 cm in length although this varies according to the height of the individual and in particular the suprasternal–xiphoid distance.

## Anatomical Relationships of the Oesophagus

The oesophagus can be artificially divided from proximal to distal into cervical, thoracic and abdominal segments [3] (Figure 1.2).

### Cervical Oesophagus

This begins at the lower border of the cricoid cartilage (C6) and ends at the level of the thoracic inlet or jugular notch (T1). It lies between the trachea anteriorly and the prevertebral layer of cervical fascia posteriorly, deviating slightly to the left at the level of the thyroid gland before returning to enter the thorax in the midline (Figure 1.3). The recurrent laryngeal nerves run in a caudal direction either side of the oesophagus in the tracheo-oesophageal groove. They innervate the laryngeal muscles and surgical trauma to the nerve at this point results in an ipsilateral vocal cord palsy. More laterally lie the lobes of the thyroid gland with the inferior thyroid artery and the carotid sheath containing the carotid vessels and the vagus nerve.

### Thoracic Oesophagus

The upper thoracic oesophagus extends the length of the superior mediastinum between the thoracic inlet and the level of the carina (T5). The middle and lower thoracic oesophagus lies

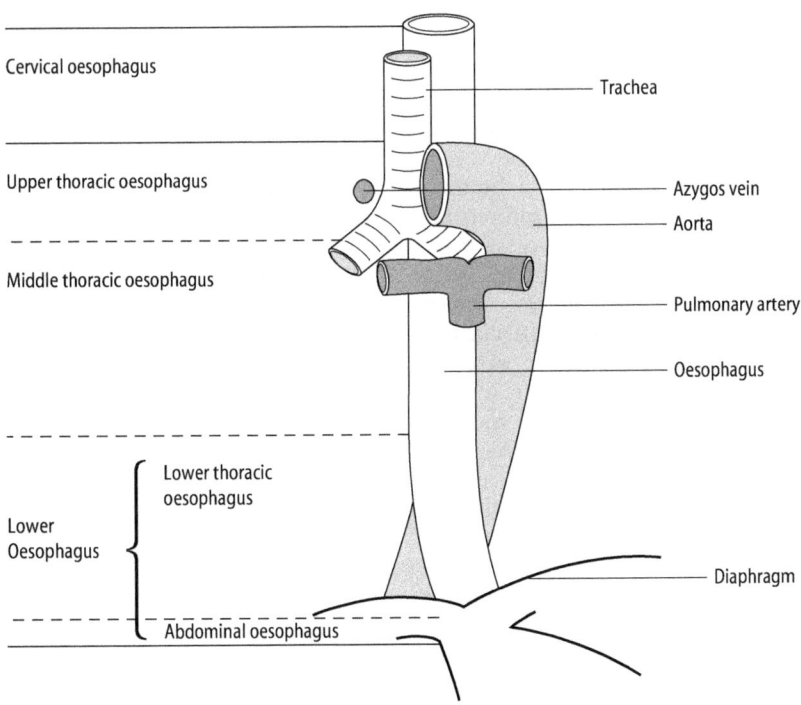

**Figure 1.2.** The divisions and anatomical relations of the oesophagus.

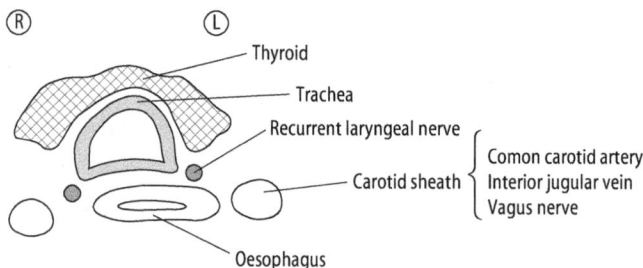

**Figure 1.3.** Cross-section of the oesophagus in the lower neck.

in the posterior mediastinum subdivided by the midpoint between the tracheal bifurcation and the oesophagogastric junction (Figure 1.2).

In the superior mediastinum the upper thoracic oesophagus maintains close contact with the left mediastinal pleura and posteriorly with the prevertebral fascia. At this level the oesophagus is indented by the arch of the aorta on its left side and crossed by the azygos vein on its right side. As it descends into the posterior mediastinum it is also crossed anteriorly and indented by the left main bronchus and crossed by the right pulmonary artery (Figure 1.2). Below this level the pericardium and left atrium lie anterior to the oesophagus.

The middle thoracic oesophagus deviates to the right, coming into close apposition with the right mediastinal pleura, which covers its right side and posterior aspect. It also moves forward with a concavity more marked than the vertebral column, allowing the azygos vein, the thoracic duct, the right upper five intercostal arteries and the descending aorta to all pass posteriorly during its course.

The azygos vein originates in the upper abdomen and enters the mediastinum via the aortic opening in the diaphragm. It ascends along the right posterolateral aspect of the oesophagus before arching over the root of the right lung to enter the superior vena cava (Figure 1.2). Resection of this arch allows improved surgical access to the oesophagus via the right chest. The thoracic duct originates in the cisterna chyli anterior to the second lumbar vertebra and passes through the diaphragmatic hiatus on the right side of the aorta posterior to the right crus. It provides lymphatic drainage for the lower body and the left half of the upper body. The duct lies on the right lateral aspect of the descending thoracic aorta in the inferior mediastinum. It is here that the duct or its radicals may be inadvertently damaged during mobilisation of the oesophagus, resulting in a chylothorax [4]. The duct then ascends, passing behind the oesophagus to lie on its left side in the superior mediastinum. The oesophagus initially lies to the right of the descending aorta but crosses it during its descent to lie anterior and on its left side as it approaches the diaphragm.

## Abdominal Oesophagus

The lower oesophagus comprises the lower thoracic, oesophagus together with the short intra-abdominal portion of oesophagus (Figure 1.2). The oesophageal opening in the diaphragm lies within fibres of the left crus inside a sling of fibres passing across from the right crus. At this point the vagal trunks lie on the anterior and posterior surface of the oesophagus having emerged from the oesophageal plexuses on its lower surface. The oesophageal branches of the left gastric artery with associated veins and lymphatics also accompany the oesophagus. The intra-abdominal portion of the oesophagus extends from the diaphragm to the gastro-oesophageal junction. It is covered by peritoneum (the gastrophrenic ligament) and lies posterior to the left lobe of the liver. It is usually 1–2 cm in length although even in the normal individual this varies according to the muscle tone, degree of gastric distension and respiration.

Although essentially a midline structure, these deviations of the oesophagus to the left in the neck, to the right in the posterior mediastinum and left and anteriorly towards the diaphragmatic hiatus have important clinical consequences. This course must be considered carefully when the surgical approach to the

# THE ANATOMY AND PHYSIOLOGY OF THE OESOPHAGUS

oesophagus is determined. For optimum exposure the cervical oesophagus should be approached from the left side of the neck, the thoracic oesophagus from the right side of the thorax and the lower oesophagus and the gastro-oesophageal junction from the abdomen or by a left thoraco-abdominal approach [5].

## Endoscopic Anatomy

These relations are also important when we consider the endoscopic anatomy of the oesophagus. By consensus endoscopic landmarks are identified by their distance in centimetres from the incisor teeth, measured with the flexible video-endoscope. The narrowest point of the oesophagus is its commencement at the level of cricopharyngeus (upper oesophageal sphincter), 15 cm from the incisors. Further indentations are caused by the aortic arch at 22 cm, the left main bronchus at 27 cm and the diaphragm at 38 cm. All distances vary according to the height of the individual. An enlarged left atrium may also indent the anterior aspect of the lower oesophagus.

The gastro-oesophageal junction is defined endoscopically as the upper margin of the proximal gastric folds. On average this is at 37 cm in females and 40 cm in males although it migrates proximally in the case of a sliding hiatus hernia. The squamocolumnar junction is also visible endoscopically as the Z-line and usually coincides with the gastro-oesophageal junction, although it may be more proximal in the presence of Barrett's oesophagus where there is columnarisation of the lower oesophagus [6].

## Attachments of the Oesophagus

The oesophagus is held in loose areolar tissue in the mediastinum, allowing sizable vertical movement during respiration. Within this are slips of smooth muscle fibres tethering it to neighbouring structures, notably the trachea, left bronchus, pericardium and aorta. The major oesophageal attachment, however, is dorsally, the phreno-oesophageal ligament. This condensation of connective tissue is an extension of the diaphragmatic and thoracic fascia. Its upper and lower limbs tether the lower few centimetres of the thoracic oesophagus and the gastro-oesophageal junction to the aorta and the diaphragmatic hiatus. It is weak anteriorly and laterally but the posterior aspect is strong and serves to maintain the intra-abdominal position of the gastro-oesophageal junction and lower oesophageal sphincter. Weakening of the phreno-oesophageal ligament allows the oesophagus to rise, resulting in a sliding type of hiatus hernia. The ligament also maintains the angle between the distal oesophagus and the proximal stomach (the angle of His), allowing a mucosal fold of the greater curve aspect of the gastro-oesophageal junction to close against the lesser curvature. The flap valve created may have a role in the antireflux mechanism of the gastro-oesophageal junction.

## Structure of the Oesophagus

### Upper Oesophageal Sphincter (UOS)

This creates a zone of high pressure between the pharynx and the proximal oesophagus, which relaxes during swallowing and prevents aerophagia during respiration. At this level horizontal fibres of the cricopharyngeus muscle pass posteriorly from the cricoid bone to join the inferior pharyngeal constrictor and create a continuous muscular band. Posteriorly just proximal to cricopharyngeus there is a relative weakness, Killian's triangle, that is the origin of a pharyngeal pouch.

### Body of the Oesophagus

Histologically this is made up of four layers: adventitia, muscle, submucosa and mucosa (Figure 1.4). In the mediastinum the oesophagus has no serosal covering and the dense connective tissue of the adventitia forms its outer layer. The muscular layer is composed of an outer longitudinal and an inner circular layer. Proximally, the longitudinal fibres originate from the dorsal aspect of the cricoid and the cricopharyngeus tendon to descend in a gentle spiral. These longitudinal muscle fibres split above the gastro-oesophageal junction creating a potential vertical weakness on the left posterolateral aspect. This is the most common site of a tear in the case of spontaneous rupture of the oesophagus (Boerhaave's syndrome). The circular muscle layer is continuous proximally with the inferior constrictor and the muscle fibre arrangement is elliptical in nature. This is designed for peristalsis, to propel food to the stomach and clear refluxed gastric contents

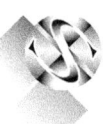

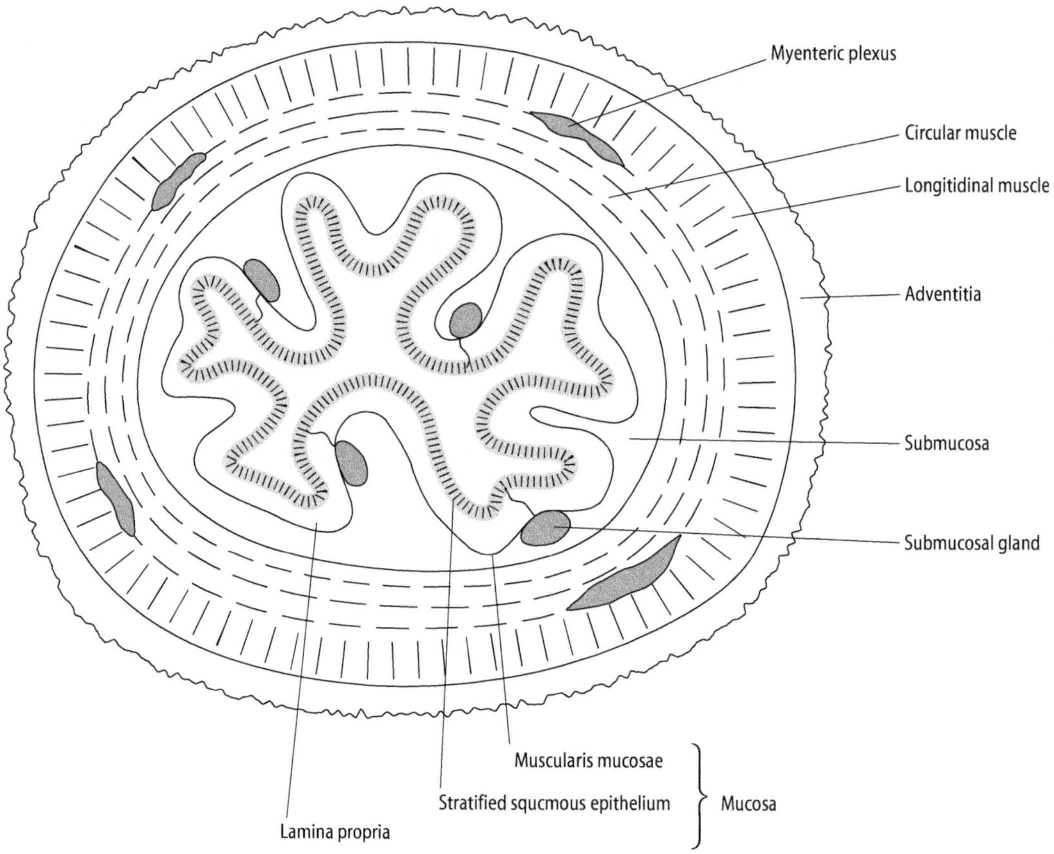

**Figure 1.4.** Histological cross-section of the oesophageal wall.

from the oesophagus. The proximal 4–6 cm of both layers of oesophageal muscle is striated. There is a mixture of striated and smooth muscle below this to around 10–13 cm and the lower half to one-third of the oesophagus contains only smooth muscle [7].

The submucosal layer consists of elastin fibres within a loose connective tissue and allows distension of the oesophagus during swallowing. The absence of a serosal layer makes oesophageal anastomosis technically difficult and reliant upon the strength of the submucosa. It transmits abundant lymphatic channels, blood vessels, and the submucosal nerve plexus. It also contains oesophageal glands, which open into the lumen via a long single duct. These secrete mucus for bolus lubrication, bicarbonate ions to neutralise refluxed acid and growth factors that help to maintain the integrity of the oesophageal epithelium.

The oesophageal mucosa is a non-keratinised stratified squamous epithelium with a basement membrane separating it from the underlying lamina propria and muscularis mucosa (Figure 1.4). This changes close to the gastro-oesophageal junction to a columnar-lined gastric epithelium at the squamocolumnar junction. In Barrett's oesophagus columnar metaplasia of the lower oesophagus occurs as a response to chronic acid and bile reflux characterised histologically by intestinal metaplasia and the presence of goblet cells [8].

## Lower Oesophageal Sphincter (LOS)

Although there is a functional high-pressure zone in the lower oesophagus, the presence of an anatomical sphincter has been disputed. There is, however, an increase in the circular muscle layer at this level and ultrastructural

# THE ANATOMY AND PHYSIOLOGY OF THE OESOPHAGUS

studies have demonstrated morphological alterations in the muscle cells of this area.

## Blood Supply and Lymphatic Drainage of the Oesophagus

### Arterial Supply

The oesophagus receives a segmental blood supply with extensive collaterals along its course (Figure 1.5). In the neck and superior mediastinum it is primarily supplied by vessels from the inferior thyroid artery, a branch of the subclavian artery. Rarely these may be supported by smaller vessels directly from the common carotid, vertebral or subclavian arteries. In the posterior mediastinum the oesophagus receives direct aortic branches. These short vessels must be carefully identified during mobilisation of the oesophagus and ligated in continuity to prevent avulsion from the aorta. They anastomose with bronchial arteries that enter the oesophagus at the tracheal bifurcation, and small branches from the intercostal arteries. The lower oesophagus receives its main supply from ascending branches of the left gastric artery, originating from the coeliac axis, aided by the left inferior phrenic artery. Although the nutrient arteries to the oesophagus are not end arteries, this segmental supply must be carefully considered during surgical reconstruction of the oesophagus to prevent ischaemic complications.

### Venous Drainage

This commences along the length of the oesophagus with the submucosal venous plexus, which drains into an extrinsic plexus on the oesophageal surface. As with the arterial supply, the precise venous drainage is variable. From the upper oesophagus it is via the inferior thyroid veins to the brachiocephalic vein and in the mediastinum it is via the azygos and hemi-azygos systems that ultimately drain into the superior vena cava. However, from the lower oesophagus it is via tributaries of the left gastric vein, which empties into the portal vein creating a portosystemic anastomosis in the lower oesophagus. In the presence of portal venous hypertension raised pressure is transmitted to the submucosal plexus of the lower oesophagus, creating fragile varicosities. These oesophageal varices are important clinically as a major cause of massive upper gastrointestinal haemorrhage. The direct communication with both the systemic and portal systems may also be important in the metastatic dissemination of oesophageal carcinoma.

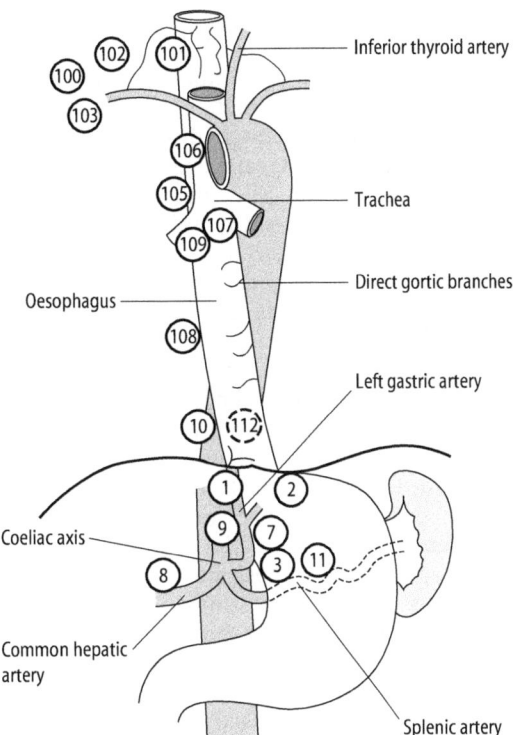

**Figure 1.5.** Arterial blood supply and lymphatic drainage of the oesophagus. *Cervical lymph nodes*: 100, lateral cervical; 101, cervical para-oesophageal; 102, deep cervical; 103, supraclavicular. *Mediastinal lymph nodes*: 105, upper para-oesophageal; 106, paratracheal; 107, carinal; 108, middle para-oesophageal; 109, left and right bronchial; 110, lower para-oesophageal; 112, posterior mediastinal. *Abdominal lymph nodes*: 1, right paracardial; 2, left paracardial; 3, lesser curve; 7, left gastric; 8, common hepatic; 9, coeliac axis; 11, splenic artery.

### Lymphatic Drainage

The lymphatic pathways draining the oesophagus are complex and the presence of lymphatics within the mucosa makes it unique within the gastrointestinal tract. These and extensive submucosal lymphatics form a complex interconnecting network extending the length of the oesophagus, intermittently piercing the muscular layers to drain into the para-oesophageal plexus. The para-oesophageal nodes lie along the oesophageal wall draining to peri-oesophageal nodes and more distant lateral oesophageal nodes. Ultimately these empty into the thoracic duct although direct connections between the oesophageal plexus and the duct may also be present. This arrangement allows for early and widespread lymphatic dissemination of oesophageal carcinoma once the basement membrane has been breached.

Lymph node status is a profound prognostic factor for oesophageal carcinoma and the pattern of dissemination derived from resected specimens suggests that the lymphatic drainage broadly mirrors the arterial blood supply. The upper oesophagus drains in a mainly cephalic direction to the cervical nodes; the middle oesophagus to the para-oesophageal, para-aortic and tracheo-bronchial stations; the lower oesophagus to both these mediastinal stations and upper abdominal stations, particularly the paracardial nodes and those along the left gastric artery (Figure 1.5). This direction of lymphatic flow has been confirmed by radionuclide studies following endoscopic injection of a radioactive tracer at different levels of the oesophagus. According to the TNM (tumour, node, metastasis) classification the regional lymph nodes are, for the cervical oesophagus, the cervical nodes including the supraclavicular nodes, and, for the intrathoracic oesophagus, the mediastinal and perigastric nodes, excluding the coeliac nodes (considered M1a nodes) [3]. The precise nomenclature differs slightly from the description by the Japanese Society [9] (Figure 1.5) although the two systems are broadly similar.

## Nerve Supply of the Oesophagus

The innervation of the oesophagus comprises an extrinsic parasympathetic and sympathetic supply and the intrinsic intramural plexuses. It is controlled by a complex swallowing centre located in the brainstem, which coordinates and interprets signals from within the brainstem and from peripheral receptors in the pharynx and oesophagus.

### Parasympathetic Supply

This provides the predominant motor and sensory innervation of the oesophagus. The fibres originate from the vagal motor nuclei and are distributed to the oesophagus via the vagus nerve to form the oesophageal plexus. The glossopharyngeal nerve and the recurrent laryngeal branches of the vagus also carry some fibres to the proximal oesophagus.

### Sympathetic Supply

This appears to play a more minor role in oesophageal function. The preganglionic fibres originate from the fifth and sixth thoracic spinal cord segments and pass to the cervical, thoracic and coeliac ganglia. The postganglionic fibres terminate in the myenteric plexus within the oesophageal wall.

### Intramural Plexuses

The myenteric (Auerbach's) plexus lies between the circular and longitudinal muscle layers and becomes more prominent in the smooth muscle portion of the oesophagus. Degeneration of the myenteric plexus in the region of the lower oesophageal sphincter results in achalasia of the cardia, a major motor disorder of the oesophagus, which is characterised by failure of the lower oesophageal sphincter to relax upon swallowing. The submucosal (Meissner's) plexus is more sparse, containing nerve fibres but no ganglia.

The neural control of the oesophagus will be covered in greater detail when the physiological control of oesophageal function is considered.

## Physiology of the Oesophagus

### Fasting State

In the fasting state the oesophageal body is relaxed and the upper and lower oesophageal sphincters are tonically contracted to prevent gastro-oesophageal reflux and aspiration. The intraluminal pressure is atmospheric in the cervical oesophagus but more distally it becomes negative and approximates with intrapleural pressure, fluctuating with respiration (−5 to −10 mmHg on inspiration, 0 to +5 mmHg on expiration). The short intra-abdominal portion of the oesophagus lies in the slightly positive

# THE ANATOMY AND PHYSIOLOGY OF THE OESOPHAGUS

(0 to +5 mmHg) environment of the abdominal cavity. Unlike the smooth muscle of the stomach and intestine, oesophageal smooth muscle does not normally exhibit spontaneous phasic slow wave activity and is therefore highly dependent on its external and internal nerve supply.

## Swallowing

During fasting the normal individual swallows on average 70 times/hour whilst awake and 7 times/hour during sleep, which may increase to 200 times/hour during eating. The act of swallowing is a complex reflex involving many muscles, which it shares with other reflex activities (retching, vomiting, belching and speech). The hyoid muscles are active throughout elevating the hyoid bone, drawing it forward and then descending it through an elliptical pathway. Swallowing consists of an oropharyngeal phase, which is partly voluntary, and an involuntary oesophageal phase. It may be initiated either voluntarily or as a reflex following stimulation of oropharyngeal receptors or the oesophagus itself.

### Oropharyngeal Phase

During the oral stage ingested food is broken down and lubricated with saliva by mastication before being pushed into the posterior oropharynx by the tongue. During the pharyngeal stage there is conversion from a respiratory to a swallowing pathway, pharyngeal filling, passive emptying and active pharyngeal peristalsis. Involuntary expulsion and clearing of the food bolus into the pharynx takes around 0.5 seconds and in anticipation of its arrival respiration is suppressed and the apertures to the nasal cavity and the larynx are closed. Elevation of the hyoid bone allows the epiglottis to cover the larynx. However, the most effective barrier to aspiration is provided by adduction of the true vocal cords. Simultaneously there is relaxation of the upper oesophageal sphincter allowing most pharyngeal emptying to occur before the onset of pharyngeal peristalsis. Pharyngeal contraction then creates a pressure differential between the pharynx and the proximal oesophagus clearing any residual bolus.

*Upper Oesophageal Sphincter (UOS)*

This provides a 2–4 cm zone of high pressure between the pharynx and the upper oesophagus. The resting sphincter pressure prevents aerophagia and the aspiration of refluxed gastric contents and is asymmetrical, being higher in an anteroposterior direction (100 mHg) than laterally (35 mmHg) [10]. This high resting tone results from a combination of continuous myogenic activity in the cricopharyngeus and inferior constrictor muscles together with the inherent elasticity of these tissues. A vagally mediated increase in UOS pressure occurs secondary to oesophageal distension or acid exposure particularly of the proximal oesophagus, whilst a decrease occurs during sleep or general anaesthesia. A swallowing-initiated pressure drop occurs prior to a bolus entering the pharynx and comprises both sphincter muscle relaxation due to neural inhibition and sphincter opening secondary to forward displacement of the hyoid bone. Once a bolus has passed into the oesophagus the UOS exhibits rebound hypertension to coincide with the initiation of oesophageal peristalsis and prevent reflux back into the pharynx.

### Oesophageal Phase

This is characterised by coordinated muscular contractions that propel a bolus through the oesophagus, and relaxation of the lower oesophageal sphincter allowing it to pass into the stomach. Peristalsis will normally completely clear the oesophagus of a food bolus in 8–10 seconds. When liquids are swallowed in the upright position, gravity draws a bolus into the stomach within a few seconds with its tail being propelled by the peristaltic wave. A combination of intrinsic and extrinsic neural factors interacts with the myogenic properties of striated and smooth oesophageal muscle to produce these organised waves of contraction.

*Primary Peristalsis*

This is the oesophageal peristaltic wave triggered by swallowing. It commences in the proximal oesophagus following pharyngeal peristalsis and relaxation of the UOS. The longitudinal muscle layer contracts first to shorten and fix the oesophagus. There is then a progressive lumen-occluding circular contraction that proceeds distally through the striated and smooth muscle of the oesophageal wall, preceded by a wave of inhibition. As it does so the lower oesophageal sphincter (LOS) relaxes and then closes after the bolus with a prolonged contraction [11]. Normally the oesophagus responds with one primary peristaltic wave for each swallow. However, during rapidly repeated swallowing oesophageal activity is inhibited and only the final swallow is followed by a peristaltic wave. This property of deglutitive inhibition is vital to allow the passage of swallowed food through the oesophagus.

*Secondary Peristalsis*

This is localised to the oesophagus and is not preceded by pharyngeal contraction or UOS relaxation. It accounts for approximately 10% of all oesophageal motor activity. Secondary peristalsis is triggered by oesophageal distension by residual bolus following ineffective primary peristalsis or by refluxed gastric contents [12]. Both these events may also initiate swallowing-induced primary peristalsis in an attempt to clear the oesophagus.

*Tertiary Contractions*

These are localised non-propagating contractions of the oesophageal body. They are not related to swallowing or oesophageal distension, do not help to propel a bolus and if present in a significant number may be considered pathological.

## Investigation of Peristalsis

Due to its accessibility oesophageal peristalsis has been extensively investigated. Manometric techniques have been used to characterise the peristaltic wave and video-fluoroscopy has been used to visualise bolus movement. These techniques have demonstrated that the primary peristaltic wave travels fastest in the mid-oesophagus, slowest immediately above the LOS, and at an average velocity of 4 cm/s. The muscular contraction itself lasts for 2–7 seconds and is most prolonged in the distal oesophagus. The mean peak amplitude of contraction ranges from 35 to 70 mmHg along the oesophagus. It is lowest at the junction of striated and smooth muscle in the mid-oesophagus and increases progressively towards the lower oesophagus [13] (Figure 1.6). Peristaltic amplitude below

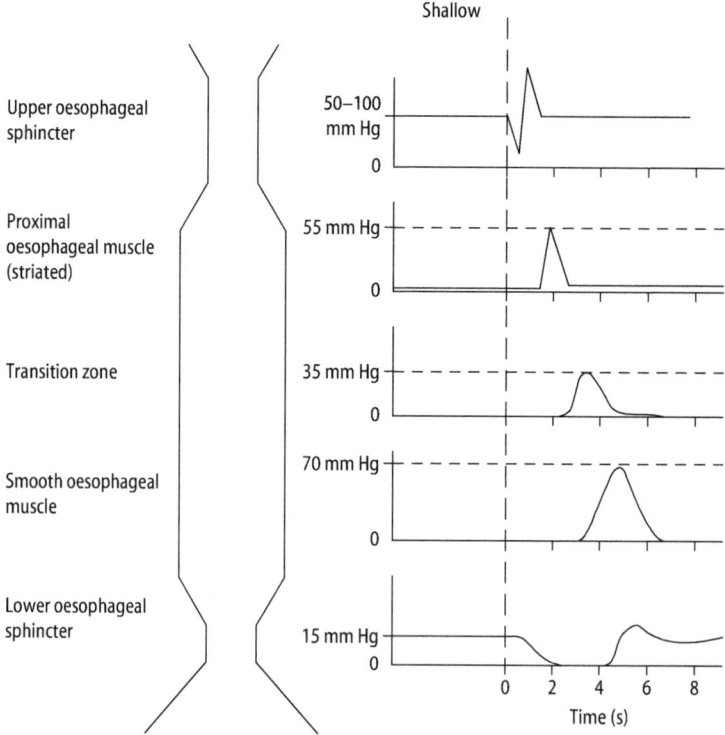

**Figure 1.6.** Manometric properties of the primary peristaltic wave.

30 mmHg is considered hypotensive, as these contractions are often associated with retrograde escape of a liquid bolus and incomplete oesophageal clearance. Although there is no defined upper limit, peristaltic contractions greater than 200 mmHg in the distal half of the oesophagus are usually considered hypertensive. This condition is termed 'nutcracker oesophagus' and is often associated with symptoms of chest pain and dysphagia. The nature of the bolus itself can influence the primary peristaltic wave with larger boluses triggering a stronger contraction. Bolus temperature is also important; warm boluses enhance whereas cold boluses inhibit peristalsis.

Secondary peristalsis is stimulated by oesophageal distension and can be reproduced by balloon occlusion of the lumen. Phasic, tonic contractions of the circular and smooth muscle develop above the balloon whilst the oesophagus relaxes below. This proximal propulsive force consists of simultaneous multipeaked contractions and is reflex mediated. It is strongest when the occlusion is sited in the distal oesophagus. When the obstruction is cleared a peristaltic wave progresses distally. The velocity and amplitude of secondary peristalsis resemble that of primary peristalsis.

## Control of Peristalsis

Peristalsis in the striated muscle of the proximal oesophagus is stimulated by sequential vagal excitation directed from the brainstem, and carried to the oesophagus by the recurrent laryngeal branches of the vagus. Peristalsis in oesophageal smooth muscle is more complex and requires integration of central and peripheral neural mechanisms with smooth muscle properties. Swallow-induced primary peristalsis is dependent on activation of the swallowing centre and vagal pathways and is abolished by bilateral cervical vagotomy. There is also some central control over coordinating the activity of striated and smooth muscle and initiating activity in the smooth muscle portion.

The propagation of peristalsis in the smooth muscle segment involves two peripheral vagal pathways. One pathway mediates cholinergic excitation (depolarisation) of both longitudinal and circular smooth muscle whilst the other mediates nonadrenergic non-cholinergic inhibition of circular muscle (hyperpolarisation), via the inhibitory neurotransmitter nitrous oxide (NO). Upon swallowing there is almost simultaneous activation of the inhibitory pathway followed by a delayed sequential activation of the excitatory pathway. This creates a wave of mechanical inhibition (latency) followed by contraction along the oesophagus, constituting peristalsis [11]. The excitatory cholinergic influence is more prominent proximally whilst the inhibitory influence increases in the distal oesophagus. These neural gradients along the oesophagus cause the velocity of propagation to decrease distally. Because cholinergic excitation decreases the delay to the onset of contraction the gradient also helps to coordinate the aboral progression of peristalsis.

When there is adequate cholinergic excitation a local myogenic control system also becomes stimulated. Oesophageal muscle may then exhibit slow wave type action potentials and coupling of the smooth muscle cells so that the whole tissue becomes a functional unit. As a consequence peristaltic progression can occur at a myogenic level once there is adequate neural excitation.

## Lower Oesophageal Sphincter (LOS)

The lower oesophageal sphincter is responsible for a 2–4 cm zone of high pressure at the gastro-oesophageal junction. It creates a resting pressure of 10–25 mmHg that is asymmetrical, being highest distally and to the left side. In the absence of a hiatus hernia the sphincter has both an intra-abdominal and an intrathoracic component. During respiration these are subjected to the different pressure changes of these two cavities and are directly influenced by contraction of the crural diaphragm.

The three major factors controlling LOS pressure are its myogenic properties and the inhibitory and excitatory neural influence [14]. The basal pressure is primarily a result of myogenic properties as within the muscle fibres continuous electrical spike activity stimulates $Ca^{2+}$ influx and maintains a depolarised state at rest. Neural activity can modulate sphincter pressure and the myenteric plexus here is innervated by both vagal preganglionic and sympathetic postganglionic fibres. Nitrous oxide is the primary inhibitory and acetylcholine the primary excitatory neurotransmitter. A large number of

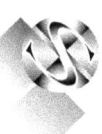

neurotransmitters, hormones, drugs, foods and lifestyle factors have been shown experimentally to alter LOS pressure, although the physiological importance of many remains to be established (Table 1.1).

Deglutitive relaxation of the LOS occurs less than 2 seconds after swallowing and is initiated whilst the peristaltic contraction is in the cervical oesophagus. Relaxation occurs to intragastric pressure, lasts for 8–10 seconds, and is followed by an after-contraction in the proximal portion of the sphincter. Swallowing-stimulated relaxation is vagally mediated and coincides with a cessation in spike activity in the sphincter muscle. During repeated swallowing the LOS remains relaxed until after the final swallow.

Failure of the LOS to relax on swallowing is characteristic of achalasia, a major motor disorder of the oesophagus. It is associated with degeneration of the myenteric plexus in the region of the sphincter and a decrease in nitric oxide synthase and consequently levels of the inhibitory neurotransmitter nitric oxide.

In addition to primary and secondary peristalsis, LOS relaxation also occurs during belching, vomiting and rumination. In the first two reflexes it is not associated with oesophageal contraction whereas in the case of rumination there is reverse oesophageal peristalsis.

## Transient Lower Oesophageal Sphincter (tLOS) Relaxation

There is now evidence that transient relaxation of the LOS is responsible for most episodes of the reflux of gastric contents, both in normal controls and in patients with gastro-oesophageal reflux disease [15]. This relaxation is unrelated to swallowing and is facilitated by pharyngeal stimulation and gastric distension, particularly following fatty meals and in an upright position. The drop in sphincter pressure occurs more slowly than with swallowing-related relaxation and is prolonged, typically lasting for 10–60 seconds until a swallow intervenes. This is frequently but not invariably associated with reflux, which occurs with 15–90% of episodes depending upon the precise study conditions. There is often also reflux of gas and this forms part of the belch reflex. Transient relaxation of the LOS is a vagally mediated reflex and as with swallowing-induced relaxation nitrous oxide (NO) is the efferent neurotransmitter.

**Table 1.1.** Factors causing relaxation or contraction of the lower oesophageal sphincter

| Factor type | Decrease LOS pressure | Increase LOS pressure |
| --- | --- | --- |
| Hormones | Glucagon<br>Cholecystokinin<br>Progesterone<br>Oestrogens | Gastrin<br>Histamine<br>Motilin<br>Pancreatic polypeptide |
| Neurotransmitters | Nitrous oxide (NO)<br>Vasoactive intestinal peptide (VIP)<br>Dopamine ($D_2$) | Acetylcholine<br>Substance P<br>Histamine |
| Prostaglandins | $E_1, E_2, A_2$ | $F_2$ |
| Drugs | Calcium antagonists<br>Atropine<br>Nitrates<br>Tricyclic antidepressants | Metoclopramide<br>Domperidone<br>Cisapride<br>Erythromycin<br>Cholinergic drugs |
| Foods | Fats<br>Chocolate<br>Caffeine<br>Alcohol | Protein meal<br>Red pepper |
| Other | Cigarette smoking | |

## Physiology of the Antireflux Mechanism

### The Oesophagogastric Junction

The reflux of small quantities of gastric fluid and air into the oesophagus particularly after meals is considered a normal physiological event. This process is limited by a number of factors comprising the antireflux barrier at the oesophagogastric junction, and by the response of the oesophageal body to clear the refluxate (Figure 1.7). A failure of these mechanisms results in the spectrum of gastro-oesophageal reflux disease (GORD).

A combination of the intrinsic smooth muscle LOS and the extrinsic pinchcock-like action of the crural diaphragm form the sphincter mechanism at the oesophagogastric junction [16]. The crural diaphragm surrounds the proximal half of the intrinsic LOS and contraction of both contributes to the intraluminal pressure at this level. Simultaneous, transient relaxation of both sphincters is responsible for the majority of reflux episodes in normal controls. Gastric sling fibres that maintain the angle of His at the oesophagogastric junction augment this antireflux mechanism. Together with the distal oesophageal mucosa this forms a flap valve that is closed by a rise in intragastric pressure. The presence of an intra-abdominal segment of oesophagus, subject to changes in intra-abdominal pressure, also serves to prevent reflux (Figure 1.7).

Pressure monitoring has demonstrated a continuous variation in the intraluminal pressure at the junction secondary to fluctuations in LOS and crural pressure. The intrinsic LOS is linked to the activity of the migrating motor complex in the stomach, and increases prior to the onset of gastric contraction preventing reflux. Contraction of the crural diaphragm is linked to respiration, increasing by 10–20 mmHg with tidal inspiration and up to 150 mmHg with forced inspiration. A sustained crural contraction is also induced by any action that increases intra-abdominal pressure, preventing reflux along the pressure gradient created between the stomach and oesophagus. Measurement of the end-expiratory sphincter pressure therefore reflects the activity of the intrinsic LOS alone. At this point of the respiratory cycle the pressure gradient between the stomach and oesophagus is only 5 mmHg and the resting intrinsic LOS tone is sufficient to prevent reflux.

The crural diaphragm also has the ability to act independently of the costal diaphragm during certain activities including vomiting when it relaxes whilst the remainder of the diaphragm contracts. Its activity is linked to that of the intrinsic sphincter because it responds to oesophageal distension, swallowing and transient LOS relaxation by relaxing itself. Both the left and right phrenic nerves supply the crural diaphragm, and this relaxation probably represents a vagophrenic inhibitory reflex.

### Investigation of Gastro-oesophageal Reflux

Physiological reflux predominantly occurs in the upright position during the postprandial period as a result of tLOS relaxation, and rarely takes place at night. It has been investigated in normal controls by 24-hour ambulatory pH monitoring whereby a pH sensor is introduced transnasally and positioned 5 cm proximal to the manometrically determined upper border of the LOS. By convention acid reflux is defined as a pH <4; normally there are fewer than fifty episodes of acid reflux during 24 hours and the total time pH <4 is less than 4% of the study period [17]. This technique has demonstrated that the majority of reflux episodes are asymptomatic. However, it only measures acid reflux

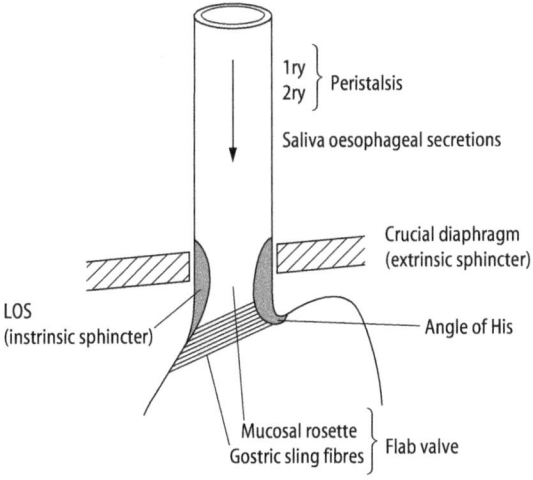

**Figure 1.7.** Mechanisms for the prevention and clearance of gastro-oesophageal reflux.

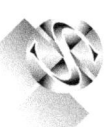

and not non-acid or gaseous reflux. More recently it has become possible to measure ambulatory bilirubin levels in the distal oesophagus as a marker of bile reflux, although normal values for this procedure are less well established. Techniques such as oesophageal impedance testing are currently being developed to assess non-acid and gaseous reflex in greater detail.

### Oesophageal Response to Reflux

When physiological reflux does occur there are a number of responses that help to clear the oesophagus of refluxate and prevent mucosal damage. Refluxed gas is either returned to the stomach by peristalsis stimulated by oesophageal distension or vented to the pharynx as a belch. The primary response of the oesophageal body to reflux is peristalsis [12]. One or two peristaltic waves will clear 90% of the reflux volume and deliver swallowed saliva to deal with the remaining 10%. The initial response to acid reflux is swallowing-associated primary peristalsis in 45–60% of cases. Secondary peristalsis is less common although it becomes the initial response in 90% of episodes during sleep when swallowing and saliva production is suppressed. Following peristalsis any residual acid refluxate lining the mucosa is neutralised by bicarbonate ions in saliva and secretions from the oesophageal submucosal glands.

### Physiology of Gastro-oesophageal Reflux Disease

Any failure of the protective antireflux mechanism can result in gastro-oesophageal reflux disease (GORD). It appears that most patients with mild/moderate reflux disease exhibit normal sphincter pressures and that as with physiological reflux it results from transient relaxation of the sphincters [15]. Some patients do have a hypotonic intrinsic sphincter and this correlates with increased acid exposure and severity of disease. Fifty per cent of patients demonstrate impaired peristaltic clearance resulting in prolonged reflux episodes although it is unclear whether this represents a primary motor disorder or is secondary to acid-induced damage. The presence of a hiatus hernia helps to destroy the normal antireflux mechanism by disrupting the crural diaphragm and flap valve at the oesophagogastric junction. In addition, upon swallowing gastric contents within the hernia are able to reflux through the relaxed LOS and on inspiration they are propelled upwards by contraction of the crural diaphragm below.

### Oesophageal Sensation

Mechanoreceptors within the myenteric ganglia both activate subconscious reflexes and transduce painful sensations. Progressive balloon distension of the oesophagus initially stimulates secondary peristalsis but at higher volumes causes a pressure and then a painful sensation. Involuntary physiological reflexes such as peristalsis are mediated by low threshold receptors via vagal pathways. Nociception is mediated by higher threshold receptors and involves splanchnic sympathetic pathways under vagal modulation. There are also intraepithelial nerve endings in the oesophagus that act as thermo-, chemo- and osmoreceptors.

## Summary

A clear understanding of the normal anatomy and physiology of the oesophagus is fundamental to comprehending the rationale behind surgical and medical decision-making in what is a complex specialty. The anatomical relationships of the oesophagus together with its blood supply and lymphatic drainage determine the surgical approach and extent of resection required for oesophageal malignancy and the technique to be used for reconstruction. The primary function of the oesophagus is as a conduit for passage of swallowed food and fluid and its structure is integrally linked to this. Our knowledge of the control of swallowing and physiology of the antireflux barrier continues to evolve. This has led to a better understanding of the pathophysiology of oesophageal motility disorders and gastro-oesophageal reflux disease and to the development of pharmacological and surgical options for their management.

# THE ANATOMY AND PHYSIOLOGY OF THE OESOPHAGUS

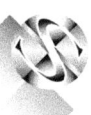

## Questions

1. Explain the development of tracheo-oesophageal fistula.
2. What are the immediate anatomical relationships of the oesophagus in the posterior mediastinum?
3. Which neural pathways control the propagation of peristalsis?
4. Which factors cause a decrease in lower oesophageal sphincter pressure?
5. What is the response of the oesophageal body to physiological reflux of gastric contents?
6. What constitutes the antireflux mechanism at the gastro-oesophageal junction?
7. What functional differences are there between the virgin oesophagus and the transposed gastric conduit following oesophagectomy and gastric pull-up?

## References

1. Muller JM, Erasmit T, Stelsner M et al. Surgical therapy of oesophageal carcinoma. Br J Surg 1990; 77: 845–57.
2. Moore K. Essentials of human embryology. Oxford: Blackwell Scientific Publications, 1988.
3. Sobin L, C Wittekind, UICC TNM classification of malignant tumours, 5th edn. New York: Wiley-Liss, 1997.
4. Orringer M, Bluett M, Deeb G. Aggressive treatment of chylothorax complicating transhiatal esophagectomy without thoracotomy. Surgery 1988; 10:720–6.
5. Akiyama H. Surgery for cancer of the esophagus, 1st edn. Baltimore: Williams & Wilkins, 1990.
6. Sampliner R. Practice guidelines on the diagnosis, surveillance, and therapy of Barrett's esophagus. The Practice Parameters Committee of the American College of Gastroenterology. Am J Gastroenterol 1998; 93: 1028–32.
7. Meyer G. Muscle anatomy of the human esophagus. J Clin Gastroenterol 1986; 8:131.
8. Demeester S, Demeester T. Columnar mucosa and intestinal metaplasia of the esophagus: Fifty years of controversy. Ann Surg 2000; 231:303–21.
9. Japanese Society for Esophageal Diseases. Guidelines for the clinical and pathological studies on carcioma of the oesophagus. Part 1. Clinical classification. Jpn J Surg 1976; 6:64–78.
10. Sivarao D, Goyal R. Functional anatomy and physiology of the upperr esophageal sphincter. Am J Med 2000; 108:27S–37S.
11. Diamant N. Neuromuscular mechanisms of primary peristalsis. Am J Med 1997; 103:40S–43S.
12. Holloway R. Esophageal body motor response to reflux events: Secondary peristalsis. Am J Med 2000; 108: 20S–26S.
13. Richter J. Esophageal manometry in 95 healthy adult volunteers. Variability of pressures with age and frequency of "abnormal" contractions. Dig Dis Sci 1987; 32:583.
14. Goyal R, Sivarao D. Functional anatomy and physiology of swallowing and esophageal motility. In: Castell D, Richter J, (eds) The esophagus, Philadelphia: Lippincott Williams & Wilkins, 1999; 1–32.
15. Mittal R, Holloway RH, Penagini R et al. Transient lower esophageal sphincter relaxation. Gastroenterology, 1995. 109:601-10.
16. Mittal, R, Balaban DH. The esophagogastric junction. N Engl J Med 1997; 336:924–32.
17. Demeester T, Johnson LF, Joseph GJ et al. Patterns of gastroesophageal reflux in health and disease. Ann Surg 1976; 184:459–69.
18. Walsh TN, Caldwell MTP, Fallon C et al. Gastric motility following oesophagectomy. Br J Surg 1995; 82:91–4.
19. Johansson J, Sloth M, Bajc M, Walther B. Radioisotope evaluation of the esophageal remnant and the gastric conduit after gastric pull-up esophagectomy. Surgery 1999; 125:297–303.
20. Gutschow C, Collard JM, Romagnoli R et al. Denervated stomach as an esophageal substitute recovers intraluminal acidity with time. Ann Surg 2001; 233:509–514.
21. Demeester T, Johansson KE, Franze I et al. Indications, surgical technique and long-term functional results of colon interposition or bypass. Ann Surg 1988:460–74.
22. Mathew G, Watson DI, Myerrs JC et al. Oesophageal motility before and after laparoscopic Nissen fundoplication. Br J Surg 1997; 84:1465–9.

## Further Reading

Akiyama H. Surgery for cancer of the esophagus. Baltimore: Williams & Wilkins, 1990.
Castell D Richter J (eds). The esophagus, Philadelphia: Lippincott Williams & Wilkins, 1999.
Griffin, SM, Raimes, SA. (eds) Upper gastrointestinal surgery, 2nd edn. London: WB Saunders, 2001.
Hennessy TPJ, Cuschieri A. Surgery of the Oesophagus, 2nd edn. Oxford: Butterworth Heinemann, 1992.

# 2

# The Anatomy and Physiology of the Stomach

Ian R. Daniels and William H. Allum

## Aims

To detail the anatomy and physiology of the stomach.

## Introduction

The stomach is the most dilated part of the digestive tube, having a capacity of 1000–1500 ml in the adult. It is situated between the end of the oesophagus and the duodenum – the beginning of the small intestine. It lies in the epigastric, umbilical, and left hypochondrial regions of the abdomen, and occupies a recess bounded by the upper abdominal viscera, the anterior abdominal wall and the diaphragm. It has two openings and is described as having two borders, although in reality the external surface is continuous. The relationship of the stomach to the surrounding viscera is altered by the amount of the stomach contents, the stage that the digestive process has reached, the degree of development of the gastric musculature, and the condition of the adjacent intestines. However, borders are assigned by the attachment of the peritoneum via the greater and lesser omentum, thus dividing the stomach into an anterior and posterior surface.

The principal function of the stomach is to mix the food with acid, mucus and pepsin and then release the resulting chyme, at a controlled rate into the duodenum for the process of absorption. Gastric motility is controlled by both neural and hormonal signals. Nervous control originates from the enteric nervous system as well as the parasympathetic (predominantly vagus nerve) and sympathetic systems. A number of hormones have been shown to influence gastric motility – for example, both gastrin and cholecystokinin act to relax the proximal stomach and enhance contractions in the distal stomach. Other functions of the stomach include the secretion of intrinsic factor necessary for the absorption of vitamin $B_{12}$ (Figure 2.1).

## Anatomy

### Embryology

Towards the end of the fourth week of embryonic development, the stomach begins to differentiate from the primitive foregut – a midline tube, separated from the developing pericardium by the septum transversum and dorsally to the aorta. Initially a fusiform dilation forms, beyond which the midgut opens into the yolk sac. The foregut, owing to the presence of the pleuroperitoneal canals on either side, is connected to the dorsal wall by a mesentery that is continuous with the dorsal mesentery of the mid- and hindguts. Thus a primitive mesentery extends from the septum transversum to the developing cloaca. The liver and ventral pancreas (uncinate process) develop from the

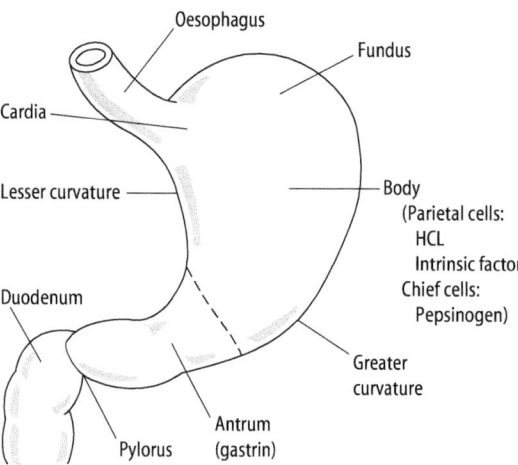

**Figure 2.1.** The regions and functions of the stomach. (With permission from Review of Medical Physiology, WF Ganong, 13th edition, Lange Medical Press, 1987.)

ventral aspect of the foregut and grow into the septum transversum, thus forming a ventral mesentery – the ventral mesogastrium. As the embryonic period continues the growth of the two "borders" becomes notably altered and the curvature of the stomach becomes apparent (Figure 2.2). The distal end rotates ventrally and with the increased growth of the dorsal border the concavity of the lesser curvature becomes apparent. With further increasing growth of the entire gut and the return of the gut to the abdominal cavity the stomach becomes rotated along its cranial-caudal plane so that the "stomach sac" rotates and the original right surface becomes dorsal and the left ventral. The position of the dorsal and ventral mesogastrium is affected by the rotation (Figure 2.3).

As the dorsal mesogastrium becomes increased in length, it folds upon itself forming the lesser omentum. This lies transverse rather than

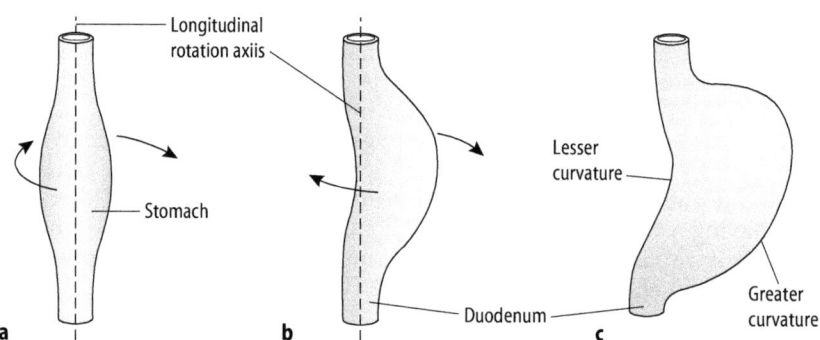

**Figure 2.2. a–c** The rotation of the stomach along its longitudinal axis.

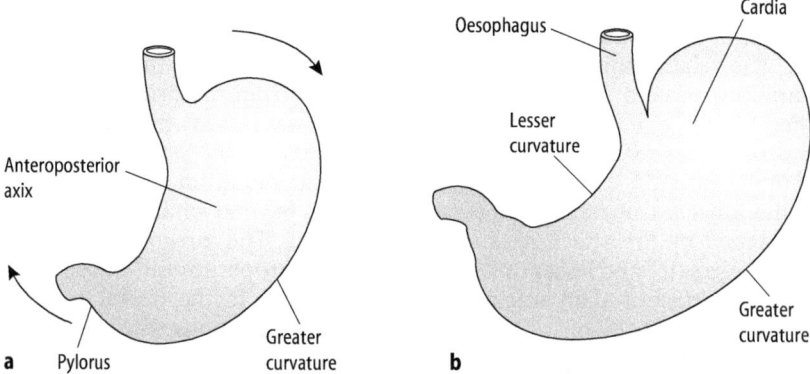

**Figure 2.3.** The rotation of the stomach along its anteroposterior axis. (With permission from Langman's Medical Embryology, 5th edition, Williams & Wilkins, Baltimore, 1985.)

# THE ANATOMY AND PHYSIOLOGY OF THE STOMACH

anteroposterior and leads to the formation of the lesser sac. This lies between the stomach and posterior abdominal wall, bounded laterally on the left by the dorsal mesogastrium, anteriorly by the stomach and laterally on the right by the developing liver. The foramen of Winslow is the only opening into the space and formed by the free border of the lesser omentum, between the stomach and liver (Figure 2.4).

With the rotation of the stomach, the duodenum is carried to the right. Initially the duodenum is fixed by a thick mesentery to the posterior abdominal wall. However, with this rotation the duodenum comes to lie on the posterior abdominal wall and the primitive mesentery disappears. This results in the duodenum coming to lie retroperitoneally. Similarly the bilary ducts and pancreas come to lie within the concavity of the duodenum, the bile duct having passed behind its proximal part.

Within the folds of the dorsal mesogastrium the spleen develops and this remains intimately attached to the stomach.

## Congenital Abnormalities

### Pyloric Atresia

Almost all cases of gastric atresia occur in the pyloric region and may present as a membrane occluding the lumen, as a gap in continuity, or as a fibrous cord intervening between patent portions at the gastroduodenal junction. There is a reported association with epidermolysis bullosa. Clinically the condition presents as upper abdominal distension and bile-free vomiting in the newborn. Maternal hydramnios occurs in approximately 50% of cases.

### Duplications

True or complete duplication of the stomach is exceedingly rare. More common (but also rare) incomplete duplications may be defined as spherical or tubular enteric formations which lie in contiguity with the normal alimentary tract and which share with it a common blood supply, and usually a common muscle coat. These cyst-like structures, or duplication cysts, usually do not communicate with the normal lumen. They may have a mucosal lining and may be pedunculated. A duplication cyst of the stomach is a communicating or non-communicating cyst lined by gastric, intestinal or pancreatic epithelium, and usually located along the greater curvature. Occasionally it may be situated in the wall of the pyloric region; in such cases encroachment on the lumen may produce gastric outlet obstruction, or an appearance resembling infantile hypertrophic pyloric stenosis. In non-communicating duplication cysts, accumulation of acid and pepsin may produce a local inflammatory reaction, perforation, abscess formation and peritonitis.

### Congenital Double Pylorus, Pyloric Membrane, Web or Diaphragm

Congenital double pylorus is an extremely rare condition. A pyloric membrane is defined as a thin, circumferential mucosal septum in the pyloric region, projecting intraluminally perpendicular to the long axis of the "antrum". It is composed of two layers of gastric mucosa, with a central core of submucosa and muscularis mucosae. It is generally regarded as a congenital anomaly and is usually associated with symptoms and signs of gastric outlet obstruction.

### Ectopic Pancreatic Tissue

Aberrant pancreatic nodules have been reported in the upper gastrointestinal tract. Although usually in the duodenum they have been reported in the stomach near the pylorus.

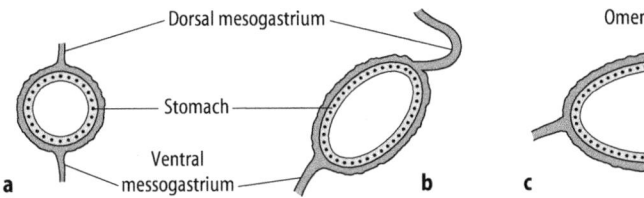

**Figure 2.4.a–c** The effect of rotation on the ventral and dorsal mesogastrium (**a, b**) and the formation of the lesser sac (omental bursa) (**c**). (With permission from Langman's Medical Embryology, 5th edition, Williams & Wilkins, Baltimore, 1985.)

## Macroscopic Anatomy

The stomach has two openings, two curvatures, two surfaces and two omenta.

## Openings

### Gastro-oesophageal Junction

The oesophagus communicates with the stomach via the cardiac orifice, which is situated on the left of the midline at the level of T10. The intra-abdominal oesophagus (antrum cardiacum) is short and conical. After passing through the diaphragm it curves sharply to the left, and becomes continuous with the cardiac orifice of the stomach. The right margin of the oesophagus is continuous with the lesser curvature of the stomach, while the left margin joins the greater curvature at an acute angle (incisura cardiaca).

### Gastroduodenal Junction

The pylorus forms the gastric outlet and communicates with the duodenum. It lies to the right of the midline at the level of the upper border of L1 and may be identified on the surface of the stomach by a circular groove (duodeno-pyloric constriction). There has long been disagreement about various aspects of the structure and function of the "gatekeeper" (Greek *pyloros*, from *pyle* = gate and *ouros* = guard). Willis (1682) introduced the term "antrum pylori" (Greek *antron* = cave) to indicate the part of the stomach adjoining the pylorus; no further demarcation was given.

## Curvatures

### Lesser Curvature (Curvatura Ventriculi Minor)

This extends from the cardiac to the pyloric orifices, thus forming the right or posterior border of the stomach. It is a continuation of the right border of the oesophagus and lies in front of the right crus of the diaphragm. It crosses the body of L1 and ends at the pylorus. A well-demarcated notch, the incisura angularis, is seen distally although its position varies with the state of distension of the stomach. Attached to the lesser curvature are the two layers of the hepato-gastric ligament (lesser omentum). Between these two layers are the left gastric artery and the right gastric branch of the hepatic artery.

### Greater Curvature (Curvatura Ventriculi Major)

This is directed mainly forward, and is four to five times longer than the lesser curvature. It starts from the incisura cardiaca and arches backward, upward, and to the left; the highest point of the convexity is on a level with the sixth left costal cartilage. It then descends downwards and forwards, with a slight convexity to the left as low as the cartilage of the ninth rib, before turning to the right, to end at the pylorus. Directly opposite the incisura angularis of the lesser curvature, the greater curvature presents a dilatation, which is the left extremity of the pyloric part; this dilatation is limited on the right by a slight groove, the sulcus intermedius, which is about 2.5 cm, from the duodenopyloric constriction. The portion between the sulcus intermedius and the duodenopyloric constriction is termed the pyloric antrum. At its commencement the greater curvature is covered at its origin by peritoneum continuous with that covering the front of the organ. The left part of the curvature gives attachment to the gastrosplenic (lineal) ligament, while to its anterior portion are attached the two layers of the greater omentum, separated from each other by the right and left gastroepiploic vessels.

## Surfaces

These change with the degree of gastric distension. When the stomach is empty they may be described as anterior and posterior surfaces, but with distension become anterosuperior and postero-inferior.

### Anterosuperior Surface

This surface is covered by peritoneum and lies in contact with the diaphragm, which separates it from the base of the left lung, the pericardium, the seventh–ninth ribs, and the intercostal spaces of the left side. The right half lies in relation to the left and quadrate lobes of the liver together with the anterior abdominal wall. The transverse colon may lie on the front part of this surface when the stomach is collapsed.

### Postero-inferior Surface

This surface is covered by peritoneum, except over a small area close to the cardiac orifice; this area is limited by the lines of attachment of the gastrophrenic ligament, and lies in apposition

# THE ANATOMY AND PHYSIOLOGY OF THE STOMACH

with the diaphragm, and frequently with the upper portion of the left suprarenal gland. Other relations are to the upper part of the front of the left kidney, the anterior surface of the pancreas, the left colic flexure, and the upper layer of the transverse mesocolon. The transverse mesocolon separates the stomach from the duodenojejunal flexure and small intestine. Thus the abdominal cavity is divided into supra- and infra-colic compartments.

The anterior boundary of the lesser sac (omental bursa) is formed by this surface. This potential space can be accessed via an opening on the free border of the lesser omentum, which contains the common hepatic artery, the common bile duct and the portal vein (the foramen of Winslow).

## Parts of the Stomach

The stomach is divided into a pyloric part and body by a plane passing through the incisura angularis on the lesser curvature and the left limit of the opposed dilatation on the greater curvature. The body is further subdivided into the fundus and cardia by a plane passing horizontally through the cardiac orifice. Distally a plane passing from the sulcus intermedius at right angles to the long axis of this portion further subdivides the pyloric portion. To the right of this plane lies the pyloric antrum. At operations, a slight groove may be seen in the serosal surface at the gastroduodenal junction. A small, superficial subserosal vein, lying within this groove and vertically across the front of the gut may be evident. This is the prepyloric vein (of Mayo) and drains into the right gastric vein. At operation, palpation of this area reveals the pyloric ring between the thick walls of the pyloric region and the thin walls of the duodenum.

## Omenta

### Lesser Omentum

This extends from the inferior and posterior surfaces of the liver to the stomach and proximal 3.0 cm of the duodenum. The free border of the lesser omentum between the porta hepatis and the duodenum contains the hepatic artery, the portal vein, the common bile duct, lymph glands, lymph vessels and nerves. Behind this free edge is the opening into the lesser sac or epiploic foramen (of Winslow). The remainder of the lesser omentum, extending from the left end of the porta hepatis to the lesser curvature, contains the right and left gastric arteries and the accompanying veins, as well as lymph glands, lymph vessels and branches of the anterior and posterior vagus nerves.

### Greater Omentum

This is formed along the greater curvature of the stomach by the union of the peritoneal coats of the anterior and posterior gastric surfaces. On its left it shortens into the gastrosplenic omentum, containing the short gastric branches of the splenic artery between its two layers. On the right it is continued for 3.0 cm along the lower border of the first part of the duodenum. From its origin the greater omentum hangs down in front of the intestines as a loose apron, extending as far as the transverse colon, where its two layers separate to enclose that part of the colon. The upper part of the greater omentum contains the greater part of the right and left gastroepiploic arteries and their accompanying veins, lymph vessels, lymph glands, nerve filaments, fat and areolar tissue.

## Blood supply

### Arterial Supply (Figure 2.5)

The coeliac artery, the artery of the foregut, supplies the stomach by its three branches. It arises from the front of the aorta between the crura of the diaphragm and is a short wide trunk, surrounded by the coeliac lymph nodes and flanked by the coeliac ganglia of the sympathetic system. The main branches are the left gastric artery, the hepatic artery and the splenic artery.

### The Left Gastric Artery.

This runs to the left, gives off an ascending oesophageal branch, and supplies the upper part of the stomach. However, it may arise directly from the aorta (5–6.7%), and may provide one or both of the inferior phrenic arteries or a common trunk for the two. Duplicate arteries have been reported and sometimes an enlarged (accessory) branch (8–25% of individuals) is found. This branch may replace the left hepatic artery (11–12% of individuals). The left gastric artery turns downwards between the layers of the lesser omentum and runs to the

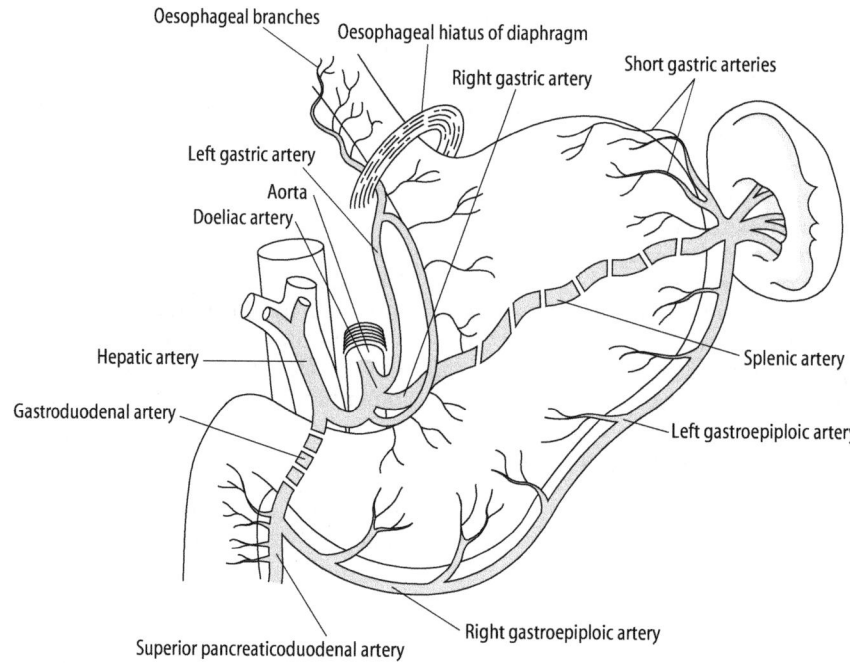

**Figure 2.5.** The arterial supply of the stomach. (With permission from Clinical Anatomy for Medical Students, 6th edition, RS Snell, p. 207, Fig. 5–14, Lippincott Williams & Wilkins, Philadelphia, 2000.)

right along the lesser curvature. Having divided into two parallel branches, these divide further supplying the anterior and posterior gastric walls. These vessels anastomose freely with arteries from the greater curvature. Around the incisura angularis, the two main branches then anastomose with the two branches of the right gastric artery. The hepatic artery may arise directly from the left gastric.

### The Hepatic Artery

This is the second branch of the coeliac trunk and passes downwards as far as the first part of the duodenum. At the opening into right border of the lesser sac it turns forwards (epiploic foramen) and curves upwards between the two layers of the lesser omentum towards the porta hepatis, to supply the liver. The gastroduodenal and right gastric arteries are given off as it turns into the lesser omentum. The right gastric artery passes to the left between the two layers of the lesser omentum, and runs along the lesser curvature of the stomach before dividing into two branches that anastomose with the branches of the left gastric artery. It also gives off branches to the anterior and posterior gastric walls, anastomosing with branches from the right gastroepiploic artery. The gastroduodenal artery descends behind the first part of the duodenum, which it supplies by multiple small branches. The terminal divisions are the superior pancreaticoduodenal artery, supplying the second part of the duodenum and head of the pancreas, and the right gastroepiploic artery. The right gastroepiploic artery passes along the greater curvature of the stomach between the layers of the greater omentum and gives off branches to the anterior and posterior gastric walls before anastomosing with the left gastroepiploic artery.

### The Splenic Artery

This passes to the left along the upper border of the pancreas, behind the peritoneum and the stomach, to supply the spleen. Division into the terminal branches close to the spleen is called a magistral splenic (~1–2 cm from the hilum), but earlier division is called a distributing splenic. During its course it gives off branches to the pancreas; just before entering the splenic hilum it gives off the short gastric arteries supplying the gastric fornix, and the left gastroepiploic artery. The latter passes downwards and to the right along the greater curvature of the stomach, between the two layers of the greater omentum, to anastomose with the right gastroepiploic artery at the mid-portion of the greater curvature. It gives off branches to the anterior and posterior gastric walls, which anastomose with branches of the gastric arteries along the lesser curvature. These arterial arcades ramify through the submucosa, forming a rich arterial network from which branches arise to supply the mucous membrane. Therefore the mucosa is not supplied by end arteries, with the possible exception of the mucosa along the lessercurvature, which appears to receive its arterial supply directly from branches of the right and left gastric arteries.

Multiple variations of the splenic artery are reported. Commonly it may divide into two branches that reunite with the splenic vein passing through the loop thus formed. It may give rise to branches normally derived from other vessels, such as the left gastric, middle colic and left hepatic. The short gastric arteries may arise from the gastroepiploic artery, the splenic artery proper, the splenic branches of the splenic artery, or any combination thereof. Similarly the left gastroepiploic artery may originate from one of the splenic branches. In a third of cases the dorsal pancreatic artery may also arise from the splenic artery.

Multiple small branches from the hepatic and gastroduodenal arteries supply the first 2 cm of the duodenum. This part of the duodenum occupies the embryological transition zone between the coeliac and superior mesenteric vascular supplies, and the vessels, which supply it vary considerably in their size and mode of origin. This variation in blood supply may partly account for the frequency of ulceration.

The coeliac trunk may lack one or more of its main branches. These may arise from the aorta or the superior mesenteric, either independently or in conjunction with another branch. The following variations have been reported:

1. Hepatosplenogastric trunk
2. Hepatosplenic trunk (hepatic and splenic)
3. Hepatosplenomesenteric trunk (hepatic, splenic and superior mesenteric)
4. Hepatogastric trunk (hepatic and left gastric)
5. Splenogastric trunk (splenic and left gastric)
6. Coeliacomesenteric trunk (superior mesenteric in conjunction with hepatosplenogastric trunk)
7. Coeliacocolic trunk (middle or accessory middle colic arising from the coeliac trunk is extremely rare).

A posterior gastric artery, a branch of the splenic, is reported to be present in 48–68% of individuals and forms another source of the blood supply to the superior portion of the posterior gastric wall. It may also supply a superior polar artery to the spleen. These vessels have a "hidden" posterior location and may be overlooked, leading to the possibility of dangerous bleeding if damaged.

## Venous Drainage

The gastric veins are similar in position to that of the arteries along the lesser and greater curvatures. These veins drain either directly or indirectly into the portal system. The major veins are:

1. *Left gastric vein.* This runs to the left along the lesser curvature, receiving the oesophageal veins below the oesophageal hiatus in the diaphragm. It usually drains directly into the portal vein at the superior border of the pancreas.
2. *Right gastric vein.* This runs along the lesser curvature to the right towards the pylorus. Posterior to the first part of the duodenum it joins the portal vein. It also receives the prepyloric vein which receives the veins from the first 2 cm of the duodenum.
3. *Left gastroepiploic vein.* This passes to the left along the greater curvature and with the short gastric veins drains into the splenic vein or its tributaries. The splenic vein is joined with tributaries from the pancreas as well as the inferior mesenteric vein; these ultimately form the portal vein with the superior mesenteric vein.
4. **Right gastroepiploic vein.** This runs to the right as far as the head of the pan-

creas. Usually it joins the superior mesenteric vein and thus drains into the portal vein. However, considerable variations may occur and the right gastroepiploic may enter the portal vein directly, or it may join the splenic vein. There is no gastroduodenal vein.

## Lymphatic Drainage

The gastric lymphatics arise in the subepithelial interglandular tissue of the mucosa. They pass outwards between the glands to communicate with each other in the periglandular plexus and from here the channels proceed into the subglandular plexus between the glands and muscularis mucosae. Short vessels passing through the muscularis mucosae form the submucous plexus. Larger vessels draining this plexus then pass through the muscular coats before communicating with the networks among the muscle fibres, and opening into the subserous plexus. From this subserosal plexus, valved collecting vessels radiate to the curvatures of the stomach to enter the omenta.

The lymphatics of the stomach can be divided into three systems:

1. *Intramural.* This consists of three networks; submucosal, intermuscular and subserosal. The submucosal lymphatic channels communicate freely throughout the submucosa of the stomach and to a lesser degree with the submucosal lymphatics of the duodenum; they also communicate freely with the intermuscular and subserosal networks.
2. *Intermediary.* This consists of numerous small channels between the subserosal network and the extramural collecting systems.
3. *Extramural.* This consists of four major zones of lymphatic drainage, corresponding to the arterial supply of the stomach. Ultimately all zones drain into the coeliac nodes around the coeliac arterial trunk on the anterior aspect of the aorta.

The lymphatic drainage of the stomach can be divided into four zones [1]. (Figures 2.6 and 2.7):

- *Zone 1.* This comprises the upper two-thirds of the lesser curvature and a large part of the body of the stomach. These drain into the left gastric nodes lying along the left gastric artery. These nodes are joined by lymphatics coming down from the lower part of the oesophagus, and their efferents proceed to the coeliac nodes.
- *Zone 2.* This is from the distal part of the lesser curvature, including the lesser curvature of the pyloric region, to the suprapyloric nodes along the right gastric artery. Efferent channels from the suprapyloric nodes drain to the hepatic and ultimately to the coeliac and aortic nodes.
- *Zone 3.* This zone includes the pyloric part of the stomach as well as the right half of the greater curvature. The lymphatics from these areas drain into the right gastroepiploic nodes in the gastrocolic ligament, lying along the right gastroepiploic vessels, and into the pyloric nodes on the anterior surface of the head of the pancreas. The direction of lymph flow is from above downwards, towards the pylorus and the nodes between the head of the pancreas and second part of the duodenum. From these groups, collectively called the subpyloric glands

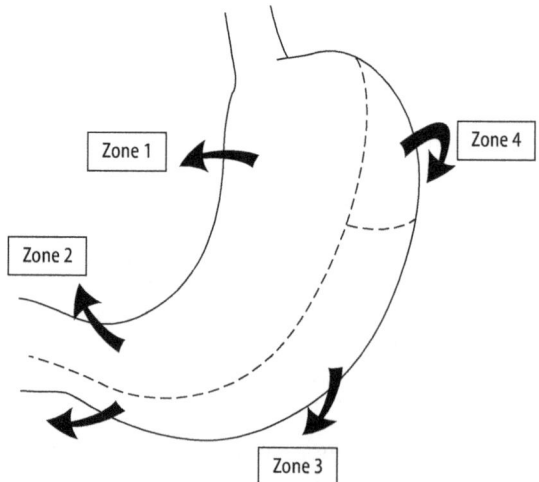

**Figure 2.6.** Zonal drainage of the gastric lymphatics. (With permission from Last's Anatomy, 10th edition, p. 245, Fig. 5.27, CS Sinnatamby (ed), Churchill Livingstone, London, 2001.)

## THE ANATOMY AND PHYSIOLOGY OF THE STOMACH

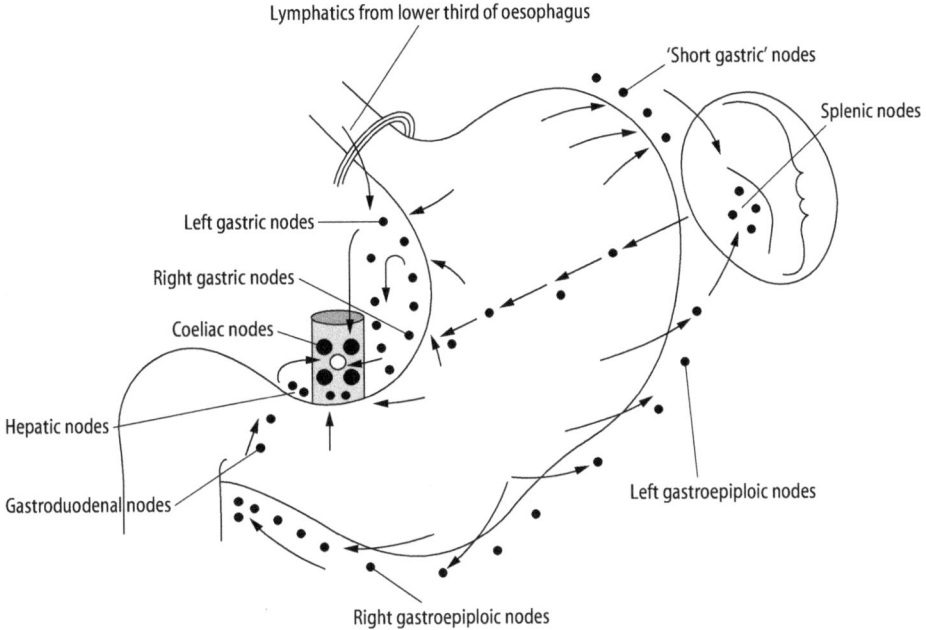

**Figure 2.7.** The nodal lymphatics. (With permission from Clinical Anatomy for Medical Students 6th edition, RS Snell, p. 207, Fig. 5–15, Lippincott Williams & Wilkins, Philadelphia, 2000.)

(which also drain the first part of the duodenum), efferent vessels pass along the gastroduodenal artery to the hepatic nodes along the hepatic artery, and thence to the coeliac nodes.

- Zone 4. This comprises the left half of the greater curvature and the gastric fornix. The lymph vessels from here pass to the left gastroepiploic nodes, lying along the left gastroepiploic artery. These drain to the pancreatico-lienal nodes along the splenic artery, before terminating in the coeliac nodes.

## Nerves

The autonomic nervous system consists of two components, cholinergic – mostly parasympathetic, and adrenergic – mostly sympathetic nerves. However, a third component of the autonomic system, which is neither cholinergic nor adrenergic, has been recognised within the gastrointestinal tract – the peptidergic system. They release a purine nucleotide as the active substance. An increasing number of peptides that are released have been recognised and this has led to the concept of a three-part autonomic control system consisting of cholinergic, adrenergic and peptidergic nerves. These peptides are unique with a dual localisation in endocrine cells and peripheral nerves in the walls of the gastrointestinal tract.

## Parasympathetic Nerve Supply

The anterior and posterior vagal trunks and their branches form the parasympathetic nerve supply to the stomach. Afferent fibres are also present in the vagi.

### Anterior Vagus

This is derived mainly from the left vagus nerve but also includes fibres from the right vagus and also some sympathetic fibres from the splanchnic nerves. It enters the abdominal cavity through the oesophageal hiatus in the diaphragm. It is usually single but may be divided into multiple trunks. Having given off several fine branches to the lower end of the oesophagus and cardiac part of the stomach, the anterior trunk breaks up into its main branches. Latarjet's classic description of the nerves is that three main sets of branches are present [2] (Figure 2.8) These are:

- Set 1. This consists of four to five direct branches, emanating "one below the other" to supply the upper part of the lesser curvature. These nerves do not form a plexus. A few filaments from the sympathetic supply join these direct branches via the coeliac plexus. One of the branches in this group is very distinct and Latarjet called it the "principal anterior nerve of the lesser curvature". It innervates the area from the cardia to the pylorus.
- Set 2. Branches from the vagal supply to the liver. There are usually three to five nerves and they descend in the lesser omentum, on to the superior margin of the pylorus and first part of the duodenum.
- Set 3. These consist of vagal filaments from the hepatic branches. These accompany the sympathetic nerves along the right gastroepiploic artery and provide vagal fibres to the inferior margin of the pylorus.

Latarjet divided the nerves of the anterior vagus into two distinct functional divisions. The first division, consisting of the direct branches, supplies the fornix and body, i.e. the "reservoir" part of the stomach. The second division, through the hepatic branches, supplies the pylorus and first part of the duodenum, i.e. the "sphincteric" part of the stomach.

*Posterior Vagus*

This is mainly formed by fibres from the right vagus nerve and enters the abdomen posterior to the oesophagus. After entering the abdomen it divides into two main branches: the coeliac and the posterior gastric. It then continues along the lesser curvature innervating the posterior gastric wall although only extending to the incisura angularis. The lowest branch is sometimes referred to as "the posterior nerve of Latarjet". These nerves do not innervate the pylorus and prepyloric region.

## Sympathetic Nerve Supply

This is derived almost entirely derived from the coeliac plexus. The gastric branches of the coeliac plexus accompany the vessels supplying the stomach – the left gastric, hepatic and phrenic arteries. Others accompany the splenic, right gastric and gastroepiploic vessels. Fibres from the coeliac plexus accompany the left inferior phrenic artery, pass anterior to the lower oesophagus and communicate with the anterior vagus before being distributed to the cardia and fornix. Other fibres travel with the left gastric artery and divide into three groups:

1. Those passing with the oesophageal and superior branches of the left gastric artery to the cardia and proximal part of the body of the stomach. These communicate with branches of the anterior and posterior vagal trunks.
2. Those passing with the main branch of the left gastric artery along the lesser curvature to supply the anterior and posterior surfaces of the body of the stomach and antrum.
3. Those passing through the lesser omentum towards the porta hepatis. These communicate with hepatic branches of the anterior vagal trunk

Fibres from the coeliac plexus pass along the hepatic artery and are distributed with its branches. They reach the pyloric region of the stomach with the right gastric and right gastroepiploic arteries.

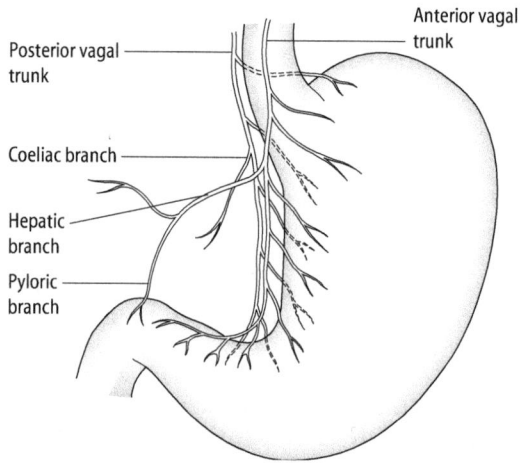

**Figure 2.8.** The anatomy of the nerves of Laterjet. (With permission from Clinical Anatomy for Medical Students, 6th edition, RS Snell, p. 246, Fig. 5–28, Lippincott Williams & Wilkins, Philadelphia, 2000.)

Preganglionic sympathetic fibres end in the coeliac ganglia. The efferent fibres emerging from the coeliac ganglia to accompany the arteries are postganglionic. Afferent visceral fibres from the stomach travel the same course in reverse, to ganglion cells in the posterior spinal nerve roots. However, these do not synapse in the sympathetic ganglia.

## Peptidergic System

Peptidergic cells are derived embryologically from neuroectoderm and are referred to as APUD cells because they synthesize monoamines through a process of amine precursor uptake and decarboxylation (APUD). They are also referred to as neuroendocrine cells. A large number of biologically active peptides have been detected in these APUD cells within the gut. These peptides include gastrin, vasoactive intestinal peptide (VIP), somatostatin, enkephalin, neurotensin and substance P.

Most of these monoamines have several molecular forms or sizes, e.g. gastrin-14, gastrin-17, gastrin-34. Some are released into the circulation, producing their biological effects in distant target organs (endocrine), whilst others act locally in the vicinity of their site of origin (paracrine) and some function as neurotransmitters (neurocrine).

## Microscopic Anatomy

The wall of the stomach and the proximal 3.0 cm of the duodenum are composed of four coats. From without inwards these are the serous, muscular, submucous and mucous coats. The mucous coat is separated from the luminal contents by a layer of gastric mucus.

## Serous Coat (Adventitia)

This is formed by the peritoneum, which is a thin layer of loose connective tissue covered with mesothelium. It is attached to the muscular coat, except at the greater and lesser curvatures, where it is continuous with the greater and lesser omentum respectively. Owing to its peritoneal attachments the proximal 3.0 cm of the duodenum, i.e. the proximal half of the first part of the duodenum, the duodenal bulb, is mobile. It shares the peritoneal covering of the pyloric region of the stomach and is unlike the remainder of the duodenum, which is retroperitoneal.

## Muscularis Externa

Since the time of Willis (1682), there has been disagreement about the muscular layers of the stomach. The muscularis externa is composed of smooth, unstriped or involuntary fibres and is made up of three layers: an external longitudinal, middle circular, and an inner oblique layer. These inner oblique fibres are arranged in inverted U-shaped bundles over the anterior and posterior gastric walls. They loop over the fornix and extend as far as the incisura angularis. Hence these fibres have no effect on the distal stomach. In this area, including the pyloric region, the muscularis externa is composed of outer longitudinal and inner circular layers.

## Submucous Coat

This is a layer of loose areolar tissue with some elastic fibres that lies between the muscularis mucosae and the muscularis externa. It is rich in mast cells, macrophages, lymphocytes, eosinophilic leucocytes and plasma cells. Within this layer the vessels and nerves divide before entering the mucous membrane. It contains arteries, veins, lymphatics and Meissner's nerve plexuses. These plexuses form part of the autonomic nervous system and contain postganglionic sympathetic fibres as well as pre- and postglanglionic parasympathetic fibres.

Unlike the duodenum (glands of Brunner), in the stomach the submucous layer does not contain any glands. However, it is wider than that of the duodenum and extends into the rugae of the stomach, forming the core of each mucosal fold.

## Mucosa

This consists of three components, the muscularis mucosae, the lamina propria, and the epithelial lining.

### Muscularis Mucosae

This is a thin layer of smooth muscle that forms the border between the mucosa and submucosa. It has outer longitudinal and inner circular fibres and fibres extend from the inner layer through the lamina propria around the gastric glands and toward the gastric lumen. These may compress the glands and aid their emptying.

## *Lamina Propria*

This layer consists of a delicate network of collagenous and reticular fibres and a few fibroblasts or reticular cells. It lies between the muscularis mucosae and the surface epithelial cells with their glands and extends into the area between the necks of the glands forming a basement membrane. It is thin in the fundus and body, where the gastric glands are numerous and closely packed, but is more prominent in the cardiac and pyloric zones. It also contains plasma cells, mast cells, eosinophilic leucocytes and lymphocytes. Local accumulations of lymphocytes may occur in the cardiac and pyloric regions. Strands of smooth muscle from the muscularis mucosae traverse this layer, which also contains fine capillaries, lymphatic vessels and nerve fibres.

## *Epithelial Lining*

A layer of simple columnar cells covers the entire luminal surface of the mucosa. However, the surface contains numerous tubular invaginations – gastric pits or foveolae. The pits are deeper in the pyloric region than elsewhere in the remainder of the stomach, extending at least halfway to the muscularis mucosae. They are V-shaped, tapering off into the glands that open into them.

The mucus-secreting columnar cells lining the luminal surface and the pits are joined by tight junctions. This may act as one of the mechanisms to protect the underlying layers against luminal acid. The supranuclear portions of the cells contain dense, homogeneous, spherical or ovoid granules consisting of a type of mucigen, which upon release into the lumen gives rise to the layer of mucus that covers the luminal surface of the mucosa. In the cells of the gastric pits, the granules become progressively less abundant at deeper levels, and in the bottom of the pits they form only a thin layer immediately beneath the cell surface. These cells continue into the necks of the gastric glands. Under physiological conditions, the surface mucous cells are continuously desquamated into the lumen and are completely replaced every 3 days. Newly formed cells appear in the deeper parts of the foveolae and in the necks of the glands; these are slowly displaced upward and continually replace those lost on the surface.

## Mucosal Zones

The mucous membrane of the entire stomach is lined by glands that open into the gastric pits. The blind ends of the glands extending into the mucosa are slightly expanded and coiled, sometimes dividing into two or three branches (Figure 2.9). The gastric mucosa can be divided into three zones, based on the predominant cell types within the glands (Tables 2.1 and 2.2).

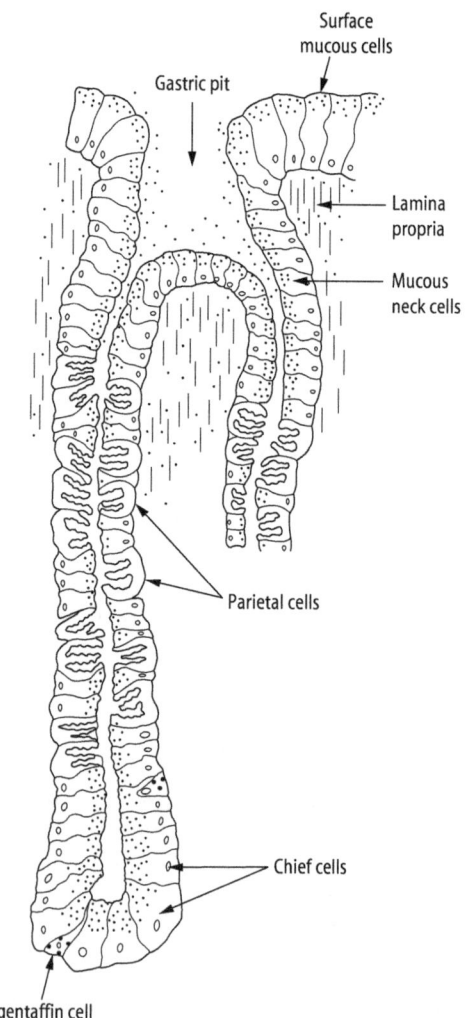

**Figure 2.9.** The gastric glands. (Reproduced with permission from Applied Physiology for Critical Care, MA Glasby, CL-H Huang, 1st Edition, 1995, Fig. 34.1, p. 337, Butterworth Heinemann Oxford.)

# THE ANATOMY AND PHYSIOLOGY OF THE STOMACH

**Table 2.1.** Summary of the mucosal zones

| | |
|---|---|
| Oxyntic zone | These glands produce nearly all the enzymes and hydrochloric acid secreted in the stomach as well as producing mucus |
| Cardiac zone | These glands secrete mucus |
| Pyloric zone | These glands secrete mucus. They also produce endocrine, paracrine or neurocrine regulatory peptides by virtue of the APUD cells contained in their glands |

**Table 2.2.** The secretory epithelial cells and their roles

Four major types of secretory epithelial cells cover the surface of the stomach and extend down into gastric pits and glands:

**Mucous cells:** secrete alkaline **mucus** that protexts the epithelium against shear stress and acid

**Parietal cells:** secrete **hydrochloric acid**

**Chief cells:** secrete **pepsin**, a proteolytic enzyme

**G cells:** secrete the hormone **gastrin**

## Cardiac Zone

This is a narrow, ring-shaped area around the gastro-oesophageal junction, containing the cardiac glands. These glands have wide lumina and shallow pits and are composed of mucus-secreting cells. This zone may contain a few APUD cells that synthesise monoamines. In the transitional area, where this zone is continuous with the oxyntic zone, a few parietal cells may be present. The glands of the cardiac zone secrete mucus.

## Oxyntic Zone

This comprises the proximal two-thirds or more of the stomach. The glands are known as fundic glands, proper gastric glands or principal gastric glands. One of their most important properties is the secretion of gastric acid. The term oxyntic (Greek: acid- forming) is also used as an indicator of this glandular zone. The mucosa here is much deeper than in the cardiac zone and contains a greater number of glands. The pits are shallow, but the glands extending from the bottoms of the pits are longer than the pits are deep.

Each principal gastric gland is composed of four kinds of cells:

1. Chief, zymogenic or peptic cells. Their secretory granules contain the precursors of pepsin.
2. Parietal or oxyntic cells. These are most numerous in the necks of the glands, but do not border directly onto the lumen, being separated from it by the peptic cells. They are triangular in shape, with the apex projecting towards the lumen between the sides of two peptic cells. These cells are intensely acidophilic, and contain the gastric proton pump mechanism that produces the hydrochloric acid. They may also contain intrinsic factor.
3. Neck mucous cells. These cells resemble the mucous cells of the cardiac and pyloric zones. They lie between the parietal cells in the necks of the glands but are smaller than the surface mucous cells. Their mucigen granules are larger and less dense than those of the surface cells.
4. Neuroendocrine cells. These are small, granulated cells that occur sporadically within the gastric mucosa. They synthesise and store serotonin (5-hydroxytryptamine, 5-HT). They are much more numerous in the pyloric zone.

## Pyloric Zone

This comprises the distal third of the stomach and extends further along the lesser curvature than the greater. The pits are the deepest within the stomach and extend into the mucous membrane for half its thickness. These glands branch more extensively and the tubules are coiled. They contain the following types of cells:

1. Mucous cells. These are similar to the neck mucous cells of the oxyntic glands and constitute the majority of cells in the pyloric glands. They have a pale cytoplasm containing indistinct granules, the nucleus is often flattened against the base of a cell, and short microvilli covered by a layer of mucus are present on the luminal surface.
2. Parietal cells. A few isolated parietal cells may be present among the mucous cells. Parietal cells also occur in the transitional region between the pyloric and oxyntic zones.

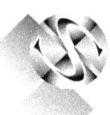

3. Neuroendocrine cells. These cells are much more numerous in the pyloric than in the cardiac and oxyntic zones although when compared with the mucous cells they are still relatively few in number. With light microscopy they have been called enterochromaffin cells. With electron microscopy their cytoplasmic granules are clearly visible after staining with chromium or silver salts. On the basis of their staining reactions, the cells have been divided into two types: argentaffin cells, in which the granules reduce silver without pretreatment, and argyrophilic cells, in which a reducing substance is required before the granules will react with silver.

The mucosal zones of the stomach are not sharply defined, the glands of one region mingle with those of the adjoining region and intermediate glands may be present between the mucosal zones.

# Physiology

## Gastric Secretions

The cells of the gastric glands secrete about 2500 ml of gastric juice daily. This contains a variety of substances and gastric enzymes, whose role is to kill ingested bacteria, aid protein digestion, stimulate the flow of biliary and pancreatic juices and provide the necessary pH for pepsin to begin protein degradation (Table 2.3).

## Mucus Secretion

The most abundant epithelial cells are mucus-secreting columnar cells, which cover the entire luminal surface and extend down into the glands as "mucous neck cells". These cells secrete bicarbonate-rich mucus that coats and lubricates the gastric surface, and serves an important role in protecting the epithelium from acid and other chemical insults. It is made up of glycoprotein subunits bound by disulphide bonds and forms a water-insoluble gel that is impermeable to $H^+$ ions. Production is stimulated by luminal acid and vagal activity, and is increased by prostaglandins. Therefore aspirin non-steroidal anti-inflammatory drugs (NSAIDs) increase the damage to the stomach by inhibiting prostaglandin formation as well as by crystallising out in the gastric cells. Bicarbonate is also secreted from parietal cells. These epithelial barrier cells are very adherent due to tight junctions between them. After epithelial disruption the cells migrate along the exposed basement membrane to fill in the defect and then stick tightly together. Gastric cells also can turn over rapidly in response to injury, as there is a rich mucosal blood flow providing oxygen, bicarbonate and nutrients and removing acid. Blood flow is normally increased simultaneously with acid secretion and is reduced by aspirin and alcohol.

## Pepsinogen Secretion

The chief cells secrete pepsinogens, contained in zymogen granules. These are the precursors of the pepsins (proteases) in gastric juice. Once secreted, pepsinogen I is activated by the presence of gastric acid into the active protease pepsin. This is an endopeptidase that is largely responsible for the initiation of protein digestion into smaller peptides and polypeptides. It splits the long amino acid chains in the region of peptide bonds containing aromatic amino acids. It acts at pH 1.5–2.5 and above pH 5.4 is inactivated. It is released mainly by vagal stimulation but also by histamine gastrin secretion, alcohol, cortisol, caffeine and acetazolamide. Pepsinogen release may also occur during periods of hypoglycaemia and prolonged increased intracranial pressure.

## Hormone Secretion

The principal hormone secreted from the gastric epithelium is gastrin, a peptide that is important in control of acid secretion and gastric motility (see below).

## Other Secretions

Gastric epithelial cells secrete a number of other enzymes, including an acid-resistant lipase and

**Table 2.3.** Contents of normal (fasting) gastric juice

| | |
|---|---|
| Cations: | $Na^+$, $K^+$, $Mg^{2+}$, $H^+$ |
| Anions: | $Cl^-$, $HPO_4^{2-}$, $SO_4^{2-}$ |
| Pepsins: | I–III |
| Gelatinase | |
| Mucus | |
| Intrinsic factor | |
| Water | |

## THE ANATOMY AND PHYSIOLOGY OF THE STOMACH

gelatinase. The lipase hydrolyses triglycerides of medium- and short-chain fatty acids into glycerol and free fatty acids.

Intrinsic factor, a glycoprotein secreted by parietal cells, is necessary for intestinal absorption of vitamin $B_{12}$. It acts by combining with the vitamin $B_{12}$ and is necessary for its attachment to receptors in the terminal ileum. Lack of intrinsic factor due to reduction in parietal cell mass following gastric surgery, or the production of antibodies to the cells, called pernicious anaemia, leads to megaloblastic anaemia. Secretion of intrinsic factor occurs following vagal, gastrin or histamine stimulation of the parietal cells.

## The Formation and Secretion of Gastric Acid

Stimulation of the parietal cells results in acid secretion (Figure 2.10). These cells contain multiple tubulovesicular structures within their cytoplasm that on stimulation move to the mucosal membrane and fuse with it, producing a microvillous appearance that increases the surface area. This results in the presence of the $H^+$-$K^+$ ATPase that transports the $H^+$ onto the luminal surface. This secretion is isotonic with other fluids and its pH is <1.

The $H^+$ is obtained from the ionisation of water, which is then actively transported into the gastric lumen in exchange for $K^+$ that has been recycled from the membrane. Chloride ions are also actively transported into the gastric lumen. The resulting $OH^-$ ion is neutralised by the carbonic acid buffer system to form a bicarbonate ion that diffuses into the interstitium to be replaced by a further $Cl^-$ ion. There is a $HCO_3^-$–$Cl^-$ exchange mechanism within the interstitium, but $Cl^-$ also enters the cell with $Na^+$. The carbonic acid is replenished by the hydration of $CO_2$, which is produced by cellular metabolism from the abundance of carbonic anhydrase within the mucosa. After a meal this results in the development of a negative respiratory quotient; thus arterial $CO_2$ is higher than venous and the gastric venous return is alkaline with a high $HCO_3^-$ content.

## Gastric Hormones

### Gastrin

Experiments in the early twentieth century using injected extract of pyloric mucosa stimulated secretion of gastric acid and pepsinogen. This action was thought to be hormonal in origin and the active substance was called gastrin [3]. However, this theory was initially disputed because this action was similar to that of histamine and the isolation of gastrin was not performed until the late 1960s when two related heptadecapeptides were identified from hog antral mucosa. These heptadecapeptides were isolated in the pyloric zone. The highest density of gastrin-producing G cells occurs in the distal 3.0 cm of the stomach, where the concentration of gastrin is 500 times higher than in the body of the stomach. The first part of the duodenum also contains a significant level of G cells. These cells originate from neuroectoderm together with other cells of the APUD series.

Microscopically they are piriform in shape and located in the mid and deep zones of the pyloric mucosal glands. Electron microscopy shows that they possess microvilli extending into the lumen and that secretory granules are present in the basal parts of the cells. This allows for secretion of hormone into the bloodstream in response to luminal stimuli.

There are two main types of gastrin, gastrin I and gastrin II, produced predominantly by the

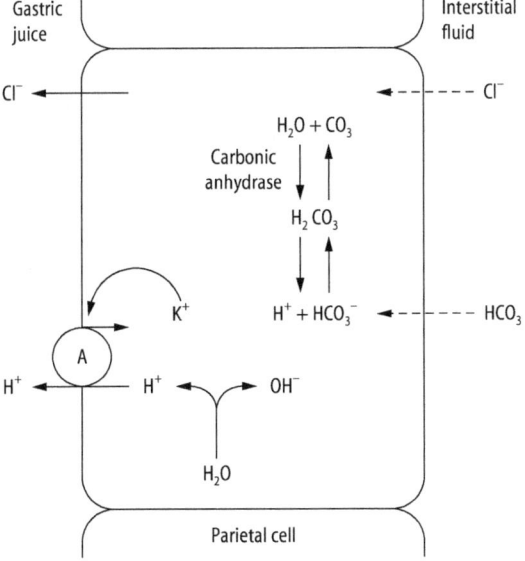

**Figure 2.10.** Hydrochloric acid production from the parietal cell.

G cells of the pyloric mucosal zone. Other sources are the duodenal G cells, D cells in the islands of Langerhans in the pancreas, and isolated G cells in the proximal-acid-producing region of the fornix and body of the stomach.

Gastrin 17 (17 amino acids) is the predominant form in the pyloric antrum, and is further subdivided into a non-sulphated gastrin I and a sulphated gastrin II form. There is also a "big" gastrin (G34) containing 34 amino acids and a "big big" gastrin with many more amino acids. "Mini" gastrin containing 14 amino acids can also be isolated, but is less active than G17. The common factor in all the molecules is the C-terminal tetrapeptide Tyr-Met-Asp-Phe-NH$_2$.

Fasting levels of gastrin are increased by achlorhydria associated with pernicious anaemia, any form of surgical vagotomy, Zollinger–Ellison syndrome (gastrinoma), chronic renal failure and massive small bowel resection.

Its physiological and pharmacological effects are summarised in Table 2.4.

## Somatostatin

Somatostatin is a tetradecapeptide that was initially found to inhibit the release of growth hormone (GH) from the pituitary gland. However, it has subsequently been identified widely in the central nervous system, the gastrointestinal tract and other organs, with the highest concentration being found in the pancreas. In the stomach it is found in the pyloric and oxyntic mucosal zones but not in the cardiac zone. Within the pancreas it is isolated from the islet D cells.

**Table 2.4.** The physiological and pharmacological effects of gastrin

| Gastrin causes: | Parietal cells to stimulate acid secretion |
| --- | --- |
| | Pepsin and intrinsic factor secretion |
| | Increased mitotic activity in the stomach and small bowel mucosa |
| | Contraction of the lower oesophageal sphincter |
| | The release of insulin, glucagon and calcitonin |
| | Pancreatic stimulation and bile flow |
| | Small bowel secretion |
| | Gastric and small bowel motility to increase |
| | The gastrocolic reflex |

Although initially thought only to suppress the secretion of growth hormone, it also possesses a wide variety of inhibitory actions on other pituitary and extrapituitary secretions. It suppresses the release of thyroid-stimulating hormone by the pituitary, the release of glucagon, insulin and exocrine secretions by the pancreas, the secretion of cholecystokinin, motilin and secretin by the intestine, and the secretion of gastrin, gastric acid and pepsin by the stomach.

Somatostatin suppresses gastric acid secretion by direct action on the parietal cells of the cardiac and oxyntic mucosal zones. Thus by lowering the pH, it also inhibits the secretion of gastrin through a feedback loop of low pH suppressing both gastric acid and gastrin secretion.

## Vasoactive Intestinal Peptide (VIP)

Vasoactive intestinal peptide (VIP) is a polypeptide with strong vascular effects isolated from small intestine. It has been subsequently demonstrated in central and peripheral neurones, suggesting a neurotransmitter function. In the peripheral autonomic system VIP nerves occur in various regions, including the superior and inferior mesenteric ganglia, and the submucous (Meissner's) and myenteric (Auerbach's) plexuses of the intestinal wall. Structures believed to exert a sphincteric function receive a particularly rich supply of VIP nerves, more so than the smooth muscle of adjacent regions. Among these are the oesophagogastric junction, the pyloric "sphincter", sphincter of Oddi, internal anal sphincter, and the openings of the ureters and urethra into the trigonum of the bladder.

In the stomach these nerves are found around oxyntic and pyloric mucosal glands. In the duodenum VIP (and substance P) is present in nerves in the villi and muscularis mucosae and around blood vessels and between the lobules of Brunner's glands. Its actions include vasodilatation, thus lowering blood pressure, increased cardiac output, glycogenolysis and relaxation of smooth muscle. In the stomach there is significant inhibition of gastric secretion associated with VIP release. It probably acts as a neurotransmitter in a paracrine, rather than in an endocrine, way. The VIP neurones have been shown to be under dual (both vagal and splanchnic) control of the autonomic system.

## Substance P

In the gastrointestinal tract nerve fibres and neurones containing substance P (11-amino-acid peptide) are encountered along its entire length. However, they are least prominent in the oesophagus and upper part of the stomach, but the highest concentrations occur in the duodenum. These neurones are located mainly in the myenteric plexuses. Here the nerve fibres richly innervate the circular musculature. However, the longitudinal muscle contains only a sparse network of fibres. Substance P may also be vasoactive as the nerve fibres are also found in close contact with blood vessels.

In the stomach substance P is found in the oxyntic zone in a few, thin fibres only and in fibres interconnecting in the pyloric antrum. In the duodenum substance P (and VIP) is present in nerve networks in the villi as well as in the muscularis mucosae and around blood vessels. It has been found to cause contraction of the muscularis mucosae.

## Other Gastric Hormones

### Encephalin

These are endogenous opiate-like compounds forming two pentapeptides, endorphin and enkephalin. They can be isolated throughout the gastrointestinal tract, although the highest concentration is found in the pyloric antrum. The role of these peptides is not clear.

### Galanin

Galanin may act as a regulatory factor in the control of gastrointestinal motility. It is usually found in close association with VIP-containing nerves.

### Neurotensin

This is secreted by N cells in ileal mucosa. However, small traces occur in the pyloric mucosal zone. The neurotensin level rises after a meal, but its function is still unclear. It may inhibit pentagastrin-stimulated gastric acid and pepsin secretion after a meal as well as delaying gastric emptying, resulting in the controlled release of chyme into the small intestine.

## Absorption from the Stomach

The stomach absorbs very few substances. Fats are not absorbed. Polypetides are absorbed only slightly. Sugars are absorbed to an extent and this varies with the sugar and its concentration. Galactose is most readily absorbed followed by glucose, lactose, fructose and finally sucrose. Low concentrations of sugars are absorbed very slowly. Ethyl alcohol is absorbed fairly rapidly as are other lipid-soluble compounds including aspirin and other NSAIDs. These substances are also well-recognised causes of gastric irritation and their use (especially overuse) is commonly associated with development of gastritis and gastric ulcers. The stomach absorbs water readily with half the ingested volume absorbed in about 20 minutes.

## Regulation of Gastric Secretion and Motility

Gastric function is classified into three phases in which secretory and motor activities are closely linked.

### Control of Gastric Acid Secretion

Acid secretion may be divided into two phases interprandial, when acid secretion is 1–5 mmol/h, and stimulated where acid secretion is maximally 20–35 mmol/h. This is further subdivided into cephalic, gastric and intestinal phase. Normal subjects maximally secrete 0.5 mmol/h/kg body weight)

### Interprandial

Resting secretion occurs in the absence of all intestinal stimulation. However, to abolish all gastic acid secretions, a bilateral vagotomy (truncal) and excision of the pyloric antrum would be necessary.

### Stimulated Secretion

*The Cephalic Phase (Figure 2.11).* The cephalic phase is initiated by seeing, smelling and anticipating food. These influences act on the limbic system and hypothalamus and these nuclei stimulate the dorsal motor nucleus of the vagus. This stimulus is transmitted thought the vagus nerve to the enteric nervous system, resulting in release of acetylcholine in the vicinity of G cells and parietal cells. Binding of acetylcholine to its receptor on G cells induces secretion of the hormone gastrin, which, in concert with acetylcholine and histamine, stimulates parietal cells to secrete small amounts of acid. Additionally, a low level of gastric motility is induced.

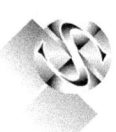

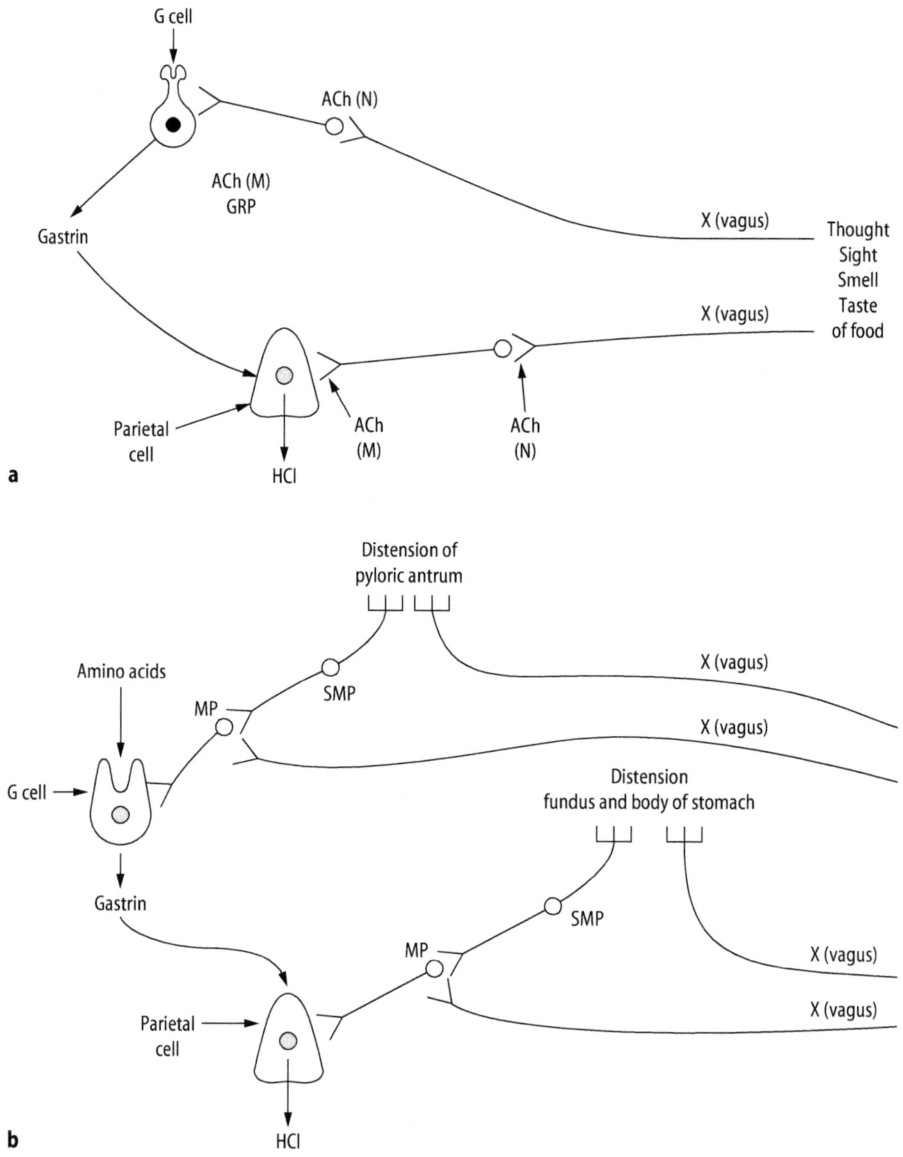

## 2 · UPPER GASTROINTESTINAL SURGERY

**Figure 2.11.** The cephalic (**a**) and gastric phases (**b**) of acid secretion. X, vagus; ACh (N), acetylcholine (nicotinic receptor); ACh (M), acetylcholine (muscarinic receptor); GRP, gastrin-releasing peptide; SMP, submucous plexus; MP, myenteric plexus. (Reproduced with permission from Applied Physiology for Critical Care, MA Glasby, CL-H Huang, 1st edition, 1995, Fig. 34.3, p. 340, Butterworth Heinemann, Oxford.)

The release of acetylcholine and bombesin (gastrin-releasing peptide) initiates gastrin release from the G cells. The gastrin passes via the portal circulation to stimulate the parietal cells. It potentiates the effect of vagal stimulation, thus resulting in increased acid secretion. The parietal cells also have $H_2$ receptors (histamine) stimulated by the release of histamine from mast cells close to the parietal cells. The histamine sensitises the parietal cell to the action of gastrin and acetylcholine. The $H_2$ receptor blockers (cimetidine and ranitidine) act on these receptors, thus reducing acid secretion.

# THE ANATOMY AND PHYSIOLOGY OF THE STOMACH

*The Gastric Phase (Figure 2.11).* When food enters the stomach several additional factors come into play, foremost among them being distension and mucosal irritation. Distension excites stretch receptors and irritation activates chemoreceptors in the mucosa. These events are sensed by enteric neurones, which secrete additional acetylcholine, further stimulating both G cells and parietal cells. Gastrin from the G cells feeds back to the parietal cells, stimulating it even further, mediated by vagovagal reflexes through the dorsal motor nucleus. Additionally, activation of the enteric nervous system and release of gastrin cause vigorous smooth muscle contractions. The net result is that secretory and motor functions of the stomach are fully turned on – acid and pepsinogen are secreted, pepsinogen is converted into pepsin and vigorous grinding and mixing contractions take place.

However, acid secretion may be inhibited during the gastric phase by local mechanisms. If the antral pH falls to 1–1.5, inhibition of gastrin release occurs. This is mediated by two mechanisms – the effect of luminal acid on the microvilli of the G cell and the stimulation of somatostatin from D cells in the antrum, which acts inhibits directly on the G cells and parietal cells by a local paracrine effect.

*The Intestinal Phase.* As chyme is emptied into the small intestine control is necessary to limit gastric emptying. This probably allows the duodenum time to neutralize the acid and efficiently absorb incoming nutrients. Hence, this phase of gastric function is dominated by the small intestine sending inhibitory signals to the stomach to slow secretion and motility. Two types of signals are used: nervous and endocrine. Distension of the small intestine, as well as chemical and osmotic irritation of the mucosa, is transduced into gastric-inhibitory impulses in the enteric nervous system – this nervous pathway is called the enterogastric reflex. Fat and carbohydrate in the chyme cause the release of GIP (gastric inhibiting peptide), which inhibits gastrin secretion. Secondly, enteric hormones such as cholecystokinin and secretin are released from cells in the small intestine and contribute to suppression of gastric activity. Gastrin also causes the release of calcitonin from the C cells of the thyroid gland, which inhibits further release of gastrin via a feedback loop.

Collectively, enteric hormones and the enterogastric reflex put a strong brake on gastric secretion and motility. As the ingesta in the small intestine is processed, these stimuli diminish, the damper on the stomach is released, and its secretory and motor activities resume.

## Gastric Motility and Hunger Contraction

### Resting Electrical Activity Within the Stomach

A pacemaker in the longitudinal muscle close to the greater curve of the cardia controls the frequency of contractions. It depolarises at a rate of 3/minute, and each wave – the gastric slow wave (or basal electrical rhythm) – increases sodium permeability across the cell membrane and the impulse spreads through the longitudinal and circular muscles via low resistance junctions. These junctions make up about 12% of the membrane surface.

In the empty stomach (approximately 50 ml volume), the resting potential is low (–50 mV) and although the waves pass at a rate of 3/minute, not all of these waves are equal in amplitude and do not set off an action potential. However, when the critical firing level is passed the resulting action potential sets off an excitation–contraction coupling and a contraction spreads throughout the stomach.

### Intragastric Pressure

Intragastric pressure remains relatively constant at 5 mmHg (0.7 kPa) because as food passes into the stomach, the musculature of the fundus and body relaxes via a feedback loop – receptive relaxation. In addition, as wall tension rises so does the radius, thus keeping the intragastric pressure constant (law of Laplace). However, above 1000 ml, the radius cannot increase in size so the wall tension and intragastric pressure rises.

Thus volumes above 1000 ml lead to stimulation of stretch receptors within the stomach wall.

### Gastric Tone

In most instances gastric hypotonicity is of idiopathic origin and presumably of little clinical significance. More severe degrees, sometimes progressing to acute gastric dilatation, may occur in a variety of conditions, e.g. postoperatively, after severe trauma and in electrolyte disturbances.

A short, transversely situated, "steerhorn" stomach, on the other hand, is now known to be the result of gastric hypertonicity. In these cases immediate emptying of liquid barium usually commences in the erect position, before the onset of peristalsis or cyclical contractions of the pyloric sphincteric cylinder.

## Control of Gastric Motility

As the volume of the stomach passes 1000 ml the intragastric wall tension rises. This activates stretch receptors, again through a vagovagal reflex arc, which cause depolarisation in the longitudinal and circular smooth muscles. However, this leads to every slow wave being above the critical firing level. An action potential is therefore propagated with each slow wave and a contraction passes from the fundus through the body to the pyloric antrum. These now occur three times per minute and the force of the contraction also increases along the stomach. Initially low in the fundus, where the muscular layer is thinnest, at the pylorus intragastric pressure may reach 40–50 mmHg (5.3–6.7 kPa).

The pyloric sphincter is not a high-pressure zone and is open in the resting phase. As a contraction wave arrives it contracts. However, since the canal was open before the rise in intragastric pressure some of the chyme passes through the pylorus (5–15 ml) before the gastric slow wave reaches it. When the slow wave reaches the antrum and pylorus they contract together – terminal contraction, and the pylorus closes. This phase of the contraction acts to recirculate or "churn" the gastric contents. Only when duodenal pressure drops due to relaxation does the pyloric pressure drop.

### Factors Modifying Gastric Motility

Both vagal stimuli and gastrin increase antral motility and influence emptying. However, after a truncal vagotomy, the force of the antral pump is reduced and gastric emptying time is prolonged, hence the need for a drainage procedure after a truncal vagotomy.

The force of the pump is also moderated by the volume and composition of the chyme. Hormonal and neuronal mechanisms also regulate gastric emptying. These include duodenal distension – via a vagal feedback loop, increased duodenal osmolarity – via osmoreceptors, the presence of acid in the duodenum – via a local enteric neuronal pathway, and the release of GIP and chalesystokinin by fat in the duodenum.

In addition, sympathetic stimuli reduce gastric emptying via the limbic and hypothalamic nuclei.

### Hunger Contractions

When the stomach is empty there can be periods of increased gastric motility several hours after a meal. With stimulation of the hypothalamus the individual feels hungry. This leads in a rise in vagal stimulation and causes increased gastric motility. Contraction of the empty stomach leads to a rise in intragastric pressure that can stimulate tension and pain receptors in the gastric wall, simulating mild pain or discomfort.

## Changes in Physiology and Function Related to Disease

### Nausea, Retching and Vomiting

The mechanism of vomiting in mammals is complex and in spite of experimental studies some aspects are still not fully understood. It is usually accepted that the vomiting sequence consists of three successive phases: nausea initially, followed by retching, often leading to forcible expulsion of gastric contents through the mouth, i.e. ejection or vomiting. During these stages a coordinated sequence of movements occurs, involving, amongst others, the upper small bowel, stomach, oesophagus, diaphragm, voluntary abdominal muscles and glottis. The complex movements of the ejection phase occur with extreme rapidity. The action is controlled by the vomiting centre present bilaterally in the medulla oblongata at the level of the olivary nuclei, and close to the tractus solitarius at the level of the dorsal vagal nuclei. A complex pathway mediated via efferents in the fifth, seventh, ninth, tenth and twelfth cranial nerves leads to contraction of the intercostal muscles, diaphragm and abdominal muscles. Afferent impulses pass via the vagus (tenth cranial nerve) and sympathetic nerves to the vomiting centre. However, other impulses reach via the labyrinth, the limbic system and the chemoreceptor trigger zone. This is situated in the lateral wall of the fourth ventricle.

Nausea is the conscious recognition of the subconscious excitation of an area known as the medulla oblongata closely associated with the vomiting centre and can be initiated by impulses from the gastrointestinal tract, the lower brain in association with motion sickness or cortical impulses. Vomiting without the prodromal phase of nausea can occur, indicating that only certain portions of the vomiting centre are associated with it.

### The Process of Vomiting

If the upper gastrointestinal tract becomes excessively irritated, over-distended or over-stimulated, vomiting may occur. Initially antiperistaltic waves begin and may occur as far down as the ileum. These waves travel at 2–3 cm/s; thus within a few minutes a large volume of intestinal contents may be pushed back into the stomach and duodenum causing distension. This may result in retching.

### Retching Phase

The retching phase is characterized by a series of violent spasmodic abdomino-thoracic contractions with the glottis closed. During this time the inspiratory movements of the chest wall and diaphragm are opposed by the expiratory contractions of the abdominal musculature. At the same time movements of the stomach and its contents take place. Whereas a patient will complain of disagreeable sensations during nausea, speech is not possible during retching. The characteristic movements furnish a ready diagnostic sign of the retching phase.

### The Vomiting Act

Once the act of vomiting has been triggered, a deep inspiratory movement occurs, with elevation of the hyoid bone, which opens the upper oesophageal sphincter and closes the glottis, the soft palate rises to close the posterior nares and then a downward contraction of the diaphragm with simultaneous contraction of the abdominal wall muscles raises intragastric pressure. With the sudden relaxation of the lower oesophageal sphincter, expulsion occurs.

## Questions

1. Outline congenital abnormalities.
2. Describe lymph drainage of stomach and relate this to surgical excision.
3. Describe nerve supply.
4. Name cells of the gastric wall and their functions.

## References

1. Eker R. Carcinomas of the stomach: investigation of the lymphatic spread from gastric carcinomas after totle and partial gastrectomy. Acta Chir Scand 1951;101: 112–26.
2. Latarjet A, Wertheimer P. L'énervation gastrique. Données expérimentales. Déductions cliniques. J Méd Lyon 1921;36:1289–302.
3. Edkins J. The chemical mechanism of acid secretion. J Physiol 1906;34:133–44.

## Further Reading

Sinnatamby CS (ed). Last's anatomy. Regional and applied. 10th edn. London: Churchill Livingstone, 2001.
Snell RS Clinical anatomy for medical students. 6th ed. Philadelphia: Lippincott Williams & Wilkins, 2000.

# 3

# The Anatomy and Physiology of the Small Bowel

David Gourevitch

## Aims

To describe the development and function of the small bowel.

## Anatomy

The length of the small intestine varies from 10 to 33 feet (3–10 metres). The average length is considered to be approximately 22 feet (6.5 metres). A considerable length of small bowel can be excised and yet this may be compatible with a normal life. In some cases up to only 18 inches (45 cm) of small bowel has been preserved and the patient has survived satisfactorily.

The mesentery of the small intestine has a 6 inch (15 cm) origin from the posterior abdominal wall and commences at the duodenal-jejunal junction, just to the left of the second lumbar vertebra. The mesentery passes downwards towards the right sacral-iliac joint. The mesentery contains the superior mesenteric vessels along with lymphatics and lymph nodes. These drain the small intestine. There are a number of autonomic nerve fibres within the mesentery.

The small bowel is divided into three sections. The first section is the duodenum, which is approximately 1 foot in length (25 cm) and extends from the pylorus to the duodenal-jejunal flexure; this point is marked by the ligament of Treitz. The duodenum is anatomically divided into four parts and curves in the shape of the letter C around the head of the pancreas. At its origin the duodenum is covered with peritoneum for about an inch (2.5 cm) after which it becomes a retroperitoneal organ.

The upper half of the small intestine is termed the jejunum and the remainder is the ileum. There is no obvious distinction between the two parts and the division is one of convention only. However, the character of the small intestine does change as it is followed distally towards the caecum.

The jejunum has a thicker wall as the circular folds of mucosa (valvulae conniventes) are larger and thicker. The proximal small bowel is of greater diameter than the distal small bowel. In addition, the jejunum tends to lie towards the umbilical region of the abdomen and the ileum to the hypogastrium and pelvis.

Mesenteric vessels tend to form fewer arcades in the jejunum with long and relatively infrequent terminal branches passing to the intestinal wall. However, the ileum tends to be supplied by shorter and more numerous vessels which arise from a number of complete arcades.

## Blood Supply to the Small Intestine

The small intestine develops from the midgut and this extends from the mid-duodenum to the

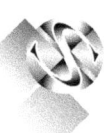

3 · UPPER GASTROINTESTINAL SURGERY

distal transverse colon and is supplied by the superior mesenteric artery, which arises from the aorta at the level of L1. The branches of superior mesenteric artery include:

1. The inferior pancreaticoduodenal artery, which supplies the pancreas and duodenum.
2. Jejunal and ileal branches of the superior mesenteric artery; these give the blood supply to the bulk of the small intestine.
3. The ileal-colic artery, which supplies the terminal ileum, the caecum and the proximal part of the ascending colon. This also goes off an appendicular branch to the appendix.
4. The right colic artery, which supplies the ascending colon.
5. The middle colic artery, which supplies the transverse colon to approximately two-thirds along its length. This vessel creates a watershed between the superior mesenteric artery and the inferior mesenteric artery.

The small intestine drains via the superior mesenteric vein and forms a confluence with the splenic vein to form the portal vein. This runs through the free edge of the lesser omentum and forms part of the superior border to the gastroepiploic foramen, before the portal vein continues to the liver.

## Histology of the Intestinal Wall

The mucosa of the small bowel is thrown into a series of folds by the plicate are the valvulae conniventes. This greatly increases the surface area available for absorption within the small bowel.

The mucosa of the small bowel contains intestinal villi which are covered by simple columnar epithelium and broken into microvilli. The wall of the small intestine is divided into the lamina propria, and this is divided from the submucosa by the muscularis mucosae. Within the lamina propria there is an extensive network of capillaries which transports respiratory gases and absorb material to the hepatoportal circulation. In addition, there are capillaries and nerve endings within the lamina propria and each villi also contains a terminal lymphatic called a lacteal.

The name lacteal refers to the cloudy appearance of the lymph contained within these channels. The lacteals themselves transport materials that fail to enter the local capillaries because they are unable to cross the capillary wall. Examples would be of fatty acids and proteins which are too large to diffuse into the bloodstream. These lipoproteins form small partials called chylomicrons which pass through the lymphatic system and account for the milky appearance within the lacteal.

## Intestinal Crypts

Within the columnar epithelium there are goblet cells which produce mucus onto the intestinal surfaces. At the base of the villi there are also found entrances to the intestinal crypts. These extend deep into the underlying lamina propria. Within the intestinal crypts there are a number of different cell populations including stem-cell divisions which continue to produce new generations of columnar and goblet cells. These new cells are continuously displaced towards the intestinal surface and within a few days will reach the tip of the villi, where they will be shed or exfoliated into the intestinal lumen. It is this process of exfoliation of the intestinal cells which ensures that the epithelial surface continues to be renewed. This also adds intracellular enzymes to the intestinal contents. One of these enzymes would be *enterokinase*, which although it does not does not directly participate in the digestion of food, is important because it activates proenzymes secreted by the pancreas.

Cells within the intestinal crypts also contain enteroendocrine cells. These are responsible for the production of several intestinal hormones including cholecystokinin and secretin.

# Physiology

## The Duodenum

The duodenum has very little absorptive function and acts mainly to neutralise the acidic contents delivered to it by the stomach. The duodenum receives the chyme from the stomach and its essential function is to buffer the gastric acid and enzymes before delivering the contents to the jejunum.

# THE ANATOMY AND PHYSIOLOGY OF THE SMALL BOWEL

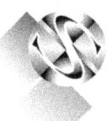

The histological characterisation of the duodenum reveals abundant presence of mucus-secreting glands. These submucosal glands, known as *Brunner's glands*, assist in the production of copious amounts of mucus. The secretion of this mucus is to protect the duodenal mucosa and also to neutralise the acid pH of the chyme. The submucosal glands are most abundant in the proximal duodenum and decrease in number towards the jejunum. The pH of the duodenal contents rises from a pH of 1–2 to 7–8 by the time it is delivered to the jejunum. In addition, the chyme is diluted by mixing with the intestinal, pancreatic and hepatic secretions.

The duodenal ampulla lies within the wall of the second part of the duodenum and allows for the delivery of bile and pancreatic enzymes to initiate the digestion and breakdown of the chyme. Absorption may occur; it is more effective under these conditions and the increase in the surface area of the duodenum in its third and fourth parts supports this increased absorptive capacity.

## The Jejunum and Ileum

The anatomy of the jejunum is a testament to the absorptive capacity. The valvulae conniventes and villi remain most prominent over the proximal half of the jejunum and it is over this area that most absorption occurs. As the ileum is approached the valvulae conniventes and villi become smaller and less numerous; they continue to diminish in size along the length of the small bowel. Under normal circumstances all absorption occurs before the chyme reaches the terminal ileum. It is squirted into the caecum where the mucosal villi are less numerous and reduced in height.

One of the major differences between the large and small intestine is the presence of bacterial activity. Bacterial presence in the large bowel is normal. However, the epithelium and underlying cells of the immune system protect the small bowel from the bacteria migrating from the large bowel. Within the ileum there are concentrations of lymphatic tissue in the submucosa called *Peyer's patches*. These represent aggregations of lymphatic tissues and they may extend for an inch or more in length. The patches are most abundant in the terminal ileum although they are seen occasionally in the duodenum.

These aggregating lymphatic follicles are placed lengthways in the intestinal wall and are usually found towards the ante-mesenteric border. Each Peyer's patch is formed by a group of solitary lymphatic follicles covered with columnar epithelium, but as a rule, the patches do not possess villi on their free surfaces. There is an abundance of lymphoid vessels around these patches. Ulceration of these lymphatic follicles may occur in typhoid fever where oval ulcers are formed in the long axis of the bowel. Perforation may occur following infection with *Salmonella* Typhi.

## Small Bowel Peristalsis

The absorptive capacity of the small bowel is enhanced by the surface area and the peristaltic movements within the small bowel. The individual villi and microvilli are manipulated by the underlying muscularis mucosae and this increases the environment around the small bowel mucosa, thereby maximising the opportunity for absorption throughout its length. At least 80% of absorption takes place within the small intestine and only a small amount within the stomach and the large intestine.

Absorption occurs as the chyme is moved along the length of the small bowel by peristaltic contractions. These contractions are myenteric reflexes associated with the splanchnic nerves and are not under the control of the central nervous system. The effect of this nerve plexus is limited to a short length of the small bowel at the site of the stimulus for peristalsis. However, there are more elaborate and coordinated reflexes and two examples are the gastroenteric reflex and the gastroileal reflex.

## Gastroenteric and Gastroileal Reflexes

The gastroenteric reflex is initiated by distension of the stomach and this stimulates an increase in the rate of glandular secretion and peristalsis activity in the duodenum and the small bowel. This increased peristalsis allows for chyme to move through the duodenum and into the small bowel.

The gastroileal reflex is a combination of a neural mediated gastroenteric reflex and a response to circulating levels of the hormone

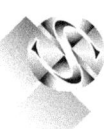

### 3 · UPPER GASTROINTESTINAL SURGERY

gastrin. The entry of food into the stomach triggers the release of gastrin and this relaxes the sphincter at the ileocaecal junction allowing for increased ileal peristalsis and the passage of chyme into the caecum. This reflex is often associated with the experience of dull, lower abdominal discomfort and a person's desire to open their bowels.

## Intestinal Secretions

There is a large flow of secretions cross the small bowel mucosa which is estimated to be between 1.5 and 2.5 litres of fluid within a 24-hour period. The fluids pass into the intestinal lumen and the vast majority will be re-absorbed before the contents enter the caecum. This movement of fluid across the intestinal mucosa is called *succus entericus*. Some of this fluid enters the intestinal lumen through osmosis because of the relatively concentrated chyme. The remaining fluid is produced by the intestinal glands and stimulated by activity of touch and stretch receptors within the wall of the intestine.

The intestinal juice assists in buffering the acids and dissolves the digestive enzymes and the products of digestion.

Regulation of the secretory output of the larger digestive and accessory glands is via the central nervous system and hormonal control. These mechanisms tend to occur in the region of the duodenum where acids are neutralised and enzymes released. The submucosal glands within the duodenum protect the duodenum from the gastric acid output and the local secretion of enzymes.

There are local reflexes mechanisms which stimulate the secretory activity of the duodenum and this activity is enhanced by the parasympathetic (vagal) stimulation. It is recognised that duodenal glands begin secreting before chyme reaches the pylorus. This is considered the cephalic phase of gastric secretion. Stimulation of the sympathetic chain inhibits secretory activity leaving the duodenal mucosa unprepared for receiving chyme, and this may have some part to play in the production of duodenal ulcers.

## Intestinal Hormones

The enteroendocrine cells within the duodenum produce hormones which coordinate the secretory activity of the stomach, duodenum, liver and pancreas. Enterocrinin is a hormone which is released by the duodenal mucosa when the acid chyme from the stomach enters the small intestine. There are many other hormones secreted which have both primary and secondary effects, and which act in a complementary fashion. The three most important hormones involved in the regulatory activity of the small intestine are *secretin*, *cholecystokinin* and the glucose-dependent *insulinotropic peptide*.

### Secretin

Secretin is produced in response to the presence of acid within the duodenum. The primary effect of secretin is to increase the production of water and buffers by the pancreas and liver. It also has an effect on stimulating the duodenal submucosal glands.

### Cholecystokinin (CCK)

The duodenal mucosa is stimulated to produce cholecystokinin when chyme arrives within the lumen of the duodenum and particularly when it contains lipids and partially digested proteins. This hormone has a target effect both on the pancreas and on the liver. The pancreas is stimulated to produce and secrete digestive enzymes, and the hormone also increases the passage of bile by stimulating the gall bladder to contract.

The net effect of cholecystokinin is to increase the secretion of pancreatic enzymes and stimulate the production of bile. However, in high concentration both secretin and cholecystokinin have the additional effect of producing gastric motility and secretions.

### Glucose-dependent Insulinotropic Peptide (GIP)

This peptide is released by the duodenal mucosa in response to fats and glucose entering the duodenum. This peptide stimulates the release of insulin from the pancreatic islet cells, although at high concentration it can also inhibit gastric activity. (Originally this was named the gastric inhibitory peptide.)

### Vasoactive Intestinal Peptide (VIP)

Several other hormones are produced in small quantities in response to chyme entering the duodenum. For example, relatively large amounts of undigested proteins will stimulate the release of gastrin by the duodenal cells. Vasoactive intestinal peptide or VIP is also produced and it stimulates the secretion of the intestinal glands whilst inhibiting acid production within the stomach. Previously, it was considered that the enzyme called enterogastrin was responsible for inhibiting gastric activity. However, it is now considered that this inhibition of gastric motility is the product of GIP and VIP.

The number and diversity of the hormones produced by the small bowel are well recognised, but poorly understood. Many of the hormones have a similar chemical structure and it is difficult to differentiate the primary effects of these various hormones. Analysis has led to an increased number of hormones being identified, although their specific functions are poorly understood.

## The Embryology of the Small Intestine (Midgut)

In the adult the midgut starts immediately distal to the point where the bile duct enters the duodenum and it terminates at the junction of the proximal two-thirds of the transverse colon with a distal third. The superior mesenteric artery supplies the entire length of the midgut.

Within the 5-week-old embryo the midgut is suspended by a short mesentery from the posterior abdominal wall and it communicates with the yolk sac by way of the vitello-intestinal duct. At the apex of the midgut loop there is a connection with the yolk sac via the vitelline duct. The proximal or cephalic limb of the loop becomes the distal part of the duodenum, the jejunum and part of the ileum, and the cordal or distal portion of the loop becomes the ileum, caecum, appendix, ascending and proximal transverse colon.

With the rapid growth and expansion of the liver and the elongation of the midgut, the abdominal cavity becomes too small to contain the intestinal loops. For a period during the sixth week of development, the intestinal loops enter an extra-embryonic cavity within the umbilical cord; this is considered to be a physiological umbilical herniation.

By the tenth week the herniated intestinal loops are returning to the abdominal cavity. The precise factors responsible for this are not known although as the mesonephric kidney regresses and there is a reduced growth of the liver with some expansion of the abdominal cavity, space becomes available to allow for the return of the midgut to the abdomen. As the midgut retracts into the abdomen it also rotates and with the expansion of the caecal bud, which appears around the sixth week, the characteristic placement of the midgut within the abdominal cavity occurs. The distal midgut expands and there is some separation into the small and large intestine. A small narrow diverticulum is formed from the caecal bud which develops into the appendix.

The mesenteries of the intestinal loops are produced during the changes and rotation of the midgut around the superior mesenteric vessels. With fusion of the mesenteric layers the small intestine retains a long and mobile mesentery; however, the caecum and ascending colon become fused with the posterior abdominal wall.

Associated with the embryological development of the small intestine a number of abnormalities can occur. Abnormal rotation of the intestinal loop may occur and this results in a volvulus where the blood supply to the loop is compromised, particularly when the base of the small bowel mesentery is shortened. On occasions there can be reverse rotation of the intestinal loop and the small intestine is found towards the right side of the abdomen, with the caecum and the large intestine to the left. Further abnormalities may include duplication of the intestinal loop with cysts. These cysts are most frequently found within the region of the ileum and they may vary from a long segment to a short one with a small diverticulum.

Other abnormalities of the small intestine may be associated with defects within the abdominal wall. An omphalocele (exomphalos) involves the herniation of the abdominal viscera through a defect within the umbilical ring. This defect often contains small bowel, and liver, stomach, spleen and gall bladder may also be included. The defect is thought to be caused by failure of the bowel to return to the body cavity following its physiological herniation between the sixth and tenth week of development. This defect may occur in up to 2.5 per 10 000 births and it is associated with a high mortality.

A further abnormality which can be confused with the omphalocele is gastroschisis. This defect is characterised by an abnormality within the abdominal wall and occurs lateral to the umbilicus. The viscera are found within the aminotic cavity and are not covered with the peritoneum. It is thought that this abnormality occurs in approximately 1 in 10 000 births and there has been some increase in its frequency among babies born to young women who are using cocaine. Unlike the omphalocele, in which 50% of infants have a chromosome abnormality, gastroschisis is not usually associated with any specific chromosomal abnormality.

More commonly vitello-intestinal duct abnormalities occur in 2–4% of people. These abnormalities may consist of a small out-pouching of the ileum with the development of a Meckel's diverticulum, but other abnormalities may occur and include a vitelline ligament or a cyst within the ligament, and occasionally a fistula is formed which connects the small bowel with the umbilicus. With this last defect there is usually a small faecal fistula present at the time of birth. These abnormalities are usually easy to correct surgically, although the patient can be quite ill and present with an intestinal obstruction, often at a young age.

Other common abnormalities within the small bowel may include atresias or stenoses. These can occur at any point along the intestine, although they occur most frequently within the duodenum. These abnormalities are likely to be the result of "vascular accidents". They may occur as a result of malrotation, volvulus, and can be associated with an omphalocele or gastroschisis, when the blood supply to the bowel is compromised and this results in fibrosis and narrowing of the bowel. On occasions, a small segment of bowel can be lost and replaced with a fibrous cord, or more simply, there can be a length of narrowing within the small bowel, and children present with subacute intestinal obstruction.

## Questions

1. Describe the anatomy of the midgut.
2. Name the important hormones of the small bowel and describe their function.
3. What abnormalities can occur in development?

## Further Reading

Sadler TW. Langman's medical embryology, 9th edition. Philadelphia: Lippincott Williams & Wilkins, 2003.

# 4

# The Anatomy and Physiology of the Diaphragm

George R. Harrison

## Aims

To describe development, anatomy and physiology of the diaphragm.

## Anatomy

### The Shape of the Diaphragm

The diaphragm is a musculo-fibrous sheet separating the thorax and the abdomen. It takes the shape of an elliptical cylindroid capped with a dome [1]. This short description of the shape of the diaphragm is not adequate to explain the way in which the structure and function are related, and a further expansion of this description is necessary. The use of the word dome in itself introduces a degree of inaccuracy, as it gives the impression that there is a curved structure rising equally from the sides to a central point, whereas a more accurate description is of a pair of cupolas either side of a central plateau.

This elliptical shape is determined by the thoracic outlet, which will also have an influence upon the function of the diaphragm, as it will determine the anatomical structure of it. This is because the thoracic outlet is set obliquely to the coronal plane, being superior anteriorly and inferior posteriorly.

The skeletal attachments of the diaphragm to the thoracic outlet commence at the xiphoid process and symphysis centrally, and, moving laterally, the ventral ends and costal cartilages of the seventh to twelfth ribs, the transverse processes of the first lumbar vertebra, and the bodies and symphyses of the first three lumbar vertebrae. As the periphery of the diaphragm is attached to the thoracic outlet anteriorly and laterally, and beyond it posteriorly, it will follow that the anterior portion of the diaphragm will be shorter than the lateral and posterior parts.

The presence of the viscera in the thorax and abdomen causes the part of the diaphragm separating them to be roughly horizontal, but will determine the shape of the unstressed dome. This may be considered as a separate zone from the other part of the diaphragm, and will be referred to as the diaphragmatic zone. The other part of the diaphragm will be referred to as the apposition zone, because it assumes a roughly vertical direction. It is also the area through which the rib cage is apposed to the abdominal contents and thus exposed to abdominal pressure (see below).

### Diaphragmatic Attachments

The sternal part is attached by two slips to the back of the xiphoid process, although these slips may be absent (Figure 4.1). The costal part is attached to the internal surfaces of the lower six costal cartilages and their adjoining ribs, the vertical fibres of the diaphragm interdigitating with the horizontal fibres from the transversi abdominis. The lumbar part is attached to the aponeurotic medial and lateral arcuate

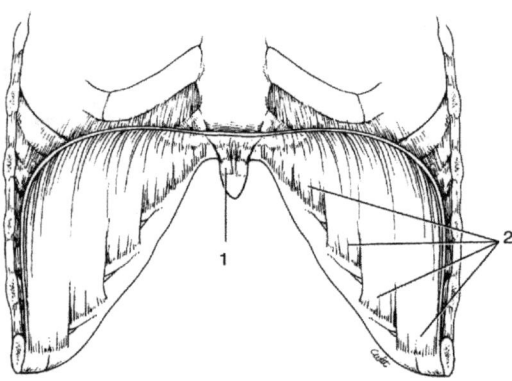

**Figure 4.1.** The inner anterior surface of the diaphragm. (Reproduced with permission from Gluzel P, Similowski T, Chartrand-Lefebvre C et al. Diaphragm and chest wall: assessment of the inspiratory pump with MR imaging – preliminary observations. Radiology 2000;215:574–83. Copyright Radiological Sciety of North America.)

ligaments (lumbocostal arches) and to the upper three lumbar vertebrae by crura. The sternocostal and lumbar portions are distinct developmentally and in 80% of the population are separated by a hiatus in the muscular sheet – the vertebrocostal trigone. This gap lies above the twelfth rib so that the upper pole of the kidney is separated from the pleura by loose areolar tissue only.

The lateral arcuate ligament is a thickened band in the fascia of quadratus lumborum, which arches across the muscle and is attached medially to the front of the first transverse process and laterally to the inferior margin of the twelfth near its midpoint.

The medial arcuate ligament is a thickened band in the fascia covering psoas major. Medially it blends with the lateral tendinous margin of the corresponding crus and is thus attached to the side of the first or second lumbar vertebrae. Laterally it is attached to the front of the first lumbar transverse process at the lateral margin of psoas. The arcuate ligaments allow the contraction of quadratus lumborum and psoas to occur without interfering with diaphragmatic activity.

The crura are tendinous at their attachments, blending with the anterior longitudinal vertebral ligament. The right crus is broader and longer and arises from the anterolateral aspect of the bodies and discs of the first three lumbar vertebrae, the left crus from the corresponding parts of the upper two. As with the anterior longitudinal ligament, the main area of attachment is at the level of the intervertebral discs and the adjacent margins of the vertebral bodies. Between these attachments the upper lumbar arteries separate the fibres from the bodies of the vertebrae. The fibres ascend and run anteriorly to cross the aorta in a median arch, where the tendinous margins converge to form the median arcuate ligament. This ligament is often poorly defined, but when it occurs it is at the level of the thoracolumbar disc.

The fibres of the crura continue in their passage anteriorly and superiorly, but divide into medial and lateral bundles. The lateral fibres continue laterally to reach the central tendon. The medial fibres from the right crus ascend to the left of the oesophageal opening. Sometimes a muscular fasciculus from the medial side of the left crus crosses the aorta and runs obliquely through the fibres of the right crus towards the vena caval opening but does not approach the oesophageal opening. The right margin of the oesophageal opening is covered by the deeper medial right crural fibres. From part of the right crus near the oesophageal opening originates the suspensory muscle of the duodenum, which goes to connective tissue near the coeliac artery. Here it joins with a fibromuscular band of non-striated muscle originating along the third and fourth parts of the duodenum and the duodenojejunal flexure. The exact nature and function of this muscle has been the subject of discussion over many years, and will not be considered here.

## The Central Tendon of the Diaphragm

All the muscular fibres converge upon the central tendon of the diaphragm (Figure 4.2). The central tendon is a thin, strong aponeurosis of interwoven collagen fibres, with its anterior margin closer to the front of the diaphragm. This results in the longer fibres being lateral and posterior. The longest fibres of the diaphragm arise from the ninth costal cartilage.

## Embryology

The diaphragm develops from four main structures, the septum transversum, the pleuroperi-

# THE ANATOMY AND PHYSIOLOGY OF THE DIAPHRAGM

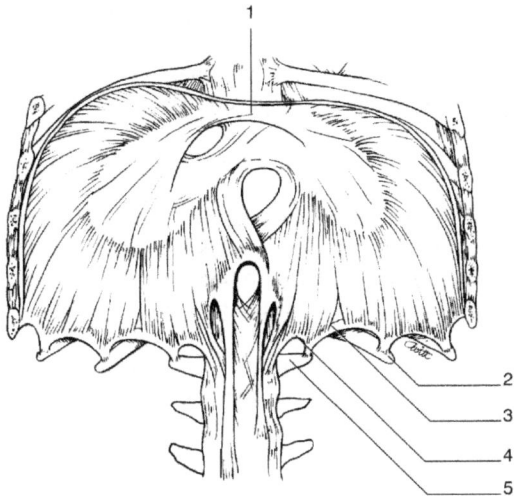

**Figure 4.2.** Inner posterior aspect of the diaphragm. 1, The central tendon. 2, Attachment of lateral arcuate ligament to end of the twelfth rib. 3, Lateral arcuate ligament. 4, Medial arcuate ligament. 5, Transverse process first lumbar vertebra. (Reproduced with permission from Gluzel P, Similowski T, Chartrand-Lefebvre C et al. Diaphragm and chest wall: assessment of the inspiratory pump with MR imaging – preliminary observations. Radiology 2000;215:574–83. Copyright Radiological Sciety of North America.)

toneal membranes, the dorsal oesophageal mesentery and the body wall.

The septum transversum forms the bulk of the diaphragm, namely the central tendon and the majority of centrally placed muscle. It starts off as a plate of mesoderm developing at the end of the fourth week of gestation in a position between the heart and the yolk sac. At this time the headfold and tailfolds form, and the heart and pericardial cavities move ventrally below the foregut. They open dorsally into the pericardioperitoneal canals, which lie above the septum transversum on each side of the foregut connecting the thoracic and abdominal portions of the intraembryonic coelom.

The septum transversum is initially at the level of the second cervical segment, but with the growth of the embryo it moves in a caudal direction, and at the level of the fourth cervical segment it receives the phrenic nerve and cells destined to differentiate into muscular tissue from the corresponding myotomes. It migrates caudally during flexion and comes to lie at the level of the junction between the thoracic and lumbar segments. At this site it forms a ventral mass of tissue which then extends dorsally and medially towards the dorsal body wall, to meet the dorsal mesentery of the foregut. As it grows it leaves two dorsolateral gaps, which are the orifices of the pleuroperitoneal canals.

The pleuroperitoneal membranes are a pair of membranes which gradually separate the pleural and peritoneal cavities. They are attached dorsolaterally to the body wall with their free edge projecting into the caudal end of the pericardioperitoneal canals. At about the sixth week of gestation they grow medially and ventrally away from the body wall towards the septum transversum. By the end of that week they have come to fuse with the dorsal mesentery of the oesophagus and the septum transversum to separate the pleural and peritoneal cavities. The closure of the openings is further enhanced by the growth of the liver and muscle tissue extension into the membranes. The right pleuroperitoneal canal closes before the left one, the latter being the more common site of persistent communication between the pleural and peritoneal cavities. The pleuroperitoneal membranes are believed only to produce a small dorsolateral part of the diaphragm in adult life.

The dorsal mesentery of the oesophagus fuses with both the septum transversum and the pleuroperitoneal membranes. This mesentery forms the medial portion of the diaphragm. The crura of the diaphragm develop from muscle fibres that grow into the oesophageal mesentery.

The contribution of the muscular body wall to the diaphragm is the result of the expansion of the pleural cavities between the ninth and twelfth weeks of gestation. To expand, the pleural cavities extend into the mesoderm dorsal to the suprarenal glands, the gonads and the mesonephric ridges, causing somatopleuric mesoderm to be peeled away from the dorsal body wall to form a substantial area of the dorsolumbar part of the diaphragm. As a result of the extension of the pleural cavities into the body wall, the costodiaphragmatic recesses are formed.

It is described variously as trifoliate, trefoil or like the club in a pack of cards, the three parts being partly separated by slight indentations. This description does not seem to agree with the pictures that are reproduced in many textbooks, which make it look far more like a boomerang. There is a middle part, which is an equilateral triangle, its apex towards the xiphoid process.

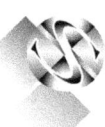

This central area is beneath and partly blended with the pericardium above, and relates to the triangular ligament of the liver in the abdomen. The right and left parts posteriorly are longer and linguiform, curving posterolaterally, the left being the narrower. These are related to the parietal pleura above and the peritoneum below. In the central area can be recognised four diagonal bands, which expand from a thick node where decussation of compressed tendinous strands occurs in front of the oesophageal aperture and left of the vena caval opening.

## The Diaphragmatic Apertures

As the diaphragm separates the abdominal and thoracic cavities, there are several structures which will either pass through it, or between it and the body wall including blood vessels, nerves and the oesophagus. There are various apertures to allow the passage of these, three of which are large and constant, and various others which are smaller and sometimes variable.

*The aortic opening*, the most inferior and posterior, lies at the level of the lower border of the twelfth thoracic vertebra and the thoracolumbar intervertebral disc, slightly to the left of the midline. This is not a true opening, rather it is a vertical osseo-aponeurotic and symphysio-aponeurotic channel between the crura laterally and the vertebral column posteriorly and the diaphragm anteriorly. Therefore it is actually behind the diaphragm or the median arcuate ligament. On occasions there are some tendinous crural fibres which pass behind the aorta, forming a fibrous ring. It transmits the aorta. Along with the aorta, generally to the right of the midline, runs the thoracic duct, posterolateral to which are the azygos vein on the right, and the hemi-azygos vein on the left. Sometimes the azygos and hemi-azygos veins will pass through the right and left crus respectively. Lymphatic trunks also descend through the opening from the lower posterior thoracic wall.

*The oesophageal aperture* is elliptical and lies at the level of the tenth thoracic vertebra, where its long axis lies obliquely, ascending to the left of the midline in the muscular part of the right crus which has by now crossed over the midline. Its lower end lies anterosuperior to the aortic opening, its upper end being further anterosuperior and a short distance to the left. It transmits the oesophagus, the trunks of the vagus nerves, and the oesophageal branches of the left gastric vessels and lymphatic vessels.

The muscle of the oesophageal wall and the diaphragm remain separate. However, the inferior diaphragmatic fascia, which is a thin areolar stratum rich in elastic fibres, lying between the diaphragm and the peritoneum, and continuous with the transversalis fascia, ascends through the opening. It does so like a flattened cone to blend with the oesophageal wall about 2 cm above the gastro-oesophageal junction. Some of the elastic fibres penetrate to the submucosa. This fascial expansion, which forms the phreno-oesophageal ligament, connects the oesophagus and the diaphragm in a flexible manner which allows some freedom of movement during breathing and swallowing.

*The vena caval aperture* is the highest of the three, and lies approximately at the level of the disc between the eighth and ninth thoracic vertebrae. It is quadrilateral and sited within the central tendon, at the junction of its right leaf with the central area. Therefore the margin is aponeurotic, to which the vena cava is adherent as it traverses the opening. With it run branches of the right phrenic nerve. The left phrenic nerve runs off the pericardium to pierce the muscular part of the diaphragm in the form of the left limb of the central tendon.

There are various minor apertures. Two lesser apertures in each crus transmit the greater and lesser splanchnic nerves. The ganglionated sympathetic trunks run from the thorax to the abdomen behind the medial end of the medial arcuate ligament. Posterior to the lateral arcuate ligament runs the subcostal nerve.

Between the sternal and costal margins of the diaphragm run the superior epigastric arteries and veins, prior to entering the rectus sheath, along with lymph vessels from the abdominal wall and liver. Similarly the musculophrenic artery and vein run between the attachments of the diaphragm to the seventh and eighth costal cartilages. The neurovascular bundles of the seventh to eleventh intercostal spaces pass between the digitations of transversus abdominis with the diaphragm into the neurovascular plane of the abdominal wall.

Extraperiteoneal lymph vessels on the abdominal surface pass through the diaphragm to nodes lying on its thoracic surface, mainly in the posterior mediastinum. Finally, openings for small veins are frequent in the central tendon.

## Nerve Supply

The diaphragm receives its nerve supply predominantly from the phrenic nerve. This arises mainly from the ventral root of the fourth cervical nerve, with contributions from the third and fifth cervical nerve roots. The intrathoracic course of these nerves will not be discussed here.

The right phrenic nerve reaches the diaphragm just lateral to the inferior vena cava (IVC). The left phrenic nerve joins the diaphragm just lateral to the border of the heart, in a slightly more anterior plane than the right phrenic nerve. The nerves divide at the level of the diaphragm, or just above it into several terminal branches, the right being the mirror of the left. Apart from small twigs to the serosa of the diaphragm, there are three main branches: a sternal or anterior branch, an anterolateral branch and a posterior branch which divides into a posterolateral branch and a crural branch that runs posteromedially to the region of the crus. They are usually deep within the muscle rather than lying exposed on the undersurface of the diaphragm [2,3].

The phrenic nerve provides the only motor supply to the diaphragm. The crural motor supply comes solely from the phrenic nerve, but all crural fibres (regardless of the side of origin) right or left of the oesophageal opening are supplied by the ipsilateral phrenic nerve. The phrenic nerve also supplies the majority of sensory fibres including muscle spindles [4]. There are some sensory fibres to the diaphragm from the lower six or seven intercostal nerves in the area where the diaphragm is attached to the ribs.

## Blood Supply

The arterial supply varies above and below the diaphragm. The superior surface is supplied by the musculophrenic, pericardiacophrenic and superior epigastric arteries, all of which are branches of the internal thoracic mammary artery, and the phrenic branches of the lower thoracic aorta. There is also a supply from the lower five intercostal and subcostal arteries. The inferior surface is supplied by the inferior phrenic arteries, which are branches of the abdominal aorta, although sometimes they may be derivatives of the coeliac trunk.

The venous drainage mirrors the blood supply. The superior surface drains through the pericardiacophrenic veins, musculophrenic veins and superior epigastric veins which all drain into the internal thoracic vein. The inferior surface of the diaphragm drains through the inferior phrenic veins. The right drains to the IVC. The left is often double, the anterior branch going to the IVC, the posterior branch to the left renal vein or left suprarenal vein. The two veins may anastomose with each other.

## Lymphatic Drainage

The diaphragmatic lymph nodes on the thoracic surface of the diaphragm form three groups. An anterior group comprises two or three small nodes posterior to the base of the xiphoid process draining the convex hepatic surface, and one or two nodes on each side near the junction of the seventh rib and cartilage which receive anterior lymph vessels from the diaphragm and drain to the parasternal nodes.

A lateral group on each half of the diaphragm comprises two or three nodes, close to the site at which the phrenic nerves enter the diaphragm, and on the right some of the nodes may lie anterior to the intrathoracic end of the IVC within the pericardium. They receive afferents from the central diaphragm (bilateral) and from the convex surface of the liver (right side), and send efferents to the parasternal, posterior mediastinal nodes, and brachiocephalic nodes.

A posterior group consists of a small number of nodes on the back of the crura, connected with the lateral aortic and the posterior mediastinal nodes.

## Lymph Vessels of the Diaphragm

An extensive lymph plexus is present in each surface of the diaphragm, and the two plexuses are united by numerous vessels that pierce the diaphragm. The thoracic plexus unites with vessels of the mediastinal and costal pleura. Anterior efferents pass to the anterior diaphragmatic nodes near the junction of the seventh ribs and cartilages, the middle efferents to nodes on the oesophagus and around the inferior vena cava, and posterior efferents to nodes around the aorta as it leaves the thorax. The abdominal plexus anastomoses with hepatic lymphatics and with subperitoneal tissue peripherally.

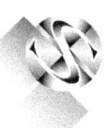

Efferents on the right end up either in a group of nodes on the inferior phrenic artery or in the right lateral aortic nodes. Efferents on the right go to preaortic nodes, lateral aortic nodes and nodes at the lower end of the oesophagus.

## Relations of the Diaphragm

Superiorly the diaphragm is associated with serous membranes. On either side is the pleura, which separates the diaphragm from the lung bases, and in the middle is pericardium separating it from the heart. The middle part of the central tendon is slightly lower, flatter and more horizontal than the other parts, which form rounded cupolas. The inferior surface is covered with peritoneum, that of the right cupola being in contact with the convex right lobe of the liver, the right kidney and suprarenal gland. The peritoneum of the left cupola is in contact with the left lobe of the liver, the gastric fundus, the spleen, left kidney and adrenal gland.

# Physiology

The main function of the diaphragm is ventilation, but there is also a non-ventilatory role of the diaphragm. This will be considered at the end of this section. Prior to that, this section will concentrate upon the ventilatory function of the diaphragm, looking at three different areas, firstly the elastic properties of the diaphragm, then the effects of contraction, followed by an examination of the importance of relaxation in maintaining normal ventilation.

## Elastic Properties of the Diaphragm

As the diaphragm is a composite structure the elasticity will vary with the type of tissue. The collagenous central tendon is relatively inelastic. The muscular component will vary in its elasticity dependent upon the state of expansion of the chest wall, as this will have an impact upon the resting length of the muscle groups.

Muscle is composed of a contractile component, and an elastic component. The elastic component can be divided into a series component and a parallel component. Elasticity of resting muscle is usually described in terms of its tensile properties, characterised by measurements of relationships between tension and muscle elongation. This relationship is non-linear, as a result of the muscle becoming stiffer as it is stretched, and is believed to represent a recruitment phenomenon within the muscle; that is, as the muscle is stretched, fibrous elements that are unstressed at low extension are progressively recruited, contributing their elasticity in parallel with increasing extension [5].

The collagenous central tendon is less extensible than the muscle. Collagen has a high modulus of elasticity, such that a high stress is necessary for a small amount of extension. It is believed that the central tendon has a function similar to that of a normal muscular tendon, namely transmitting the stress generated by the muscle, and allowing this to be converted into movement.

## Contraction of the Diaphragm

During quiet breathing, the zone of apposition represents one-quarter to one-third of the total surface of the rib cage. In an average human in the upright position the axial extent of the zone of apposition from costal insertion to the diaphragmatic reflection increases from nearly 0 to 5 cm as the lung volume is reduced from total lung capacity to functional residual capacity, and increased further to 10 cm at residual volume [6].

When the diaphragmatic muscle shortens during inspiration, the axial length of the cylindrical portion diminishes and the dome descends relative to its costal insertions. The zone of apposition of the diaphragm cannot change shape during breathing, unless the shape of the rib cage does. The dome part of the diaphragm is able to change, but does not normally do so during quiet breathing.

During quiet breathing the decrease in axial length of the apposed diaphragm is about 2 cm, whereas the increase in sagittal and coronal diameters of the rib cage is only approximately 0.3 and 0.5 cm, respectively. Therefore the most important change in diaphragmatic shape, responsible for the majority of volume displacement during normal quiet breathing, is the piston-like axial displacement of the dome of the diaphragm by the contraction of the axial length of the zone of apposition.

The pressure difference across the diaphragm (the transdiaphragmatic pressure (Pdi)) is

# THE ANATOMY AND PHYSIOLOGY OF THE DIAPHRAGM

related to the orthogonal tensions and radii of curvature by Laplace's law, but in the zone of apposition the radius of curvature in the axial direction is large, and so local Pdi would be related to circumferential tension and curvature. Pdi is therefore the total axial force developed by the apposed diaphragmatic fibres divided by the cross-sectional area at the zone of apposition. Because the number of fibres contracting is probably fairly consistent, the Pdi is directly related to the tension developed within the fibres and inversely related to the thoracic cross-sectional area. As recent radiological studies have shown that the area of the dome of the diaphragm varies very little between residual volume and functional residual capacity, this may not need to be considered in assessing the Pdi [7].

The shape of the dome does not vary significantly during quiet breathing as mentioned above, and therefore the radius of curvature of the diaphragmatic dome also does not need to be considered in assessing the Pdi. This is an advantage because the shape of the diaphragm is complex as described above, and has many radii of curvature, all of which will conspire to make estimates of Pdi from Laplace's law difficult.

The piston analogy breaks down when the diaphragm has shortened enough to eliminate the zone of apposition. Under these conditions the transdiaphragmatic pressure has to be analysed by considering the radii of curvature and the anisotropic (i.e. varying with position) tension within the muscular sheet of the diaphragm. A major variable for determining the force generated by the diaphragmatic muscle is the length–tension behaviour of the muscle. Generally the greater the initial length of the muscle fibre, the greater the force developed, and therefore the greater the transdiaphragmatic pressure. When considering the diaphragm, one of the determinants of fibre length will be the lung volume; the lesser the volume the greater the fibre length.

## Effect of Diaphragmatic Contraction on Abdomen and Rib Cage

The descent of the dome of the diaphragm, which occurs during inspiration, will increase the subdiaphragmatic pressure and cause displacement of the abdominal viscera caudally. As the contents of the abdomen are virtually incompressible (apart from a small amount of gas within the bowel), there must be an equal and outward displacement of the abdominal wall. In the human the abdomen is bounded by the lumbar spine posteriorly and pelvis inferiorly, which are not readily displaced, and by the rib cage, which nearly meets the iliac crest at the side. The free abdominal wall is therefore limited to the ventral abdominal wall, and contraction of the diaphragm should displace it. However, if the rib cage expands sufficiently the diaphragm may contract during inspiration without producing any abdominal displacement.

There is evidence in humans to demonstrate that there are changes in the rib cage that occur as a result of diaphragmatic activity. This work has been done by studying the breathing patterns in patients who have had transections of the cervical spine, so that there is an active phrenic nerve, but no intercostal muscle activity [8]. Measurements were made in sitting subjects at the third and seventh costal interfaces, and demonstrated a difference between the two parts of the rib cage. During inspiration the abdominal wall moves out, associated with an increase in the sagittal and coronal diameters of the lower rib cage. In contrast, at the upper rib cage the movement in both planes is inward.

Thus the contraction of the diaphragm appears to have two actions on the rib cage. Firstly, the decrease in pleural pressure that it produces would tend to displace the rib cage inwards. This is an effect predominantly on the upper ribs, although in the non-tetraplegic patient the scalene and intercostal muscles tend to prevent this. Secondly, it also has an inspiratory action, which tends to affect the lower ribs. The inspiratory action has two components to it, one being related to the force developed through the insertion into the ribs (insertional component), the second being the force exerted through the zone of apposition by the increase in abdominal pressure that occurs during diaphragmatic contraction (appositional component). The net action of the diaphragm at this level will depend upon the balance between the insertional and appositional inspiratory forces and the expiratory force generated by the fall in pleural pressure. In general inspiration is the greater force.

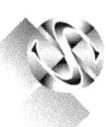

The insertional component of the inspiratory action of the diaphragm relates to the manner of insertion of the costal fibres, namely into the lower ribs. As these fibres are directed upwards and parallel to the rib cage axis, their contraction exerts a force that tends to raise the ribs, and therefore move them outwards. This is dependent upon forces resisting the descent of the diaphragm. Part of this resistance is provided by the abdominal pressure, as well as by the solid elements in the abdomen, the latter providing resistance by resisting displacement, which is not reflected in the abdominal pressure. That the abdominal viscera provide a fulcrum on which the diaphragm acts to raise the lower ribs has been confirmed in canine experiments, which demonstrate that evisceration of the animal causes the costal fibres of the diaphragm to contract rather than to expand the rib cage [9].

The appositional component of lower rib cage expansion relates to changes in abdominal pressure. This increase in abdominal pressure that occurs during diaphragmatic contraction will act through the zone of apposition. There are several variables that will affect the appositional component, the main two being the abdominal pressure and the size of the zone of apposition, but the compliance of the abdominal wall will also have an impact upon it.

If there is a large zone of apposition, the increase in abdominal pressure will be transmitted to the rib cage over a large area, and will act by causing outward movement of the ribs. This will be greater if the abdominal compliance is low. This is the situation occurring during normal tidal breathing. However, if the zone of apposition is greatly reduced, which occurs at lung volumes approaching vital capacity, the pressure generated upon the abdominal contents will not have such a great inspirational component.

## Influence of Posture

In normal upright subjects quiet breathing occurs in such a manner that with inspiration there is an increase in the anteroposterior diameters of both the abdomen and the rib cage which is reversed on expiration. In the supine subject there is a greater increase in the abdominal component than the rib cage during inspiration. Although the effect of diaphragmatic contraction on the rib cage has been discussed above, the situation in the normal subject is complicated by the fact that there are inspiratory muscles other than the diaphragm, including the intercostals and scalenes. These appear to be automatically brought into play with the diaphragm.

However, even when these are taken into consideration, it has been demonstrated that the diaphragm expands the lower rib cage less in the supine position than the erect. This evidence comes from tetraplegic patients, in whom, during inspiration in the upright posture, the lower rib cage moves outwards [10]. However, in the supine position, during inspiration the lower rib cage moves inwards, whilst the abdominal diameter increases. The rib cage then moves outwards during expiration. Thus the diaphragm has an inspiratory activity in the erect posture, but expiratory effect in the supine position.

The explanation for the mechanism behind these differences in posture is not fully elucidated. Whatever the position of the body, the effect of diaphragmatic contraction is to cause a fall in pleural pressure, and therefore for the same increase in lung volume the expiratory force of the rib cage would be assumed to be equal. Thus the differences in rib cage movement between supine and erect posture are considered to be related to differences in appositional and/or insertional forces. The zone of apposition is known to vary between erect and supine posture, both in shape and size, the dorsal component being greater when supine, the ventral component being less. In transferring between the upright and horizontal position the abdominal contents are displaced cephalad and the lung volume at functional residual capacity is reduced by approximately 15% of the vital capacity. The diaphragmatic muscles are lengthened and develop appreciable passive tensions at relatively higher lung volumes. Also, the diaphragmatic dome is subject to varying transmural pressures, increasing from the uppermost to the lower surfaces, as a result of gravitational effects. The gradient of pleural pressure is probably less than that of the abdominal side, and in humans the difference in transmural pressure between the upper and lower surfaces is about 10 cmH$_2$O. This will give the dome an increase in curvature in the direction of gravity.

The latter may have an impact upon the insertional component of the ventral part of the diaphragm, possibly as a result of converting the axial tension, which would be created in the erect posture, to a radial tension, which would cause the ribs to be drawn in. On top of this there will be an increase in abdominal compliance in the supine position, which will also cause the ribs to move inwards, the opposite to the changes occurring in the erect posture.

The effects of diaphragmatic contraction on the upper part of the rib cage are unrelated to posture. When the rib cage muscles are inactive the diaphragm causes the upper rib cage to move inwards in both erect and supine postures. This has been demonstrated not only in tetraplegic patients [8] but also in normal subjects during rapid-eye-movement sleep [11], when there is a reduction of electrical activity in the parasternal area, allowing a paradoxical movement of the rib cage with inspiration.

### Influence of Lung Volume

Lung volume will have a marked influence on the action of the diaphragm on the rib cage. As lung volume decreases below functional residual capacity the zone of apposition will increase. Thus the area of the rib cage exposed to abdominal pressure will increase while the area exposed to the pleural pressure decreases. Conversely, with an increase in lung volume, there will be a reduction in the zone of apposition. From this it will be seen that there is a reduction in the diaphragm's inspiratory activity with increasing lung volumes. Furthermore, when the lung volume approaches total lung capacity, the zone of apposition disappears completely, and the muscle fibres at their insertion into the ribs are orientated radially towards the body axis rather than axially along the body axis. The insertional component then enhances rather than opposes the expiratory force related to a fall in pleural pressure, and contraction of the diaphragm therefore deflates the lower rib cage.

The ability of the diaphragm to generate pressure is also strongly dependent upon lung volume. As lung volume increases, the transdiaphragmatic pressure created for a given stimulation of the phrenic nerve decreases almost linearly. This relationship, demonstrated in humans [10], is related to the force length characteristic of the diaphragmatic fibres, the greater the lung volume, the lesser the length of the muscle fibre, placing them on a less advantageous portion of the length/tension curve. It has also been shown that for a given electrical stimulation of the phrenic nerve, the transdiaphragmatic pressure increases as the abdominal anteroposterior diameter decreases (i.e. as the diaphragm is more cephalad with its fibres longer). At high lung volumes when the zone of apposition has disappeared and the muscles are no longer inserting into the ribs tangentially, the transdiaphragmatic pressure will be less because of the increasing radius of curvature of the diaphragm (Laplace's law). Finally, near total lung capacity phrenic nerve stimulation is expiratory to the lungs, as a result of both the rib cage constricting activity of the diaphragm at high lung volumes and the inability of the flattened dome to expand the abdomen.

## Relaxation of the Diaphragm

Muscle relaxation is the process by which the muscle actively returns, after contraction, to its initial conditions of length and load. The diaphragm contracts and relaxes continuously throughout life, and must return to a relatively constant resting position at the end of each contraction–relaxation cycle. There is evidence to support the hypothesis that rapid and complete relaxation of the diaphragm plays an important role in adaptation to changes in respiration load and breathing frequency [12]. Relaxation abnormalities may contribute, in part, to impaired contractile performance. This may occur at various levels from the molecular level upwards.

### Molecular Aspects of Relaxation in Diaphragm Muscle

There is a complex interplay between inactivation (mainly at the molecular and cellular level) and loading conditions (forces affecting muscle length and tension). The rate of inactivation is limited by various mechanisms, which will be described below.

Firstly there is active $Ca^{2+}$ pumping by the sarcoplasmic reticulum (SR). The SR is a specialised form of agranular endoplasmic reticulum, which forms a plexus of anastomosing membranous channels filling much of the space between the myofibrils. The arrival of the action potential causing contraction is responsible for the release of large amounts of calcium from the SR, which triggers the development of actin-myosin cross-bridges and hence muscle contraction. The reverse is essential for relaxation, the cytosolic $Ca^{2+}$ being transported into the SR, an active process assisted by $Mg^{2+}$- $Ca^{2+}$-activated ATPase. Thus the rate of uptake will be a function of the number of pumping sites and the rate at which they operate.

There are variations in the SR of the different muscle types described elsewhere in this chapter. There is a higher capacity of SR $Ca^{2+}$ uptake in fast- compared with slow-twitch fibres, which is mirrored by the higher relaxation rate. This is related to differences in the density of active pumping sites. There are also molecular differences, particularly in the sarco(endo)-plasmic reticulum $Ca^{2+}$-ATPase (SERCA), of which two isoforms have been found in the human diaphragm, namely SERCA1 and SERCA2a. SERCA1 is found only in fast-twitch skeletal fibres, whereas SERCA2a is expressed in slow-twitch skeletal fibres as well as in cardiac and smooth muscles.

It should also be noted that there are age-associated changes within the muscle fibres, as an age-related decline in SR $Ca^{2+}$ pump function has been described in skeletal muscles. This decline, presumably due to impaired coupling between ATP hydrolysis and $Ca^{2+}$ transport into the SR, may contribute to the slowing of the diaphragm relaxation rate in older persons.

Secondly there is $Ca^{2+}$ removal from troponin C (TnC). The binding of $Ca^{2+}$ to TnC acts as a switch to allow cross-bridge formation, hence contraction of the muscle, whilst removal inhibits cross-bridge attachment and hence relaxation. The movement will depend in part on the affinity of $Ca^{2+}$ for TnC, which increases with sarcomere length and decreases with a decline in intracellular pH. Thus the capacity of TnC to release $Ca^{2+}$ and the SR to reuptake it explains the length dependence of relaxation in the diaphragm. At heavy load sarcomere shortening is moderated so that the high affinity of TnC for $Ca^{2+}$ impedes $Ca^{2+}$ removal from the myofibrils, whilst at short sarcomere length and/or low load, the low affinity of TnC to $Ca^{2+}$ promotes the dissociation of the two. Therefore as long as the $Ca^{2+}$ can be sequestered into the SR, relaxation is faster as the sarcomere shortening increases.

Thirdly there are other mechanisms which may be relevant. It has been suggested that parvalbumin, a high affinity $Ca^{2+}$-binding protein, may modulate the relaxation rate of skeletal muscle by facilitating $Ca^{2+}$ transport from the myofibrils to the SR. In mammalian skeletal muscle the relaxation rate has been found to correlate with the parvalbumin concentration.

Another possibility is that changes in membranous ionic conductances play a role in the slowing of relaxation in fatigued diaphragm by slowing of action potential repolarisation.

## Mechanical Aspects of Relaxation in Diaphragm Muscle

Although much work has been done on relaxation of the diaphragm after isometric contraction, and has demonstrated that there are various factors which can impair the relaxation rate, such as ageing, maturation, denervation, malnutrition, cardiomyopathy and fatigue, this is not the normal situation, as the in vivo diaphragm contracts and relaxes against various levels of load. During afterloaded contraction, the muscle relaxation phase classically consists of isotonic lengthening, followed by isometric tension decay.

Isotonic relaxation is an increase in length at constant tension. It has been shown that the maximum extent of muscle shortening, $\Delta L$ is the main mechanical determinant of peak lengthening velocity [13]. Peak lengthening velocity (VL) physiologically increases with the extent of muscle shortening, irrespective of initial muscle length and of the load imposed on the muscle during the lengthening process. The slope of the VL–$\Delta L$ relationship is lower in twitch than in sustained mode and/or when the lengthening process is delayed. In myopathic models, VL is slowed and the overall duration of isotonic lengthening is prolonged. The myopathic process modifies the coupling between $\Delta L$ and VL.

Isometric relaxation is a falling tension at constant length. When tension decay occurs at initial length, the peak rate of tension decline is mainly determined by the afterload, and except at approximately isometric load levels an increase in afterload linearly accelerates the peak rate of tension decline [14].

Relaxation of the diaphragm, like the heart, is load sensitive, that is, the overall time course of relaxation is strongly affected by the afterload level. A contraction loaded with light or moderate load terminates earlier than a full isometric contraction, so that a muscle that is allowed to shorten has a shorter contraction–relaxation cycle. This is a manifestation of the shortening-induced deactivation phenomenon described above.

Although the muscle appears to relax in two stages, sarcomeres relax auxotonically, i.e. changes in sarcomere length and tension occur simultaneously. Because loading conditions have opposite effects on isotonic and isometric relaxation rates, it has been suggested that different intracellular mechanisms regulate the diaphragmatic muscle-lengthening rate on the one hand, and the isometric relaxation rate on the other [14]. It may be that the sarcomere length (SL) at the start of the relaxation phase is important.

As has been observed in cardiac muscle, sarcomere relaxation in the afterloaded diaphragm displays two consecutive phases: an initial phase of rapid sarcomere lengthening corresponding to the isotonic relaxation phase followed by a second, slower relaxation phase corresponding to the isometric relaxation phase [15]. It has also been shown, in studies that have examined both muscle length and SL, that as the load level increases, isotonic muscle lengthening occurs at progressively longer SL, which will correspond to the SL at peak shortening. In contrast, at the end of the isotonic phase, when the muscle has finished shortening, the sarcomere has not yet returned to its resting length. At that stage isometric contraction begins, and it is demonstrated that the SL is constant at that time, regardless of the external load.

Thus there is a complex equilibrium modulated by the capacity of TnC to liberate $Ca^{2+}$ and SR to recapture $Ca^{2+}$ and by length-dependent changes in myofilament lattice spacing, which may help to explain why relaxation occurs earlier and faster at low loads than it does at heavy loads. Provided SR is efficient, length-dependent changes in the affinity of TnC and in myofilament lattice spacing may favour rapid and early muscle lengthening when the muscle length is notably shortened (i.e. at low loads).

## Relaxation of the Diaphragm In Vivo

Although much is learnt about the function of the diaphragm from in vitro studies, it is only when applied in vivo that it starts to have clinical relevance. As mentioned above, it is known that changes in relaxation occur with fatigue of the diaphragm, and that a suitable means to measure this clinically would be an advantage. Various means have been tried, which involve deriving the relaxation rate from various pressure curves, measuring either the transdiaphragmatic pressure (Pdi) oesophageal, mouth or nasal pressures. These rely on the assumption that the chest wall and lungs will not have a significant effect upon the pressure curves, and that the pressure decay coincides with the start of diaphragmatic relaxation. The latter may not be true, as studies have demonstrated that the diaphragm continues to receive motor output during the early part of expiration [16].

Two main measures have been derived from the pressure decay curves. The first is the maximum relaxation rate (MRR), which is the negative peak of the pressure derivative as a function of time, and measures the initial part of the pressure decay. The latter portion of the curve is described in terms of its time constant, as it is normally a mono-exponential curve. The MRR varies with Pdi, such that relaxation is accelerated when Pdi increases.

It has been shown in the in vivo diaphragm that respiratory muscle fatigue slows the relaxation rate, as demonstrated by an increase in the time constant and/or a decrease in the MRR. Slowing of relaxation is an early signal of the onset of fatigue as it precedes failure of the diaphragm to generate a previously attainable Pdi. A slowing of relaxation has been shown in normal subjects who have undergone fatiguing contractions of the diaphragm, and in patients with chronic obstructive airways disease walked to dyspnoea. Slowing of inspiratory muscle relaxation has been proposed as a predictive index of weaning failure in mechanically ventilated patients.

New techniques have enabled measurements to be made in intact animals, and it has been demonstrated that the decay of pleural pressure ends before the crural and costal parts of the diaphragm have returned to their initial muscle length [17]. Thus pleural pressure swings during relaxation do not totally coincide with diaphragm muscle relaxation. Also it is noted in supine animals that the peak lengthening velocity of the crural diaphragm, which has a greater extent of shortening, exceeds that of the costal part, suggesting that VL is related to ΔL in vivo as well as in vitro.

## Role of Diaphragm Relaxation in Respiratory Function

The ventilatory performance of the diaphragm depends upon its resting length, which also depends upon the relaxation and compliance of the muscle. The optimal resting length ($L_o$) of the diaphragm is at or slightly below functional residual capacity (FRC) [18]. During inspiration between FRC and total lung capacity the human diaphragm will shorten by 25–35% $L_o$. It is necessary for the diaphragm length to return to $L_o$ by the end of expiration. If this does not occur, due to incomplete or delayed relaxation, there will be incomplete expiration to FRC. This will cause multiple problems, as the lungs will move up the lung compliance curve, potentially increasing the work of breathing, while the diaphragm moves down its passive length–tension relation, is placed at a mechanical disadvantage for optimal force generation, and its inspiratory shortening capacity is curtailed. This will increase the risk of ventilatory failure.

As in other skeletal muscle, contractile performance is dependent upon adequate energy supplies, hence an adequate blood supply. The relaxation phase is responsible for accommodating most of the changes in blood perfusion brought about by increased diaphragmatic work. Diaphragmatic blood flow is reduced during inspiration and can be completely abolished during forceful contractions [19]. Blood flow restriction has been attributed to intramuscular pressure acting on the blood vessels between muscle fibres. The pressure in turn depends upon the load to which the diaphragm is subjected and the degree of muscle shortening. However, the zone of apposition is known to increase greatly in thickness during inspiration, which may have a beneficial effect upon the regional blood flow by minimising the pressure surrounding the microvasculature [20]. During relaxation intramuscular pressure declines to baseline, thus allowing diaphragmatic perfusion to occur. At a low respiratory rate the duration of relaxation is long and the blood flow can increase to meet the metabolic demands. At higher rates the relaxation period may be insufficient to meet diaphragmatic oxygen requirements. Thus delayed or slowed relaxation may further limit diaphragmatic perfusion, especially at high breathing frequencies [21].

## Non-ventilatory Properties of the Diaphragm

The concept that the diaphragm had functions other than that of ventilating the lungs originated in the work of Bartelink [22]. This study looked at the load placed upon the lumbar intervertebral discs when lifting heavy objects, and calculated that the load applied to the discs would be greater than that required to rupture them (as measured in vitro). Thus there must be some form of protective mechanism available to the body. Bartelink further demonstrated that the intra-abdominal pressure increased with lifting heavy weights, but also that the pressure was much greater as the trunk was flexed, in comparison with the erect position. He postulated that the abdominal contents acted as a fluid ball, surrounded by muscles, namely the diaphragm, the transverse abdominal muscles and the muscles of the pelvic floor. He suggested that if there were such a ball present between the costal margin and the pelvis, the lumbar spine could be removed, and the body would not collapse as a result thereof. In the presence of the lumbar spine, the increase in intra-abdominal pressure will serve to unload the spine and increase trunk stability.

It was recognised that the abdominal and thoracic cavities upon which the diaphragm acts are involved with the stability of the trunk and postural control [23]. Other respiratory muscles acting upon the rib cage and abdomen perform a postural function which is integrated with their respiratory role, for example the intercostal muscles stabilise the rib cage [24]. Contraction of the abdominal muscles contributes to trunk stability prior to and during movement of the limbs, an action which is increased when respiratory demands increase [25].

Contraction of the pelvic floor muscles and abdominal muscles, in particular transversus abdominis, correlates closely with the increase in intra-abdominal pressure in a variety of postural tasks [23]. When the stability of the trunk is challenged by reactive forces due to limb movement, transversus abdominis contracts before the agonist limb muscle, which suggests that the response might be pre-programmed by the central nervous system [25,26].

More recent studies have demonstrated that the diaphragm contributes to the increased intra-abdominal pressure prior to the initiation of movements of large segments of the upper limb. This contraction is independent of the phase of respiration [24]. This evidence suggests that the diaphragm has a function in the maintenance of the postural control of the human trunk. The same paper also showed that the preparatory contraction of the diaphragm is associated with initial shortening of its muscle fibres and occurs simultaneously with activation of transversus abdominis.

The argument in favour of this conclusion relates to the fact that any movement of a limb is associated with reactive forces imposed upon the trunk which are equal and opposite to those producing the movement, and that the diaphragm in itself is unable to move the trunk directly to oppose these forces.

Moreover, the contraction of the diaphragm increases pressure within the abdominal cavity, which may contribute to trunk stability. Also, diaphragmatic contraction could increase stability of the trunk by minimising displacement of the abdominal contents into the thorax, maintaining the hoop-like geometry of the abdominal muscles, which could then increase spinal stability through tension in the thoracolumbar fascia. This study also demonstrated that there was co-activation of the costal and crural portions of the diaphragm [24], which suggests that for postural reasons the two parts of the diaphragm may function together, although there have been previous studies which demonstrate that the two portions of the diaphragm may function independently [27].

Unlike other muscles that are involved with the maintenance of posture, the diaphragm has to continue to act in its primary role as a muscle of ventilation. That it is able to do so is demonstrated in studies looking at the activity of the diaphragm during repetitive arm activity [28]. This modifies diaphragmatic activity in two ways unrelated to ventilation. First, unlike breathing at rest, the diaphragm contracted tonically throughout the respiratory cycle. If this were accompanied by abdominal muscle activity, the intra-abdominal pressure would be elevated. As well as this, phasic modulation of diaphragm activity at the frequency of limb movement was superimposed on its ventilatory and tonic activation. Therefore ventilation can continue uncompromised by the activity of other muscle groups whilst the diaphragm is acting as a spinal support.

Further studies of a similar nature have demonstrated that there is a reciprocal activity of transversus abdominis with the diaphragm during breathing under conditions of repetitive arm action. With the initiation of movement the diaphragm and abdominal muscles contract simultaneously to increase abdominal pressure. Breathing is facilitated by the relaxation of transversus abdominis during diaphragmatic contraction, to allow displacement of the abdominal contents, and vice versa during expiration [29].

That the diaphragm acts tonically with activity in other parts of the body is consistent with earlier findings, which demonstrate the sustained elevation of transdiaphragmatic pressure during lifting [30]. More recent studies have demonstrated that the greatest increase in transdiaphragmatic pressure is seen during sit-ups and power lifts, and studies in weight-lifters has demonstrated an increase in the diaphragmatic mass in these people [31]. This is further evidence to support the proposition that the diaphragm is recruited in non-ventilatory activities. As well as supporting the spine, it is important in maintaining ventilation. With lifting of heavy objects, or even upper limb movement, there is an increase in intra-abdominal pressure. If there were no diaphragmatic recruitment, the elevated intra-abdominal pressure would be transmitted to the thorax, provoking the unwanted effects of raised intrathoracic pressure (raised central venous, intracranial and systemic blood pressures).

In patients with phrenic nerve paralysis there is often a difficulty in breathing with bending or lifting. Measurements made within such patients [31] demonstrate that there is a rise in intra-abdominal pressure with lifting, but there is no transdiaphragmatic pressure, i.e. the pressure in the abdomen is transmitted directly to the thorax. Thus these patients become dyspnoeic on exertion, as they are only able to breathe in between bouts of activity, unlike the normal person who is able to breathe and lift or move at the same time.

It will be apparent from this section that there is still a great deal of uncertainty about the

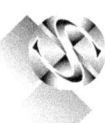

complete function of the diaphragm, and that there is a lot of work ongoing investigating the activity of the diaphragm in health and disease, utilising newer and more sophisticated techniques. It will be interesting to see what more will be learned about this fascinating organ in the coming years.

## Questions

1. Which structures pass through the diaphragm?
2. Describe the nerve supply.
3. What is the function of the diaphragm?

## References

1. De Troyer A, Loring SH. Action of the respiratory muscles. In: Fishman AP, Mackelm PT, Mead J, Geiger SR (eds). Handbook of physiology Section 3: The respiratory system Volume III. Mechanics of breathing, part 2. Bethesda, MD: American Physiological Society, 1986; 443–62.
2. Fell SC. Surgical anatomy of the diaphragm and the phrenic nerve. Chest Surg Clin N Am 1998;8:281–94.
3. Merendino KA, Johnson RJ, Skinner HH, Maguire RX. The intradiaphragmatic distribution of the phrenic nerve with particular reference to the placement of diaphragmatic incisions and controlled segmental paralysis. Surgery 1956;39:189–98.
4. Muller N, Volgyesi L, Bryan MH, Bryan AC. Diaphragmatic muscle tone. J Appl Physiol 1979;47:279–84.
5. Smith JC, Loring SH. Passive mechanical properties of the chest wall. In: Fishman AP, Mackelm PT, Mead J, Geiger SR (eds). Handbook of physiology Section 3: The Respiratory System Volume III. Mechanics of breathing, part 2. Bethesda, MD: American Physiological Society, 1986; 429–42.
6. Braun NMT, Arora NS, Rochester DF. Force-length relationship of the normal human diaphragm. J Appl Physiol 1982;53:405–12.
7. Cluzel P, Similowski T, Chartrand-Lefebvre C et al. Diaphragm and chest wall: assessment of the inspiratory pump with MR imaging preliminary observations. Radiology 2000;215:574–83.
8. Mortola JP, Sant'Ambrogio G. Motion of the rib cage and the abdomen in tetraplegic patients. Clin Sci Mol Med 1978;54:25–32.
9. De Troyer A, Sampson M, Sigrist S, Macklem PT. Action of costal and crural parts of the diaphragm on the rib cage in dog. J Appl Physiol 1982;53:30–9.
10. Danon J, Druz WS, Goldberg NB, Sharp JT. Function of the isolated paced diaphragm and the cervical accessory muscles in $C_1$ quadriplegics. Am Rev Respir Dis 1979; 119:909–19.
11. Tusiewicz K, Moldofsky H, Bryan AC, Bryan MH. Mechanics of the rib cage and diaphragm during sleep. J Appl Physiol 1977;43:600–2.
12. Coirault C, Chemla D, Lecarpentier Y. Relaxation of diaphragm muscle. J Appl Pysiol 1999;87:1243–52.
13. Coirault C, Chemla D, Pery N et al. Mechanical determinants of isotonic relaxation in isolated diaphragm muscle. J Appl Physiol 1993;75:2265–72.
14. Coirault C, Chemla D, Pery-Man N et al. Isometric relaxation of isolated diaphragm muscle: influences of load, length, time and stimulation. J Appl Physiol 1994;766: 1468–75.
15. Coirault C, Chemla D, Suard I et al. Sarcomere relaxation in hamster diaphragm muscle. J Appl Physiol 1996;81:858–65.
16. Easton PA, Katagiri M, Kieser TM, Platt RS. Postinspiratory activity of costal and crural diaphragm. J appl Physiol 1999;87:582–9.
17. Newman S, Road J, Bellemare F et al. Respiratory muscle length measured by sonomicrometry. J Appl Physiol 1984;56:753–64.
18. Margulies SS, Farkas GA, Rodarte JR. Effects of body position and lung volume on in situ operating length of the canine diaphragm. J Appl Physiol 1990;69:1702–8.
19. Bellemare F, Wight D, Lavigne CM, Grassino A. Effect of tension and timing of contraction on the blood flow of the diaphragm. J Appl Physiol 1983;54:1597–1606.
20. Wait JL, Johnson RL. Patterns of shortening and thickening of the human diaphragm. J Appl Physiol 1997;83: 1123–32.
21. Hu F, Comtois A, Grassino AE. Optimal diaphragmatic blood perfusion. J Appl Physiol 1992;72:149–57.
22. Bartelink DL. The role of abdominal pressure in relieving the pressure on the lumbar intervertebral discs. J Bone Joint Surg 1957;39B:718–25.
23. Grillner S, Nilsson J, Thorstensson A. Intra-abdominal pressure changes during natural movements in man. Acta Physiol Scand 1978;103:275–83.
24. Hodges PW, Butler JE, McKenzie DK, Gandevia SC. Contraction of the human diaphragm during rapid postural adjustments. J Physiol 1997;505:539–48.
25. Hodges PW, Richardson CA. Contraction of the abdominal muscles associated with movement of the lower limbs. Phys Ther 1997;77:132–44.
26. Hodges PW, Richardson CA. Feedforward contraction of transversus abdominis is not influenced by the direction of arm movement. Exp Brain Res 1997;114:362–70.
27. De Troyer A, Sampson M, Sigrist S, Macklem PT. The diaphragm: two muscles. Science 1981;213:237–8.
28. Hodges PW, Gandevia SC. Activation of the human diaphragm during a repetitive postural task. J Physiol 2000;522:165–75.
29. Hodges PW, Gandevia SC. Changes in intra-abdominal pressure during postural and respiratory activation of the human diaphragm. J Appl Physiol 2000;89:967–76.
30. Hemborg B, Moritz U, Löwing H. Intra-abdominal pressure and trunk muscle activity during lifting. IV. The causal factors of the intra-abdominal pressure rise. Scand J Rehabil Med 1985;17:25–38.
31. Al-Bilbeisi F, McCool F. Diaphragm recruitment during nonrespiratory activities. Am J Respir Crit Care Med 2000;162:456–9.

# 5

# The Spleen

Hugo W. Tilanus

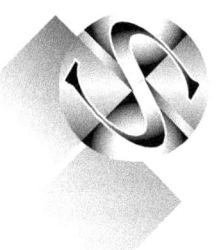

## Aims

To describe the development and anatomy of the spleen. To describe the effects of a splenectomy.

## Embryology

The spleen starts to develop in the fourth week of gestation as a mesenchymal condensation in the dorsal mesogastrium of the lesser sac. In the following weeks these early mesenchymal cells differentiate to a vascular lymphatic pedicle that eventually forms the spleen. Smaller condensations that develop near the hilum of the spleen form accessory spleens. When the embryo is about 10 cm in length the dorsal mesogastrium can be divided into a posterior part and an anterior part. The posterior part, from the posterior abdominal wall to the spleen, is eventually invaded by the pancreatic bud, which grows as far as the hilum and later fuses with the peritoneum of the posterior abdominal wall ventral to the left kidney to form the *splenorenal ligament*. In this dorsal structure the splenic artery and vein develop. The anterior part of the dorsal mesogastrium develops into the *gastrosplenic ligament* and contains the short gastric vessels. It is now clear that the spleen is of mesenchymal origin and does not originate from the embryonic entodermal gut.

The splenic condensation forms a trabecular structure resulting in a mesh and ending up in the connective supportive structure of the spleen. The isolated free cells in this network differentiate into hematopoietic cells in the next months of gestation. Other cells derived from the sinusoids of the splenic artery specialize to participate in the reticuloendothelial system [1].

## Anatomy

The normal spleen cannot be palpated as it lies at the dorsal side of the left upper quadrant of the abdomen and its surface covers an oval area of the diaphragm, the hilum being projected ventrally depending on the distension of the stomach. As the tail of the pancreas is the Achilles heel of splenectomy, detailed knowledge of the peritoneal reflections of the spleen is essential. Starting from the gastrosplenic ligament it divides at the hilum. The anterior sheet covers the surface of the spleen and reflects to the anterior surface of the left kidney. The posterior sheet encloses the splenic vessels and reflects to the dorsal peritoneum. The inferior part rests upon the phrenicocolic ligament and is, if connected with this ligament, a preferential place for rupture of the capsule and bleeding.

The abundant arterial vasculature of the spleen arises from the splenic artery and comes from the celiac trunk, running, sometimes tortuously, all along the upper border of the pancreas and ending in a number of smaller branches that vascularize the spleen. Two branches, the superior polar artery and the left gastroepiploic artery, serve a special function. The superior polar artery is one of the early branches of the splenic artery and divides into the short gastric vessels before entering the spleen. The intrasplenic arterial supply in divided into three segments, creating a superior, middle and inferior segment.

The left gastroepiploic artery, one of the most inferior branches of the splenic artery, vascularizes the greater curvature distal to the short gastric vessels and mostly anastomoses with the right gastroepiploic artery.

Some large veins join at the splenic hilum to form the splenic vein, which runs a straight course to the portal vein, and receiving the inferior mesenteric vein.

The spleen is created in units called the red pulp and the white pulp. The red pulp contains the vascular structures: the pulp sinuses and pulp cords that are lined by reticuloendothelial cells and filled with blood. The white pulp consists of arterioles surrounded by periarteriolar T lymphocytes. A zone of B lymphocytes that also contain the germinal centers made up of B cells and macrophages surrounds this central area of the white pulp. The most peripheral layer of the white pulp is another B-cell layer, the marginal zone.

Once inside the spleen, the blood flow from the branches of the splenic artery enters firstly the trabeculae and from there goes into the small central arteries dividing into the arterial capillaries. The periarteriolar lymphoid sheet of T cells surrounded by B cells continues along the arterial vessels until they become small arterioles. Red blood cells pass from the central arteries to pulp cords and further through critical small openings in the sinus endothelium to the spleen sinuses and the spleen venous system. During this passage through the white pulp, aged red blood cells, nuclear material, denaturated hemoglobin and other debris are retained in the pulp cords and phagocytosed by macrophages [2].

## Physiology and Function

The role of the spleen as an important functional organ, not only in childhood but also in adults, should not be underestimated. For the surgeon this should lead to careful handling of the spleen in elective abdominal surgery in order to avoid injury, preventing splenectomy and to a conservative approach in case of trauma of the spleen without jeopardizing the patient's health. It is therefore important to remember the four major physiologic functions of the spleen.

1. The spleen is an important organ in the clearance of microorganisms and unwanted antigens from the circulation. Moreover it generates immune responses to foreign antigens, especially by the production of IgM antibodies. Opsonic proteins produced in the spleen promote phagocytosis and initiate complement activation, resulting in destruction of bacteria and foreign or abnormal cells. Especially against bacteria in the bloodstream that are not recognized by the host's immune system, the spleen is a major second line of defense. When a specific antibody in the liver is missing for bacterial removal, the spleen becomes the site for this action.

2. In addition to sequestration and removal of older normal red blood cells, the spleen is able to remove abnormal red blood cells, e.g. morphologically abnormal erythrocytes such as spherocytes and sickled cells. As the spleen removes immunoglobin-coated blood cells it is the place of destruction in a variety of autoimmune diseases. Intraerythrocytic parasites as in malaria are also removed in the white pulp. In addition, the blood flow rate plays an important role in the filtering function of the spleen. In splenic vein thrombosis resulting in stasis this leads to increased red cell removal.

3. The spleen has a "buffer-like" function in regulation of the portal flow and in pathological conditions like portal hypertension.

4. The spleen has an important auxiliary function in the production of red blood cells when normal hematopoiesis in bone marrow fails as in hematological diseases [3].

## Splenomegaly

Enlargement of the spleen is a symptom of a large variety of diseases. The enlargement is due to an increase in cellularity and vascularity and the most important groups of diseases are:

1. Infections like bacterial septicemias, viral and parasitic infections and splenic abscess.
2. Diseases related to abnormal red blood cells like spherocytosis and sickle cell anemia.
3. Infiltrative enlargement as seen in benign amyloidosis and Gaucher's disease or in malignant leukemias and lymphomas.
4. Altered splenic blood flow. This group of diseases can be divided into an isolated outflow obstruction of the splenic vein only as in splenic vein thrombosis or enlargement of the spleen as in generalized portal hypertension.
5. Immune disorders like rheumatoid arthritis or systemic lupus erythematosus.
6. Hypersplenism. The spleen removes excessive quantities of blood cells from the circulation leading to anemia and platelet reduction. Hypersplenism occurs in the course of an underlying disease or is idiopathic.

The degree of the splenomegaly and the symptoms vary with the underlying disease. A fast increase in diameter provokes upper abdominal discomfort and local tenderness becoming extreme pain when splenic infarction occurs in acute disease. Massive enlargement can be completely asymptomatic as in portal hypertension or hemolytic anemias or other more chronic diseases. At physical examination splenomegaly can easily be missed if the examination is not started in the left lower quadrant of the abdomen with the patient in a left-sided position. Other techniques to assess the size of the spleen are ultrasound scanning, computed tomography and $^{99}$Tc-colloid liver-spleen scan [4].

## Indications for Splenectomy

The indications for splenectomy can be arbitrarily divided into two large groups – hematologic disorders or trauma. The hematologic disorders comprise platelet disorders like idiopathic thrombocytopenic purpura, thrombotic thrombocytopenic purpura and hypersplenism in which low platelet count is accompanied by depression of one or more of the formed elements of blood, red cells white cells and platelets. Splenectomy for staging of Hodgkin's and non-Hodgkin's lymphoma has decreased over the last 10 years and is no longer the most important diagnostic test for these diseases. Splenectomy for trauma can be divided into surgical trauma of the spleen, especially during upper abdominal surgery leading to accidental splenectomy, and accidents involving blunt trauma of the spleen.

## Splenectomy for Hematologic Disorders

### Immune Thrombocytopenic Purpura (ITP)

ITP is caused by a circulating antiplatelet factor identified as an IgG antibody directed towards a platelet-associated antigen. There is no evidence for a clear autoimmune entity. Most patients are women in their late thirties but the percentage of men is increasing, as is the total incidence. Spontaneous and easy bruising and bleeding are the most common first symptoms. Petechiae, epistaxis, mucosal bleeding and menorrhagia are often seen and reflect the number of platelets being mostly under 20 000/mm$^3$ in serious blood loss. ITP is diagnosed after exclusion of other underlying illnesses or medications like sulfonamides and quinine, which can induce thrombocytopenia. An otherwise normal blood count, a normal bone marrow aspirate and a not enlarged spleen support the diagnosis. There is an increased megakaryocyte mass in combination with a greatly shortened platelet survival. The amount of circulating antiplatelet-associated antibodies mirrors the

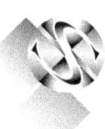

severity of the disease. These antibodies are preferentially produced in the spleen: liver and bone marrow are less involved. One-third of the total circulating platelets are harbored within the spleen so most platelets are destroyed there.

Prednisone therapy does not prevent destruction but the increased platelet count is the result of increased platelet production. Most patients improve with corticosteroid therapy but complete and sustained remission of ITP is only achieved in up to 25% of patients. Splenectomy is performed in patients who are completely or partially refractory to corticosteroids. Sustained remission is more probable in patients who showed an initial response to corticosteroid therapy. Most patients are referred after failure of the initial corticosteroid therapy, which should be continued during surgery. Immunization with polyvalent pneumococcal vaccine should be administered preferably 10 to 14 days before splenectomy. High dose intravenous gammaglobulin is effective in increasing the platelet count in patients refractory to corticosteroids especially in urgent cases such as intracranial hemorrhage. Nearly 80 to 90% of patients develop a normal sustained platelet count after splenectomy [5–7].

## Thrombotic Thrombocytopenic Purpura (TTP)

In thrombotic thrombocytopenic purpura platelet microthrombi depositions occlude arterioles and capillaries resulting in intravascular depositions of hyaline material consisting of platelets and fibrin. The etiology is unknown but the disease may be initiated by connective tissue disorders like lupus erythematosus, bacterial and viral stimuli, malignancies and AIDS.

The clinical picture is dominated by hemolysis. Anemia occurs in association with fragmented red blood cells in the peripheral blood, an elevated reticulocytes and thrombocytopenia. As the disease progresses over weeks or months, patients, primarily young adults and more often women, die of progressive renal failure and brain involvement with a 1-year survival of less than 10% in untreated patients. Treatment consists of plasmapheresis with infusion of fresh frozen plasma, antiplatelet agents and high dose corticosteroids in combination with removal of a normal to moderately enlarged spleen. The explanation of the response to splenectomy is not clarified but the majority of long-term survivors have undergone this procedure [8].

## Hodgkin's Disease

Hodgkin's disease, described by Thomas Hodgkin in 1832, usually presents with localized lymphomas that spread to lymphoid structures elsewhere in the body. Half of the patients present with lymph nodes in the neck or the supraclavicular region and half of them present with mediastinal lymphadenopathy. The disease is characterized by the unique multinuclear giant cell, the Sternberg–Reed cell.

Most patients are asymptomatic at first presentation but weight loss, fever, night sweats and pruritus, the so-called B symptoms, sometimes accompanied by the characteristic intermittent high, Pel–Ebstein fever, are signs of widespread disease and carry a bad prognosis. Anemia, leucocytosis, and eosinophilia are common. In 1966 the Rye classification was introduced and has been unaltered since then. There are four histologic subgroups identified in decreasing order of prognosis: the lymphocyte predominant group, the nodular sclerotic group, the mixed cellular group and the lymphocyte depleted group. Staging is based on the lymph node region involved. In stage 1 disease, the lymph nodes of one region, above or below the diaphragm, are involved. Stage 2 includes two affected lymph node regions on one side of the diaphragm. Stage 3 refers to lymph node involvement above and below the diaphragm and stage 4 describes disseminated disease to extranodal organs on both sides of the diaphragm. It is important to remember that treatment and prognosis in Hodgkin's disease are dependent on stage of the disease whereas in non-Hodgkin's lymphoma, treatment and prognosis are largely based on histologic subtype.

Controversy exists regarding the role of staging laparotomy and splenectomy in the diagnosis and treatment of Hodgkin's disease as the introduction of non-invasive diagnostic tests and less toxic chemotherapy make this procedure less and less indicated. Today, staging laparotomy is indicated in selected patients only and includes splenectomy, liver biopsy, intra-abdominal and retroperitoneal lymph node sampling according to clinical findings and the outcome of preoperative diagnostics. A review of the different therapeutical strategies for the different stages of Hodgkin's disease is beyond the scope of this chapter [9].

## Non-Hodgkin's Lymphomas

Non-Hodgkin's lymphomas (NHL) are mostly detected as an abdominal mass or as hepatic and/or splenic enlargement in addition to mediastinal and peripheral lymphadenopathy and in combination with general symptoms such as night sweats, weight loss and fever. NHL spreads fast to distant nodal and extranodal sites through the bloodstream.

Chemotherapy and radiation are the first-line therapeutic options based on histologic features and the stage of the disease. Splenectomy is only indicated in patients with primary NHL in the spleen presenting with symptomatic splenic enlargement due to parenchymal tumor infiltration or in order to correct hypersplenism, which is the result of hematological depression with anemia and thrombocytopenia. In this situation splenectomy relieves the discomfort of splenomegaly and the systemic effects of hypersplenism [10].

## The Spleen in Chronic Leukaemia

The spleen is often involved in different forms of leukemia like chronic lymphocytic, chronic myeloid and hairy cell leukemia.

In chronic lymphocytic leukemia (CLL) lymph node enlargement is the most common finding and progressive splenomegaly is present in most patients. There is as yet no curative therapy but due to effective medical treatment with chemotherapeutic agents and corticosteroids combined with irradiation most patients can be palliated for up to 10 years or more. In later stages CLL is often complicated by autoimmune hemolytic anemia, which is an indication for the removal of an often very large spleen, up to more than 6 kg in severe cases. This leads to hematologic improvement in the large majority of patients but does not improve survival.

In chronic myeloid leukemia splenomegaly is a common finding together with lymphadenopathy, hepatomegaly and sternal tenderness. A myeloblastic crises results in death from infection or bleeding within weeks or months. Splenectomy is only indicated in a small group of patients with severe thrombocytopenia and anemia or for relief of pain due to splenomegaly or infarction.

Hairy cell leukemia (HCL) is an uncommon form of leukemia presenting with moderate splenomegaly, hepatomegaly and lymphadenopathy. It is characterized by malignant cells with "hairy" cytoplasmic filamentous projections in the peripheral blood. The majority of patients are elderly men presenting with moderate to severe pancytopenia resulting in anemia, thrombocytopenic bleeding, neutropenia and recurrent infections. For patients with diffuse manifestations of HCL especially in bone marrow and severe cytopenia, interferon in combination with pentostatin is remarkably effective. Splenectomy especially in an early stage of the disease leads to improvement of symptoms in half of the patients [11,12].

## Hereditary Hemolytic Anemias

Hemolysis resulting in hemolytic anemia must be quite severe as the normal bone marrow can produce erythrocytes up to eight times the normal production. Congenital disorders have an intrinsic defect involving different metabolic functions and structures of the red cell. The clinical picture consists of pallor and/or jaundice and biliary complications due to the excessive amount of bilirubin to be disposed of by the biliary system. Mild to moderate symptoms often already manifest at a young age. Hereditary spherocytosis, sickle cell anemia and thalassaemia are the most common hereditary disorders that benefit from splenectomy [13,14].

## Autoimmune Hemolytic Anemias

Autoimmune hemolytic anemia (AIHA) is an acquired disease caused by antibody production against the own red cells. A positive direct Coombs test is discriminating for AIHA. There are two forms, which are classified as warm or cold reactive depending on the affinity of the antibody to the red cell at 37°C and at temperatures approaching 0°C. Warm antibodies are usually IgG whereas cold antibodies mostly concern IgM immunoglobulins. The latter bind to red cells in the peripheral, cold circulation leading to immediate or delayed hemolysis.

AIHA may be associated with drugs especially penicillins, with viral infections such as infectious mononucleosis and with leukemias and lymphoproliferative disorders. Treatment directed at the hemolytic anemia consists of transfusion of blood, corticosteroids and splenectomy when conservative medical therapy fails. The response rate to splenectomy is high, up to 80% of patients, especially when there is a high degree of sequestration in the spleen [15].

## Principles of Elective Splenectomy

Before elective splenectomy is planned, patients should receive polyvalent pneumococcal vaccine, polyvalent meningococcal vaccine and *Haemophilus influenzae* vaccine. Blood products should be ordered at an early stage, as cross-matching is sometimes difficult, especially in acquired haemolytic anemias and isoantibodies. Some patients may have developed cold hemagglutinins so blood and blood products should be warmed before transfusion.

## Open Splenectomy

The midline upper abdominal incision is preferred in virtually all splenectomies. Neither in very large spleens, nor in trauma, are thoracoabdominal incisions necessary. The lateral surface is palpated carefully in order to rule out adhesions. If present they can be divided sharply. In rare cases the spleen can be firmly adhered to the lateral abdominal wall and laceration of the capsule should be prevented by sharp division of its posterior attachments. During splenectomy it is important to remember the local anatomy. The gastrosplenic ligament covers the vascular structures at the ventral side, divides at the hilum and covers the surface of the spleen. The dorsal part envelops the vessels and reflects to the dorsal peritoneum. After division of this dorsal part of the splenic ligament the spleen can be mobilized in most cases, leaving the tail of the pancreas in place. Thereafter the splenic artery and vein and the short gastric vessels can be divided. The tail of the pancreas is the Achilles heel of the procedure.

Mobilization of the tail can lead to pancreatitis and injury to the pancreatic duct of the tail can lead to pseudocyst formation. Special care should be taken of the stomach fundic vessels. A ligature can very easily catch a small part of the stomach wall leading to perforation. Especially in very large spleens some authors prefer an early and more central ligation of the splenic vessels in order to prevent massive hemorrhage during the splenectomy phase. Draining of the left upper abdominal space is not routinely advised and should be restricted to cases with large blood loss or pancreatic damage [16].

## Laparoscopic Splenectomy

Laparoscopic splenectomy has gained wide acceptance since the first reports in 1999. There is no longer an absolute contraindication and some large series highlighted the many advantages of the laparoscopic procedure especially in adults and children with hematological disorders. There are relative contraindications, e.g. a higher complication rate is seen in patients with or after portal hypertension or splenic abscess predisposing for perisplenitis. Massive spleens remain a challenge with a high failure rate in early series. Successful laparoscopic removal of spleens with a diameter over 30 cm has been reported; but rather than the absolute diameter, the relationship between the patient's body size and the size of the spleen, the splenic index, is the limiting factor. A splenic index of 0.2 being normal, a patient with an index exceeding 0.76 is unlikely to benefit from a laparoscopic approach. In a series of over 200 splenectomies for mostly hematologic disorders the laparoscopic procedure was successful in 97% of patients.

In the right decubitus position, open insertion of the first trocar is advised and pneumoperitoneum is obtained. three to four ports are placed along an arch concentric to the spleen and 3 cm distal to the costal margin. The lateral splenic attachments are divided leaving the uppermost fibrous bands intact to facilitate exposure. The two layers of the gastrosplenic ligament are opened and the short gastric vessels are elevated and divided. Not before the spleen is completely mobilized is the hilum divided with an endoscopic linear stapler, avoiding damage to the tail of the pancreas. This last step is more difficult in large spleens as they tend to turn dorsally, which complicates placement of the stapler. A nylon bag is manipulated around the spleen after which the last superior fibers are severed. The spleen is morcellated or completely retrieved through the largest trocar opening [17].

## The Spleen in Trauma

In cases of blunt and especially high velocity trauma information regarding direction of the force, vertical or horizontal, and the nature of the force, compression or deceleration, is of the utmost importance. Information should be obtained about prior operations or diseases of the spleen, as the enlarged spleen is especially prone to injury.

Splenic injury produces vague abdominal symptoms with occasionally left shoulder pain caused by free intra-abdominal blood which causes only a mild irritation of the peritoneum. Skin lesions may be helpful in the diagnosis, as are lower left rib fractures and pelvic fracture. Shock and hypotension are late symptoms that are seen after major loss of circulating volume of 30% or more. Physical findings are more often than not disappointing, especially in the polytraumatic patient with multiple fractures that provide another explanation for sometimes major blood loss and instability.

Effective resuscitation in the shock room is mandatory before evaluation is performed. Direct laparotomy is performed in persisting unstable patients but mostly there is time for further evaluation with diagnostic peritoneal lavage to confirm intra-abdominal blood loss, ultrasound and or CT scan. Delayed symptoms in case of rupture of a subcapsular hematoma can develop days or weeks after the primary trauma. Splenic injury is classified according to a number of grading systems in order to standardize the impact and to formulate therapeutic guidelines. The most current of these is the Organ Injury Scaling of the American Association for the Surgery of Trauma, which grades the injury from grade 1: subcapsular haematoma, to grade 5: a completely shattered spleen.

Non-operative management by observation alone is historically associated with a mortality approaching 90%. With current diagnostic modalities, however, there is a place for conservative treatment which should be weighed against the grading of the injury, the age of the patient, the risk of mortality of the asplenic condition and the risk of blood transfusion [18–20].

Planned observation in children with splenic injury has gained acceptance. The juvenile spleen contains more connective tissue than the spleen in adults, which is a possible explanation for the relative resistance of the parenchyma to hematoma formation. Several series report success rates for conservative treatment in children of 90% or more. Furthermore, due to their expected long lifespan they are more patient-years prone to overwhelming post-splenectomy infection as compared to adults, which is a further argument for conservative treatment or spleen-saving surgery [21].

## Splenectomy after Trauma

Splenectomy in trauma follows essentially the same guidelines as in elective splenectomy. A midline upper abdominal incision should suffice in virtually all patients. Close collaboration with the anesthesiologist is mandatory before entering the abdominal cavity as the sudden drop in intra-abdominal pressure due to the evacuation of a large quantity of blood may lead to sudden hypotension. The large amount of free intra-abdominal blood should be removed carefully: injury to other organs should be prevented at this sometimes rather hectic stage. After removal of the free and clotted blood the left upper abdomen is packed before careful assessment of the splenic injury is performed and other causes of major bleeding are excluded. Splenic injury is graded from grade 1, injury of the splenic capsule to grade 4, complex splenic fractures. Total splenectomy should be performed in all patients who remain in shock or who have other life-threatening injuries intra- or extra-abdominally. In the absence of extrasplenic sources of bleeding the choice of treatment is mainly dictated by the grading of the bleeding. Grade 1 bleedings are better left alone in most cases, but if hemostasis is needed direct pressure with the addition of topical hemostatic material like thrombin fleece will suffice. Grade 2 injuries include larger hematomas and deeper lacerations and are initially also treated with compression and hemostatic agents. The procedure can be repeated once or twice, evaluating the blood loss in between. Grade 3 bleeding is not stopped with the above-mentioned measures and needs careful suture transfixion over protecting Gelfoam or Surgicel pledgets. The firmer capsule and parenchyma in children permits direct suturing in most cases. In grade 3, multiple deep lacerations and extensive capsule loss, the bleeding may be treated by wrapping the spleen in an absorbable woven polyglycolic acid mesh. The mesh is wrapped around the spleen under controlled tension and the vascular inflow and outflow in the hilum is left uncompromised by a keyhole in the wrap to prevent, especially venous, obstruction that could add to the bleeding. In grade 4, complex splenic fractures, partial resection is possible with suturing of the cutting edge over Teflon pledgets, but total splenectomy is performed in most cases. All efforts to prevent total splenectomy in trauma of the spleen should be weighed against the possibility of persistent bleeding or rebleeding and the possibility of post-splenectomy infection [22,23].

## Post-splenectomy Complications

Rebleeding after splenic repair or splenectomy results from inadequate hemostasis of the short gastric vessels or the splenic hilar vasculature and occurs in 1.5–2.5% of cases, repair being more prone to persistent bleeding than excision. Early re-operation is advised in most cases.

Thrombocytosis of more than 400 000/cm$^3$ occurs in half of the patients after splenectomy, suggesting an increased risk of deep venous thrombosis and pulmonary embolism, but antiplatelet therapy is not recommended unless the platelet count exceeds 1 million/cm$^3$.

Pneumonia, pleural effusion and subphrenic abscess are the most frequent complications after splenectomy. The rate of abscess formation is possibly higher in patients with bowel perforation after trauma and after drainage of the left upper quadrant.

Postoperative infections are possibly less frequent after a splenic salvage procedure than after total splenectomy but splenectomy alone may not be an independent risk factor for the development of postoperative infectious complications.

The risk of overwhelming post-splenectomy infection, first suggested by Morris and Bullock in 1919, is considered the greatest in children under 5 years of age and during the first years after splenectomy but it is in fact a lifelong one. It is estimated to be between 0.8% and 0.026% in children and adults but the mortality rate is extremely high. A recent survey by Waghorn [24] suggests that the increased risk of life-threatening post-splenectomy sepsis persists in adults and that the mortality rate varies between 50 and 70%. The majority of patients are under 50 years of age and in good health without further underlying disease. In contrast to earlier findings, which suggest that there is a decreasing risk with increasing interval, this analysis showed that the increased risk is indeed lifelong.

The clinical picture is typified by the onset of nausea, vomiting and confusion leading to coma and death within hours after the onset of symptoms. Disseminated intravascular coagulation, hypoglycemia and electrolyte disturbances are symptoms of progressive and often fatal septicemia. *Streptococcus pneumoniae*, *Meningococcus*, *Escherichia coli*, *Staphylococcus* and *Haemophilus inflenzae* are the most common microorganisms in decreasing order of frequency [24]. The recommendations for prevention include splenic autotransplantation, immunization with, at least, pneumococcal vaccine, antibiotic prophylaxis before surgery and prevention of animal and tick bites.

Splenic autotransplantation was thought to prevent overwhelming post-splenectomy infection but remains controversial as, experimentally, the critical amount of splenic tissue needed to keep its function is at least 30%. Although splenic tissue can be autotransplanted successfully, the number of transplanted splenocytes seems insufficient to function against microbial challenge.

The current pneumococcal vaccines, although not completely protecting, cover the serotypes responsible for 90% of bacteremias. Protection is not lifelong and revaccination is recommended possibly best based on antibody measurements. Moreover the protection by vaccination is not complete and prophylaxis with penicillin has been recommended, especially in children under the age of 5 years, gradually changing to antibiotic therapy at the first signs of infection in patients over 18 years of age [25,26].

# Conclusion

The normal spleen is, in infancy and in adulthood, an important and immunocompetent organ that should be preserved in elective and in trauma surgery. Removal of a diseased spleen especially in hematologic disorders carries a high morbidity, although this has dramatically decreased with the introduction of laparoscopic splenectomy, which is now the treatment of choice. Overwhelming post-splenectomy sepsis is a lifelong risk that requires adequate prevention and treatment.

# Questions

1. What is the tissue of origin of the spleen?
2. Describe the vascular supply of the spleen.
3. What is the risk of a splenectomy?

# References

1. Mollit DL, Dokler ML. Surgery of infants and children: Scientific principles and practice. Philadelphia: Lippincott-Raven Publishers, 1997.
2. Sheldon GF, Croom RD, Meyer AA. The spleen. Sabiston textbook of surgery. Philadelphia: WB Saunders, 1997.
3. Eichner ER. Splenic function: normal, too much and too little. Am J Med 1979; 66:311.
4. Kraus MD, Fleming MD, Vonderheide RH. The spleen as a diagnostic specimen: a review of 10 years experience at two tertiary care institutions. Cancer 2001; 91(11): 9.
5. George JN, Woolf SH, Raskob GE et al. Idiopathic thrombocytopenic purpura: a practice guideline developed by explicit methods for the Am. Soc. of Hematology. Blood 1996; 88:3.
6. Bourgeois E, Caulier MT, Rose C et al. Role of splenectomy in the treatment of myelodysplastic syndromes with peripheral thrombocytopenia: a report on six cases. Leukemia 2001;15(6):950.
7. Kuhne T, Imbach P, Bolton-Maggs PH et al. Newly diagnosed idiopathic thrombocytopenic purpura in childhood: an observational study. Lancet 2001;358(9299): 2122.
8. Liu J, Hutzler M, Li C, Pechet L. Thrombotic thrombocytopenic purpura (ttp) and hemolyt uremic syndrome (hus): the new thinking. J Thromb Thrombolysis 2002;11(3):261.
9. Brandt L, Kimby E, Nygren P et al. A systematic overview of chemotherapy effects in Hodgkin's disease. Acta Oncol 2001;40(2–3):185.
10. Kimby E, Brandt L, Nygren P et al. A systematic overview of chemotherapy effects in non-Hodgkin's lymphoma. Acta Oncol 2001;40(2–3):198–212.
11. Hamblin TJ. Achieving optimal outcomes in chronic lymphocytic leukemia. Drugs 2001;61(5):593.
12. Mesa RA, Elliott MA, Tefferi A. Splenectomy in chronic myeloid leukemia and myelofibrosis with myeloid metaplasia. Blood Rev 2000;14(3):121.
13. Al-Salem AH, Naserullah Z, Qaisaruddin S et al. Splenic complications of the sickling syndromes and the role of splenectomy. J Pediatr Hematol Oncol 1999;21(5):401.
14. Olivieri N. Thalassaemia: clinical management. Baillières Clin Haematol 1998; 11(1):147.
15. Dacie SJ. The immune haematolytic anaemias: a century of exciting progress in understanding. Br J Haematol 2001;11(4):770.
16. Schwartz DI, Adams JT, Bauman AW. Splenectomy for hematologic disorders. Chicago: Yearbook Medical Publishers, 1971.
17. Park AE, Birgisson G, Mastrangelo MJ et al. Laparoscopic splenectomy: outcomes and lessons learned from over 200 cases. Surgery 2000;128(4):660.
18. Esposito TJ, Gamelli RL. Injury to the spleen. Trauma, 4th edn. New York: McGraw-Hill, 1999.
19. Brasel KJ. DeLisle CM, Olson CJ, Borgstrom DC. Splenic injury: trends in evaluation and management. J Trauma 1998;44:283.
20. Rutledge R, Hunt JP, Lentz CW et al. A statewide, population-based time-series analysis of the increasing frequency of nonoperative management of abdominal solid organ injury. Ann Surg 1995;222:311.
21. Pranikoff T, Hirschl RB, Schlesinger AE et al. Resolution of splenic injury after nonoperative management. J Pediatr Surg 1994;29:1366.
22. Powell M, Courcoulas A, Gardner M et al. Management of blunt splenic trauma: significant differences between adults and children. Surgery 1997;122:654.
23. Pachter HL, Guth AA, Hofstetter SR, Spencer FC. Changing patterns in the management of splenic trauma: the impact of nonoperative management. Ann Surg 1998;227:708.
24. Waghorn DJ. Overwhelming infection in asplenic patients: current best practice. Preventive measures are not being followed. J Clin Pathol 2001;54(3):214.
25. Kassianos GC. Uncertainty exists over frequency of blood tests to test antipneumococcal immunity. BMJ 1996;312:1360.
26. Spickett GP, Bullimore J, Wallis J et al. Northern region asplenia register-analysis of first two years. J Clin Pathol 199;53:424.

# 6

# Benign Disease of the Oesophagus

Stephen E.A. Attwood and Christopher J. Lewis

## Aims

- To describe the pathology and management of gastro-oesophageal reflux.
- To describe the pathology and management of non-reflux disease.
- To describe the pathology and treatment of motility disorders.
- To outline the nature and management of uncommon oesophageal disease.

The common benign diseases of the oesophagus are gastro-oesophageal reflux disease and dysmotility disorders. The other conditions that are found are unusual and include various types of inflammation, anatomical abnormalities, benign tumours and perforation.

## Gastro-oesophageal Reflux Disease

### Definition

Heartburn (feeling of a burning sensation moving up from the epigastrium through the central retrosternal area towards the neck), regurgitation (the effortless appearance of material of gastric content in the mouth or throat) and dysphagia are the classical symptoms of gastro-oesophageal reflux disease (GORD). When these are present with sufficient frequency and degree to disrupt a patient's quality of life more than a few times a week, it is relatively easy to define the circumstance in terms of a clinically significant disease. However, the definition of GORD is difficult because the symptoms may be present in much lesser degree, and heartburn, in particular, may be part of the normal human experience. Other less typical symptoms may contribute significant clinical problems relating to gastro-oesophageal reflux, and these include respiratory symptoms such as nocturnal aspiration, with episodes of choking and coughing, or exacerbation of asthma, pneumonitis or the development of a chronic cough. Dentists may find erosion of dental enamel, ENT surgeons may find chronic laryngitis, and patients may suffer hoarseness and water brash (the collection of saliva or fluid in the mouth that is not related to regurgitation) and these may all be related to significant gastro-oesophageal reflux. Patients who have gastro-oesophageal reflux may also suffer significant abdominal discomforts including epigastric pain, left and right hypochondrial pain, and it is frequent for patients to have significant reflux while also suffering gallstones, irritable bowel syndrome or diverticulitis. The symptoms of gastro-oesophageal reflux may also be confused with the symptoms of peptic ulcer disease, although it is unusual for patients to present with both.

## Aetiology

Reflux occurs because of a failure of the lower oesophageal sphincter mechanism. The resting pressure may be too low, the position of the pressure zone may be in the thorax, or there may be inappropriate transient lower oesophageal sphincter relaxation. GORD may be congenital and can result in serious problems with infant nutrition and respiratory function. Usually, however, the condition is acquired and presents in the fourth and fifth decades of life without any particular precipitating event or illness. It is now realised that there are strong genetic predispositions to GORD. There are also environmental and dietary factors, which may aggravate the condition. Agents that lower the lower oesophageal sphincter tone include coffee, fat and gastrointestinal hormones such as cholecystokinin. Obesity aggravates reflux, as does the consumption of acidic fluids such as white wine. Unfortunately the strict control of these dietary factors by lifestyle modification is not sufficient to control reflux symptoms; definitive therapy, in the form of medication or surgery, is needed if the symptoms occur frequently enough to disturb a patient's life. As a guide, symptoms that require medication or disturb lifestyle twice a week are sufficient to warrant assessment by a primary care physician.

## Management

### Primary Care

The majority of patients with GORD will be managed by their primary care physician using acid suppression medication inhibiting the proton pump with intermittent courses, continuous therapy or possibly by "on-demand" medication. Endoscopy is mandatory in the assessment of new onset symptoms in patients over the age of 50. In other patients referral may result from the patient's dissatisfaction with the quality of their medical therapy and the quality of their life [1].

### Secondary Referral

In secondary care, it is important to identify the reason for assessing patients with GORD before embarking on specific investigations. Identify if a patient has alarm features of cancer such as weight loss, gastrointestinal bleeding, known risk factors such as a family history of gastric carcinoma, or the presence of a previously diagnosed Barrett's oesophagus. The degree of interference of the symptoms or disease with a patient's occupation, sporting and social activities should be determined before considering investigation and therapeutic strategies.

In the hospital setting, gastroscopy and oesophageal manometry and pH studies are critically important in giving advice to patients with GORD. It must be emphasised that these investigations are not needed for the majority of patients in primary care. (Chapter 21 details diagnostic and therapeutic endoscopy.) The findings on endoscopy in GORD are commonly normal. In endoscopy negative reflux disease, it is useful to be able to reassure the patient that there is no tissue damage, and no other serious diseases, but the patient should not be made to feel that the absence of endoscopic findings indicates normality. If there is clinical doubt about the presence of acid reflux in this circumstance, 24-hour pH studies, preceded by oesophageal manometry, are useful in defining the severity of acid reflux and guiding future management. The diagnosis of oesophagitis at endoscopy reveals the degree of tissue injury. These are graded using a variety of grading systems, the most important of which currently is the Los Angeles system grade A to D [1] (Figure 6.1). Previously, it had been common to use the Savary–Miller grading system (Table 6.1) and much of the current literature is based on that system. Endoscopy may also reveal the presence, size and type of hiatus hernia, or the presence of complications, such as Barrett's oesophagus or a stricture (for details of endoscopy see Chapter 21).

When endoscopy or pH monitoring shows no abnormality in the oesophagus with the presence of symptoms strongly suggestive of them arising in the oesophagus, further investigation with physiological testing is sometimes worthwhile. New impedance reflux monitoring systems (Sandhill/Gaeltec) identify the presence of reflux regardless of its acidic content. Extended pH testing over longer than 24 hours is feasible using a more comfortable method of pH testing than the standard nasal oesophageal intubation by clipping a hook to the lining of the oesophagus, and obtaining extended telemetry recordings over

# BENIGN DISEASE OF THE OESOPHAGUS

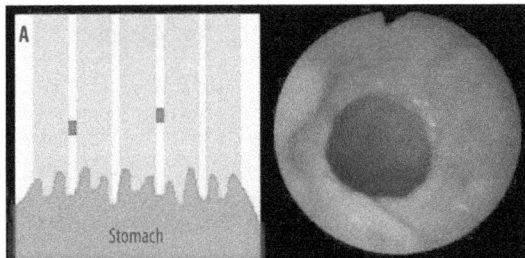
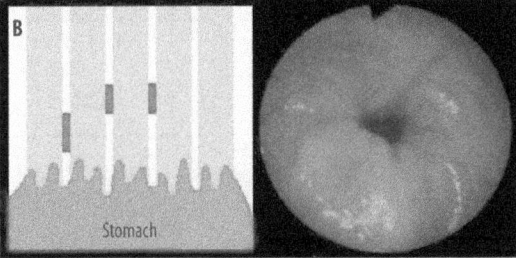
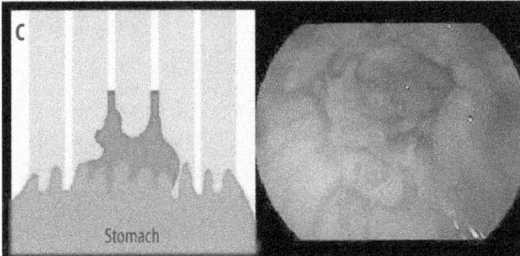
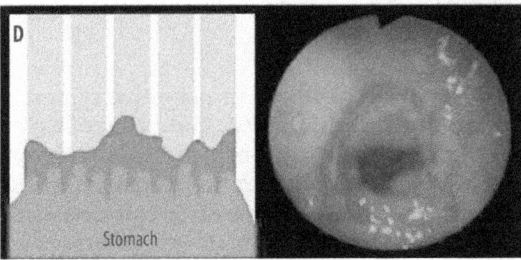

**Figure 6.1.** L.A. grading (A–D) for endoscopic assessment of oesophagitis. (Reproduced with kind permission of Astra-Zeneca, Ltd, UK.)

48–72 hours (Figures 6.2 and 6.3). Balloon testing of the oesophageal reaction to distension may identify abnormal motility or a low threshold of pain perception. Balloon distension studies do not give precise information physiologically about the sensation of the oesophagus to distension unless the actual cross-sectional area of the balloon is measured during these investigations, and this can be done using impedance stimulated manometry

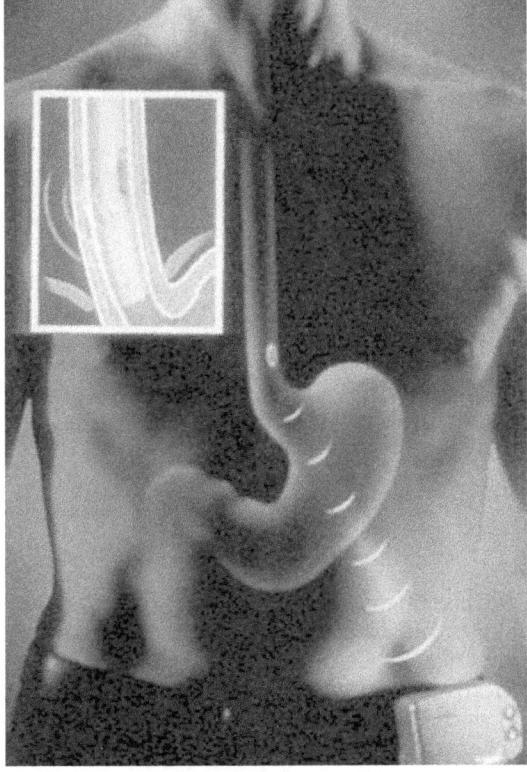

**Figure 6.2.** pH probe clipped to oesophagus. (Reproduced with kind permission of Endonetics Inc, USA.)

**Table 6.1.** Savary–Miller grading for endoscopic assessment of oesophagitis

| Grade | Appearance |
|---|---|
| I | Non-confluent red patches or streaks proximal to Oesophagogastric junction, single or multiple non-confluent superficial linear erosions |
| II | Distal confluent patches which do not extend around the entire oesophageal circumference. Confluent non-circumferential erosions. Proximal inflammation |
| III | Confluent patches extending around entire circumference, oedema, friable mucosa, circumferential erosions |
| IV | One or more ulcers with or without strictures/stenosis |

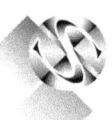

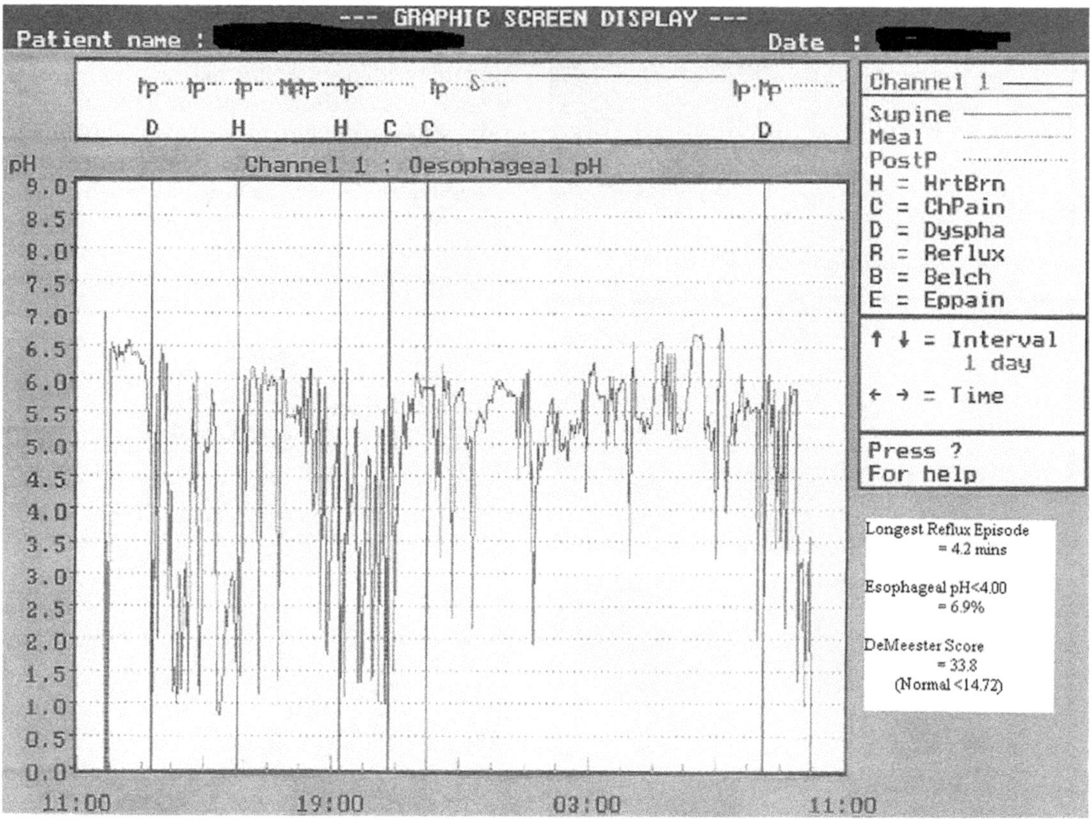

**Figure 6.3.** Graph of refluxing pH trace.

or clinemetry. Sensory testing can also be done with electrically induced potentials and motor neurone integrity can be assessed using electromagnetic resonance stimulation. All these investigations are useful in a difficult case, where the standard investigations and therapies have been unsuccessful.

## Hiatus Hernia

The presence or absence of a hiatus hernia is not important in the distinction of the diagnosis of GORD, but is important in the decision about potential treatment strategies. Hiatus hernia may be present as a sliding or rolling hernia (Figure 6.4). Sliding hernias (type 1) are very common, and may contribute to the symptoms of dysphagia. The remaining symptoms in sliding hiatus hernia are usually due to the presence of acid reflux rather than the presence of the hernia itself. In contrast, a rolling (type 2) hiatus hernia will present definitive symptoms of vomiting, regurgitation, chest pain of a character different to heartburn, pressure symptoms within the chest, which if related to a large hernia may cause dyspnoea. A combination of both sliding and rolling or para-oesophageal hiatus hernia (type 2b) can also occur, but this is rare.

## Complications of GORD

The complications of reflux include oesophagitis, with varying degrees of ulceration (see Figure 6.1, LA grading), stricture formation in the oesophagus, and Barrett's oesophagus with a growth of intestinal metaplasia in the lower oesophagus. Barrett's columnar lined lower oesophagus occurs in 10% of patients with GORD. In contrast to reflux itself, which does seem to have a genetic familial tendency, the development of Barrett's oesophagus does not,

# BENIGN DISEASE OF THE OESOPHAGUS

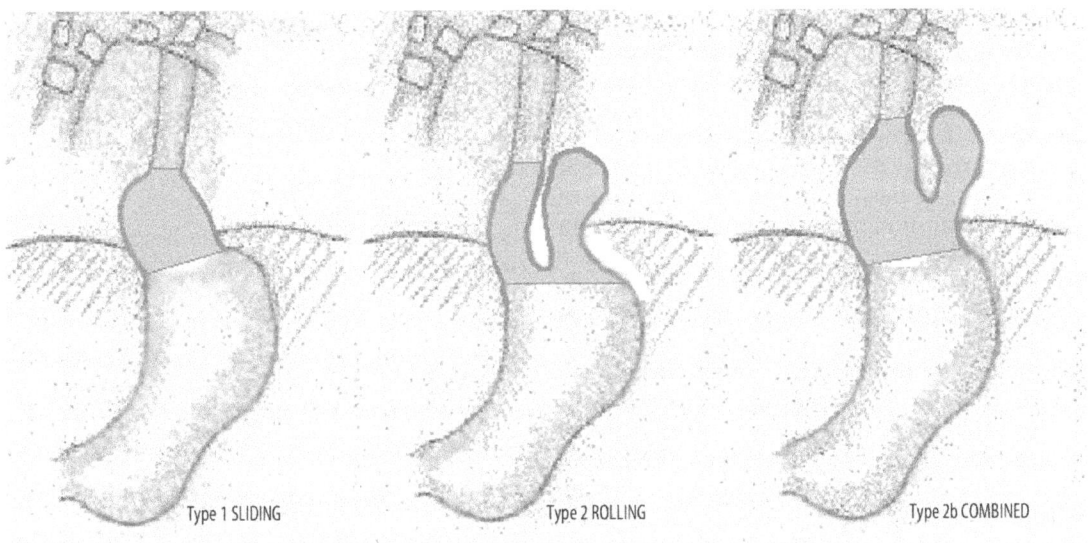

Figure 6.4. Diagram illustrating differing types of hiatus hernia.

and seems to occur sporadically. The degree of reflux in Barrett's oesophagus is usually severe when measured. Paradoxically, some patients with Barrett's oesophagus have little in the way of reflux symptoms despite severe acid exposure. The presence of Barrett's oesophagus appears to reduce the sensitivity of the oesophagus to acid reflux. For a detailed review of the malignant potential of Barrett's oesophagus refer to Chapter 26.

In both symptomatic reflux disease and Barrett's oesophagus, there is a significant increase in the risk of adenocarcinoma of the oesophagus. In symptomatic refluxers this risk has been defined in a Swedish epidemiological study. Lagergren and co-workers [2] identified that a patient who refluxes daily for more than 20 years is 43 times more likely to develop adenocarcinoma than someone who has had no reflux. Complications also include aspiration pneumonitis and chronic laryngitis, and in children there can be significant malnutrition and failure to thrive.

## The Role of Antireflux Surgery

The only continuous therapy for GORD is the repair of the valve mechanism of the gastro-oesophageal junction [3,4]. Currently, this is done by a formal surgical operation at the gastro-oesophageal junction, usually by a laparoscopic approach [5]. It should be remembered that antireflux surgery provides continuous protection to the lower oesophagus from the noxious effects of reflux [3]. Antireflux surgery has no effects on normal digestion, it allows normal acid protection against ingested bacteria, and it has no carcinogenic side effects. When it is successful, it can provide continuous complete symptom control, and allows the patient the psychological benefit of being restored to normal. It has no long-term potential systemic effects [4,6,7]. There is the possibility that it provides cost-effective care, although this depends on the true costs of long-term or even lifelong medication and the subsequent development of complications [8,9].

## Indications for Antireflux Surgery

### Patient Desire

Antireflux surgery is indicated for patients who have a justifiable desire to be free of reflux, and who are fit to undergo a surgical procedure. What is meant by a justifiable desire? Patients, who despite regular proton pump inhibitors, at full and maintenance dose, have further troublesome symptoms such as volume reflux,

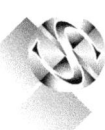

night-time aspiration symptoms with coughing or choking. Sometimes, asthma can be exacerbated by GORD and, if this is well documented, it may be an indication for surgery. Recurring heartburn or chest pain, despite being on optimum regular therapy, is relatively rare, but does occur. It also occurs in the situation of delay, interruption or dose reduction of proton pump inhibitors, which may occur because the patient forgets to take or obtain their medication. Patients with long-term side effects of proton pump inhibitors, such as diarrheoa, headache or neurological symptoms, often desire a surgical alternative [1,4]. Recently, because of the acknowledged link between gastro-oesophageal symptoms and the subsequent development of adenocarcinoma of the oesophagus, patients who are reminded of their symptoms due to symptom breakthrough, or who are anxious about the long-term effects of partially treated reflux, may wish to stop their reflux in the belief that it might influence the subsequent malignant potential. This is currently a common desire but there is no scientific data to support the particular argument that surgery might prevent cancer [6].

*Patient Fitness*

Patients should only be considered for antireflux surgery if they are truly fit. This is usually a balance of issues, which includes a physiological age of less than 70 years in most communities. There needs to be a lack of morbid obesity, no symptomatic cardiac problems, good respiratory function (unless there is controlled reversible airways disease), good mobility and an independent lifestyle. Particular problems do occur in patients who are mentally retarded and in cerebral palsy, where there are combinations of additional risks, difficulties in assessing the patients' own desires, their symptoms and their understanding of consent. There is also limited outcome data in this group, and advising their carers on the true risks is difficult to base on published material. Patients with rheumatic diseases limiting mobility vary in their outcome. People with scleroderma do benefit from antireflux surgery when carefully chosen, but those with rheumatoid arthritis often have too many other co-morbidity problems to be able to benefit from the operation without complications [10].

*Reflux Complications*

In the presence of some complications, antireflux surgery is sometimes desirable. In particular, strictures that require frequent dilatation may do better when their reflux is controlled surgically rather than with proton pump inhibitors. When Barrett's oesophagus is present, there may be additional problems with symptoms, bleeding or failure to heal ulceration and, in this circumstance, surgery may be considered a better method of controlling of reflux injury. It is important again to emphasise that there is no data to support any attempts at cancer risk reduction in Barrett's oesophagus by antireflux surgery.

## Long-term Medication vs Surgery

For the majority of patients who are well controlled on proton pump inhibitors, there is no clear benefit in changing the strategy to antireflux surgery. Lundell et al, in 1998, [11] identified in a prospective randomised study with 5 years of follow-up that if patients were well controlled on proton pump inhibitors at the beginning of the study, randomising them to medical treatment or surgery resulted in the same quality of life, as long as they were allowed to adjust the dose of their proton pump inhibitors to deal with any recurrent symptoms when medically treated. Thus, if patients are very satisfied with their medical therapy, there is little to be gained with an operation. In stark contrast, when patients have a particular desire, and when there are clear indications for them to consider surgery, there is often a dramatic improvement in their quality of life [7]. The surgeon should consider specifically the patient's own risks and potential benefits, and also the surgical unit's own experience and outcome figures.

## Contraindications

Contraindications to antireflux surgery may include patients who do not have reflux. Patients who fail to show acid reflux on pH monitoring are unlikely to benefit. Patients who have a primary motility disturbance, such as achalasia or nutcracker oesophagus on manometry, will not benefit from antireflux surgery unless it is an adjunct to a myotomy [10]. Patients with significant irritable bowel

# BENIGN DISEASE OF THE OESOPHAGUS

syndrome, gas bloat preoperatively, fibromyalgia and arthritis are relatively contraindicated. Clearly patients who have no desire for surgery should remain on medical therapy.

## Fundoplication and Hiatas Hernia Repair

Antireflux surgery usually requires correction of any hiatus hernia by reduction of the oesophagogastric junction into the abdominal cavity [3], identification of the diaphragmatic crura, and separation of the oesophagus from these. A window is usually created behind the oesophagus if a fundoplication is to be performed. Repair of the diaphragmatic crura is undertaken with non-absorbable sutures, approximating the left and right diaphragmatic crural pillars, and leaving sufficient space for the oesophagus to expand during the swallowing of a bolus of food. Some operators place a 50 or 60 French bougie at this stage of the operation, in order to gauge the size of their hiatal repair. The second part of the operation is fundoplication, taking part of the fundus of the stomach around the lower oesophagus just above the oesophagogastric junction. There are a number of different ways of doing this, and these include a Nissen fundoplication [12] (a 360° wrap, requiring mobilisation of the short gastric arteries) and the Nissen Rosetti modification, in which the anterior wall of the gastric fundus is brought behind the oesophagus and sutured to the greater curvature of the stomach brought across the front without mobilisation of the short gastric vessels. Other variations of fundoplication include the Toupet [13,14], which is a 240° posterior wrap, leaving the anterior part of the oesophagus uncovered (Figure 6.7). The wrap is fixed both to the lateral walls of the oesophagus, and to both diaphragmatic crura. A claimed advantage of the Toupet operation is that it is less constricting, and therefore suffers less early postoperative dysphagia [14]. Other variations include the Watson anterior fundoplication, the Lind fundoplication, and the Hill gastropexy [15–17].

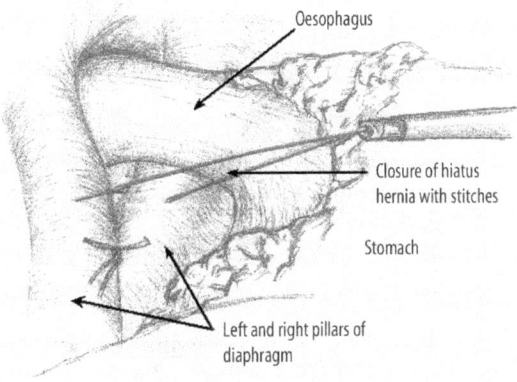

**Figure 6.5.** Diagram of laparoscopic hiatal repair.

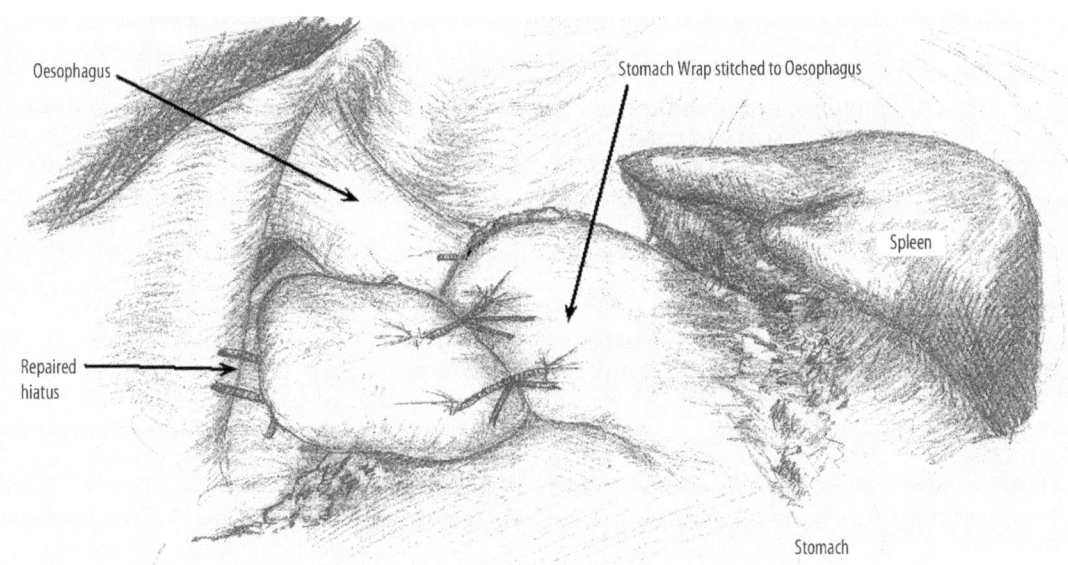

**Figure 6.6.** Diagram of laparoscopic fundal wrap.

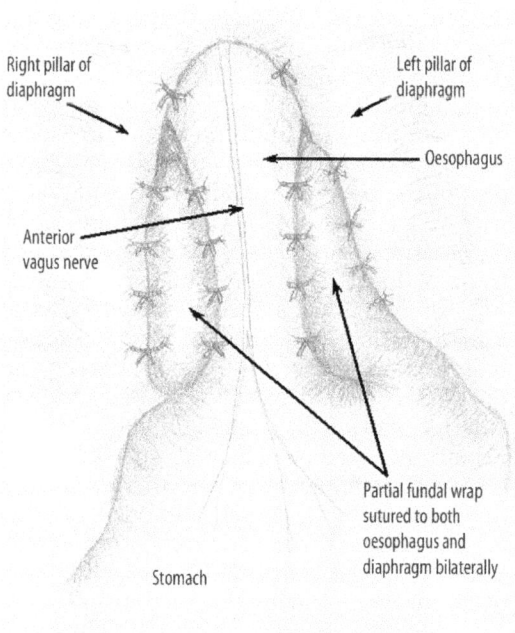

**Figure 6.7.** Diagram of Toupet fundoplication.

### Outcomes and Complications

With good case selection, 90% of patients who undergo antireflux surgery have a good or excellent outcome, with relief of their symptoms of regurgitation, dysphagia and potentially other less typical manifestations of gastro-oesophageal reflux disease. For patients who have atypical symptoms, such as asthma, laryngitis, cough, and variations of chest and abdominal pain, the outcomes are less predictable. In most studies dysphagia is common in the early postoperative period, but resolves in all except approximately 5%, by 3 months postoperatively. A graded introduction of solid diet is required during this period. In the 10% of patients in whom there is a less satisfactory outcome the problems include disruption of the wrap (3–5%), persistent dysphagia (3–5%), and persistent symptoms of bloating that are a disturbance to quality of life. There are occasionally more serious complications such as para-oesophageal herniation, splenic injury at the time of surgery requiring splenectomy, oesophageal or gastric perforation, and possibly other more unusual problems. Reoperation rates in large reported series vary between 3 and 10% [5–7,14,18].

For the 90% who do well there is often a significant quality of life improvement including improvement of sleep disturbance, allowance of physical activities and exercises previously restricted, restoration of normal social eating habits and the feeling of being free of a previous label of disease [7]. The outcome in relation to oesophagitis shows almost universal healing of ulceration. Barrett's oesophagus, however, does not regress completely, and usually persists although it remains asymptomatic. It is not known what the effect on cancer risk is in relation to reflux protection either by medication or by antireflux surgery. [6]

## Non-reflux Oesophagitis

Inflammation of the mucosa of the oesophagus, although most commonly caused by reflux of gastric contents, can be associated with several other pathologies.

### Caustic Injury

Injury by ingestion of caustic substances can be significant, and have long-term consequences. The degree of damage is dependent on two main factors: firstly, the caustic potential of the substance involved, for example pH, and secondly, the transit time of the relevant substance. The commonest substances involved are household cleaners, such as bleach, and other acid or alkaline solutions. In liquid form the transit time in the oesophagus is often short. The rapid action of these caustic substances means that attempts to dilute the solution, and therefore reduce injury, are usually unsuccessful. Gastric injury and perforation may also occur. Caustic crystals may also be ingested and cause localised burns. These rarely enter the oesophagus, as the caustic action usually occurs in the pharynx, causing burns proximal to the oesophagus. The alkaline anode of disc batteries can cause very localised but significant burns to any area of the gastrointestinal (GI) tract should they become lodged at any time. Tablets, such as potassium chloride, can have a similar effect, and the resulting burns are often deep and may cause perforation.

After ingestion, prevention of significant caustic injury is difficult. Treatment is primarily supportive with a primary role of preventing stricture formation, reducing inflammation, and reducing the risk of perforation. Steroids can be used in mild to moderate burns to reduce the inflammatory response, but are contraindicated in severe injury. Repeat dilatation is often required should a stricture develop, and antibiotics should be used in the acute phase as a prophulactic measure. Complete destruction of the oesophagus may require feeding by gastrostomy, or jejunostomy if a gastrectomy is required. Secondary reconstruction with colon or small bowel interposition is a task for specialised centres.

## Infective Oesophagitis

All forms of infective oesophagitis are uncommon in an otherwise well person. Immunocompromised patients and those with malignancy, however, do have an increased incidence. Patients present with a variety of symptoms, often non-specific, and they may present with symptoms or signs of an underlying malignant disease or other cause for immunocompromise. Common symptoms at presentation include dysphagia, odynophagia, heartburn, non-specific chest pain, and the patient may complain that they are aware of the passage of food on swallowing. In these cases, diagnosis can only be made by upper GI endoscopy and microscopy and culture of biopsies taken (Table 6.2).

*Candida* is a comensal microbe in the upper GI tract and pharynx. This can become an opportunistic pathogen if systemic antibiotic therapy is given, allowing overgrowth due to removal of regional flora.

Herpes simplex (HSV) is primarily a reactivation of a latent virus from the regional ganglion. It may, however, spread directly from the oropharynx. The patient presents with severe odynophagia often with associated retrosternal burning and/or dysphagia, or they can occasionally present with a severe upper GI bleed. Treatment is primarily with antiviral agents.

Cytomegalovirus (CMV) is more common with infection with HIV. Again, it is reactivation of a latent virus, and presents in a similar way to HSV, but dysphagia seems to be a more prominent symptom.

## Eosinophilic Oesophagitis

Eosinophilic oesophagitis is an uncommon condition first described as a distinct clinical entity in 1993 [19]. It is characterised by an intense eosinophilic infiltration of the oesophageal mucosa and symptoms of dysphagia, which are often intermittent, progressive and associated with odynophagia. Previously, eosinophilia in the oesophagus was regarded as an incidental component of GORD or a variant of eosinophilic gastroenteritis. However, the clinical syndrome of eosinophilic oesophagitis is not usually seen with either of these. Most recent literature refers to eosinophilic oesophagitis in children, but the adult phenomenon may escape diagnosis due to lack of awareness of this separate pathology. The hallmark of this condition is intermittent and often painful dysphagia, which may become constant as the disease progresses. Thorough investigations often show essentially normal or mildly abnormal oesophageal endoscopy, pH and manometry studies. Mechanical obstruction is usually absent, and unless a biopsy is taken, these patients are found to be a diagnostic enigma and management dilemma.

### Presentation

The presentation of these patients is quite variable, with some attending accident and emergency departments with acute bolus obstruction. The majority tend to be young, 20–40 years of age. Diagnosis is only confirmed by biopsy of an often normal looking oesophagus, although rings, mucosal reticulation and furrows may be seen (Figures 6.8, 6.9 and 6.10). Histology shows dense eosinophilic infiltration within the oesophageal mucosa.

### Management

Management of these patients has been made difficult by diagnostic problems, and a poor understanding of the disease pathogenesis. Acid suppression has no effect. Antihistamine medication has been used in the past with little

**Table 6.2.** Agents in infective esophagitis

| Usual pathogens | Rare pathogens |
|---|---|
| *Candida* CMV, herpes simplex | TB, HIV, HPV, *Trypanosoma cruzi* (Chagas' disease) |

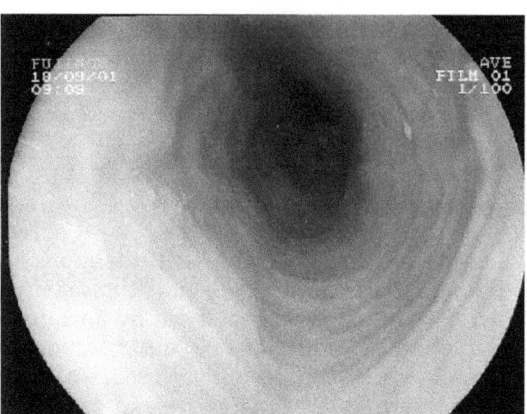

**Figure 6.8.** Endoscopic appearance of eosinophilic oesophagitis rings.

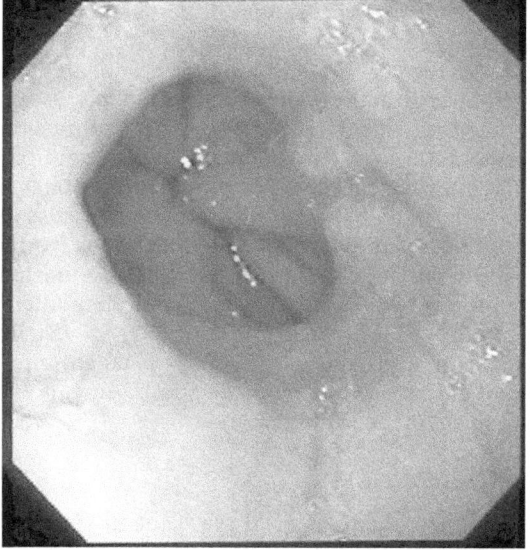

**Figure 6.9.** Endoscopic appearance of eosinophilic oesophagitis furrows.

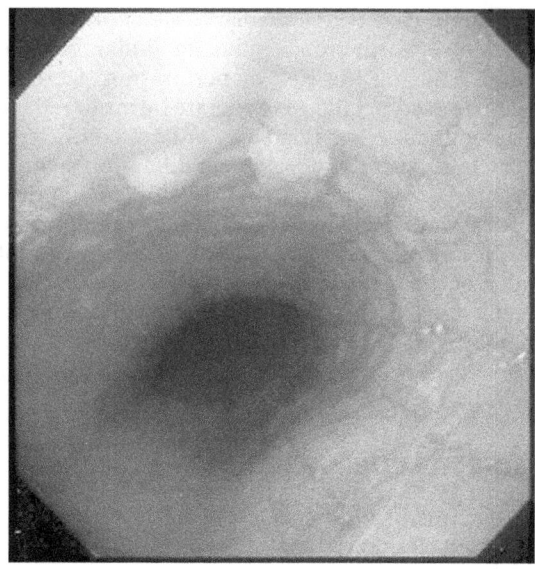

**Figure 6.10.** Endoscopic appearance of eosinophilic oesophagitis cobblestone.

reported success. Oesophageal dilatation has also been undertaken for symptomatic relief but, unfortunately, this can be very uncomfortable and only provides short-term relief. Corticosteroid therapy has shown some success in the literature. Symptoms soon relapse, however, once treatment is ceased, and the significant side effect profile of long-term steroid therapy in young patients greatly limits their value in this setting. There is some early evidence to show that eosinophil stabilisation, using montelukast (Singulair, MSD), a leukotriene D4 antagonist used in severe asthma, may allow significant symptom relief.

## Inflammatory Bowel Disease

Crohn's disease may manifest with oesophageal involvement, although this is uncommon. In the typical fashion, skip lesions can be present and fistulation has been reported. Treatment is unchanged from that of intestinal Crohn's disease, with steroid therapy, stricture dilatation and resection all being described.

## Irritable Bowel Syndrome (IBS) and Functional Foregut Disorders (FFD)

A spectrum of GI symptoms is perceived by patients to relate to the upper GI tract. In relation to the lower abdomen and a variable bowel habit the irritable bowel syndrome is a commonly diagnosed condition, where no specific pathology is identified. It is often associated with symptoms of upper GI dysfunction, and the term functional foregut disorder has been coined. The range of symptoms includes reflux-like sensations, central chest pain and even dysphagia, when no abnormality can be found

# BENIGN DISEASE OF THE OESOPHAGUS

on endoscopy, biopsy, manometry or 24-hour pH monitoring. Functional testing with impedance plethysmography and sensory tests may show levels of mucosal hypersensitivity. Our understanding of the brain–gut axis is now growing and while there are clear relationships between the brain and the mucosal and mural sensitivity of the oesophagus [20], there are no clear therapeutic strategies yet defined. The use of tricyclic antidepressants may modulate central responses, and identification of the neurotransmitters of hypersensitivity may, in the future, allow specific strategies of management.

## Motility Disorders

### Achalasia

This is a failure of oesophageal motility and coordination that results in chronic dysphagia. The condition presents in a bimodal age distribution with peaks in the age ranges 20–40 years and 70–90 years, and is relatively rare (1/100 000 of population)

### Aetiology and Presentation

In Western societies achalasia is a sporadic, idiopathic condition. In South America it is related to the infective agent *Trypanosoma cruzi*, and is called Chagas' disease. It is familial in 1% of cases and can be related to other neurodegenerative diseases such as Parkinson's. The usual presenting complaint is dysphagia to solids, which most patients say has been gradually progressive over several years. Misdiagnosis is common, and a label of GORD, chest pain or dyspepsia is often given. Postural regurgitation is typical of achalasia. The description by the patient is often characteristic and clearly points towards the pathology. They complain of non-acidic, undigested and non-bilious food regurgitation, which can be foul tasting or smelling due to extended fermentation in the dilated non-motile oesophagus. This occurs especially at night when the patient is lying flat; they awake coughing and choking. This classical patient may also have considerable weight loss, and complain of fear of eating due to social embarrassment from regurgitation. They will also tend to drink copious amounts of fluid with meals in an attempt to wash the food bolus down.

### Pathophysiology

Oesophageal manometry is the definitive investigation in achalasia (Figure 6.11). The distinguishing feature is failure of the lower oesophageal sphincter to relax on swallowing. The lower oesophageal pressure tends to be greater than normal (approximately × 1.5–2),

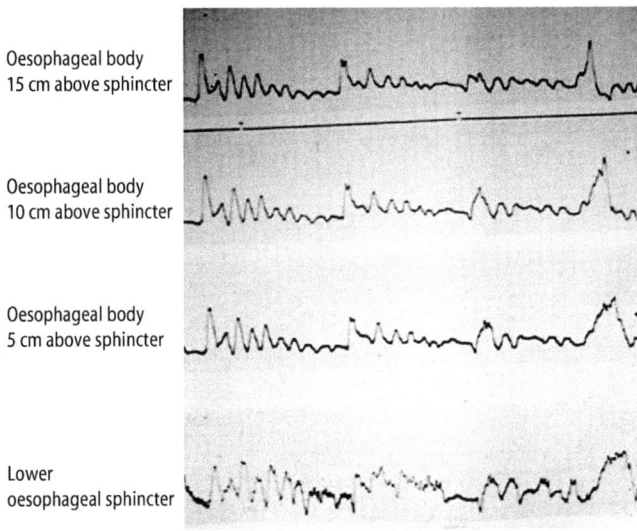

**Figure 6.11.** Manometry trace of achalasia.

although the pressure does not necessarily relate to the severity of symptoms. There is often a progressive weakening and discoordination of oesophageal peristalsis. In a small number of patients painful, strong, simultaneous contractions occur; this is sometimes called vigorous achalasia. Barium/contrast studies show a dilated lower oesophagus with a classical sigmoid shape (Figure 6.12). There is a gradual smooth tapering of the distal oesophagus. Where there is an air/fluid level in the oesophagus, it is usually dilated and in this situation the gastric air/fluid level is absent.

### Treatment

Treatment of achalasia is by dilatation or surgical myotomy. The increasingly popular *Botulinum* toxin (Botox) injection has yet to provide superior control of symptoms than the two standard therapies. Dilatation of achalasia requires the complete disruption of the lower oesophageal sphincter necessitating a balloon dilator 30–40 mm in diameter (Figure 6.13). These are usually passed over a guide wire under radiological control and may require sedation or a general anaesthetic. Success with dilatation seems to depend upon a strict protocol, and many specialised units achieve 60–80% satisfaction with long-term relief of dysphagia. Because dilatation may fail, the surgical option of Heller's myotomy is an important alternative. It is reasonable to try balloon dilatation, but repeated attempts may increase the risk of perforation and increase the difficulty of any subsequent myotomy.

In most specialist centres the access for myotomy is by laparoscopic approach. Thoracoscopy is also feasible. A Heller's myotomy requires a longitudinal incision in the lower oesophageal musculature, at least 5 cm long and including the gastro-oesophageal junction. The

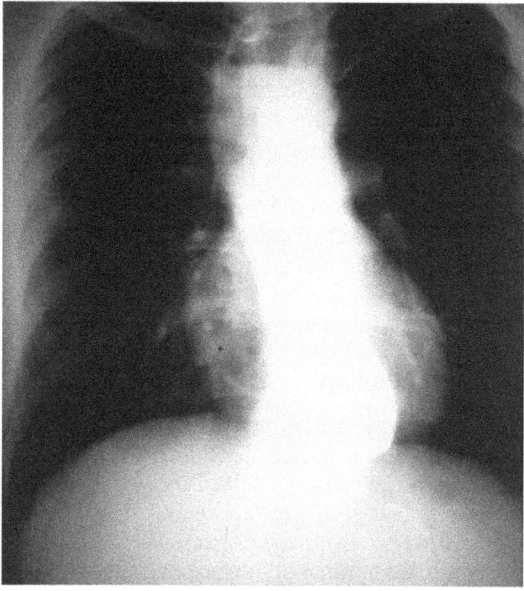

**Figure 6.12.** Achalasia on contrast radiograph.

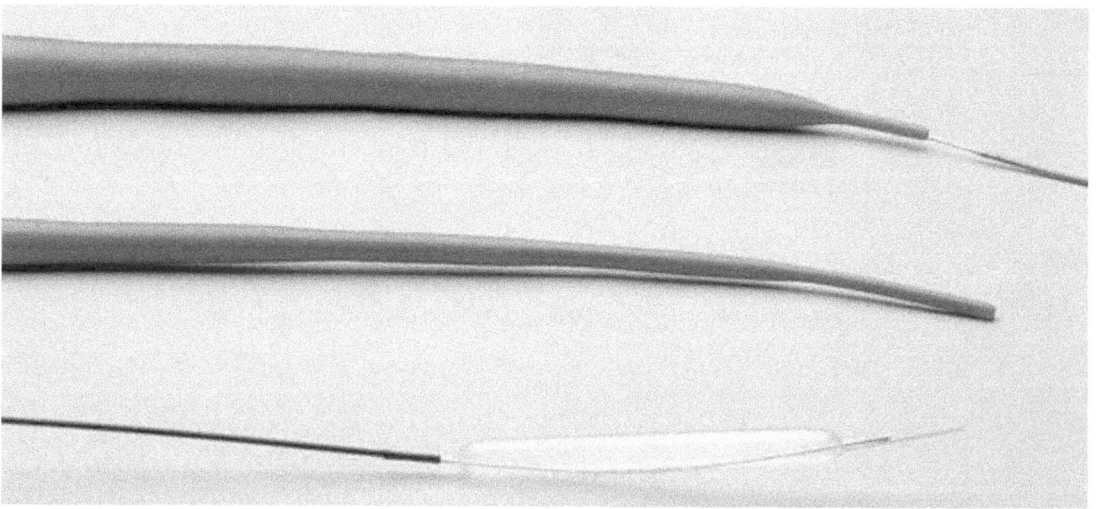

**Figure 6.13.** Celestin and balloon oesophageal dilators. (Reproduced with kind permission of Salford Royal Hospitals NHS Trust.)

## BENIGN DISEASE OF THE OESOPHAGUS

operation requires a careful technique to ensure complete sphincter disruption and avoid perforation. Some surgeons recommend the use of a fundoplication anteriorly (Dor fundoplication) to hold open the edge of the myotomy and provide some protection against reflux. The complications of surgery include perforation, sepsis, reflux and occasionally symptom recurrence.

Untreated achalasia can lead to severe malnutrition. Aspiration of oesophageal contents can occur, resulting in chest infections, and in the long term squamous carcinoma has an increased incidence. This is thought to be secondary to a chronic irritation by stagnating and fermenting oesophageal contents.

## Diffuse Oesophageal Spasm

This is characterised by diffuse powerful simultaneous contractions in the oesophagus (Figure 6.14), and is a cause of oesophageal pain sometimes found in patients labeled as non-cardiac chest pain. Lower oesophageal sphincter pressure is usually not affected and relaxes completely. The oesophageal wall may be thickened as a result, and may create dysphagic symptoms. The disease is not usually progressive and may resolve spontaneously. The presentation is frequently confused with cardiac disease, as like angina pectoris, it may even be relieved by nitrates. Gastro-oesophageal reflux disease may sometimes precipitate diffuse oesophageal spasm. There is a very variable disease profile with patients complaining of a wide spectrum of frequency, severity, duration and onset of pain. There may be occasional food bolus impaction. Manometry shows uncoordinated motility with simultaneous contractions greater than 20% of normal. Treatment is usually medical, using calcium channel blockers, such as nifedipine, along with reassurance. Balloon dilatation is occasionally used, and in exceptional cases long oesophageal myotomy is indicated.

## Nutcracker Oesophagus

This has a very similar presentation to angina pectoris and is often confused with it. It is

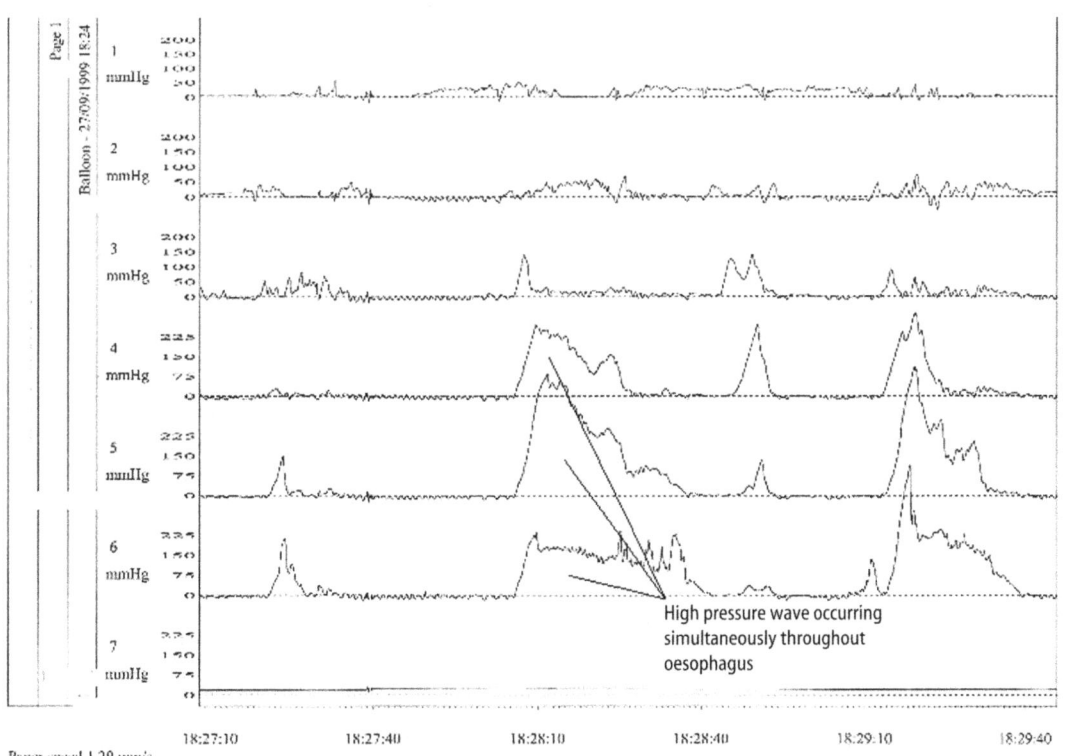

**Figure 6.14.** Manometry trace of diffuse oesophageal spasm.

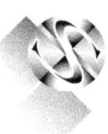

6 · UPPER GASTROINTESTINAL SURGERY

characterised by very high amplitude peristaltic contractions of greater than 180 mmHg or persistent elongated oesophageal contractions. Notable symptoms are chest pain and dysphagia, but again this is often not progressive, and may resolve spontaneously. It is distinguished from diffuse spasm by the retention of a normal peristaltic wave. Treatment, however, is identical to diffuse oesophageal spasm

## Hypertensive Lower Oesophageal Sphincter

Patients with chest pain and dysphagia who have raised lower oesophageal sphincter pressure but often a normal peristaltic activity have been described as having a hypertensive lower oesophageal sphincter. This can combine with high amplitude contractions of nutcracker oesophagus, and therefore the pathologies are closely related.

## Non-specific Oesophageal Motility Disorders

Scleroderma or systemic sclerosis affects the gastrointestinal tract in approximately 90% of patients, and its most common manifestation is in the oesophagus. The systemic effects of this disease occur via obliteration of small vessels, vasculitis and production of related fibrosis. The oesophagus characteristically develops smooth muscle atrophy and inflammatory cell infiltration. Symptoms of dysphagia, regurgitation and dyspepsia/heartburn can occur in quite mild cases of scleroderma even before there is any smooth muscle atrophy. These symptoms are thought to be secondary to motility disruption (Figure 6.15) from neurological dysfunction in Auerbach's plexus. Patients with scleroderma often have significant gastro-oesophageal reflux secondary to their hypotonic lower oesophageal sphincter. Treatment regimens for this disease concentrate on reduction

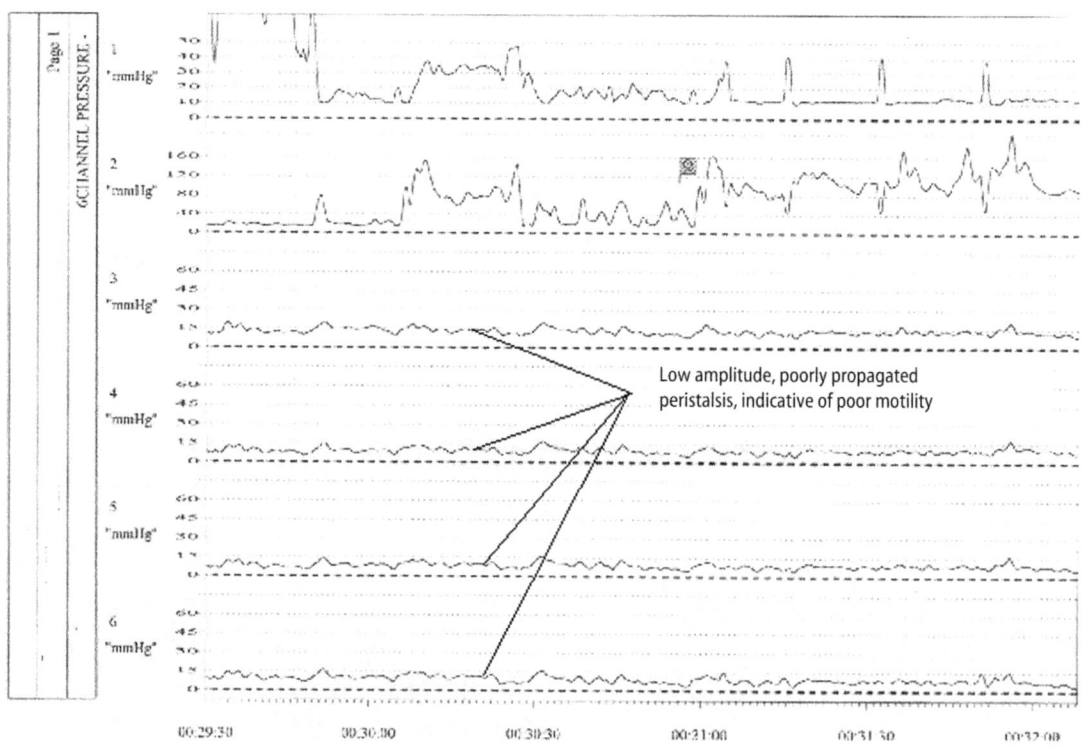

**Figure 6.15.** Manometry trace of poor oesophageal motility.

of gastro-oesophageal reflux but, at present, there is no effective treatment for the arrest of the sclerosing effect of the disease on the oesophagus, even though there have been significant advances recently in systemic immunosuppressive therapy for scleroderma. With increased GORD, there is also an increase in the incidence of Barrett's oesophagus. There is, however, no significant increase in the incidence of adenocarcinoma in these patients, and the reason for this is unclear. Motility agents do provide some symptomatic relief by increasing gastric emptying. They do not, unfortunately, affect motility in the oesophagus. Oesophageal strictures, and other complications of gastro-oesophageal reflux, can be treated by medical therapy. Decreased peristalsis, or even complete lack of peristalsis, makes these patients more likely to have dysphagia postoperatively, but in selected cases antireflux surgery is useful.

Mixed connective tissue disease has features similar to lupus, scleroderma and polymyositis. Inflammatory myositis, such as polymyositis, inclusion body myositis and dermatomyositis, affects predominantly striated muscle. This therefore affects the proximal oesophagus and cricopharyngeus. The main symptoms are regurgitation, dysphagia and occasionally aspiration. Gastric emptying is also decreased secondary to reduction in overall GI peristalsis. Lupus and rheumatoid arthritis can involve the oesophagus reducing by lowering peristaltic activity, both frequency and amplitude of contractions.

## Diverticula

### Upper Oesophageal Diverticula

Diverticula commonly occur at three separate levels in the oesophagus each with specific pathological causes. Firstly, in the upper oesophagus a diverticulum may occur proximal to the upper oesophageal sphincter (Figure 6.16). This is known as a Zenker's diverticulum, pharyngo-oesophageal diverticulum or an oesophageal/pharyngeal pouch. Uncoordinated contraction of cricopharyngeus muscle to a bolus transfer with the upper oesophageal sphincter closed during the initiation of swallowing causes the oesophagus to bulge posteriorly between the inferior constrictor muscles,

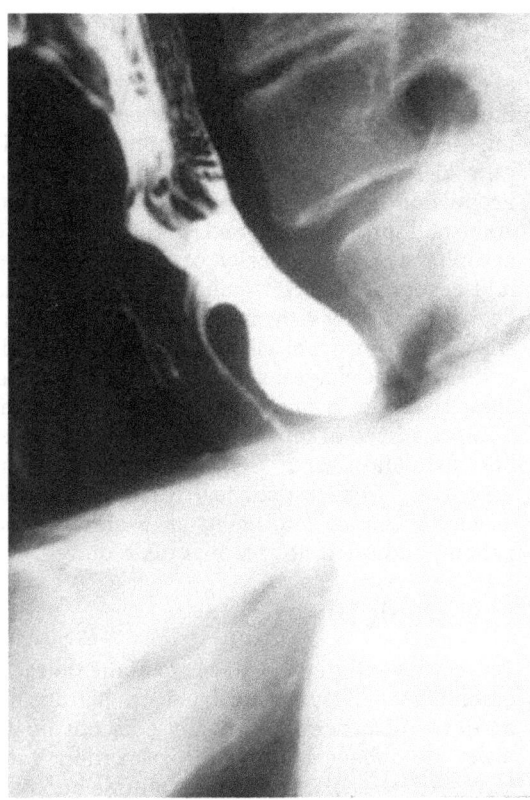

**Figure 6.16.** Pharyngeal pouch on contrast radiograph.

and over time the diverticulum develops. The characteristic presentation is of regurgitation of undigested food, which may have been eaten many hours previously. Other symptoms include persistent chronic cough, vague pharyngeal irritation, intermittent dysphagia, a gurgling sensation on swallowing, aspiration and subsequent pneumonitis. The degree of dysphagia is related to the size of the diverticulum. Successful treatment is through surgical myotomy of the cricopharyngeus muscle. This can be performed endoscopically or via open technique [21]. Complications of pharyngeal pouches are fairly uncommon. There is an increased association with squamous carcinoma, occasionally fistula formation can occur or there may be bleeding from within the diverticulum. Without a prior diagnosis of pharyngeal pouch, identification of this bleeding area can be quite difficult. The presence of a pharyngeal pouch increases the risk of instrumental perforation during flexible upper GI endoscopy.

## Mid-oesophageal Diverticula

Mid-oesophageal diverticula may occur from traction of surrounding fibrotic tissue, involving the full thickness of the oesophagus (classically described in relation to tuberculosis). Propulsion related diverticula occur due to abnormal propagation and peristalsis in the oesophagus. The majority of patients with a mid-oesophageal diverticulum will have some degree of motility disorder detected via manometry. Symptoms from associated disorders, such as diffuse oesophageal spasm, i.e. dysphagia and chest pain, are a more common presentation. Complications of this phenomenon are rare, but fistulation and perforation have been described. Mid-oesophageal diverticulum is usually a chance finding in an asymptomatic patient, and often no treatment is required.

## Epiphrenic Diverticula

These arise within the distal 4 cm of the thoracic oesophagus. They are related to significant motility disorders, especially discoordinate lower oesophageal sphincter relaxation with increased peristalsis or high amplitude peristalsis, such as diffuse oesophageal spasm, achalasia, or nutcracker oesophagus. Epiphrenic diverticula only become symptomatic when large. Management of these diverticula can be quite difficult and is dependent on primary pathological cause. If excision is performed, a myotomy of the lower oesophageal sphincter is needed, possibly with partial fundoplication.

## Intramural Pseudodiverticulosis

The pseudodiverticula have no clear aetiology. Commonly, they occur proximal to a stricture or in association with chronic inflammation, which causes submucosal glandular pseudocystic dilations. Symptomatic presentation tends to be dysphagia, often difficult to distinguish from that caused by related strictures. Dilatation of strictures usually gives good symptomatic relief.

# Oesophageal Webs and Rings

## Webs

Webs are formed from an eccentric mucosal fold, and can arise anywhere in the oesophagus, but usually in the anterior post-cricoid region. It is difficult to establish the true incidence of oesophageal webs, as the majority are asymptomatic. They are usually described as incidental findings on endoscopy performed for an unrelated problem.

In iron-deficiency anaemia when a web is associated with glossitis and koilonychias, it is known as Plummer–Vinson/Patterson–Kelly syndrome. In this circumstance upper GI endoscopy is indicated to exclude other causes of anaemia, especially in the stomach or oesophagus [22]. Other less common causes of oesophageal webs are in relation to thyroid disease, inflammatory states, as part of an embryonic or congenital malformation, in association with diverticula, and also occasionally as sequelae of graft versus host disease.

Patients present with long-standing dysphagia, which is not generally progressive. Treatment, when related to iron-deficiency anaemia, is by dietary manipulation in mild cases. In cases where the web is significant and causing significant distress, a disruption may be required. This can be performed by Bougie, laser or balloon dilatation.

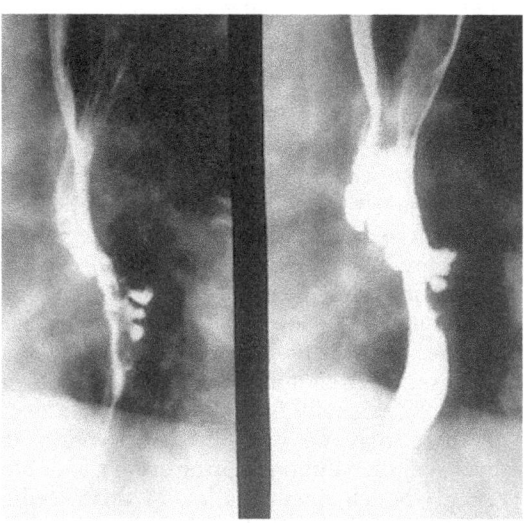

**Figure 6.17.** Multiple oesophageal diverticulae on contrast radiograph.

BENIGN DISEASE OF THE OESOPHAGUS

## Rings

Oesophageal rings tend to arise in the distal oesophagus. Most appear to be related to GORD, (Schatzki ring; Figure 6.18). Whereas a web is a mucosal fault, an oesophageal ring often contains submucosal tissue, and may have smooth muscle fibres included. When a significant stenosis is present it causes dysphagia. Intermittent obstruction, from meat or bread, can occur. Such complete bolus obstruction requires urgent endoscopy for retrieval. The treatment of oesophageal rings is primarily through ring destruction by dilatation.

## Vascular Ring (Dysphagia Lusoria)

A vascular ring is a rare condition caused by abnormal embryological development. Forming from the branchial arches, mediastinal vasculature encircles both trachea and oesophagus. This is usually diagnosed in childhood and symptoms include aspiration, stridor, lower respiratory tract infections, and dysphagia.

## Congenital Oesophageal Disease

### Oesophageal Atresia and Tracheo-oesophageal Fistulas (TOF)

Oesophageal atresia is a condition of embryological origin where the formation of the oesophagus is arrested. This may be at variable levels of the oesophagus and may, in fact, be of highly variable length. The lumen of the oesophagus fails to form, creating a blind end. Tracheo-oesophageal fistulas are often related to atresia. Detailed neonatal management of these conditions is beyond scope of this chapter. The various anatomical variations are shown in Figure 6.19.

It is important to maintain nutritional support for the neonates, while preparing for repair of the TOF or atresia at the appropriate time. In atresia, this can be enteric, usually through a radiologically placed gastrostomy. In tracheo-oesophageal fistula, the fistula may involve the distal oesophagus. This can create respiratory difficulties. Preoperative care is vital and involves optimising oxygenation, continuing nutritional support, and drainage of the upper oesophagus. This can be performed in a supine, head-up position, and using an oesophageal drainage system.

Repair is optimal by direct closure of the fistula or, if present, re-anastomosis of the oesophagus. If the length discrepancy is significant, myotomy or bouginage can be used to proximate the ends. If this discrepancy is still present, colonic interposition or gastric tube formation can be performed. This is a

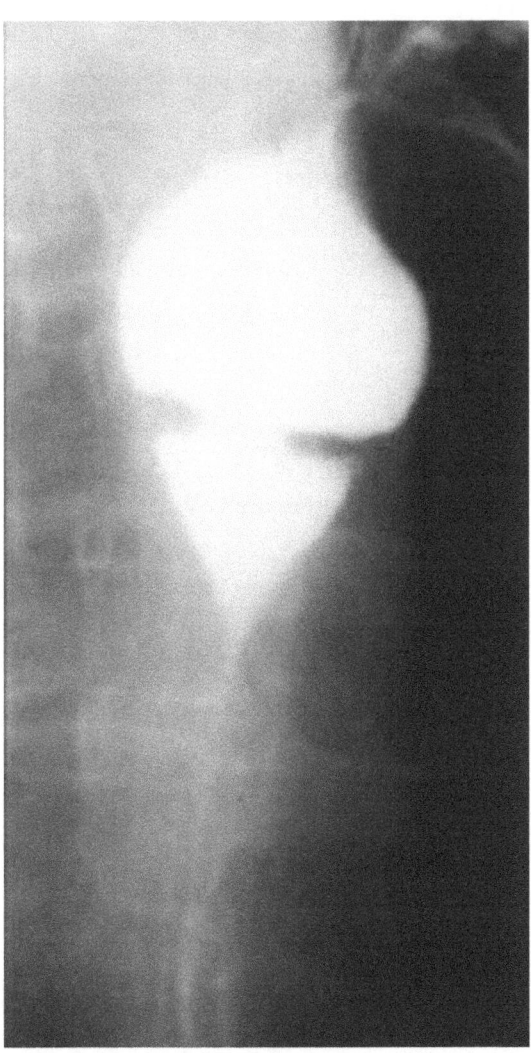

**Figure 6.18.** Schatzki ring on contrast radiograph.

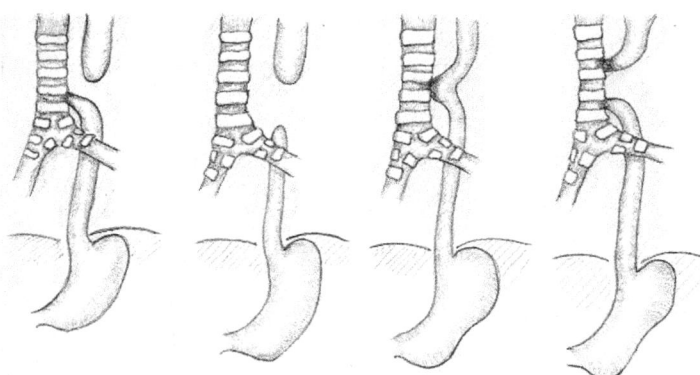

1. Oesophagus atresia with distal tracheo-oesophageal fistula. Incidence 87%
2. Isolated Oesophageal atresia. Incidence 8%
3. Isolated tracheo-oesophageal fistula. Incidence 4%
4. Oesophageal atresia with proximal and distal tracheo-oesophageal fistula. Incidence 1%

**Figure 6.19.** Types of oesophageal atresia and tracheo-oesophageal fistulas.

contentious issue among neonatal surgeons as to the best method to use with a significant gap. However, adult patients will have motility problems after having neonatal surgery.

## Duplications, Rests and Cysts

These are secondary to developmental abnormalities of the embryological oesophagus, which may only present in adulthood. Duplication is where the oesophagus has two separate lumens throughout any part of its length. An embryological diverticulum is patent at one end only, which could be at the proximal or distal end. If both ends are closed, this is called an oesophageal cyst. Oesophageal rests are ectopic areas of epidermal tissue in the mesodermal layer, which creates cysts, usually in the oesophageal wall.

# Benign Tumours of the Oesophagus

## Classification

Benign tumours of the oesophagus can be classified by two separate methods.

1. Intramural, extramural or intraluminal.
2. Nemir's classification of epithelial, non-epithelial and heterotrophic.

### Intramural Tumours

These consist of:

- leiomyoma (70–90% of all benign tumours) (Figure 6.20)
- myoma
- fibroma
- lipoma
- neurofibroma
- osteoclastoma
- granular cell tumours.

### Intraluminal Tumours

These consist of:

- polyps
- papillomas
- adenomas
- haemangiomas (very rare).

## Presentation

Symptoms of lower oesophageal tumours are entirely dependent on size and site of the lesion. Dysphagia is the most common presenting complaint but this only occurs after a considerable size has been reached. When a patient presents, it is often difficult to distinguish via endoscopy alone whether a lesion may be

# BENIGN DISEASE OF THE OESOPHAGUS

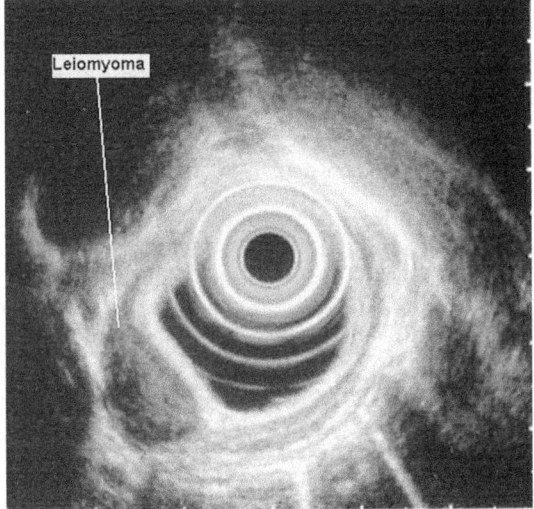

**Figure 6.20.** Endoscopic ultrasound of leiomyoma.

intramural, extramural or due to external compression on the oesophagus. In these cases, further definitive radiological investigation is necessary. In very rare cases, where a large proximal polyp has been described, this has the potential to cause asphyxia.

## Treatment

Intra luminal polyps or tumours may be removable using an endoscopic snare or by thermal ablation using laser or argon beam plasma coagulation. If they reach significant proportions, this may be impossible and formal resection may be required. This will involve oesophagotomy, performed in the opposite luminal wall to the origin of the tumour, or its pedicle. Intra/extramural tumour requiring operative treatment can create significant problems. Approach is dependent on the site of the tumour, i.e. cervical, abdominal or thoracic approach. Once the procedure has commenced, it may be difficult to identify the tumour from the external perspective. It may therefore be advisable to perform endoscopy at the same time to identify the site of the tumour, or by preoperative Indian ink injection.

# Oesophageal Perforation

## Presentation

Pain is the most common presenting complaint, which can be generalised in the abdomen, in the epigastrium, in the chest, or even in the neck, back and between the shoulders. If there has been significant passage of time since the perforation the patient can present in a severely unwell state with signs of generalised sepsis. These include tachycardia, pyrexia, peritonitis, tachypnoea and other related symptoms. Conversely the patient may simply complain of symptoms such as dysphonia, shortness of breath, and may have signs of surgical or mediastinal emphysema. Diagnosis can sometimes be difficult if no obvious cause for a perforation can be elicited from the history. On examination clinical signs may include Hamman's mediastinal crunch (when the heart beats against mediastinal emphysema) or there may be Mackler's triad, which is vomiting, chest pain and subcutaneous emphysema.

## Causes of Oesophageal Perforation

### Spontaneous Oesophageal Perforation

Boerhaave first described this in 1723. It is characterised by spontaneous oesophageal perforation following severe violent emesis, affecting the lower third of the oesophagus on the left-hand side.

### Iatrogenic Oesophageal Perforation

This is the commonest cause of perforation and usually occurs during interventional endoscopy.

Dilatation of stricture, especially if it is malignant, may cause a perforation. The incidence has been variably reported in the literature (0.5–2%) but does appear to be related to method of dilatation and disease process involved. Balloon dilatation under direct vision, using through the scope balloons, may be safer than endoscopic bougie. A careful technique of dilation will minimise the risk [23].

With increasing use of therapeutic endoscopy and use of thermoablative techniques special care must be taken to avoid perforation. Modalities such as laser, diathermy, endoscopic

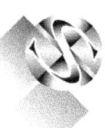

resection, and argon beam plasma coagulation have all been found to cause oesophageal perforation. Photodynamic therapy for tumours or other lesions has also been described as a cause of perforation, as has oesophageal stent insertion. Again an agitated retching patient is the most common candidate. Ligation and sclerotherapy of oesophageal varices may also cause perforation. This classically presents 5-10 days following the procedure as pressure necrosis of the oesophageal wall over a delayed period can cause significant perforation.

### Surgical Perforations

Any surgery conducted in the region of the oesophagus has the ability to cause a perforation. This is, however, most common in surgery involving the oesophagus itself such as Heller's myotomy and leiomyoma resection. Thoracic surgery, such as pneumonectomy, aortic repair or tracheostomy, can also cause perforation, although providing surgical technique is careful this is rare.

### Traumatic Perforation - Penetrating Injury and Blunt Disruption

Due to the anatomical position of the oesophagus in relation to other structures penetrating injury involving the oesophagus alone is extremely rare. Blade or gunshot injury most commonly affects the structure with more dramatic response (such as vascular injury). However, oesophageal injury in such cases must be excluded. The cervical oesophagus is most commonly affected, again due to position, but in a suspicious case contrast studies are recommended. Blunt disruption is rare and usually associated with other, often fatal, significant injuries.

### Other Causes of Oesophageal Perforation

There are numerous other causes of oesophageal perforation; all are uncommon.

1. Infection - *Candida*, CMV and herpes simplex, usually in immunocompromised host.
2. Ulceration related to reflux disease, or Zollinger-Ellison, or Barrett's oesophagus.
3. Tumour, both primary and secondary.
4. Caustic injury (including pill ingestion) (KCl, tetracycline, NSAIDs).
5. Foreign body perforation usually around cricopharyngeus.

### Treatment

This is quite a controversial subject and is highly dependent upon site, severity, time elapsed since perforation, and the patient's general health. In every case it is important to identify the site and size of the perforation, usually radiologically. In small and early perforation, without significant contamination of mediastinum, thorax or abdomen, conservative treatment may be appropriate. This is also the case in a patient with poor general health. Supportive nutrition and antibiotic therapy is the mainstay of this treatment. Surgical repair of oesophageal perforation enables evacuation and dilution of any significant contamination, whether this is in the thorax or in the abdomen, and is indicated when contrast shows free leakage into the thorax. If surgery is to be successful, early exploration within 24 hours is advantageous. Stenting of the leak is not indicated in benign disease. Despite significant advances in surgical technique and antibiotic therapy the mortality for oesophageal perforation is still described as 15-30%, even in specialist centres.

## Questions

1. Describe the systems for grading oesophagitis.
2. Compare and contrast medical and surgical management of GORD.
3. What are the advantages of surgical management of achalasia?
4. How would you manage an iatrogenic oesophageal perforation?

## References

1. Dent J, Brun J, et al. An evidence based appraisal of reflux disease management - The Genval Workshop Report. GUT 1999;44(Suppl 2):S1-16.
2. Lagergren J, Bergstrom R et al. Symptomatic gastroesophageal reflux as a risk factor for esophageal adenocarcinoma. N Engl J Med 1999;340(11):825-31.

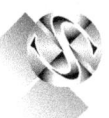

3. Jamieson GG. Anti-reflux operations: how do they work? Br J Surg 1987;74:155–6.
4. Spechler SJ. VA Study Group. Comparison of medical and surgical therapy for complicated gastroesophageal reflux disease in veterans. N Engl J Med 1992; 326:786–91.
5. Watson DI, Jamieson GG. Antireflux surgery in the laparoscopic era. Br J Surg 1998;85:1173–84.
6. Attwood, SE, Barlow AP et al. Barrett's oesophagus: the effects of anti-reflux surgery on symptom control and development of complications. Br J Surg 1992;79: 1021–4.
7. Blomqvist A, Lonroth J et al. Quality of life assessment after laparoscopic and open fundoplications: Results of a prospective, clinical study. Scand J Gastroenterol 1996;31:1052–8.
8. Blomqvist AMK, Lonroth H et al. Laparoscopic or open fundoplication? A complete cost analysis. Surg Endosc 1998;12:1209–12.
9. Lundell L, Dalenback E et al. Comprehensive 1-year cost analysis of open antireflux surgery in Nordic countries. Br J Surg 1998;85:1002–5.
10. Beckingham IJ, Cariem AK et al. Oesophageal dysmotility is not associated with poor outcome after laparoscopic Nissen fundoplication. Br J Surg 1998;85: 1290–93.
11. Lundell L, Dalenback J et al. Outcome of open antireflux surgery as assessed in a Nordic multicentre prospective clinical trial. Nordic GORD-Study Group. Eur J Surg 1998;164(10):751–7.
12. Donaghue PE et al. Description of anti-reflux surgery. Arch Surg 1985;120:663.
13. Toupet A. Technique d'oesophago-gastro-plastie avec phrenogastropexien appliquée dans la cure radicale des hernies hiatales et comme complément de l'opération d'Heller dans les cardiospasmes. Mem Academ Chir 1963;89:384–9.
14. Lundell L, Abrahamson H et al. Long-term results of a prospective randomised comparison of total fundic wrap (Nissen–Rosetti) or semifundoplication (Toupet) for gastro-oesophageal reflux. Br J Surg 1996;83:830–5.
15. Hill LD, Tobias JA. An effective operation for hiatal hernia: an eight year appraisal. Ann Surg 1967;166:681–8.
16. Lind JF, Burns CM et al. "Physiological" repair for hiatus hernia – manometric study. Arch Surg 1965;91: 233–7.
17. Watson A. A clinical and pathophysiological study of a simple effective operation for the correction of gastrooesophageal reflux. Br J Surg 1984;71:991–5.
18. Hunter JG, Swanstrom L et al. Dysphagia after laparoscopic anti-reflux surgery. The impact of surgical technique. Ann Surg 1996;224:51–7.
19. Attwood SE, Smyrk TC, Demeester TR et al Esophageal eosinophilia with dysphagia. A distinct clinicopathologic syndrome. Dig Dis Sci 1993;38(1):109–16.
20. Aziz Q, Thompson DG. Brain–gut axis in health and disease. Gastroenterology 1998;114(3):559–78.
21. Mattinger C, Hormann K. Endoscopic diverticulotomy of Zenker's diverticulum: management and complications. Dysphagia 2002;17(1):34–9.
22. Miller G. Patterson–Kelly, Plummer–Vinson syndrome. Dig Dis Sci 1980;25(10):813–2.
23. Talley NJ. Dyspepsia: management guidelines for the millennium. Gut 2002;50 Suppl 4:IV72–IV78.

# 7

# Benign Diseases of the Stomach

Robert C. Mason BSc

## Aims

To discuss

- the most appropriate management of peptic ulcer disease.
- to describe the role of surgery in peptic ulcer disease – primary treatment and complications.
- to present the indications for surgery in upper GI haemorrhage.
- To discuss the management of complications of previous peptic ulcer surgery.
- to consider the role of gastric surgery in morbid obesity.

## Introduction

Surgery for benign diseases of the stomach has undergone changes in the last 15 years as radical as those promoted by Billroth and Dragstedt, who popularised surgery for uncomplicated peptic ulcer. Operations such as highly selective vagotomy, selective and truncal vagotomy and drainage and gastric resection as primary treatment for peptic ulcer have been largely assigned to history by the discovery of *Helicobacter pylori* and the realisation that long-term cure of ulcers can be achieved by eradication therapy. This does not mean that there is no role for surgery in peptic ulcer disease. There is still a major role in the treatment of complications, namely bleeding and perforation and rarely obstruction. The role of surgery in the management of the complications of previous peptic ulcer surgery is ongoing.

## Congenital Disorders of the Stomach (see also Chapter 2)

With the exception of hypertrophic pyloric stenosis, these are rare although cases of diverticula and reduplication are found in the literature. Hypertrophic pyloric stenosis can present in adult life and may be treated by balloon dilatation or pyloromyotomy. Care must be taken to exclude pyloric canal cancer.

## Peptic Ulcer Disease

### Aetiology

It is now accepted that there are two main factors in the aetiology of peptic ulcers – non-steroidal anti-inflammatory drugs (NSAIDs) and *H. pylori*.

### NSAIDs

The link between these drugs and peptic ulcers is well established [1]. This is a major problem in the elderly where the consumption of these

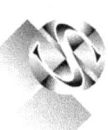

drugs is associated with a two- to four-fold increase in the incidence of gastrointestinal haemorrhage. The probable mechanism by which NSAIDs cause peptic ulcers is by disruption of the "mucosal barrier". The effect is mediated via prostaglandins and the microcirculation, which sweeps hydrogen ions away and buffers them with bicarbonate, rather than an effect on the mucus layer.

## H. pylori

This organism lives in the epithelium and mucus of the stomach and duodenum. It is transmitted by the oral route and infection probably occurs in childhood.

The prevalence of *H. pylori* mirrors the prevalence of peptic ulcer and accounts for at least 95% of non-NSAID peptic ulcers. The incidence of peptic ulcer in patients with *H. pylori* infection is less than 10%. Once eradicated, the risk of reinfection in western countries is less than 0.5% per annum. The mechanism by which *H. pylori* causes peptic ulceration is a combination of a direct effect on epithelial cells due to cytokine release, and increased release of gastrin and pepsinogen as a result of antral gastritis [2].

Confirmation of infection can be obtained by gastric antral biopsy and histological examination or CLO test for urease in biopsy tissue. Non-invasive confirmation can be obtained by a carbon isotope urea breath test or by measurement of *H. pylori* antibodies in the blood. This latter test can remain positive for up to one year post eradication. The accuracy of these tests exceeds 90%.

## Diagnosis of Peptic Ulcers

The main means of diagnosis is endoscopy. This should be undertaken in all cases in suspected gastric ulcers along with biopsy to exclude malignancy. In young patients (<45 years) with symptoms of duodenal ulceration it is probably safe to treat expectantly and only endoscope if there is no response to medical treatment or recurrence of symptoms following a course of medical treatment. To treat on the basis of positive serology or breath test alone is contentious, as only a minority of positive cases will have ulcers. As there is an association of *H. pylori* and antral cancer [3] it could be argued that this would be preventative. This is, however, a "disappearing cancer" and it is recognised that eradication of *H. pylori* is associated with increased gastro-oesophageal reflux, which is a precursor of Barrett's cancer at the gastro-oesophageal junction – an "increasing cancer". If the patient is symptomatic it is best to treat; if not then eradication should probably be withheld.

## Treatment of Peptic Ulcers

The mainstay of treatment of peptic ulcer is medical as outlined below. Surgery as primary treatment of uncomplicated disease has been consigned to history. The operations described for duodenal ulcer [4] together with mortality and recurrence rate are shown in Table 7.1. For comparison, the success of eradication therapy is also included.

The basis of these procedures is reduction of acid secretion by either vagotomy, resection of the antrum removing gastrin or resection of acid-secreting mucosa. As can be seen these procedures did not heal all ulcers and had a significant recurrence rate associated with them. This compares with eradication therapy with a healing rate of >98% and recurrence rate at 7 years of <5% [5]. As similar rates of healing of gastric ulcers can be achieved medically, Billroth I gastrectomy has gone a similar route. The complications of surgery are dealt with later in this chapter.

It is still important to modify lifestyle to maximise success of treatment. Smoking should be stopped and diet adjusted. Any ingestion of NSAIDs should be stopped if at all possible. If

**Table 7.1.** Operations for peptic ulcer

|  | Mortality (%) | Recurrence rate (%) |
|---|---|---|
| Bilroth I gastrectomy (GU) | 1 | 1 |
| Gastrojejunostomy (DU) | <1 | 40 |
| Truncal/selective vagotomy and drainage(DU) | <1 | 8–10 |
| Highly selective vagotomy (DU) | <1 | 10–20 |
| Bilroth II Gastrectomy (DU) – stomal ulcer | 2 | 2 |
| Truncal vagotomy and antrectomy (DU) | 2 | 0.5 |
| Eradication therapy | 0 | <5 |

GU, gastric ulcer; DU, duodenal ulcer.

# BENIGN DISEASES OF THE STOMACH

this is not possible then lifetime treatment with either an $H_2$ receptor antagonist (ranitidine 150 mg twice daily) or proton pump inhibitor (lansoprazole 15 mg daily) is indicated.

In all other cases a course of eradication therapy for *H. pylori* is indicated.

Many such regimens exist but a common one is "HeliClear" – a 7-day course of lansoprazole 30 mg twice daily, clarithromycin 500 mg twice daily, and amoxicillin 500 mg twice daily for 7 days. This eradicates *H. pylori* in over 90% of cases. Eradication should be confirmed by breath test 6 weeks later. If eradication has not been achieved, a further course is given with the possible addition of metronidazole 400 mg twice daily.

The role for maintenance therapy with either $H_2$ receptor antagonists or proton pump inhibitors is reserved for those with early recurrence of symptoms or ulcers resistant to healing. Care must be taken to ensure eradication and exclude Zollinger–Ellison syndrome although there are several causes of raised serum gastrin (Table 7.2) and other multiple endocrine adenopathies. Repeat biopsy to exclude malignancy is mandatory, especially in cases of gastric ulcer.

## Recurrent Peptic Ulcers

These should be investigated as for primary ulcers to exclude *H. pylori* or NSAIDs and treated appropriately. There is a case for long-term low dose proton pump inhibitors in such cases.

## Complications of Peptic Ulceration

### Bleeding

This potentially is the most serious and common complication of peptic ulcers. Bleeding can be both overt, presenting with haematemesis, melaena or overt rectal bleeding, or occult blood loss, presenting with iron-deficient anaemia. In the latter situation, it is vital also to investigate the lower gastrointestinal (GI) tract as a second source of bleeding may be found in up to 20% of cases [6]. All common causes of upper GI haemorrhage are shown in Table 7.3 and peptic ulceration (acute and chronic) can be seen to be the major cause.

### Management of Gastrointestinal Bleeding

This commences with full resuscitation, followed by investigation to determine the site of bleeding and then treatment to arrest haemorrhage and prevent rebleeding and promote ulcer healing. Investigation is primarily upper GI endoscopy with rigid sigmoidoscopy if there is evidence of bleeding per rectum. If the source is not identified then further investigation with selective angiography and/or labelled red cell scan and colonoscopy is indicated.

The majority of bleeds are small and the patient stabilises rapidly. Such individuals should have endoscopy on the next available elective endoscopy list after a period of fasting to enable the stomach to empty. If the patient requires early endoscopy due to haemodynamic instability or continued haemorrhage or rebleeding, then the endoscopy should be undertaken in theatre under crash general anaesthesia to protect the airway and prevent aspiration. Such individuals are going to require an intervention either endoscopic or surgical to arrest bleeding and this is best achieved with an anaesthetised and stable patient. In all such patients, ingestion of NSAIDs should be stopped and a course of eradication therapy commenced. There is no evidence that the acute administration of intravenous $H_2$ receptor antagonists is beneficial although this may change with the advent of intravenous proton pump inhibitors.

**Table 7.2.** Conditions resulting in increased levels of serum gastrin

- Pernicious anaemia
- Atrophic gastritis
- Medical treatment of peptic ulcers by acid supression
- Previous surgery for peptic ulcers
- Excluded gastric antrum
- G cell hyperplasia

**Table 7.3.** Causes of upper gastrointestinal bleeding

| 1. Peptic ulcers and erosions | 80% |
| 2. Oesophageal varices | 8% |
| 3. Oesophagitis | 5% |
| 4. Gastro-oesophageal cancer | 5% |
| 5. Angiodysplasia | 2% |

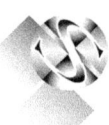

## Arresting Haemorrhage from Peptic Ulcers

This can be achieved both endoscopically and surgically.

Endoscopic techniques [7] are based on injection into and around the ulcer bed. This can be performed by the injection of adrenaline (epinephrine) 1 in 10 000 through a varices injection needle. The main benefit is probably from the tamponading effect of the fluid rather than vasospasm induced by the adrenaline. This technique is also indicated in patients who are not actively bleeding but are at high risk of a rebleed – visible vessel or clot on the ulcer base. Other endoscopic techniques include the use of a heater probe, laser, argon beam photocoagulation, or the placement of clips on the vessel. As in all such cases, the simplest technique is the best and that is injection treatment, which requires no specialised equipment. Following cessation of bleeding, eradication therapy is administered as soon as oral intake can commence. There may be a role for parenteral proton pump inhibitors in the time between arrest of bleeding and commencement of oral intake.

## The Role of Surgery in Bleeding Peptic Ulcers

Surgery is indicated when the patient is actively bleeding and the source cannot be seen or controlled endoscopically. Timing for surgery is contentious [8], but experience teaches us that we tend to intervene too late when the patient has had at least 6 units of blood, is unstable and is entering a state of coagulopathy. This probably explains why the mortality from bleeding peptic ulcer has changed little in the past 20 years. Active intervention (endoscopic or surgical) is required when the fourth unit of blood goes up and the threshold needs to be lower in older infirm patients, especially if they have a known chronic ulcer and are on NSAIDs. Those on anticoagulation are a special case and need rapid reversal in cooperation with the haematologists.

Which operation should be undertaken [9]? The principle is to do the quickest and safest procedure to arrest bleeding and then treat with appropriate eradication therapy. In the case of duodenal ulcers this is a duodenotomy and oversew of the vessel and if possible ulcer exclusion with interrupted 2/0 vicryl sutures. If the pylorus is intact, the duodenotomy can be closed longitudinally. If it has been divided, then closure is in the form of a Heineke-Mikulicz pyloroplasty. If there is significant pyloric scarring, an anterior gastrojejunostomy can be performed. There is probably now little role for adding a truncal vagotomy initially as this does not improve ulcer healing over medical treatment nor for performing a partial gastrectomy due to the high morbidity/mortality associated with this operation. If rebleeding does occur, however, some form of resection will be required. Bleeding gastric ulcers are best treated by Billroth II gastrectomy if this can be performed quickly and safely. If not then oversewing the bleeding vessel followed by medical therapy is indicated.

## Other Gastric Causes of Bleeding

Oesophageal and gastric varices secondary to portal hypertension are dealt with elsewhere. Bleeding gastric cancer should be treated as for all gastric cancer but if resection is not indicated and bleeding persists then external beam radiotherapy should be considered. A rare cause of upper gastrointestinal bleeding is Dieulafoy syndrome – a vascular malformation in which a jet of blood appears to come from normal epithelium. This can be controlled by either endoscopic injection or thermal ablation or simple suture if open surgery is indicated. Wide spread angiodysplasia can affect the distal stomach – watermelon stomach. This usually presents with chronic blood loss and anaemia and is treated with photocoagulation rather than resection. A rare cause of occult bleeding is leiomyoma which can ulcerate on its surface. If small they may be snared but if larger they will require resection.

## Perforation

As the incidence of bleeding peptic ulcer has increased, the incidence of perforation has decreased. It is now most commonly seen in elderly patients taking NSAIDs and/or steroids. In such individuals such perforations may be occult and only diagnosed as the presence of free gas on a chest X-ray taken for other reasons. It is important to recognise that up to a third of perforations, especially of duodenal ulcers, may not have free gas under the diaphragm due to

# BENIGN DISEASES OF THE STOMACH

the loss through the perforation being liquid only. This is rare in perforated gastric ulcer as this is a gas-filled organ. In patients with free gas the site of perforation will be colonic diverticular disease in a significant proportion.

## Diagnosis of Perforation

This is a combination of history, clinical examination revealing peritonitis and the presence of free gas on an erect chest X-ray or lateral decubitus abdominal X-ray. There is no role for endoscopy or barium study in such patients and the decision to operate is largely made on clinical grounds.

## Treatment of Perforation

In those patients with occult perforation picked up on X-ray, who are stable with no physical signs, management is conservative. This involves stopping NSAID ingestion and treatment with eradication therapy and maintenance therapy if the patient is on long-term steroids or requires NSAIDs for other pressing reasons. Such patients should be investigated at some stage to confirm the diagnosis, exclude gastric cancer and colonic diverticular disease.

For all other patients with a symptomatic presentation, the treatment is surgical after a short period of aggressive resuscitation. The approach can be by open surgery or laparoscopically if appropriate skills exist. The basis of treatment of duodenal ulcer is closure of the perforation with an omental plug and thorough peritoneal lavage. If the ulcer is large with pyloric obstruction a gastrojejunostomy is advised. There is little role for gastric resection. The patient should be given intravenous proton pump inhibitors or $H_2$ receptor antagonists until oral intake can commence followed by eradication therapy. It is crucial in such patients to ensure eradication has been achieved. Future ingestion of NSAIDs and steroids should be reviewed.

In the case of gastric ulcer, care must be taken to exclude cancer. In fit patients with large perforated lesser curve gastric ulcers, the treatment is Billroth II type gastric resection. If the patient is frail or the expertise does not exist, closure with sutures ± omental plug and biopsy of the ulcer margin should be undertaken. It is important to recognise that the base of such ulcers is frequently the pancreas with the splenic artery clearly visible.

It is vital to exclude at some stage gastric cancer. Such patients should have intravenous proton pump inhibitors or $H_2$ receptor antagonists followed by eradication therapy as for duodenal ulcers. Emphasis is placed on the importance of thorough peritoneal toilet in all cases of perforation.

The advent of the laparoscope has led to experimental treatments gluing and plugging perforations. These should be treated with extreme caution and only performed with informed consent as patients do not suffer from a short midline incision and conventional suture.

# Pyloric Stenosis

In all cases of gastric outlet obstruction secondary to presumed duodenal ulcer, every attempt must be made to exclude cancer either of the distal stomach or pancreas. If doubt exists on endoscopy and biopsy, CT scan, endoluminal ultrasound and even laparoscopy may need to be performed. This is now a rare complication. Such patients may if chronic have electrolyte disturbances, the classical picture being a hypokalaemic metabolic alkalosis. This needs correction before any therapy is given.

In cases where the diagnosis is made with confidence, the first-line treatment is with endoscopic or radiological balloon dilatation [10] associated with eradication therapy. In the few cases where this is not successful, surgery in the form of a gastrojejunostomy or pyloroplasty can be undertaken. It is now accepted that there is no need to perform a truncal vagotomy as medical treatment is so good and with eradication of H. pylori the risk of stomal ulceration is largely a thing of the past. In patients with chronic obstruction there may be some considerable delay before gastric emptying occurs. It is vital not to rush in with revisional surgery but to support with parenteral nutrition until emptying occurs. To reassure the clinician a gentle endoscopy at 2 weeks will demonstrate a patent gastrojejunostomy.

There is no role for gastric resection in such cases unless there is obstruction of the gastric body by scarring from giant gastric ulcers. These are now a thing of the past.

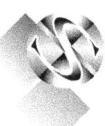

## Malignant Change in Peptic Ulcers

It is now accepted that malignant change never occurs in benign duodenal ulcers. If malignancy is detected on biopsy of a non-healing ulcer it is likely to be either a primary duodenal carcinoma or pancreatic cancer growing through the duodenal wall. These must be staged and treated appropriately.

If a risk occurs of malignant change in a benign non-healing gastric ulcer it is less than 1%. The likelihood is that it was primary gastric cancer all along as both are associated with infection with *H. pylori*. It emphasises the importance of multiple biopsies of non-healing gastric ulcers, and if doubt exists CT scanning and endoluminal ultrasound. Gastric ulcers situated other than on the incisura of the lesser curve should be treated as cancer and treated by resection. Non-healing benign gastric ulcers on the incisura do occur. They are often associated with long-term steroid or NSAID ingestion and reflect a defect in the cytoprotective aspect of the gastric mucosa. Once malignancy and *H. pylori* infection have been excluded by repeat biopsy and breath test, these ulcers are treated by long-term maintainance proton pump inhibitor therapy. If doubt exists or risk factors for haemorrhage are present they must be resected by either a Billroth I or II resection.

## Complications of Previous Gastric Surgery

These can be classified as the six Ds: dumping, diarrhoea, deficiencies, delayed emptying, duodenogastric reflux and dysplasia/cancer.

Any operation on the stomach whether it be a vagotomy, resection (partial or total) or even a gastrojejunostomy/pyloroplasty (bypass or damage the pylorus) exposes the patient to any or all of the above, the magnitude depending on the degree of insult. In general, surgery has little to offer any of these complications and should only be embarked upon when all medical therapies have been exhausted and the patient's quality of life is unacceptable. Many of the complications post gastric surgery will improve with time and it is unwise to intervene in less than 1 year from the original surgery.

### Dumping

This falls into two categories, early and late.

Early dumping results from early emptying of a hyperosmolar meal into the jejunum. This results in a shift of fluid into the gut lumen producing hypotension and feeling of lightheadedness. This can usually be controlled by eating smaller meals, separating liquids and solids.

Late dumping is due to hypoglycaemia secondary to hyperinsulaemia resulting from a high glucose peak rather than the sustained rise seen in normal individuals. This occurs a few hours after eating and responds to oral glucose.

### Diarrhoea

This was common following truncal vagotomy and drainage and is mainly due to rapid intestinal transit. It can be usually be managed by GI sedatives and dietary modification. Operations designed to slow transit by reversal of jejunal loops or reversed jejunal patches have been largely unsuccessful [11]. With the disappearance of vagotomy this complication, which can be disabling, is now a rare problem.

### Deficiencies

These result from both the loss of gastric mucosa following resection and/or from intestinal hurry resulting in malabsorbtion.

The loss of a gastric reservoir following total gastric or high subtotal resection can restrict intake to such a degree that weight cannot be maintained. This is best treated by strict dietetic supervision with small regular high calorie/protein intake. In rare cases nocturnal supplementation with a jejunostomy may be needed. Similarly following Billroth II resection duodenal secretions may never "catch up " with gastric contents. If such an afferent loop syndrome exists an enterostomy below the gastrojejunostomy may help.

The usual means of reconstruction post total gastrectomy is by oesophagojejunostomy and Roux-en-Y. In a small group maintenance of weight can be a problem. Conversion to a jejunal pouch between the oesophagus and first part of the duodenum has been advocated as a preferred means of reconstruction [12]. It is, however, more complicated and should be reserved for rare cases of malnutrition resistant to all other means.

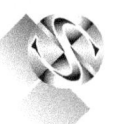

The stomach is crucial for the absorption of vitamin $B_{12}$ and all cases of total gastrectomy will require lifetime replacement therapy. The stomach is also important for the reabsorption of iron and calcium and all cases of total and high subtotal resection are advised to take regular mineral and vitamin supplements.

## Delayed Gastric Emptying

Any case of truncal vagotomy is subject to delayed emptying. In one-third of cases this will be significant resulting in severe gastric stasis. This was the reason why operations involving truncal vagotomy were combined with a drainage procedure – gastrojejunostomy or pyloroplasty. These additional procedures ameliorate this problem in cases other than those with pre-existing pyloric stenosis when poor emptying can persist. The other operation associated with delayed gastric emptying is truncal vagotomy, antrectomy and Roux-en-Y reconstruction performed to combat severe duodenogastric or gastro-oesophageal reflux when a fundoplication cannot be performed or has failed. It is not uncommon for patients having undergone this operation to fail to empty their stomachs for many weeks. They require prolonged intravenous or enteral feeding. It is important to exclude a technical problem by gentle endoscopy but resist the temptation if all anastomoses are patent to reoperate. It will improve with time.

Truncal vagotomy will also influence gall bladder motility and is associated with an increased incidence of gallstones.

## Duodenogastric Reflux

In any operation in which the pylorus is resected or bypassed, duodenogastric reflux will occur. In most cases the patient is asymptomatic and requires no treatment. In a few however, there will be associated postprandial pain and bilious vomiting. Confirmation that this is due to duodenogastric reflux can be achieved by either a HIDA scan [13] or a provocation test. This involves the passage of a nasogastric tube into the afferent limb or duodenum. Cholecystokinin is given and duodenal contents aspirated. The tube is withdrawn into the stomach and the patient given either saline, duodenal secretions or acid "blind". If the symptoms are reproduced only by the duodenal secretions then revisional surgery can be undertaken with some degree of success. In cases of pyloroplasty, this can be reversed, a gastrojejunostomy can be taken down and a Billroth II gastrectomy converted to a Roux-en-Y. In cases associated with a truncal vagotomy, at least 1 year should elapse before reversal to allow normal gastric emptying to occur.

## Dysplasia and Carcinoma

There is now a well-established association between duodenogastric reflux consequent upon a gastrojejunostomy alone or associated with partial gastric resection and an increase incidence of gastric cancer [14]. These tumours are found at the site of the afferent limb and have a latent period of at least 20 years. The duodenogastric reflux produces chronic irritation of the anastomosis leading to a hyperplasia/dysplasia/carcinoma sequence. Although the prognosis for these so-called gastric stump carcinomas is poor they should be staged and treated as for primary cancer of the stomach.

The only other significant complication of gastric surgery is an increased incidence of tuberculosis and fungal infection due to the loss of the gastric acid barrier.

## Inflammation of the Stomach

Acute gastritis can follow any insult on the gastric mucosa by such things as drugs, spicey foods and acute infection with *H. pylori*. This will usually heal when the irritant is removed.

In patients on the intensive care unit, gastrointestinal haemorrhage can occur from acute gastritis which can progress to superficial widespread gastric erosions. This is the result of mucosal ischaemia failing to sweep away the hydrogen ions which have penetrated the epithelial cells. Prevention of this complication is achieved by maintaining a high intraluminal pH by either intravenous $H_2$ receptor antagonists, proton pump inhibitors, coating the mucosa with sucralfate or neutralising the gastric pH with antacids via a nasogastric tube. A total gastrectomy may be required if the bleeding becomes torrential although the mortality of this is in excess of 80%.

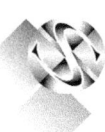

## 7 · UPPER GASTROINTESTINAL SURGERY

In contrast, chronic gastritis is characterised by a mucosal infiltration with lymphocytes and plasma cells. It is usually persistent and progressive to atrophic gastritis. In most cases this is associated with infection with *H. pylori*. If this progresses to intestinal metaplasia (type 3) in which differentiation is lost and which can be regarded as a form of dysplasia, an increased risk of gastric cancer appears.

The link between the immune system and chronic gastritis has been established in those patients with pernicious anaemia in whom anti-intrinsic factor and anti-parietal cell antibodies can be demonstrated. These patients have a fourfold increase in gastric cancer and should have regular surveillance by gastroscopy.

Other forms of gastritis include granulomatous gastritis from Crohn's disease involving the stomach and hyperplastic gastritis in Ménétrier's disease which may present with hypoproteinaemia.

## Gastric Volvulus

This condition is frequently symptomless and is a chance finding on a barium meal examination. When symptoms occur they are usually of sudden onset of vomiting and severe epigastric or retrosternal pain. It is invariably associated with a para-oesophageal hiatus hernia especially if of the organoaxial type. Treatment is surgical and involves repair of the diaphragmatic defect and fixing the greater curve of the stomach to the anterior abdominal wall by means of sutures or by performing a high greater curve gastrostomy and posterior gastrojejunostomy.

## Acute Gastric Dilatation

This usually presents as a complication of upper abdominal surgery especially splenectomy. The patient complains of shoulder tip pain and hiccoughs. If not recognised, the patient can rapidly become shocked and may die from a vomit and massive aspiration. Treatment is by passage of a wide bore nasogastric tube. This condition can occur in patients suffering from anorexia nervosa and other psychiatric conditions such as depression, especially when they are prescribed large doses of psychotropic drugs.

## Gastric Bezoars

These can be composed of hair – trichobezoars, or vegetable matter – phytobezoars which can be precipitated by gastric stasis post vagotomy. Attempts can be made to break them up endoscopically or with pancreatic enzymes. If large, however, they will need removal by open surgery.

## Trauma to the Stomach and Duodenum

These organs are at risk from both sharp and blunt injury, particularly when the stomach is full. In all cases of gastric and duodenal trauma, care must be taken to exclude injury to other organs, especially the pancreas.

## Gastric Surgery for Morbid Obesity

Morbid obesity is defined as a body weight 100% greater than the ideal weight. Before contemplating surgery, endocrine disorders and hypothalamic lesions which cause obesity must be excluded. The need to reduce weight is based on the major increase in mortality associated with morbid obesity. There is a 14-fold increase if the patient is 100% above ideal weight.

The success of diet and psychological modification of eating habits is disappointing in this group. Early surgical procedures to help weight loss are either disappointing (jaw wiring) or have an unacceptable morbidity and mortality (jejunoileal bypass). Current surgical approaches focus on the stomach and are based on suppressing appetite by producing early fullness using a vertical banded gastroplasty or placement of an inflatable cuff. These can be performed using minimal access techniques. An alternative approach involves a combination of reduced gastric capacity with malabsorption produced by a Roux-en-Y gastric bypass and biliopancreatic bypass.

The importance of full medical and psychological preparation cannot be overstated, and in the postoperative period the patients need careful monitoring as they are at high risk of respiratory and thromboembolic complications. Patients often end up with a degree of malabsorbtion, and the haemoglobin, iron, Vitamin $B_{12}$ and calcium should be regularly monitored. Gastroplasty leads to weight reduction to within 50% of the ideal weight in 23% of cases compared with 55% for gastric bypass, although evidence from long-term follow-up is poor [15].

## Questions

1. Is there a role for surgery in the primary treatment of peptic ulceration?
2. Should all patients with suspected peptic ulceration have endoscopy before commencing therapy? If not who should?
3. Should *H. pylori* be eradicated in the asymptomatic patient?
4. What are the indications for maintenance therapy in patients with peptic ulcer?
5. When should patients with upper GI haemorrhage be endoscoped?
6. What is the best means to control bleeding endoscopically?
7. What are the indications for surgery in upper GI bleeding and what operation should be performed?
8. How should chronic peptic ulcers be managed?
9. When considering revisional surgery for the complications of previous gastric surgery what factors should be considered in the timing of such procedures?
10. What is the interval for the genesis of gastric stump cancer, and how should at-risk patients be followed up?
11. What are the indications for surgery for gastric volvulus and what operation should be undertaken?
12. What are the indications for surgery in morbid obesity and what are the risks associated with it?

## References

1. Faulkner G, Pritchard P, Sommerville K et al. Aspirin and bleeding ulcer in the elderly. Br Med J 1998;297: 1311–13.
2. Dunn B. Pathenogenic mechanisms of Helicobacter pylori. Gastroenterol Clin North Am 1993;76:219–25.
3. Eurogastric study group. An international association between Helicobacter pylori infection and gastric cancer. Lancet 1993;341:1359–62.
4. Taylor TV. The current surgical management of chronic duodenal ulcer. In: Irving M, Beart RW (eds) Gastroenterological surgery. London: Butterworth International Medical Reviews, 1983;33–50.
5. Forbes GM, Glaser MI, Cullen DJE et al Duodenal ulcer treatment with Helicobacter pylori eradication: seven year followup. Lancet 1994;343:258–60.
6. Cook IJ, Pavli P, Riley JW et al. Gastrointestinal investigation of iron deficiency anaemia. Br Med J 1986;292: 1380–2.
7. Steele RJC. Endoscopic haemostasis for non-variceal upper gastrointestinal haemorrhage. Br J Surg 1989; 76:219–25.
8. Morris DL, Hawker PC, Brearley S et al. Optimal timing of operation for bleeding peptic ulcer: prospective randomized trial. Br Med J 1984;288:1277–80.
9. Poxon VA, Keighley MRB, Dykes PW et al. Comparison of minimal and conventional surgery in patients with bleeding peptic ulcer: a multicentre trial. Br J Surg 1991;78:1344–5.
10. Griffin SM, Chung SCS, Leung JWC et al. Peptic pyloric stenosis treated by endoscopic balloon dilatation. Br J Surg 1989;76:1147–8.
11. Cuschieri A. Surgical management of severe intractable postvagotomy diarrhoea. Br J Surg 1986;73:981–4.
12. Cuschieri A. long term evaluation of a reservoir jejunal interposition with an isoperistaltic conduit in the management of patients with the small stomach syndrome. Br J Surg 1982;69:386–8.
13. Donovan IA, Fielding JWL, Bradby H et al. Bile diversion after total gastrectomy. Br J Surg 1982;69:389–90.
14. Clarke CG, Fresini A, Gledhill T. Cancer following gastric surgery. Br J Surg 1985;72:591–4.
15. Renquist KE, Cullen JJ, Barnes D et al. The effect of followup on reporting success for obesity surgery. Obes Surg 1995;5:285–92.

## Further Reading

Burnand KG, Young AE (eds). The new Aird's companion in surgical studies 2nd edn. London: Churchill Livingstone, 1998.

Griffin SM, Raimes SA (eds). Upper gastrointestinal surgery London: WB Saunders, 1997.

# 8

# Benign Disease of the Small Bowel

Ling S. Wong, Emmanuel A. Agaba and Michael R.B. Keighley

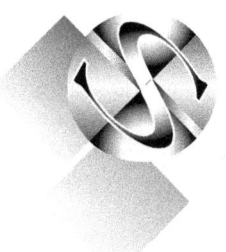

## Aims

To identify the benign conditions of small bowel and the principles of surgical management.

## Crohn's Disease (Regional Ileitis)

Crohn's disease is a chronic non-specific, transmural inflammation of the gastrointestinal tract of unknown aetiology. It may affect any part of the gastrointestinal tract from the mouth to the anus and may be associated with extraintestinal manifestations. In the gastrointestinal tract, involvement of the ileum is the most common pattern of presentation. The disease commonly affects people between 15 and 30 years of age. Both sexes are equally affected. The disease affects urban dwellers more than rural dwellers and is associated with higher socio-economic class.

## Epidemiology

Crohn's disease occurs worldwide, although there is wide variation in the actual incidence. The worldwide prevalence is estimated to be 10–70 cases per 100 000, with an incidence of 4–6 cases per 100 000 populations per year.

The disease is more common among whites, among Jewish people. Even among Jews, Ashkenazi Jews born outside of Israel are four times more likely to develop the disease than Askenazi Jews born in Israel (16.69 per 100 000 compared with 4.19 per 100 000) [1]. Similarly, the incidence of Crohn's disease among Afro-Caribbean and Asian communities in the United Kingdom is higher than in their native country [2]. These findings suggest the impact of varying environmental influences within these communities.

## Aetiology

The aetiology of Crohn's disease remains unknown despite several decades of investigation. Current theories implicate the role of genetic, immunological, microbial, dietary and vascular as potential causative agents. It has been suggested that Crohn's patients have an inherited susceptibility for an aberrant immunological response to one or more of these provoking factors.

### Infection

The presence of non-caseating granulomas in affected segments of small bowel suggests an infective cause for Crohn's disease. To date, specific infections such as *Mycobacterium paratuberculosis* and measles have not been substantiated.

## Genetics

There is evidence to suggest Crohn's disease is a polygenic disorder without any single Mendelian pattern of inheritance. The risk for Crohn's disease is increased 30 times in siblings of patients with the disease and 13 times for first-degree relatives. There is also a high degree of concordance in monozygotic twins.

The first susceptibility locus for Crohn's disease is on the pericentrometric region of chromosome 16 and is designated IBD1 locus [3,4]. Mutations of the NOD2 gene in this region have been shown to be associated with Crohn's disease. NOD2 acts as a cytosolic receptor for bacterial lipopolysaccharides and activates nuclear factor κB, which is a key transcriptional factor involved in initiation of the inflammatory response (Figure 8.1). About 20% of Crohn's disease is attributable to NOD2 mutations; other IBD genes must exist. Susceptibility loci for the disease have now been reported on chromosomes 12 (IBD2), 6 (IBD3) and 14 (IBD4).

In patients with heterozygous and homozygous defects in the NOD2 gene, there is a 3- and 40-fold increased risk respectively of developing Crohn's disease compared with the general population [5].

## Pathogenesis

The pathogenesis of Crohn's disease involves an excessive activation of mucosal T cells leading to transmural inflammation, which is amplified and perpetuated by the release of proinflammatory cytokines and soluble mediators [6]. In normal circumstances, the gastrointestinal tract is able to modulate the inflammatory response to dietary, microbial and other antigens that are in contact with the intestinal mucosa.

It is widely believed that a reduced T-suppressor cell (Ts cell) activity to antigens leads to uninhibited immune response resulting in tissue damage due to cell-mediated, humoralan, and lymphokines factors. Intestinal mucosal damage occurs as a bystander since it is not the primary target. There is marked increase in the total lymphocytes especially B cells in the lamina propria of Crohn's patients. B cells produce IgG, which facilitates the antigen-specific effector response leading to inflammatory tissue damage. The presence of marked inflammatory mediators such as interleukin (IL1, IL2, IL6), tumour necrosis factors (TNF), platelet-activating factor (PAF), transforming growth factor and macrophages in the circulation may be responsible for the systemic and local effects of Crohn's disease.

## Pathology

Crohn's disease may affect any part of the gastrointestinal tract but has a particular preference for the ileocolic region. Other regions commonly affected in order of frequency are: small bowel alone, perianal region, colon alone, stomach and duodenum. Characteristically, it is a segmental disease in which the involved segments are sharply demarcated from the contiguous normal bowel (skip lesions).

### Macroscopic Features

Grossly, the early sign of Crohn's disease is aphthoid ulceration, which is visible endoscopically. These ulcers are often multiple and as they grow; they coalesce to form large areas of ulceration of the mucosa with intervening areas of oedematous mucosa. This gives the mucosa its characteristic cobblestone appearance. Sloughing and linear ulceration of the oedematous mucosa may occur along the mesentery border (Figure 8.2). Deep fissuring from linear ulceration may lead to formation of fistulas, sinus tracts, abscess formation, adhesion and localised perforation. Fistulous tracts are possible between the diseased segment and

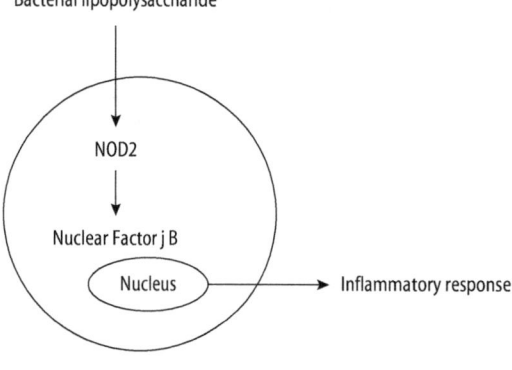

**Figure 8.1.** NOD2 acts as a cytosolic receptor for bacterial lipopolysaccharides and activates nuclear factor κB, which is a key transcriptional factor involved in initiation of the inflammatory response.

# BENIGN DISEASE OF THE SMALL BOWEL

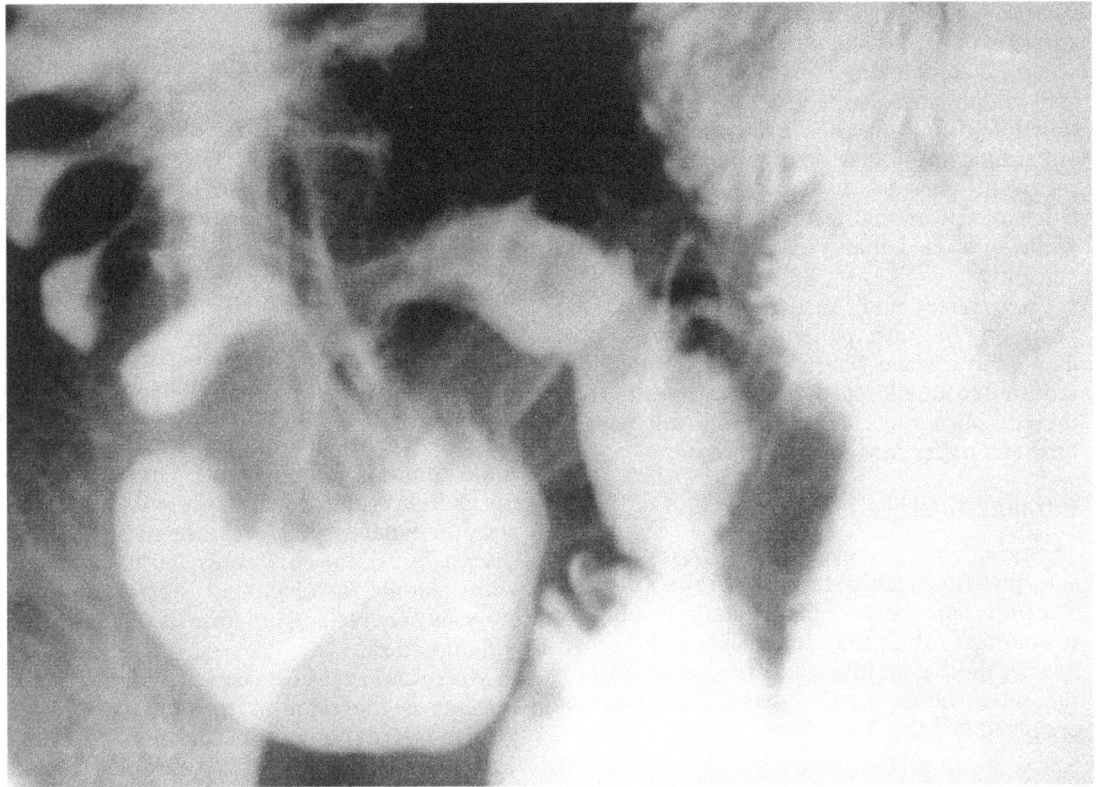

**Figure 8.2.** Small bowel enema showing linear fissures extending through the bowel wall.

any intra-abdominal or extra-abdominal structures or organs. In severe disease, pseudopolyps and mucosa bridges may occur. Typically, the serosal surface of the affected segment is granular and inflamed. This inflamed segment is often wrapped in mesenteric fat, a process called "fat wrapping". As a result of the transmural inflammation, the involved segment feels firm, thickened and heavy (hosepipe) and this may lead to narrowing.

## Microscopic Features

In Crohn's disease, the inflammation involves the full thickness of the bowel wall. Early in the disease process, there is accumulation and attack of the base of crypts by inflammatory cells. This leads to formation of aphthoid ulcers, crypt ulcers and abscess. Non-caseating granulomas are found from aggregations of epithelioid histiocytes surrounded by lymphocytes and Langhan's giants cells and are the hallmark of Crohn's disease. Connective tissue changes occur in all the layers of the affected segment producing the hosepipe appearance. Fistulas and sinus tracts develop from confluence of crypt abscesses and transmural inflammation. Transmural inflammation leads to serositis, which causes adhesion to adjacent loops of bowel.

## Clinical Features

### Gastrointestinal Features

The clinical presentation varies depending on the site of the disease. Ileal disease may mimic acute appendicitis whilst colonic disease may present as a fulminating colitis. Abdominal pain is a common feature of Crohn's disease. The pain is colicky in nature and is due to distension and peristaltic movement induced by partial or complete blockage of the bowel.

Diarrhoea occurs in most patients and it may result from several causes such as mucosal inflammation, bacterial overgrowth, fistulation between loops of bowel and bile salt malabsorption due to terminal ileitis. The presence of complex carbohydrate in the colon may also lead to diarrhoea. Rectal bleeding is rare in terminal ileitis but may occur in colonic disease.

Perianal lesion may be in the form of fissure, recurrent perianal fistulas and weight loss. Other constitutional features are malaise, low-grade pyrexia, lethargy, anorexia, nausea and vomiting.

Progressive and recurrent episodes are common. In most patients, the disease progresses to a stage where surgical treatment is required to ameliorate the symptoms or to treat the complications. Many patients will require further surgery for recurrent disease.

## Extraintestinal Features

The skin, joints and eyes are the most common extraintestinal manifestation of Crohn's disease. The prevalence of these manifestations is higher in colonic Crohn's than in small bowel disease. Rarely, these extraintestinal manifestations are the initial feature of the disease. These features are listed in Table 8.1.

**Table 8.1.** Extraintestinal features

| Manifestation |
| --- |
| *Eyes* |
| Episcleritis |
| Conjunctivitis |
| Uveitis |
| *Joints* |
| Arthritis |
| Ankylosing spondylitis* |
| Sacroilitis* |
| *Skin* |
| Pyoderma gangrenosum |
| Erythema nodosum |
| Aphthous stomatitis |
| Vasculitis |
| *Renal* |
| Calculi* |
| *Liver* |
| Sclerosing cholangitis |
| Chronic active hepatitis |
| Cirrhosis |
| Gallstone |
| *Others* |
| Amyloidosis |

*These manifestations are unrelated to disease activity.

## Physical signs

Physical signs are often few and many patients may appear normal with no signs. In a number of patients, there may be signs of weight loss, anaemia, pyrexia, finger clubbing, peripheral oedema, aphthous ulceration of the mouth and a general feeling of ill health. In most patients, abdominal examination is often normal, although tenderness and a mass in the right iliac fossa are occasionally found. Some patients may present with perianal fissures, abscesses or large perianal skin tags. Multiple perianal fistulas producing "watering can perineum" may occur in some patients. Enterocutaneous fistula may occur in all patients with Crohn's disease but is more common in patients who have had previous surgery and usually presents through a scar. Perianal lesions are rare in small bowel disease but occur commonly (80%) in patients with colonic involvement. Rectal and anal stenosis may result from fibrosis due to chronic inflammation.

The course of the disease in children and adolescents is the same as in adults except that growth retardation occurs commonly. In young women, the disease reduces fertility. Spontaneous abortion and preterm delivery are common in the presence of active disease but in the absence of active disease, the outcome of pregnancy equals that of matched controls.

## Investigations

### Blood Tests

Full blood count, erythrocyte sedimentation rate (ESR), biochemical profile and serum proteins are always necessary. Decreased serum albumin, hypochromic, microcytic anaemia and low serum iron and/or folate are present in half of the patients. There is often an elevated ESR and C-reactive protein (CRP). Abnormal liver biochemistry may occur but persistent elevation requires further investigation. Low serum calcium, magnesium, zinc, selenium and vitamin A may occur in severe or established disease.

### Radiology

Small bowel enema is the investigation of choice for detection of small bowel Crohn's disease. Radiological features of small bowel Crohn's

# BENIGN DISEASE OF THE SMALL BOWEL

disease consist of alteration in the mucosal pattern with deep ulceration, thickening of the ileocaecal valve and areas of narrowing of the lumen ("strings sign" of Kantor) (Figure 8.3). Skip lesions with intervening normal bowel are also seen.

Large bowel Crohn's disease can be investigated using double contrast barium enema. The changes in the colon are similar to those in the small bowel. As the disease progresses, there is shortening and lost of haustral markings. It is important to perform a large bowel study for two reasons: as a baseline for future comparison and in order to assess the severity and extent of the disease.

## Medical Treatment

Medical treatment is usually symptomatic and empirical and often followed by remission and exacerbation until complications prompt intervention by the surgeons. Medical treatment aims at control of distressing symptoms such as abdominal pain, diarrhoea, infections and correction of nutritional deficiencies. Symptomatic treatment includes the use of antidiarrhoeal agents such as loperamide, codeine phosphate and diphenoxylate with atropine. Cholestyramine is required for patients with bile salt diarrhoea. Anaemia may be corrected with iron supplements. For most patients and those with severe disease, specific anti-inflammatory agents and immunosuppressive agents may be required.

### Aminosalicylates

Sulfasalazine consists of a sulphonamide moiety, sulfapyridine linked to the aspirin analogue 5-aminosalicylate (5-ASA). In the terminal ileum and colon, intestinal bacteria break the compound into sulphonamide and 5-ASA.

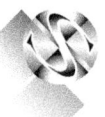

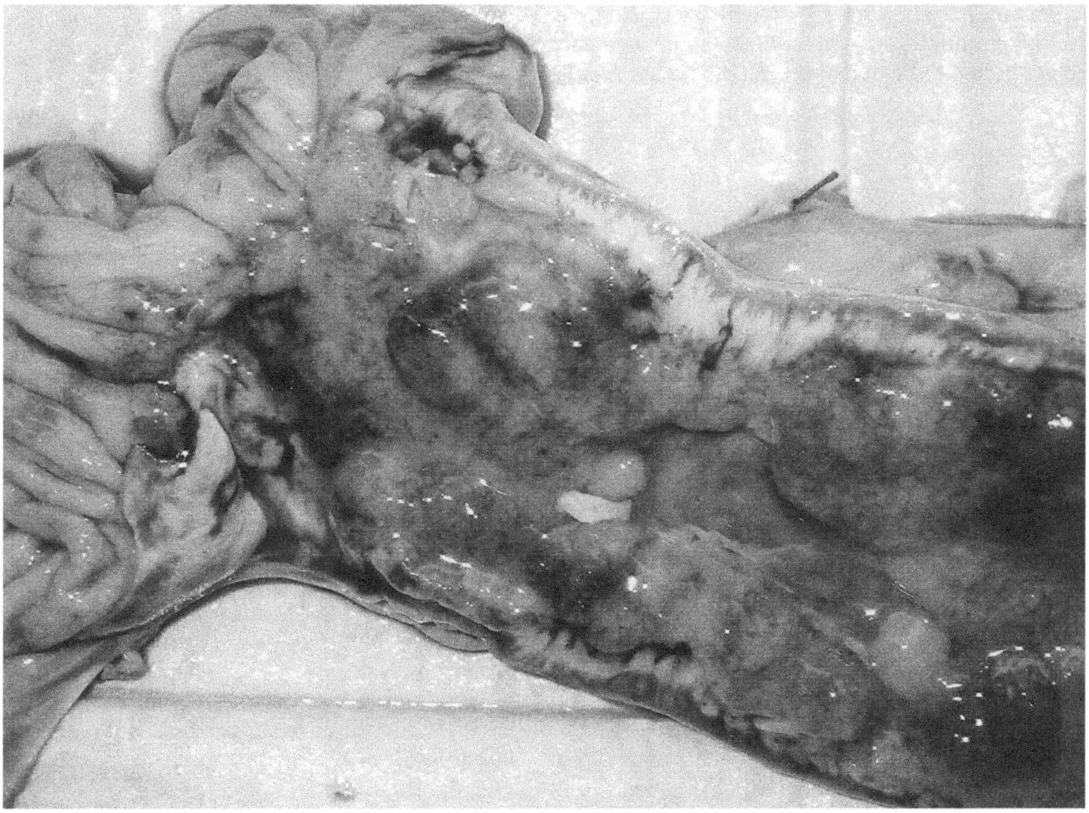

**Figure 8.3.** Resection specimen of ileal Crohn's disease. Note the fat encroachment of the mesentery, hosepipe thickening of the terminal ileum, and the relative normality of the caecum.

Most of the sulphonamide is absorbed whilst only 20% of 5-ASA is absorbed. The rest is excreted unchanged in the stool. The mechanism of action is unknown but it is believed to be due to its inhibitory effect on cyclooxygenase. The side effects include rash, headache, nausea, diarrhoea, pancreatitis, or blood dyscrasias in up to 55% of patients; interstitial nephritis occurs in around 1 in 500.

The newer oral 5-ASA formulations such as Pentasa and olsalazine that release 5-ASA in the distal small bowel secondary to pH changes are more useful in patients with small intestinal Crohn's disease. Given in high doses for up to 4 months, these drugs can induce remission in about 40% of patients with moderately active ileocaecal Crohn's disease.

## Steroids

Systemic steroids are the most effective agents for moderate to severe disease. In 70–80% of patients this will induce remission. Long-term maintenance therapy either with steroid alone or in combination with sulfasalazine has not been shown to be of benefit in preventing recurrence.

## Antibiotics

Antibiotic therapy is only indicated when there is an infective complication. It does not affect the course of the primary disease. Metronidazole is particularly of value in the presence of perianal disease.

## Immunosuppressive Agents

The agents in use include azathioprine, 6-mercaptopurine, methotrexate and cyclosporins. Immunosuppressive agents are useful in patients whose disease relapses once steroid therapy is withdrawn completely or reduced to a critical dose (15 or 10 mg daily). It is also useful in patients with refractory disease. Most patients response to this treatment and in most centres the treatment is continued for 1–2 years before it is withdrawn.

## Infliximab (Remicade)

Infliximab is a mouse–human chimeric monoclonal antibody (cA2), which inhibits the proinflammatory cytokine, tumour necrosis factor-alpha. This preparation was launched in the United States in 1988 and in the United Kingdom in September 1999 [7,8]. It was introduced for the treatment of severe, active Crohn's disease that is refractory to corticosteroid or immunomodulating agents and for the treatment of refractory fistulas of Crohn's disease. At present, it is not licensed for maintenance treatment.

Infliximab is given as an intravenous fusion of 5 mg/kg body weight over at least 2 hours. For an average adult patient with Crohn's disease, the average cost for a single infusion at 5 mg/kg is approximately £1350.00. Recent data from the Accent 1 trial indicated that the mean duration from a single dose may be as long as 24 weeks.

Infliximab has been associated with severe risk of development of tuberculosis, usually at extrapulmonary sites, and for this reason should only be used by a gastroenterologist experienced in the management of Crohn's disease. Infliximab is also contraindicated in patients with moderate to severe heart failure and in patients with a history of sensitivity to other murine proteins or infliximab. A delayed hypersensitivity has been observed in 25% of patients with Crohn's disease who were retreated with infliximab after a 2- to 4-years drug-free period.

## Nutritional Therapy

Severe disease is characterised by malnourishment and requires both nutritional replacement and support during acute phase of the disease. Such support may be in the form of enteral feeding using a fine-bore nasogastric tube or by the parenteral route in the form of total parenteral nutrition (TPN) or peripheral nutrition.

Parenteral nutrition has no primary effect on the disease process, but by eliminating intraluminal dietary antigen, which may be driving the inflammatory response, it is hoped that the patient may progress to a state of remission. Several trials have confirmed that elemental diets are as effective as corticosteroids in obtaining remission. The relapse rate is high. Total parental nutrition is less effective in isolated colonic disease. There is no added benefit in combining TPN with steroid over using only one agent.

Vitamin $B_{12}$ supplementation is not routinely advised provided a regular monitoring of serum vitamin $B_{12}$ is carried out. In patients with

# BENIGN DISEASE OF THE SMALL BOWEL

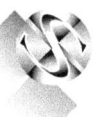

extensive disease, folic acid, iron, calcium and zinc deficiencies may occur and supplementations of these agents are required.

## Surgical Treatment

The majority of patients with Crohn's disease require one or several operations during their lifetime and for this reason surgery should be as conservative as possible. In the modern era, since Crohn's disease is a diffuse disease that can affect any segment of the gastrointestinal tract, surgery should involve resecting the least amount of bowel to re-establish satisfactory intestinal function. Operative indications are the same no matter where the disease manifests itself.

The indications are:

- failure of medical treatment
- complications, e.g. intestinal obstruction, fistula or abscess, perforation, bleeding
- some extraintestinal manifestation (e.g. pyoderma gangrenosum, erythema nodosum – others are rarely influenced by surgical excision)
- Growth retardation (paediatric patients)
- Malignant transformation.

## Preparation for Surgery

The nutritional status of the patient should be optimised prior to elective or semi-elective surgery. Severe malnutrition is best served by enteral nutrition over a course of 5–7 days. Anaemia should be treated by blood transfusion, and potential electrolyte problems and other co-morbid conditions corrected.

## Bowel Preparation

Full bowel preparation should always be made in all elective cases, as there is always a potential for colonic involvement with small bowel Crohn's disease. Mechanical bowel preparation is not suitable for patients with obstructive symptoms; instead a low residue diet over several days prior to surgery may be more appropriate in these patients.

## Anti-thrombus Prophylaxis

Routine deep vein thrombosis prophylaxis using thromboembolic deterrence stockings and low dose heparin should be instituted until the patient is fully mobile. Pneumatic compression boots should be used during surgery to reduce the risk of deep vein thrombosis.

## Steroid Therapy

For patients who are currently receiving steroid therapy, intravenous hydrocortisone 100 mg thrice daily should be given until the patient is able to resume oral intake.

## Preoperative Marking of Stoma Site

Preoperative marking of the stoma is essential if there is any indication that a stoma may be required. Certain groups of Crohn's patients are more likely than others to have stomas. They include the malnourished and those with intra-abdominal sepsis. Stoma patients benefit from a preoperative visit by a stoma nurse.

## Technical Aspect of Surgery

It is important to remember that Crohn's disease affects the entire gastrointestinal tract; surgery is unlikely to be curative and the long-term outlook for the patient should be kept in mind. Surgery is therefore directed towards the segment of the bowel that is severely diseased or presenting with complications. Non-obstructing, non-bleeding segments do not require resection. In order to prevent the development of short small bowel syndrome, resection of diseased segments should be kept to the minimum, as recurrence is almost inevitable (15% per year). If a stricture is identified at operation, this segment should be excised or subjected to stricturoplasty as it likely to be symptomatic in future. Stricturoplasty is particularly useful for recurrent disease, especially if earlier operations have involved substantial small bowel resection. Microscopic and endoscopic evidence of the disease at the resection margins does not appear to increase recurrence rates or compromise safe anastomosis. Frozen section examination of resected margins is unnecessary.

Any part of the bowel can be involved, so it is best to place the patient in the Lloyd Davies position in case pelvic dissection should be required. When incising the abdomen, the incision should be planned with attention given to previous incisions and to the siting of a stoma.

We prefer the midline abdominal incision because it preserves the right and left lower quadrants, which can be used in future for siting of stoma. As a rule, we prefer to reopen previous incisions rather than creating new one. At each operation, a full laparotomy should be carried out to assess the extent and severity of the disease and to measure the length of the remaining small bowel. Spillage during construction of anastomosis should be kept to a minimum.

## Surgical Procedures for Small Bowel and Ileocolic Crohn's Disease

### Ileocolic Disease

This is the most common disease pattern in Crohn's disease. The ideal treatment is a limited ileocaecal resection in which a few centimetres (10 cm) of macroscopically normal bowel at both ends are included and an anastomosis fashioned. The type of anastomosis depends on individual preference and ranges from hand-sewn to stapling anastomosis. The type of anastomosis does not affect recurrence rates. Reoperation rates are 20–25% at 5 years after the first operation and 35–40% at 10 years. After operation, recurrence tends to occur on the ileal side of the anastomosis and represents new disease rather than an inadequate resection margin. Patients with small bowel disease should be encouraged to stop smoking as this will reduce the risk of recurrence.

### Jejunal and Ileal Disease

About 10–20% of small bowel Crohn's disease affects the jejunal ileal region. This can cause obstructive strictures throughout the small intestine. Depending on the clinical settings, these lesions may be excised and anastomosed primarily. If multiple sites are involved there is a real danger of short small bowel syndrome if the whole of the affected segments are excised. In such situations, stricturoplasty is the preferred procedure. Stricturoplasty is also suitable for patients with extensive short fibrotic strictures and in patients with stricture in the presence of short bowel syndrome.

Stricturoplasty involves making a linear incision on the antimesenteric border of the affected segment of bowel and the enterotomy closed in a transverse manner. A Heineke–Mikulicz type stricturoplasty is better suited for short strictures whilst the Finney type or a combination of the two is more suited for longer strictures. Strictureplasty is a safe and effective procedure. The long-term follow-up is very promising. Relief from obstructive symptoms occurred in 98% of patients and two-third of patients on steroids were successfully weaned off their drugs. Reoperative recurrence occurred in 28%, and 78% of those requiring reoperation had new strictures at a location remote from the original stricturoplasty. The reoperation rate was statistically similar between stricturoplasty alone (31%) and stricturoplasty with resection (27%). The complications of stricturoplasty include bleeding and intra-abdominal sepsis.

### Gastroduodenal Disease

Symptomatic gastroduodenal Crohn's disease is rare, affecting 1–7%, and is usually associated with Crohn's disease in other sites. Commonly, the first and second parts of the duodenum are affected and the disease may extend upwards to affect the gastric antrum. Obstructive symptoms are the most frequent complaint and occasionally, a few patients present with bleeding. Distinguishing between Crohn's disease and peptic ulceration at endoscopy is very difficult and a trial of medical ulcer therapy may be diagnostic. Gastrojejunostomy is the standard procedure for duodenal or pyloric stenosis. In a stricture that renders itself amenable to stricturoplasty, this is preferred to bypass.

## Outcomes

Crohn's disease is characterised by high morbidity and low mortality. Most patients lead a full and active life despite recurrences and several operations. The standardised mortality rates are high for patients whose disease started early. As the disease affects the young and economically productive age group, the socioeconomic implications are significant. Many patients report increased unemployment, and problems with missed schooling, recreation and sexual relationships. Many patients adapt to their disability.

# Tuberculous Enteritis

In the Western world, tuberculous enteritis is rare because of the pasteurisation of milk, tuberculin testing of herds, improved standards of living and effective antituberculosis therapy. It is still common among immigrant communities, especially those from Indian subcontinent.

Tuberculous enteritis occurs in two forms. Primary infection results from ingestion of milk contaminated with *Mycobacterium bovis*. This accounts for less than 10% of reported cases. Secondary infection is caused by *M. tuberculosis* and is the result of swallowing infected sputum from a cavitating primary focus in the lungs. Tuberculous enteritis commonly affects the ileocaecal region. Intestinal tuberculosis can assume any of the three macroscopic forms: hypertrophic, ulcerative and fibrotic.

The *hypertrophic* form is the least virulent type and occurs in an individual with a high resistance from previous exposure to tuberculous infection. It commonly affects the ileocaecal region and is characterised by marked thickening of submucous and subserosal layers and lack of gross caseous necrosis. Typically, the patient is not very ill, although they may exhibit the systemic features of TB. Intestinal TB may unmask itself by the presence of a mass in the right iliac fossa or recurrent episodes of subacute intestinal obstruction.

The *ulcerative* form affects the terminal ileum where it causes multiple transverse deep ulcers. These ulcers may extend to the serosal surface and may perforate. The serosal surface is often studded with tuberculin and is usually thickened. Healing of these ulcers leads to formation of strictures. The symptoms include altered bowel habit and colicky lower abdominal pain. Sometimes, the diagnosis can be made on small bowel enema in a patient with known pulmonary TB. Surgery is contraindicated unless there is a perforation, obstruction or bleeding.

The *fibrotic* form affects the terminal ileum, caecum and ascending colon. It is associated with marked shortening and long stricture. It also leads to plastic peritonitis.

In the ascitic form of tuberculous peritonitis, there is marked pale, straw-coloured fluids within the peritoneal cavity. Frequently, there is a history of weight loss, general malaise and facial pallor. The patient presents with a distended abdomen. Pain is often absent; there is also a history of change in bowel habit. Umbilical hernia is common because of increased abdominal pressure. At operation, the peritoneum is studded with tubercles and the omentum is rolled up and infiltrated with tubercles (Figure 8.4).

Preoperative diagnosis is rarely made even in places where TB is endemic. The Mantoux test is negative in 45% of cases. Gastric washing made on three consecutive mornings should be attempted in order to culture the organism. The organism may also be cultured from stool, peritoneal fluid and from lymph node biopsy. Chest X-ray may show a cavitating lesion in pulmonary TB. Plain abdominal X-ray may show extensive calcifications. Barium enema may reveal stenotic areas indistinguishable from colonic Crohn's disease. Laparoscopy may provide an opportunity to obtain tissue and ascitic fluid for establishing the diagnosis.

## Treatment

If diagnosis is confirmed and in the absence of intestinal obstruction and perforation, the treatment is conservative with adequate rest, nutrition and anti-tuberculous chemotherapy. The treatment includes a 12-month course of rifampicin, isoniazid and ethambutol.

Surgical treatment is indicated if there are complications such as perforation, bleeding, obstruction or failure of medical treatment. Ileocaecal resection or right hemicolectomy is the procedure of choice for ileocaecal TB. Segmental resection is indicated in the treatment of isolated TB in the small intestine. The early results are encouraging provided patients continue their anti-tuberculous chemotherapy long after the operation.

# Typhoid Enteritis

Typhoid fever is an acute, systemic infection caused by *Salmonella* Typhi. Although salmonellas have a worldwide distribution, they usually result in disease in places with poor sanitation and overcrowding. Transmission is by ingestion of contaminated foods (especially eggs and poultry products). Following ingestion, the organism colonises the small intestine where it multiplies in Peyer's patches. From

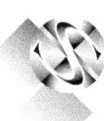

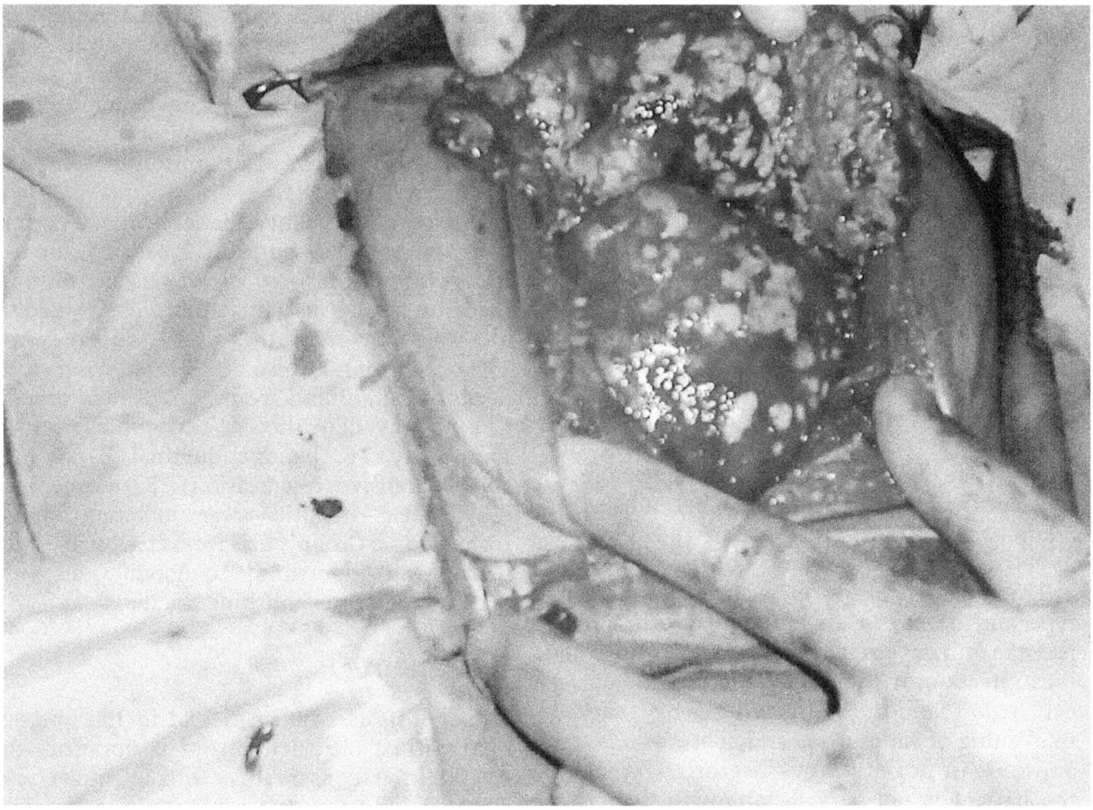

**Figure 8.4.** Operation showing rolled-up greater omentum infiltrated with tubercles.

here, they are carried by the lymphatics into the bloodstream and are then transported to the reticuloendothelial system. The terminal ileum bears the brunt of intestinal infection with formation of a longitudinal ulcerating lesion along the antimesenteric border, situated within 45 cm of the ileocaecal valves. This ulcer may perforate or bleed profusely. In the majority of patients, the ulcer is solitary.

The organism can be cultured from stool, blood, urine and bone marrow. Of the serological tests, the Widal test, which measures serum agglutinins against the O and H antigens, is most helpful. A fourfold increase in titre in sequential blood samples indicates *Salmonella* infection.

Chlorampenicol is the drug of choice despite the growing incidence of resistant strains and bone marrow depression. Other drugs that are helpful in the management of typhoid enteritis include Ciproxin, ampicillin and cotrimoxazole. Ampicillin is particularly helpful in the carrier state as it is excreted in its active form.

Gross haemorrhage occurs in 10–20% of hospitalised patients. Perforation occurs in 2% of patients. Operative treatment is indicated for perforation as localisation or walling off of the perforation is uncommon. Although simple oversewing of the perforation is possible, the experience from Zaria in Nigeria where such perforations are common suggests that segmental resection is the preferred option.

# Pneumatosis Cystoides Intestinalis

This is a rare condition in which gas-filled cysts are found in the submucosal and subserosal planes of the intestine. The cysts may range in size from a few millimetres to several centime-

# BENIGN DISEASE OF THE SMALL BOWEL

tres in diameter. The jejunum is the commonest site followed by the ileocaecal and colon. The condition probably results from lymphatic stasis with the filling of the lymph space with gas. It is associated with chronic obstructive airway disease. In 85% of cases, it is associated with other gastrointestinal lesions. The cysts are thin-walled and can rupture spontaneously, producing pneumoperitoneum. The symptoms are non-specific. Diagnosis is usually made radiologically.

No active treatment is required but treatment by administering high flow oxygen over 3–4 days has had some success.

## Small Bowel Diverticular Disease

Generally speaking, small bowel diverticular disease is not as common as large bowel diverticular disease. Diverticula may be congenital (true) or acquired (false). A congenital diverticulum is called a true diverticulum because it is composed of all layers of the bowel wall whereas a false diverticulum is made up of only mucosal and the submucosal layers. Duodenal diverticula are the commonest form of acquired diverticula of the small intestine whilst Meckel's diverticulum is the commonest form of true diverticulum of the small intestine.

### Duodenal Diverticula

Diverticular disease of the duodenum is common but the true incidence remains unknown. Most of these diverticula are asymptomatic. The male:female ratio is 1:2. Up to 75% of diverticula occur in the periampullary region and usually project from the medial wall of the duodenum. Duodenal diverticulum is important because it can precipitate pancreatitis, cholangitis and recurrent common bile duct stone in patients who have had cholecystectomy. The diverticulum may bleed, perforate or even obstruct.

Treatment is usually directed toward the control of the complication. Diverticulectomy can be considered if there is bleeding or obstruction. In the presence of perforation, a gastrojejunostomy and duodunojejunostomy should be performed. Serosal patch using jejunal loop is advocated by some.

### Jejunal and Ileal Diverticula

Diverticula of the jejunum and ileum are rare and account for less than 1%. Jejunal diverticula are larger in size, often multiple and are more common than ileal diverticula. These diverticula are found on the mesenteric border unlike Meckel's diverticulum, which is found on the antimesenteric border. Most of these diverticula are asymptomatic. The symptomatic ones often present with incomplete intestinal obstruction, malabsorption due to bacterial overgrowth in the diverticulum or perforation.

Treatment is usually directed toward the control of the complication. Complication such as bleeding or obstruction require segmental resection. Malabsorption due to bacterial overgrowth requires antibiotic therapy.

### Meckel's Diverticulum

Meckel's diverticulum represents the remnant of the vitello-intestinal tract. It occurs in 2% of the population, measures about 2 inches (5 cm) in length and arises from the antimesenteric border of the ileum, approximately 2 feet (60 cm) from the ileocaecal valve. It may contain gastric, pancreatic or duodenal tissues. Meckel's diverticulum may be associated with peptic ulceration, which may give rise to profuse gastrointestinal haemorrhage or perforation.

Technetium pertechnetate is the investigation of choice in patients bleeding from a Meckel's diverticulum. Surgery in the form of wedge resection of the ileum and closure of the defect transversely or segmental resection is indicated in symptomatic patients. Removal of uninflamed Meckel's diverticulum found incidentally during laparotomy is ill advised and should be discouraged.

## Miscellaneous Problems

### Non-specific Small Bowel Ulceration

Most ulcerations of the small bowel are due to known causes such as drugs, Crohn's disease, infection or tumours. In a few cases non-identifiable causes are responsible for such ulcers. These ulcers are called non-specific ulcers and

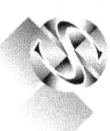

occur frequently in the terminal ileum. Often the ulcer is solitary although multiple ulcers are not uncommon. Most ulcers are self-limiting and occur on the antimesenteric border. These ulcers are associated with fibrous scar formation, which may lead to obstruction. Preoperative diagnosis is rare. Treatment is directed towards the complications. Bleeding and intestinal obstruction are best managed by segmental resection.

## Blind Loop Syndrome (Stagnant Loop Syndrome)

The term blind loop refers to bacterial overgrowth in a stagnant loop of small bowel caused by fistula, blind pouch, stricture, stenosis or diverticula. Bacterial colonisation leads to damage to the mucosa. The affected segment becomes inflamed, swollen and dilated. Bacteria utilise vitamin $B_{12}$ for their own metabolism and also deconjugate bile salts leading to formation of deoxycholate and lithocholate.

Clinically, the characteristic features are diarrhoea, anaemia, abdominal pain, steatorrhoea, weight loss, vitamin $B_{12}$ and fat-soluble vitamin deficiencies as well as neurological disorders. Schilling's test is usually diagnostic.

Surgical removal of the offending segment is recommended. In some cases surgical excision is not possible (e.g. extensive jejunal diverticulosis), and treatment with antibiotics such as tetracycline and metronidazole is beneficial.

## Small Bowel Fistulas

A fistula is an abnormal communication between two epithelial surfaces. The majority of small bowel fistulas are caused by anastomotic dehiscence or unrecognised injury during operation. Others causes include Crohn's disease, colonic diverticulitis, cancer radiation enteritis, intestinal tuberculosis and mesenteric vascular disease.

The effect of the fistula depends on the site and what is responsible for it. Sepsis, skin necrosis, malnutrition and fluid and electrolyte abnormalities are the major complications of intestinal fistulas.

Fistulas can be classified into high or low fistula depending on their location and daily output. This classification is important because these factors determine the type of treatment as well as morbidity and mortality.

Generally, the more proximal the fistula, the greater the output, the more serious the problem. A fistula that puts out 500 ml or more in 24 hours is regarded as high. High output fistulas are associated with marked fluid and electrolyte losses as well as malnutrition.

Investigations are required to outline the pathological anatomy. Commonly, a small bowel enema, barium enema and a fistulogram are performed to define the abnormality. The outlook for intestinal fistulas has been improving since the introduction of total parenteral nutrition and better skin stoma care. With modern conservative management, spontaneous closure occurs in 70–80% of cases and the mortality averages 6–10%.

### Conservative Management

*Nutritional Support*

Safe nutritional therapy has had a major impact on the management of small bowel fistula. The aim is to deliver 40–50 kcal/kg per day, together with 300–400 mg of nitrogen/kg of body weight. Total parenteral nutrition and restricted oral intake has also been associated with a rapid reduction in the volume of fistula discharge [9]. Enteral nutrition may be used as an alternative to total parenteral nutrition in certain circumstances. The enteral nutrition takes 3–5 days to become established; the fistula output is not immediately reduced and may actually increase in volume.

*Control of Sepsis*

The use of sump suction helps to control sepsis and provide drainage for the associated intra-abdominal abscess. The use of a nasogastric tube in patients with ileus helps to reduce the output from the fistula. Somatostatin, which inhibits intestinal secretion and motility, is helpful in reducing the output from a fistula. Systemic antibiotics should be administered until the sepsis is controlled.

*Skin-stoma care*

The protection of skin around the fistula is important, as the effluents from a high output fistula are very rich in enzymes capable of digesting the skin. Nowadays, stoma adhesive appliances are used, but there is still a role for silicone-based barrier creams in the initial period.

A fistula may not close spontaneously if there is a distal obstruction, an undrained abscess, high output, or the affected segment has active granulomatous disease, cancer, a foreign body in the tract or radiation enteritis. If there is still a significant output after 4–6 weeks of conservative management, then operative intervention is indicated. Surgery involves reopening the previous scar and gentle mobilisation of the bowel with resection of the affected segment. If the ends of the bowel appear healthy, end-to-end anastomosis is performed, if not the bowel should be exteriorised. Operative management is associated with a high mortality rate (20%).

## Short Bowel Syndrome

Short bowel syndrome is the severest form of intestinal decompensation resulting from massive resection of the small bowel. The commonest reasons for such an extensive resection are:

- Crohn's disease
- small bowel tumours
- superior mesenteric infarction
- multiple small bowel fistulas
- midgut volvulus
- radiation enteritis.

The critical length of residual small bowel that can comfortably support nutrition is variable, and the more distal the resection the greater is the complication. Generally, resection of up to 70% of the small bowel can be tolerated provided the terminal ileum and the ileocaecal valve are preserved. Resection of the terminal ileum and ileocaecal valve, which accounts for 25% of the total length of small bowel, leads to marked vitamin $B_{12}$ and bile salt malabsorption.

Proximal small bowel resection is better tolerated than distal resection because the ileum exhibits a greater adaptive capacity than the jejunum. The presence of an intact ileocaecal valve slows the transit time and also prevents bacterial overgrowth in the small bowel. With massive resection, there is a sudden reduction in the absorptive surface required for the absorption of carbohydrates, fat, protein, vitamins, water and trace elements. Invariably, there is malabsorption of all nutrients but its severity varies with the length and site of the residual bowel. Of all the nutrients, carbohydrate absorption is the least affected and normality returns within 4–6 weeks. Protein absorption continues to improve over several months but fat absorption remains impaired due to disruption of enterohepatic circulation of bile. As some of the bile salts are lost in the stool, hepatic synthesis is unable to compensate for such losses. In the large bowel, primary bile salt that spilled over is deconjugated into secondary bile salts. These salts contribute to the diarrhoea of short bowel syndrome. Accompanying malabsorption of fat is the malabsorption of fat-soluble vitamins, calcium and magnesium.

Although the small bowel has an intrinsic capacity to adapt, it does so by dilatation of the remaining intestine, enlargement of the villi and the enterocytes. Adaptation is brought about by luminal and humoral factors. Luminal factors such as luminal nutrients, pancreatico-biliary and gastroduodenal secretions are necessary for complete adaptation to occur. Duodenal juice is an important source of epidermal growth factor required for the proliferation of the intestinal mucosa. In animal studies, the long-term use of TPN following massive small bowel resection may maintain nutrition, but intestinal adaptation does not occur because of the lack of luminal nutrients. Thus luminal nutrition by oral ingestion is an essential factor for adaptive response. Of the humoral factors, enteroglucagon is the most important factor. This adaptive mechanism is better developed in neonates and infants than in adults. Adaptation may take several weeks or months to complete and it is heralded by decreasing diarrhoea and improved absorption of glucose and vitamin $B_{12}$. In massive resection, this adaptive mechanism may be overwhelmed leading to the intestinal decompensation. Short gut syndrome is characterised by diarrhoea, fluid and electrolyte deficiency and malnutrition.

Massive small bowel resection is associated with gastric hypersecretion, renal stone formation, impaired renal function, cholesterol gallstone formation, hepatic disorder and metabolic bone disease.

### Treatment

In situations where the viability of the small bowel is in question, resection of the barest

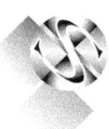

minimum is advocated. A second look operation should be performed within 24–48 hours to allow demarcation of the ischaemic region. Early treatment includes total parenteral nutrition, control of diarrhoea, fluid and electrolyte replacement.

### Total Parenteral Nutrition

The regime should be administered over a 12-hour period, preferably via a Hickman line. It must provide the following:

- calorie 40 kcal/kg body weight
- nitrogen 300 mg/kg body weight
- vitamins, trace elements and electrolytes.

### Fluid and Electrolytes

Fluid loss in excess of 5 litres/day is not uncommon in the early period. Strict input and output records must be maintained and replacement of the losses must be instituted. $H_2$ blockers or proton pump inhibitors are useful in reducing gastric secretion and by implication the need for nasogastric tube. Diarrhoea may be controlled by judicious use of antidiarrhoeal agents, e.g. loperamide, codeine, Lomotil. These agents inhibit gut motility, thereby worsening ileus.

### Reintroduction of Oral Feeding

When adaptation has occurred (usually 4–6 weeks after the resection) oral diet can be reintroduced in those with adequate length of residual small bowel. In those with residual length greater than 1 m, normal or near-normal oral diet can be commenced but these patients are unlikely to have the normal number and consistency of stool. In those with less than 100 cm of residual bowel, long-term enteral feeding is required. Commonly enteral feeding is commenced gradually, initially in iso-osmolar concentration. Afterwards, either an elemental (Vivonex) or polymeric feed (Ensure, Isocal) is introduced. Enteral feeding is administered via a nasogastric tube and gradually increased to full strength. Milk products should be avoided as they worsen the diarrhoea.

During the early period of introduction of enteral feeds, diarrhoea is a significant problem and often requires treatment with antidiarrhoeal agents. Somatostatin may be useful in those with intractable and life-threatening diarrhoea. In those with an intact colon after ileal resection, cholestyramine may be used as a bile salt binder to prevent the cathartic effect of unabsorbed bile salts on the colon.

Steatorrhoea occurs in patients with massive small bowel resection and usually indicates the presence of excess dietary fat. Fat provides twice as many calories per gram as carhohydrate or protein. Medium chain triglycerides are absorbed directly into the portal vein and do not require bile salts for their absorption. Whenever possible, fat should be administered as medium chain triglycerides. Calcium, magnesium, zinc, iron, and fat-soluble vitamins must be provided.

Three monthly-injection of vitamin $B_{12}$ is required in those with ileal resection.

### Surgical Treatment

Surgery is rarely indicated in adults and is considered only in the event of failure of conservative management. Surgery is designed to reverse the effect of decreased absorptive surfaces and rapid transit time. Intestinal lengthening procedures have been developed and seem useful in neonates and infants. The early results seem promising. Other procedures described include reversed segments and serosal patch. None of these procedures has been effective and in the UK, they are rarely performed. Truncal vagotomy and pyloroplasty was used extensively in the past to control gastric acid hypersecretion. In the modern era of potent proton pump inhibitors, there is no longer any justification for this practice.

## Ingested Foreign Bodies

The majority of ingested foreign bodies occur accidentally and often the victim is a child. The objects range from toys, coins, pencils, pins, needles, whistles, toothpicks, fish bones to pieces of metal.

Treatment is expectant. The progress of radiopaque objects can be monitored by serial pain abdominal X-rays. Sharp objects can penetrate the bowel wall and if the patient experiences abdominal pain associated with fever and raised white cell count, surgical removal of such an object is indicated. The use of laxatives to facilitate the expulsion of ingested foreign bodies should be discouraged as it is counterproductive.

## BENIGN DISEASE OF THE SMALL BOWEL

## Questions

1. Outline the genetics of Crohn's disease.
2. What are the clinical features of Crohn's disease?
3. Summarise benign conditions of the small bowel.
4. Outline the surgical principles of benign small bowel disease.
5. Discuss the critical length of small bowel to support nutrition.

## References

1. Schraut WH, Medich DS. Crohn's Disease. In: Greenfield LJ, Mulholland MW, Oldham KT et al. (eds) Surgery: scientific principles and practice, 2nd edn. Lippincott-Raven: Philadelphia, 1997; 831–43.
2. Langman NJS. Epidemiology of inflammatory bowel disease. In: Allan R, Keighley M, Alexander-Williams J, Hawkins C (eds) inflammatory bowel disease, 2nd edn. Edinburgh: Churchill Livingstone, 1990.
3. Hugot JP, Laurent-Puig P, Gower-Rousseau C et al. Two-stage genome-wide search in inflammatory bowel disease provides evidence for susceptibility loci on chromosomes 3, 7 and 12. Nat Genet 1996;14:199–202.
4. Rioux JD, Daly MJ, Silverberg MS, et al. Genetic variation in the 5q31 cytokine gene cluster confers susceptibility to Crohn's disease. Nat Genet 2001;29:223–8.
5. Cho JH. The Nod2 gene in Crohn's disease: implications for future research into the genetics and immunology of Crohn's disease. Inflamm Bowel Dis 2001;7:271–5.
6. Fiocchi et al. 1998
7. Targan SR, Hanauer SB, van Deventer SJH et al. A short-term study of chimeric monoclonal antibody cA2 to tumor necrosis factor alpha for Crohn's disease. N Engl J Med 1997;337:1029–35.
8. Present DH, Rutgeerts P, Targan SR et al. Infliximab for the treatment of fistulas in aptients with Crohn's disease. N Engl J Med 1999;340:1398–405.
9. Wolfe BM, Keltner RM, Williams VL. Intestinal fistula output in regular, elemental and intravenous elementation. Am J Surg 1972;124:803–6.

# 9

# Benign Disease of the Diaphragm

Juliet E. King and Pala B. Rajesh

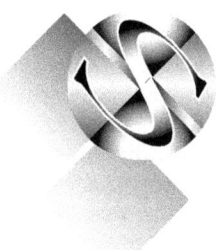

## Aims

- To describe diaphramatic eventration and phrenic nerve palsy.
- To describe the diagnosis and management of traumatic diaphragmatic hernias.
- To discuss diagnosis and management of congenital diaphragmatic hernias.

## Surgical Anatomy of the Diaphragm

The diaphragm consists of peripherally placed muscular elements that radially insert into the domed, trefoil-shaped central fibrous tendon. The muscular portion consists of three parts, lumbar, costal and sternal, which are separated by muscle-free gaps. These gaps consist of little more than loose connective tissue, pleura and peritoneum. The lumbar muscular part is the strongest and arises from the anterior surface of the upper lumbar vertebrae and intervertebral discs, the crura and arcuate ligaments. The costal part originates from the cartilages of the lower six ribs anterolaterally, interdigitating with muscular slips from the transversus abdominis muscles. The gap between the lumbar and costal elements represents the site of the lumbocostal (Bochdalek's) foramen. The sternal origin arises from the posterior part of the rectus sheath and xiphoid process. The gap between the sternal and costal elements is referred to as the foramen of Morgagni. These foramina are illustrated in Figure 9.1.

The position of the central tendon depends on many factors. These include the respiratory cycle, body habitus and the degree of abdominal distension. During full expiration the dome of the right hemidiaphragm lies approximately at the level of the fourth intercostal space

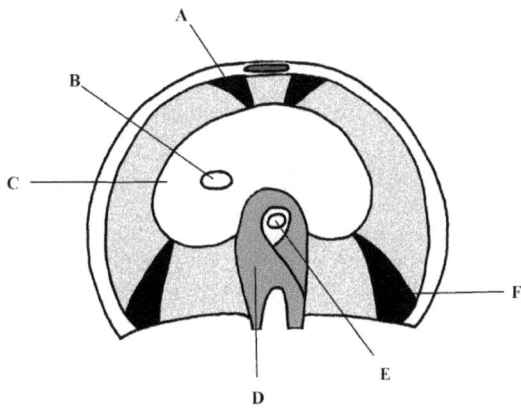

**Figure 9.1.** Diagram illustrating the position of the common congenital diaphragmatic hernias (viewed from below). A, sternocostal foramen (Morgagni hernia); B, inferior vena cava; C, central tendon of the diaphragm; D, crura and oesophageal hiatus; E, oesophagus; F, lumbocostal foramen (Bochdalek hernia).

and the left hemidiaphragm is usually a space lower. In forced inspiration the domes may move downwards by as much as two intercostal spaces, the central tendon flattens and the costodiaphragmatic recesses enlarge, enabling downwards excursion of the lungs.

The vascular supply to the diaphragm arises from several sources. The peripheral muscular parts are supplied by branches from the lower five intercostal and the subcostal arteries. The pericardiacophrenic arteries, which are terminal branches of the internal mammary artery, supply the fibrous pericardium, phrenic nerve and a small portion of the central tendon. Further blood supply is via the musculophrenic and superior phrenic arteries, all of which supply the cranial aspect of the diaphragm. The posterior aspect is directly vascularised by small branches of the descending thoracic aorta, whilst the caudal aspect is supplied from the inferior phrenic arteries and direct branches from the coeliac trunk.

The nerve supply to the diaphragm reflects its origin as a cervical structure. The primary motor innervation is via the right and left phrenic nerves (C3–5). Both phrenic nerves supply the diaphragm from below, the right passing through the caval foramen, and the left piercing the muscular part anterolateral to the pericardium. The nerves branch into sternal, anterolateral, posterolateral and crural branches that spread radially to the peripheral musculature. The lower intercostal nerves also supply branches to the peripheral muscular parts, but these are primarily proprioceptive rather than motor.

## Diaphragmatic Incisions

The radial arrangement of the diaphragmatic neurovascular supply has implications for the placement of incisions. Peripheral circumferential incisions should be placed approximately 3 cm from the costal margin to avoid the radially-placed neurovascular bundle (Figure 9.2). Radial incisions should be limited to the anterolateral portion of diaphragm and not extended back to the hiatus if possible, as this can compromise a significant proportion of phrenic nerve branches. Incision through the central tendon must be located well away from the main phrenic nerve [1,2].

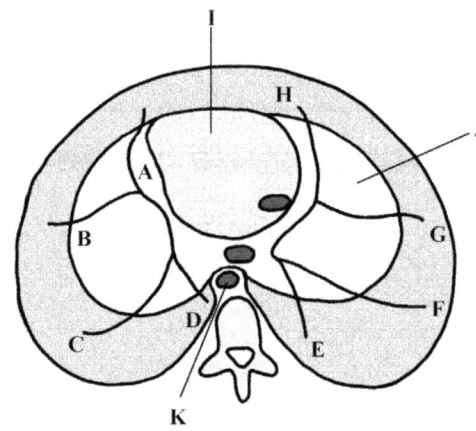

**Figure 9.2.** Diagram illustrating the branches of the phrenic nerve (viewed from above). A, left sternal; B, left anterolateral; C, left posterolateral; D, left crural; E, right crural; F, right posterolateral; G, right anterolateral; H, right sternal; I, fibrous pericardium and inferior vena cava; J, central tendon of the diaphragm; K, aorta.

## Openings in the Diaphragm

There are three main openings through, or in the case of the aortic foramen, behind the diaphragm, with a variable number of other structures that pass from abdomen to thorax. The caval foramen is located on the right at the level of T8 within the central tendon. On the left is the oesophageal foramen, at the level of T10. This is formed by the right crus with contribution from the left crus anteriorly. The aortic opening lies behind the diaphragm at its lowest point, opposite the T12 vertebra. The aortic opening is bounded by the interdigitating crura and median arcuate ligament anteriorly and the vertebral column posteriorly. The contents of each foramen and a summary of other structures that traverse the diaphragm are listed in Table 9.1 [1,3].

## Congenital Diaphragmatic Hernias

The first description of a congenital diaphragmatic hernia (CDH) has been attributed to Riverius in 1679 [4,5]. Morgani and Bochdalek subsequently described their eponymous hernias in 1769 and 1840 respectively [4]. The

# BENIGN DISEASE OF THE DIAPHRAGM

**Table 9.1.** Summary of structures passing from the abdomen to thorax via the diaphragm

| Diaphragmatic foramen | Position | Contents |
|---|---|---|
| Caval | Central tendon opposite T8 | Inferior vena cava<br>Right phrenic nerve[a]<br>Lymphatic vessels |
| Oesophageal | Between right and left crus at level of T10 | Oesophagus<br>L and R vagal trunks<br>Oesophageal branches of L gastric artery + veins/lymphatics.<br>Phrenicoabdominal nerve |
| Aortic | Behind diaphragm at the level of T12 | Descending thoracic aorta<br>Aortic plexus<br>Azygos vein<br>Thoracic duct |
| Structures crossing the diaphragm via other openings | | Greater, lesser and least splanchnic nerves<br>Sympathetic trunk<br>Subcostal neurovascular bundle<br>Lower five intercostal nerves<br>Inferior hemiazygos vein.<br>Left and right* phrenic nerves<br>Superior epigastric vessels<br>Lymphatics |

\* Some texts state that the right phrenic nerve pierces the diaphragm next to the caval foramen rather than passing through it. [1,4].

first successful repair of a neonatal CDH is attributed to Gross in 1946 [6].

Congenital diaphragmatic hernias are uncommon with a prevalence of between 1 in 2000 and 1 in 5000 overall. Most occur sporadically although a few cases may be seen as part of a familial condition, Fryns syndrome [7]. The male to female ratio is equal for the more common forms of CDH. Small hernias may escape detection in the neonatal period, presenting later in life. Congenital diaphragmatic abnormalities can be classified in a variety of ways depending on whether embryological, anatomical, or clinical criteria are used. This can cause confusion: for example some texts consider pleuroperitoneal canal defects synonymous with Bochdalek's hernia. Table 9.2 summarises the more common defects and their main features.

The most common form of CDH is the posterolateral Bochdalek hernia, which involves the left side in 80% of cases. Most of what follows regarding prognosis and treatment refers to this type of CDH. Pleuroperitoneal canal and septum transversum defects are far less common. The advent of routine prenatal ultrasonography has resulted in the majority (>90%) of cases of CDH being picked up before the 25th week of gestation. The prevalence of associated congenital malformations is variable, and their presence greatly influences outcome and survival. Most common are defects affecting the heart, brain, genitourinary system and limbs [8] The incidence of potentially lethal associated chromosomal anomalies (including trisomy 13, 18 and 21) ranges between 30% and 50% in most studies, and [8]. A recent study has proposed an association between CDH and anomalies affecting the long arm of chromosome 15 (15q24–26) [9]. The chest x-ray in Figure 9.3 illustrates the appearances of a large right diaphragmatic hernia with associated pulmonary hypoplasia in a neonate.

Much of the morbidity and mortality of CDH results from induced changes in the cardiopulmonary circulation. A widely accepted explanation for these changes is that pulmonary development, particularly bronchial branching, is impeded by the mass effect of herniated abdominal viscera, resulting in alveolar hypoplasia and pulmonary hypertension. This theory is supported by the finding that the

# 9 · UPPER GASTROINTESTINAL SURGERY

**Table 9.2.** Summary of developmental anomalies affecting the diaphragm

| Condition | Anatomical Features | Epidemiology |
| --- | --- | --- |
| Diaphragmatic agenesis | Complete absence of diaphragm | Very rare defect |
| Diaphragmatocele | Failure of muscle development. Diaphragm consists of fibrous sheet only | Very rare defect |
| Eventration | Muscular part of diaphragm deficient with normal but sparsely distributed muscle cells. Phrenic nerves normal. Diaphragm sits in elevated position and attenuated muscle allows abdominal viscera to bulge into thorax | More commonly seen in males. Associated with malrotation of gut in proportion of cases |
| Pleuroperitonal canal defect | Also known as "hernia diaphragmatica spuria". The canals fail to close in week 8 leaving a defect in the lateral muscular part of the diaphragm | Rare defect |
| Bochdalek hernia | True hernia through the lumbocostal triangle. More than 85% on left. Associated with pulmonary hypoplasia, malrotation of the gut, tracheo-oesophageal fistula and cardiac defects | Approximately 1:4000 all births. Equal sex incidence |
| Morgagni hernia | Retrosternal hernia through the right sternocostal gap. Sac initially present but may regress and be difficult to identify. Commonly presents late and may be exacerbated by trauma. Left sternocostal hernia often known as Larrey's hernia | Uncommon |
| Septum transversum defects | Failure of development that affects both diaphragm and pericardium | Very rare |

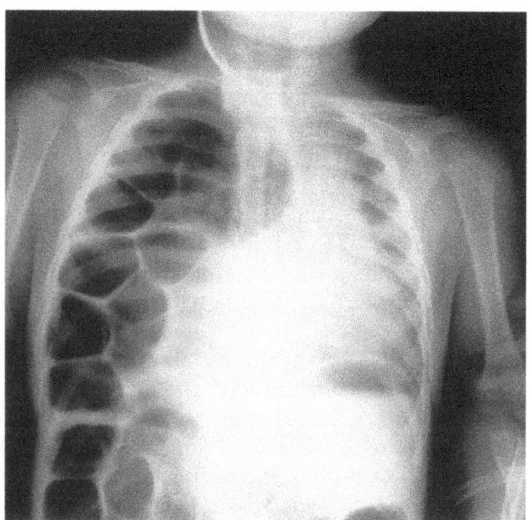

**Figure 9.3.** Chest X-ray of a large right diaphagmatic hernia in a neonate.

degree of hypoplasia and overall mortality relate to the size of the diaphragmatic defect, and the time that it develops in relation to gestational age. However, pulmonary hypoplasia is also seen in the lung contralateral to the CDH. Some animal experiments have suggested that lung hypoplasia occurs simultaneously with the diaphragmatic malformation rather than as a result of it [10]. The pulmonary circulation is also affected by the presence of a hernia. Pulmonary artery branching is intimately related to bronchial development: reduced branching results in arterial hypoplasia and excess arteriolar wall muscle development. This in turn contributes to the development of pulmonary hypertension [11].

During pregnancy fetal oxygenation is maintained by the placenta. A right to left shunt across the foramen ovale ensures that most of the lungs are bypassed. The first few gasps of air at the time of birth reduce pulmonary resistance and raise the oxygen tension in the pulmonary veins, inducing closure of the foramen ovale and ductus arteriosum. In neonates with CDH the conversion from a fetal circulation is opposed by hypoxaemic pulmonary vasoconstriction secondary to alveolar hypoplasia. Persistence of the fetal circulation induces a vicious cycle of increasing hypoxia and pulmonary hypertension that invariably results in critical respiratory failure. This may be further compounded by the presence of associated cardiac abnormalities.

## Perinatal Management and Timing of Surgery

With improvements in diagnosis, paediatric anaesthesia and intensive care the number of neonates surviving surgical repair of CDH has steadily increased [5]. There is a greater understanding of the pathophysiological cardiopulmonary changes that accompany CDH, and more effective treatments for conditions often seen in association with CDH, such as heart disease. However, the morbidity and mortality of infants with CDH remains substantial.

It was initially believed that the poor outcome associated with CDH was predominantly a result of continued compression of the lung after birth. Surgery was therefore undertaken immediately after delivery to minimise this effect. Experimental work in the 1980s suggested that some of the consequences of CDH could be further reduced if the diaphragmatic repair was undertaken prenatally. Although encouraging results were reported in animal models, the results of surgery in humans have been disappointing. The biggest obstacle was how to avoid of inducing preterm labour in the mother, which was seen in almost all pregnancies.

An improved understanding of the relationship between pulmonary hypoplasia, hypertension and outcome has led to a shift in management. It is now accepted that the optimal approach is to undertake surgery once cardiac and respiratory function has been optimised and stabilised in the first few hours of life. The primary goal is correction of hypoxaemia through ventilation without barotrauma, thereby interrupting the vicious cycle of hypoxaemia, pulmonary vasoconstriction and reduced pulmonary compliance that is otherwise seen in the immediate postnatal period.

Thoughts have also changed regarding the methods of ventilation, with a shift away from aggressive hyperventilation. Instead, the goal is to maintain oxygenation with the minimum of ventilatory pressure, and a degree of permissive hypercapnia. Introduction of this approach appears to have reduced the morbidity and mortality associated with pulmonary barotrauma [5]. Other novel ventilatory methods that have been investigated in CDH include high frequency oscillatory ventilation (HFOV) and extracorporeal membrane oxygenation (ECMO).

Extracorporeal membrane oxygenation is a method of cardiopulmonary bypass that enables arterial blood oxygenation and removal of $CO_2$ via an extracorporeal venoarterial or venovenous circuit. By reducing pulmonary hypoxaemia without the need for mechanical ventilation, the problems of pulmonary hypertension and barotrauma are avoided. Although an established treatment in other forms of neonatal respiratory distress, the use of ECMO is associated with significant morbidity and mortality in its own right, predominantly due to bleeding complications and neurological injury. There is also some controversy regarding patient selection, optimum timing and duration of ECMO treatment. Overall the impact of perioperative ECMO on survival in CDH has been investigated in several units and remains unproven [5,11].

As the vast majority of CDH are diagnosed prenatally this enables some degree of planning, as far as delivery is concerned. Clinical signs at birth include respiratory distress associated with a scaphoid abdomen, evidence of intrathoracic stomach or bowel, and signs of mediastinal shift [11]. Immediately following delivery a nasogastric tube should be passed to decompress the stomach and intestine, thereby reducing the risk of aspiration and intrathoracic strangulation of abdominal viscera. The neonate should then be intubated and ventilated to maintain arterial oxygenation, and an appropriate attention paid to fluid balance and temperature control. Prolonged ventilation via a facemask produces gastric distension and predisposes to aspiration, and should therefore be avoided. The presence of associated defects should be ascertained and investigated as appropriate. Transfer to a specialist centre is essential once the neonate is stabilised.

## Surgical Procedures and Outcome

Surgical repair involves reduction of herniated viscera into the abdomen, with resection of the hernial sac and diaphragmatic repair. Morgani hernias are usually small and can be closed without a patch. It is often more difficult to close larger defects primarily, in which case surgical mesh or autologous muscle flaps are options. Surgery is usually performed through an abdominal rather than thoracic approach, and may need to be combined with other procedures, e.g. correction of intestinal malrotation.

The results of surgery for CDH remain disappointing despite advances in perioperative management. Much of this mortality relates to the presence of other associated congenital defects. Some bias has probably been introduced by better survival of the sickest infants, who previously would have died shortly after birth. Earlier identification and better perinatal management enables these infants to survive long enough to become potential surgical candidates. Overall survival rates approach 50%, with results from centres that routinely use ECMO reported as higher, in the region of 65% [11]. Long-term complications of surgery for CDH include patch disruption, recurrent herniation, and chest wall deformity. It is also common for children with CDH to suffer with chronic gastro-oesophageal reflux disease, probably as a result of impaired diaphragmatic motility [12]. The effect of correction on pulmonary function is unpredictable and a proportion of surviving infants remain respiratory cripples [11]. Such children inevitably require long-term follow-up by a multidisciplinary team to enable effective management of their many medical problems.

# Eventration of the Diaphragm and Phrenic Nerve Palsy

Diaphragmatic eventration is an uncommon condition that can mimic both CDH and traumatic herniation. Eventration is caused by a paucity or absence of the muscular parts of one or both hemidiaphragms, which is otherwise normally innervated. The peripheral muscle is unable to contract adequately against the upward force of the abdominal viscera, gradually becoming stretched and attenuated until the dome of the diaphragm lies at an elevated position. In distinction from hernias, the muscular elements are intact and in continuity with the chest wall. Eventration is more common in males, and is associated with malrotation of the gut and possibly other congenital myopathies. The majority of cases affect the left side. The underlying cause of eventration is unclear. There appears to be an association with CDH and it has been suggested that premature return of abdominal contents during fetal development may compromise muscular growth. Complete eventration, in common with CDH, is associated with ipsilateral pulmonary hypoplasia. Histological examination of eventrated diaphragm shows muscle cells to be present but sparsely distributed with associated scarring, inflammation and fibrosis [13].

Phrenic nerve palsy can result in a clinical and radiological appearance that may be difficult to distinguish from eventration on clinical or radiological grounds. The nerve palsy may be congenital or acquired, but with time leads to atrophy of the muscular elements resulting in elevation of the central tendon. True congenital phrenic palsy is uncommon, with a reported incidence of 0.03–0.5% of neonates [4]. However, acquired palsy can result from numerous pathological processes, which include neuromuscular disorders such as poliomyelitis, neoplastic invasion, trauma and iatrogenic injury. In children phrenic nerve palsy is a recognised complication of perinatal trauma and congenital heart surgery [1].

## Symptoms and Diagnosis

Minor degrees of eventration may be asymptomatic. More severe forms usually present with breathlessness secondary to pulmonary compression, particularly in the supine position. Both eventration and phrenic palsy can have serious consequences in the newborn. The accessory muscles of respiration are poorly developed in infants, who are consequently far more reliant on diaphragmatic contraction than are adults. In addition, the thoracic cage is softer and therefore more compliant. Respiratory distress may develop rapidly and the effects of diaphragmatic paralysis are compounded by the presence of paradoxical respiration in the supine position. Abnormal outwards excursion of the lateral chest wall during inspiration due to unopposed intercostal muscle contraction may be clinically apparent. The other common presentation of eventration relates to the digestive system, with symptoms of reflux, belching and vomiting, and poor feeding in children. More serious consequences include the development of gastric volvulus or strangulation [13].

The diagnosis of eventration and/or phrenic palsy is usually suggested by the presence of an elevated hemidiaphragm on standard posteroanterior and lateral chest radiography. The diaphragmatic contour is unbroken, in distinction from CDH or traumatic hernia, and the gastric fundus is in a subdiaphragmatic position. These findings can be confirmed by computed tomography. Diaphragmatic movement is best confirmed by fluoroscopy, with normal but reduced movement seen in eventration. In contrast phrenic nerve palsy is associated with true paradoxical movement, i.e. elevation during inspiration. The diagnosis may only be confirmed beyond doubt at surgery via thoracoscopy or thoracotomy, at which point the integrity of the diaphragm can be confirmed. The phrenic nerve can also be assessed by direct stimulation.

## Surgical Management

The need for surgical intervention for either eventration or phrenic palsies depends on many factors. In infants the need for surgery is high in all but the most minor of cases, for the reasons listed earlier in this section. Acquired phrenic nerve palsies in infants are twice as likely as congenital palsies to require surgical intervention. As with CDH the priority should be stabilisation and ventilatory support in the first instance, with surgical repair undertaken once this has been achieved, usually within 2 weeks of the commencement of mechanical ventilation. In adults surgery is reserved for those with symptoms of dyspnoea or gastrointestinal disturbance after exclusion of other underlying pathologies.

Surgical treatment of eventration is primarily that of diaphragmatic plication via an open or thoracoscopic approach. The slack muscle and redundant central tendon are gathered in a series of radial pleats located to avoid the branches of the phrenic nerve [14]. The pleats are formed by the use of deep mattress sutures using heavy non-absorbable sutures. These may need to be buttressed with Teflon as the diaphragmatic tissue is often thin [15]. An alternative method that is suitable for localised eventration is to resect the affected part of the diaphragm and oppose normal edges in a two-layer repair [13]. Diaphragmatic plication has also been described via a thoracoscopic approach [16]. With both methods protection of underlying viscera and avoidance of excess tension are paramount.

## Results of Surgery

In both infants and adults it is essential to exclude other causes of dyspnoea, e.g. congenital cardiac disease or pulmonary conditions, and to correct exacerbating factors such as obesity, wherever possible. The results of surgery for eventration in infants are good with low perioperative morbidity and mortality and good functional results in the longer term [13]. In adults the results in selected patients also appear good, with demonstrable and prolonged improvement in respiratory function and symptoms [15,17,18].

# Traumatic Diaphragmatic Rupture

## Incidence and Aetiology

Diaphragmatic hernia (rupture) is a relatively uncommon and frequently undiagnosed sequel to both blunt and penetrating trauma involving the upper abdomen and thorax. First descriptions of this condition are attributed to Paré and Sennertus in the sixteenth century [19]. It was not until the nineteenth century that surgical treatments were attempted [20]. The true incidence of diaphragmatic rupture can be difficult to define because of the association with multiple injuries and tendency for late presentation. The incidence appears to be rising. However, it is unclear whether this is a true increase, or a reflection of increased awareness, improved diagnosis or better survival in polytrauma patients. Mansour cites an incidence of 0.8–1.6% in blunt thoracoabdominal trauma, rising to between 4 and 6% in those undergoing laparotomy or thoracotomy for trauma [19]. Rosati cites an incidence of up to 7% in blunt trauma, rising to 10–15% in penetrating thoracoabdominal trauma [20]. An injury scoring system specific to the diaphragm has been devised by the Organ Injury Scaling Committee of the American Association for the Surgery on Trauma. This grades the injury on a scale I–V depending on the nature of the injury (contusion versus laceration), the size of the defect and the total amount of tissue loss [21].

There are two potential mechanisms of injury in blunt trauma. One is the forceful herniation of contents through one of the weaker areas of the diaphragm, e.g. lumbocostal foramen. The other is a radial tear at the musculotendinous boundary of the diaphragm secondary to a sudden increase in intra-abdominal pressure against a closed glottis. Under normal circumstances a pressure differential of up to 20 mmHg exists across the diaphragm. However, during coughing or straining, the transdiaphragmatic pressure difference can rise to more than 100 mmHg. The forces acting on the chest and abdomen during road traffic accidents or falls may momentarily reach ten times this force [4]. Once the initial tear has been caused the influence of the transdiaphrgamatic pressure gradient, combined with the effects of coughing etc., will further widen the defect, pushing abdominal viscera into the chest.

Spontaneous healing of diaphragmatic injury does not occur. However, small defects may be temporarily plugged with omentum, preventing early visceral herniation. Less commonly direct trauma produces dehiscence of the muscular parts of the diaphragm from the chest wall. Diaphragmatic ruptures appear to be far more common on the left (80–90% of reported cases) with a small percentage bilateral (1–5%) [22]. However, the incidence of right-sided ruptures is significantly higher in some series, particularly those that include post-mortem findings [23].

Most large studies have shown that up to 40% of subsequently confirmed diaphragmatic ruptures are diagnosed preoperatively, with a similar proportion found unexpectedly at the time of thoracotomy or laparotomy [22,24]. The remaining cases have a delayed presentation: a small defect enlarges with time until the signs and symptoms of pulmonary compression, visceral strangulation, perforation or haemorrhage become apparent. Herniation may also occur after penetrating injury to the central tendon. Because of the domed shape of the diaphragm, the path of a penetrating object may cause an injury in more than one place, and small tears may be easily missed at laparotomy or thoracoscopy/thoracotomy. Diaphragmatic rupture has also been described spontaneously and in pregnancy, particularly during labour.

The overall mortality for patients with diaphragmatic rupture is fairly constant in several series, at 10–20% [4,20,22,23]. The majority of early fatal cases are secondary to associated injuries, particularly those involving the thorax and abdomen, as this group of patients have been shown to have high overall injury severity scores.

## Clinical and Radiological Diagnosis

The diagnosis of traumatic diaphragmatic rupture requires careful assessment and a high index of suspicion in patients with an appropriate mechanism of injury. It can be obscured by the presence of associated injuries which can be life-threatening in their own right. It has been estimated that between 7 and 66% of patients with polytrauma have a diaphragmatic rupture which is initially missed or misdiagnosed [24]. Correct diagnosis relies heavily on radiological investigations. Chest X-ray (CXR) is the most commonly available, and is very useful as an initial screening tool. The passage of a nasogastric tube helps to confirm the position of the stomach. Radiological features range from obvious loss of diaphragmatic contour associated with displacement of the stomach or bowel into the chest, through to more subtle signs. These include irregularity or elevation of the diaphragm and lower lobe atelectasis. These features can be misinterpreted as, or concealed by, those of a loculated hydrothorax. The CXR appearances of a left traumatic diaphragmatic hernia are shown in Figure 9.4. Overall CXR is diagnostic or suggestive of diaphragmatic rupture in 28–64% of cases [25]. Ultrasonography is valuable in confirming the diagnosis of diaphragmatic rupture, and has the advantages of being safe, portable, repeatable and readily available in most hospitals. The diagnostic sensitivity of ultrasound has been estimated at up to 82% [23]. However, it is less useful in the

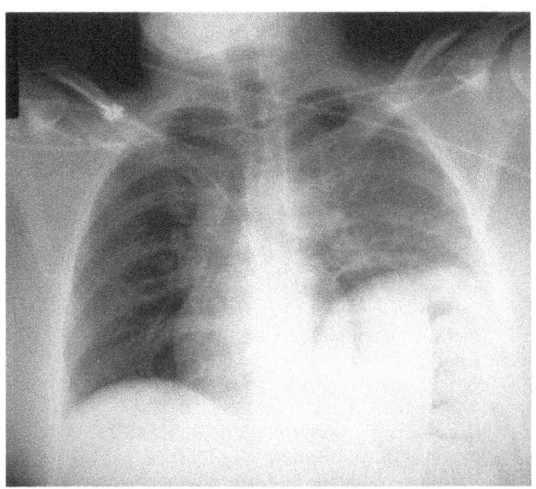

Figure 9.4. Chest X-ray of a left traumatic diaphragmatic hernia.

presence of significant chest wall trauma, surgical emphysema or pneumothorax.

Computed tomography (CT) is another diagnostic modality that is readily available in most hospitals and is commonly used to assess patients with thoracic and abdominal trauma. The main disadvantage of CT is that the diaphragm itself is difficult to directly image because of its axial position, and cannot be accurately distinguished from the liver on the right. Sagittal reconstructions and spiral CT, which are now becoming more widely available, are of greater value. Overall CT has been found to have a diagnostic sensitivity of 33–83% and specificity of 76–100%, and is considered the gold standard for diagnosing chronic herniation [4]. Magnetic resonance imaging (MRI) has the advantage of being able to produce sagittal and coronal images that facilitate the diagnosis of diaphragmatic injury. Unfortunately MRI is less available than CT in most centres, and excludes the examination of unstable patients requiring monitoring or ventilation because of the effects that the associated magnetic field has on metallic objects.

Laparoscopy and thoracoscopy have both been investigated in the diagnosis of diaphragmatic rupture. Smith and colleagues have reported their results using laparoscopy in 133 patients with thoracocabdominal injury [26]. They were able to identify and repair a diaphragmatic injury in only four cases (3%). The laparoscopy was diagnostic only, with no injury of any type identified, in over half of the cases ($n = 72$, 54%). This study excluded patients with cardiorespiratory instability and complex trauma, who are the group most likely to have sustained a significant diaphragmatic injury. The disadvantages of laparoscopy are that it requires a general anaesthetic and the induction of a pneumoperitoneum. Both of these can exacerbate cardiorespiratory instability, and the latter can precipitate tension pneumothorax in the presence of a diaphragmatic defect. The technique is expensive, operator-dependent and poor at visualising the right hemidiaphragm. Thoracoscopy has the advantage of better visualisation of either hemidiaphragm, but requires that the patient can tolerate single-lung anaesthesia, and can be hindered by the presence of pulmonary injury of intrathoracic adhesions. Overall it would seem that neither technique is of great value as a routine screening tool in the evaluation of diaphragmatic trauma per se.

## Surgical Management

In contrast to congenital hernias, diaphragmatic ruptures are better approached from the thorax [4]. The absence of a hernial sac and the presence of associated pulmonary and chest wall injuries predisposes to adhesions that may require careful dissection before the herniated organs can be returned to the abdomen. Thoracotomy or thoracoabdominal approaches are therefore recommended, and the latter has the advantage of enabling abdominal exploration at the same time. Most diaphragmatic lacerations or tears can be repaired directly with a one- or two-layer technique using nonabsorbable suture. Peripheral injuries may require reattachment of the diaphragm to the chest wall. Chronic large defects occasionally have to be repaired using a prosthetic patch.

## The Chronic Sequelae of Missed Traumatic Diaphragmatic Rupture

Despite the fact that a proportion of diaphragmatic injuries may initially be missed, most will eventually become clinically apparent in patients who survive. Symptoms may reflect pulmonary complications such as basal atelectasis, hydrothorax or mediastinal and pulmonary compression. Alternatively gastrointestinal symptoms secondary to visceral displacement, incarceration, strangulation, perforation or haemorrhage may predominate. This may produce a diagnostic conundrum as the symptoms may not localise to the abdomen. Only a small percentage of hernias will remain asymptomatic long term. Of those that do result in strangulation, the majority (85%) occur within 3 to 5 years of the initial injury [27,28]. For this reason all traumatic diaphragmatic hernias should be electively repaired once the patient's condition has been stabilised.

## Summary

Conditions affecting the diaphragm are generally uncommon in surgical practice but can affect all ages. The consequences of diaphragmatic herniation of any cause can be life-threatening, yet the diagnosis may be obscured by associated conditions and the effects of trauma. A thorough understanding of the developmental anatomy of the diaphragm aids diagnosis and facilitates surgical repair.

## Questions

1. Name the foramina of the diaphragm and structures passing through.
2. On which side do Bochdalek hernias most frequently occur?
3. Describe the cardiopulmonary changes that may be induced by a congenital diaphragmatic hernia.
4. How is the diagnosis of eventration made?
5. Describe the surgical treatment of traumatic hernias of the diaphragm.

## References

1. Fell S. Surgical anatomy of the diaphragm and the phrenic nerve. Chest Surg Clin N Am 1998;8:281–94.
2. Merendino K, Johnson R, Skinner H et al. The intradiaphragmatic distribution of the phrenic nerve with particular reference to the placement of diaphragmatic incisions and controlled segmental paralysis. Surgery 1956;39:189–98.
3. McMinn R (ed) Last's anatomy. Regional and applied, 8th edn. Edinburgh: Churchill Livingstone, 1990.
4. Schumpelick V, Steinau G, Schlüper I et al. Surgical embryology and anatomy of the diaphragm with surgical applications. Surg Clin N Am 2000;80:213–9.
5. Langer J. Congenital diaphragmatic hernia. Chest Surg Clin N Am 1998;8:295–314.
6. Gross R. Congenital hernia of the diaphragm. Am J Dis Child 1946;71:579–92.
7. Langer J, Winthrop A, Whelan D. Fryns syndrome: A rare familial cause of congenital diaphragmatic hernia. J Pediatr Surg 1994;29:1266–7.
8. Benjamin D, Juul S, Siebert J. Congenital posterolateral diaphragmatic hernia: Associated malformations. J Pediatr Surg 1988;23:899–903.
9. Schlembach D, Zenkerr M, Trautmann U et al. Deletion 15q24–26 in prenatally detected diaphragmatic hernia: Increasing evidence of a candidate region for diaphragmatic development. Prenat Diagn 2001;21:289–92.
10. Iritani I. Experimental study on embryogenesis of congenital diaphragmatic hernia. Anat Embryol (Berl) 1984;169:133–9.
11. Greenholz S. Congenital diaphragmatic hernia: An overview. Semin Pediatr Surg 1996;5:216–23.
12. Fasching G, Huber A, Uray E et al. Gastroesophageal reflux and diaphragmatic motility after repair of congenital diaphragmatic hernia. Eur J Pediatr Surg 2000;10:360–4.
13. Deslauriers J. Eventration of the diaphragm. Chest Surg Clin N Am 1998;8:315–30.
14. Schwartz M, Filler R. Plication of the diaphragm for symptomatic phrenic nerve paralysis. J Pediatr Surg 1978;13:259–63.
15. Graham D, Kaplan D, Evans C et al. Diaphragmatic plication for unilateral diaphragmatic paralysis: A 10-year experience. Ann Thorac Surg 1990;49:248–51.
16. Mouroux, J, Padovani B, Poirier N et al. Technique for the repair of diaphragmatic eventration. Ann Thorac Surg 1996;62:905–7.
17. Wright C, Williams J, Ogilvie C et al. Results of diaphragmatic plication for unilateral diaphragmatic paralysis. J Thorac Cardiovasc Surg 1985;90:195–8.
18. Ribet M, Linder JL. Plication of the diaphragm for unilateral eventration or paralysis. Eur J Cardiothorac Surg 1992;6:357–60.
19. Mansour K. Trauma to the diaphragm. Chest Surg Clin N Am 1997;7:373–83.
20. Rosati C. Acute traumatic injury of the diaphragm. Chest Surrg Clin N Am 1998;8:371–9.
21. Moore E, Malangoni M, Cogbill T et al. Organ injury scaling. IV: Thoracic vascular, lung, cardiac, and diaphragm. J Trauma 1994;36:299–300.
22. Shah R, Sabanathan S, Mearns A et al. Traumatic rupture of the diaphragm. Ann Thor Surg 1995;60:1444–9.
23. Pfannschmidt J, Seiler H, Bottcher H et al. Diaphragmatic ruptures: Diagnosis, therapy, results, experiences with 64 patients. Aktuelle Traumatol 1994;24:48–51.
24. Troop B, Myers R, Agarwal N. Early recognition of diaphragmatic injuries from blunt trauma. Ann Emerg Med 1985;p14:97–101.
25. Shackleton K, Stewart E, Taylor A. Traumatic diaphragmatic injuries: Spectrum of radiographic findings. Radiographics 1998;18:49–59.
26. Smith S, Fry W, Morabito D et al. Therapeutic laparoscopy in trauma. Am J Surg 1995;170:632–7.
27. Hood R. Traumatic diaphragmatic hernia. Ann Thorac Surg 1971;12:311–24.
28. Pomerantz M, Rodgers B, Sabiston DJ. Traumatic diaphragmatic hernia. Surgery 1968;64:529–34.

# 10

# Benign Diseases of the Spleen

Refaat B. Kamel

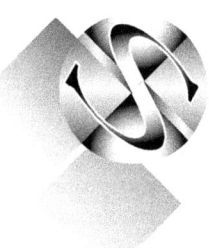

## Aims

- Identifying the value and functions of the spleen in health and diseases.
- The role of spleen in haematological disorders (sickle cell disease, thalassaemia, spherocytosis, idiopathic thrombocytopenic purpura).
- Haematological functions of the spleen (haemopoiesis in myeloproliferative disorders, red blood cell maturation, removal of red cell inclusions and destruction of senescent or abnormal red cells) and immunological functions (antibody production, removal of particulate antigens as well as clearance of immune complex and phagocytosis (source of suppressor T cells, source of opsonin that promotes neutrophil phagocytosis and production of "tuftsin").
- Effects of splenectomy on haematological and immunological functions.
- Complications and sequelae of splenectomy including overwhelming post-splenectomy infection (OPSI).
- Hyposplenism, asplenia and associated manifestations.
- Indications for splenectomy whether therapeutic or diagnostic.
- Alternatives to total splenectomy.
- Splenic conservation, various techniques.
- Splenic injuries and management.

## Introduction

The spleen has always been considered a mysterious and enigmatic organ. Aristotle concluded that the spleen was not essential for life. As a result of this, splenectomy was undertaken lightly, without a clear understanding of subsequent effects. Although Hippocrates described the anatomy of the spleen remarkably accurately, the exact physiology of the spleen continued to baffle people for more than a 1000 years after Hippocrates. The spleen was thought in ancient times to be the seat of emotions but its real function in immunity and to remove time-expired blood cells and circulating microbes, has only recently been recognised.

## Anatomy of the Spleen

The development of the spleen begins in the fifth week of intrauterine life. Mesenchymal cells, between the two mesothelial layers of the mesogastrium, aggregate and differentiate as the anlage of the spleen. Primitive vessels, during the second month of gestation, vascularise these cellular aggregates to form a lobulated embryonic spleen. Continued growth and formation occurs during fusion of the splenic lobules. From the fourth to eighth months, the spleen participates with the liver in haemocytopoiesis. After the eighth month and throughout postnatal life, the spleen resumes haemocytopoiesis only when bone marrow is incapable of meeting the demands of the body (extramedullary haemocytopoiesis), or in pathological circumstances.

The parenchyma of the spleen appears as greyish-white areas, the white pulp scattered in a spongy deep-reddish-purple substance, the red pulp. The white pulp consists of 0.2–0.8 mm masses of diffuse and nodular lymphatic tissue surrounding small arteries called central arteries. The white pulp undergoes involution between the ages of 10 and 14. After the age of 60, the spleen as a whole undergoes involution. The red pulp possesses unique *venous sinuses* supported in a spongy reticular stroma containing free erythrocytes, macrophages, reticular cells and other cells.

## Blood Supply

The blood supply to the spleen is provided by the *splenic* artery, the largest of the three branches of the coeliac artery. During its course, it sends branches to (1) the stomach (via the left gastroepiploic artery and a short gastric artery), (2) the pancreas (via the pancreatic artery) and (3) the spleen (via the end of the splenic artery). About 3.5 cm from the spleen, the splenic artery divides into superior and inferior terminal branches, each of which further subdivides into several smaller branches prior to penetrating the hilum of the spleen.

On the basis of comparative anatomy, the spleen has been divided into segments separated by fibrous septa [1]. Gupta et al. [2] inferred segmentation of the spleen on the basis of avascular planes. In one of our studies, we showed the parenchymal distribution of the splenic artery -and clarified the avascular planes in the human spleen. The mode of termination of the splenic artery was studied in 25 cadavers. Observation of the parenchymal distribution of the artery in 17 cases revealed avascular planes that divided the spleen into lobes, inside which other avascular planes separated the lobes into segments [3] (Figure 10.1).

Lymphatic vessels in the red pulp or white pulp of the human spleen are few. Lymphatic capillaries originating in the capsule and trabeculae converge on lymph nodes of the hilum and pancreaticoduodenal lymph nodes. Nodes in the splenic hilum are often involved in disease processes such as lymphoma, when the spleen is involved. Accessory spleens may be confused with these lymph nodes, whose appearance is vascular (haemolymph) on gross examination.

## Physiology

The spleen is the largest mass of lymphoid tissue in the body. Like a lymph node, the spleen provides for the storage of lymphocytes and their production; it removes foreign matter in the blood by the reticular cells; it prolongs the life of red cells by providing temporary shelter from certain ionic changes to which they are exposed in the circulation; it stores blood and can expel the contents into the circulation during haemorrhage, exercise or at high altitudes. Not only is the spleen involved in many systemic diseases but unsuspected splenic abnormalities may produce widespread effects. Unlike the lymph nodes, which are interposed in chains of lymphatic vessels to filter lymph, the spleen is situated in the course of the blood vascular system to filter blood. Added to this, the spleen receives a disproportionate amount of the circulating blood volume for its relatively small size. Hence, it becomes involved secondarily in a wide range of haematological disorders.

### Haematological Functions of the Spleen

Because of the peculiar anatomical arrangement of its blood vessels, the spleen is ideally suited as a site for fine quality control of the erythrocyte population. It removes fragmented, damaged or senescent red cells from the circulating blood, a process known as "culling". It also plays a role in remodelling the surface of the maturing erythrocytes and in preserving the normal relationship between their membrane surface area and volume. Target cells, which have a relatively high ratio of membrane to intracellular content, appear in the peripheral blood soon after splenectomy.

# BENIGN DISEASE OF THE SPLEEN

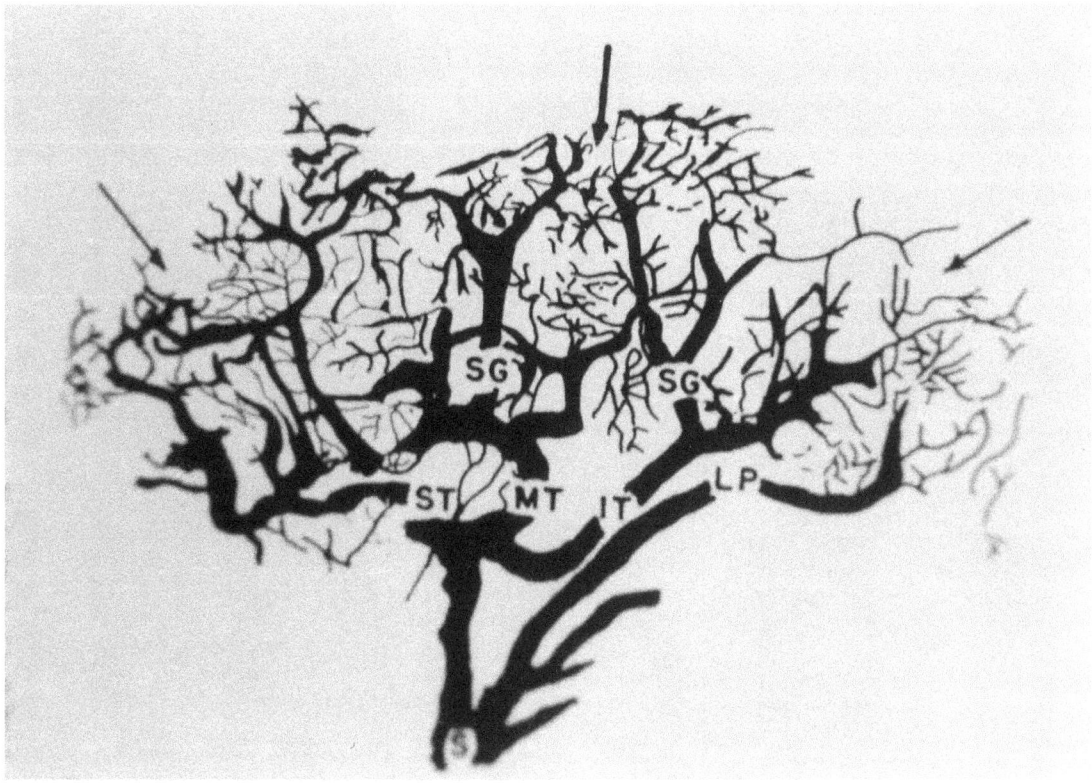

**Figure 10.1.** Arterial supply of the spleen. Arrows indicate avascular planes coinciding with surface notches. (S, Splenic; ST, superior terminal, MT, middle terminal; IT, inferior terminal, LP, lower polar; SG, segmented.)

A variety of intra-erythrocyte inclusions are removed by the spleen (through a process known as pitting), after which the red cells are returned to the circulation. Among the inclusions removed are Howell–Jolly bodies, which are probably nuclear remnants, siderotic granules, which are haemosiderin aggregates laid down during normal erythroid maturation, and Heinz bodies, which are pathological aggregates of denatured haemoglobin (normally the percentage of these abnormal cells and inclusions does not exceed 3%). Thus after splenectomy, Howell–Jolly bodies and siderotic granules may be seen in the peripheral blood and the red cells show striking changes in shape and size with the appearance of acanthocytes, irregularly crenated cells and target cells (their percentage may reach up to 20–25%) (Figures 10.2 to 10.6).

The human spleen unlike that of many animals contains relatively little blood and hence has no important storage role. It appears to sequester a significant number of platelets, however, and after splenectomy there is nearly always a transient thrombocytosis so that the need for preoperative platelet transfusion is not important. The increase in platelet count occurs intraoperatively shortly after splenic artery ligation during splenectomy.

## Splenic Pooling and Hypervolaemia

It has been known for many years that plasma volume is increased in patients with splenomegaly, while the red cell mass is normal or even increased, despite the venous haematocrit being depressed. Anaemia is to a large extent due to haemodilution. Similar observations were reported in patients with Gaucher's disease and massive splenomegaly. In patients with cirrhosis of the liver, expansion of the plasma volume is common and is not closely related to splenic enlargement. On the other hand, with

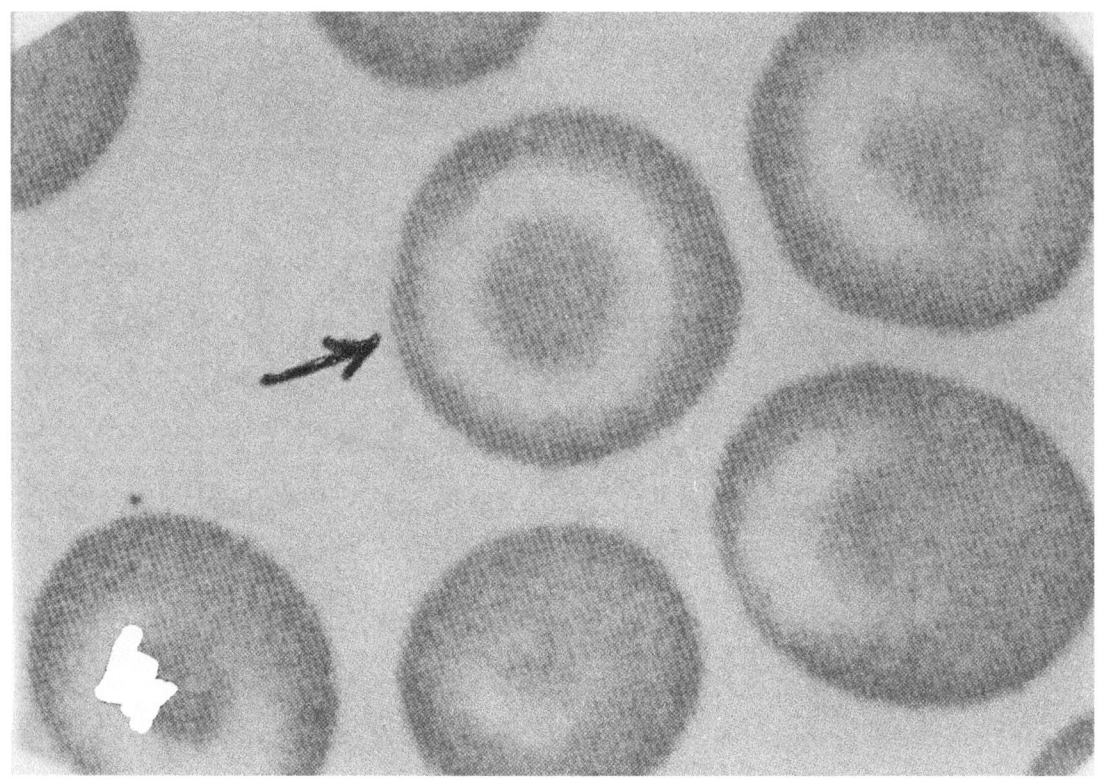

**Figure 10.2.** Target cells in the blood film.

moderate to massive splenomegaly, the spleen size does play a role, as there is a decrease in the plasma volume following splenectomy, although it may remain above normal.

Some authors have postulated that increased blood flow through an enlarged spleen acts as a functional arteriovenous shunt, the increased venous return to the heart causing a high cardiac output together with an increase in the blood volume. The increase in plasma volume has also been suggested to be the result of expansion of the intravascualr space consequent upon the development of splenomegaly.

Blood "doping" in athletes is a fairly recent innovation, but in some mammalian species the expulsion of high haematocrit intrasplenic blood, in order to raise the oxygen-carrying capacity of peripheral blood, is an effective physiological mechanism. Spleen of such species as horse, dog, cat, and diving seal are very contractile and serve as a reservoir of blood at high haematocrit. In times of "fight or flight", splenic contraction, which is produced by myoepithelial cells in the capsule or trabeculae, transfers blood from the reservoir into the circulation, and the splenic filtration function is put "on hold", since all blood flows via the fast pathways in contracted spleens, until the organ relaxes again. In the normal human spleen, this reservoir function appears to be lacking. In patients with splenomegaly, splenic contraction can increase portal venous pressure (paroxysmal portal hypertension), which can predispose to variceal bleeding, and this may have seasonal variation.

## Splenic Contraction

It is a common clinical observation that during an attack of haematemesis, the spleen diminishes in size because of contraction and

# BENIGN DISEASE OF THE SPLEEN

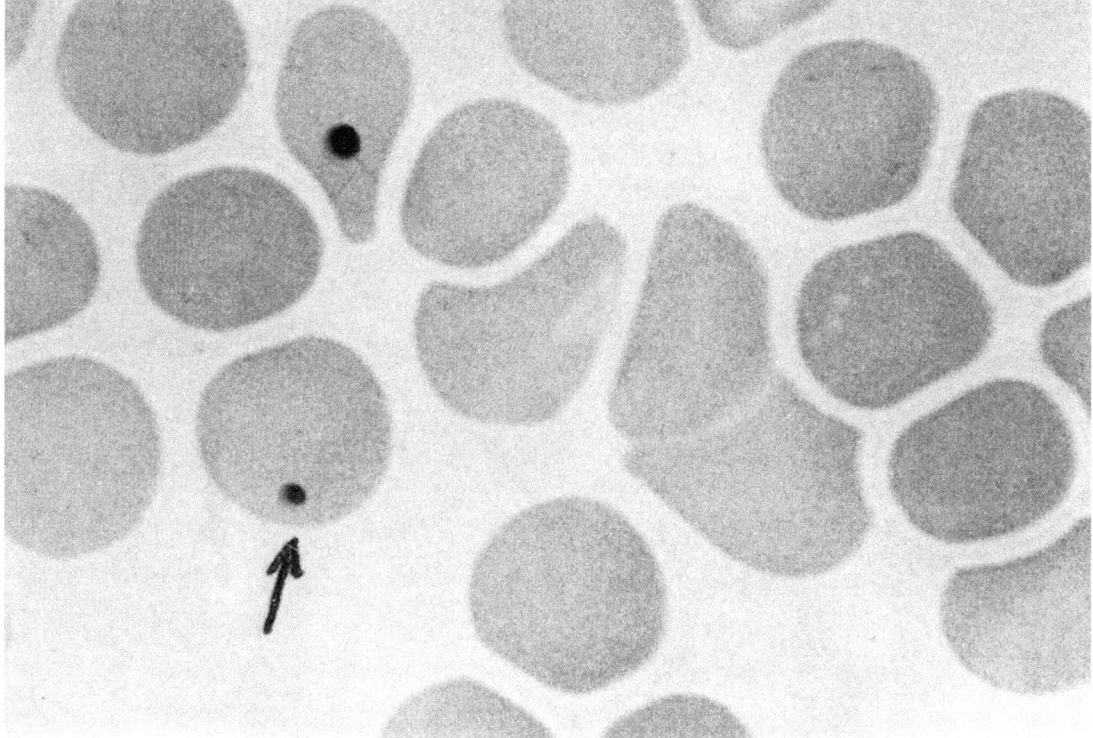

**Figure 10.3.** Howell–Jolly bodies in blood film.

the spleen may become impalpable or just palpable.

In the differential diagnosis of causes of haematemesis, the size of the spleen is usually put as a differentiating point between cases of portal hypertension and variceal haemorrhage and other causes such as bleeding peptic ulcer, but because of contraction of the spleen it is not helpful in the differential diagnosis of the cause of hematemesis.

In our experience, injection of vasoactive material into the splenic artery during surgery produces contraction of the spleen and can act as a form of autotransfasion.

## Immunological Functions

The anatomical location of the spleen in the circulatory system, and its structural organisation, provides a critical opportunity for contact with bloodborne antigens and for participation in the system of circulating lymphocytes. It has been calculated that the traffic of lymphoid cells through the spleen exceeds the combined cell traffic through all the lymph nodes of the body, with a daily exchange rate of about $5 \times 10^{11}$ lymphocytes.

The role of the spleen is relative to the liver in the clearance of particulate and is increased in the absence of opsonins. The spleen has a special role in the elimination of polysaccharide-encapsulated bacteria species. It is also an important source of antibody synthesis, particularly of the IgM class, and in the development of effector T lymphocytes. The population of lymphocytes in the spleen is in constant motion, a substantial proportion recirculating between lymph nodes and the spleen by way of the thoracic duct and bloodstream. In the case of the spleen about half of the small lymphocytes recirculate fairly rapidly.

The spleen is one of the principal sites of clearance of damaged and effete cells from the blood. It is also involved in the removal of circulating antibody-coated cells generated during autoimmune responses, which may give it a crit-

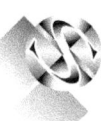

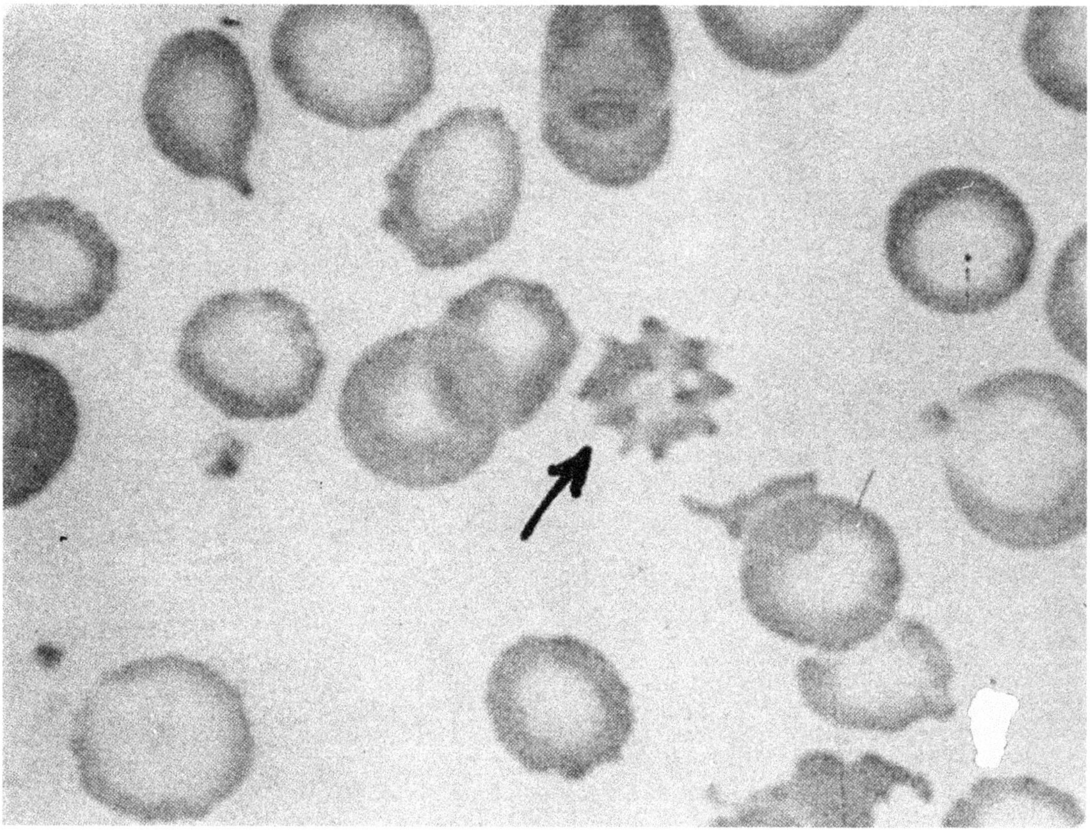

**Figure 10.4.** Acanthocytes in the blood film.

ical role in autoimmune haemolytic disease. The spleen, together with the liver, is an important site of the fixed macrophages, which remove particulate antigens from the blood.

### Tuftsin

The spleen is the normal site of one step in the production of the immunomodulatory molecule tuftsin. Among the numerous immunomodulatory molecules that have been identified, tuftsin is uniquely related to the spleen: tuftsin activity is not found in asplenic individuals. Among the biological activities attributed to tuftsin is the stimulation of phagocytosis. Tuftsin can help in management of overwhelming post-splenectorny infection (OPS1).

The main functions of the spleen are listed in Table 10.1.

## Congenital Anomalies of the Spleen

- Accessory spleens
- Splenic band
- Asplenia
- Polysplenia
- Wandering spleen that may predispose to torsion
- Splenic-gonadal fusion

## Accessory spleens

Accessory spleens are found in about 10–18% of the general population. The most common location is within the splenic hilum, along the course

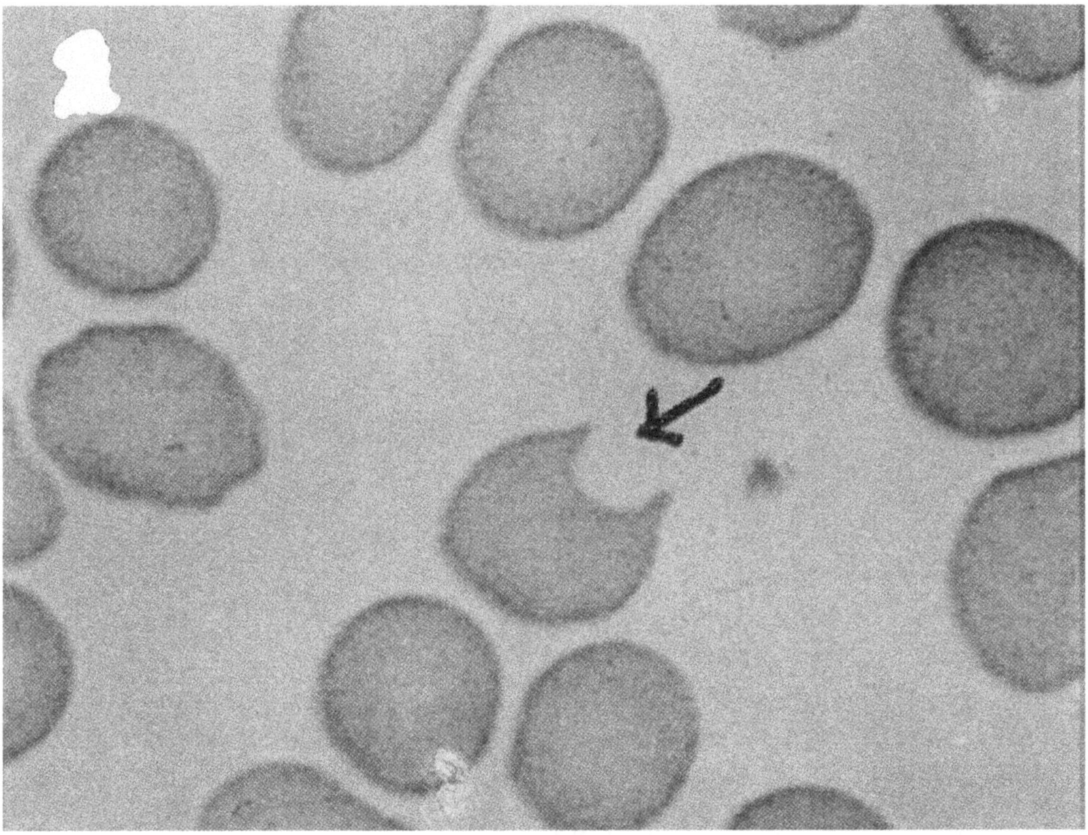

# BENIGN DISEASE OF THE SPLEEN

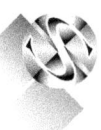

**Figure 10.5.** Pitted red blood cells.

**Table 10.1.** Main Functions of Spleen

*Immunological*
1. Antibody production and cell-mediated responses
2. Removal of particulate antigens and clearance of immune complex
3. Phagocytosis:
   - Maturation of lymphoid cells
   - Significant lympopoiesis
   - Source of suppressor T cells
   - Source of opsonins that promote neutrophil phagocytosis
   - Production of immunomodulatory molecule "tuftsin"

*Haematological*
- Haemopoiesis during intrauterine life, and compensatory haemopoiesis later in life, as in myeloproliferative disorders
- Red blood cell remodelling and maturation
- Filtration of particles from blood: non-specific or antibody coated
- Removal of red cell inclusions
- Destruction of senescent or abnormal red cells
- Storage of platelets, iron and factor VIII

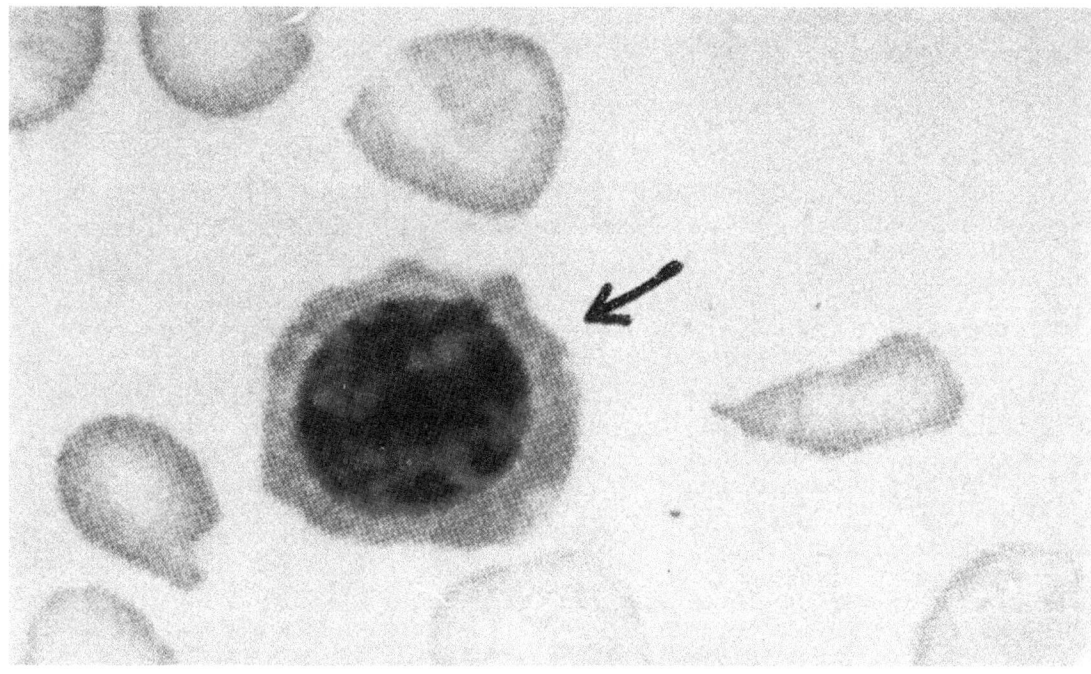

**Figure 10.6.** Normoblasts in blood film.

of the splenic artery, or within the tail of the pancreas. Other common locations include the omentum, the gastrosplenic and splenocolic ligaments, and the mesentery of the small bowel. Occasionally an accessory spleen is found in presacral, pelvic or paratesticular locations. The accessory spleen is generally involved through the same pathological process as the primary spleen.

When total splenectomy is performed for disorders such as hereditary spherocytosis, hereditary elliptocytosis or idiopathic thrombocytopenic purpura, a careful search should be made and any accessory spleens present should also be removed. After splenectomy, an accessory spleen may enlarge and cause recurrence of the symptoms for which the original surgery was performed. Howell–Jolly bodies normally appear within the erythrocytes after splenectomy; when these are absent, an accessory spleen should be suspected. The combination of CT scan and radionuclide scan provides satisfactory diagnostic accuracy in identifying the location of the accessory spleen. The treatment of choice is surgical removal, if an accessory spleen causes recurrence of a haematological disorder.

## Asplenia

The absence of the spleen (asplenia) occurs after surgical removal (iatrogenic), or it is congenital. Trauma is the most common reason for removing the spleen in children and sickle cell disease is the most common cause of functional asplenia in children. Congenital absence of the spleen is usually associated with serious malformations, primarily cardiovascular and abdominal heterotaxia.

The embryological control of splenogenesis resides in the homeobox gene, HOXDII. In humans, the spleen is the site of early haematopoietic development, particularly of erythrocytes, for the first four months of gestation. After birth, the spleen has several important functions, importantly the provision of primary immunological defensive responses. The spleen has an active role in phagocytosis, production of IgM antibodies, and complement; it also plays a significant role in the functional maturation of antibodies. It is a significant reservoir for T lymphocytes. The percentages of total T cells (CD3), T-helper cells (CD4) and the lymphoproliferative responses to mitogens

# BENIGN DISEASE OF THE SPLEEN

(concanavalin A, phytohaemagglutinin and pokeweed mitogen) may decrease in asplenic patients. However, these T-cell changes reflect the loss of the spleen as a reservoir rather than a direct T-cell abnormality.

The impaired clearance of opsonized particles, decreased IgM levels, and poor antibody production (especially to polysaccharide antigens) contribute to the increased susceptibility of these patients to serious and often fatal infections. Apart from this filtering and immunological function, the spleen is an important scavenger: it participates in the destruction of all three-blood elements – the erythrocytes, white cells and the platelets. It plays and important role in selective removal of abnormal cells (spherocytes, poikilocytes) and intracellular inclusions (Heinz bodies, Howell–Jolly bodies). These functions, known as culling and pitting respectively, and are the basis for the hematological abnormalities seen in patients with absent splenic function.

## Causes of Hyposplenism or Asplenism

*Common Surgical Causes*

1. Splenectomy
2. Partial splenectomy or segmental splenectomy (a certain volume of the spleen should be left a little larger than normal to maintain a state of eusplenism; cf. euthyroidism)

*Common Medical Causes*

1. Coeliac disease, cirrhosis, vasculitis and systemic lupus erythematosus

*Other Causes of Hyposplenism*

1. Cyanotic heart disease
2. Ulcerative colitis
3. Haemoglobinopathy
4. Splenic arterial or venous occlusion
5. HIV infection
6. High dose corticosteroid

## Polysplenia

Congenital anomalies of the spleen may be isolated, but most cases of asplenia/polysplenia result from interference of establishment of normal right–left asymmetry during embryogenesis (laterality sequences). Asplenia may be viewed as bilateral right-sidedness of which Ivemark's syndrome is an example.

Polysplenia is usually associated with other congenital anomalies of the cardiovascular or gastrointestinal systems (polysplenia syndrome) (Figure 10.7). Polysplenia syndrome is more predominant in females, whereas asplenia is more common in males.

Accessory spleens should be distinguished from polysplenia. In polysplenia, there is absence of a normal spleen along with multi-system involvement. Accessory spleens are usually located in the hilum of the spleen or the tail of the pancreas in addition to the presence of a normal spleen. Normally the accessory splenules are very small and clinically insignificant but may hypertrophy under certain situations.

## Splenic Torsion (Ectopic Spleen)

Elongation of the splenic pedicle and increase in its mass predispose the organ to torsion and subsequent infarction. This rare condition occurs in mutiparous women and in children. An elongated pedicle without torsion results in an ectopic or "wandering spleen". This is thought to be congenital and due to a persistent dorsal mesogastrium in children, but may be acquired in multiparous women.

Diagnosis of acute splenic torsion requires some clinical awareness, and is often inade only at laparotomy. Splenectomy is indicated if the spleen remains non-viable after untwisting the pedicle, and may be necessary if the mobile organ cannot be safely fixed in the left upper quadrant. Splenic preservation has been achieved by plication of the elongated pedicle with fixation of the spleen to the abdominal wall or left hemidiaphragm (splenopexy).

## Splenogonadal Fusion

Splenogonadal fusion is a rare congenital anomaly whereby the left gonad is typically fused to a segment of splenic tissue. A single case of splenogonadal fusion occurring on the right side has been reported. The clinical presentation of splenogonadal fusion is usually as a scrotal mass, left inguinal hernia, hydrocele and undescended testis. It may be associated with pain in the region of the testicles during running (due to splenic contraction).

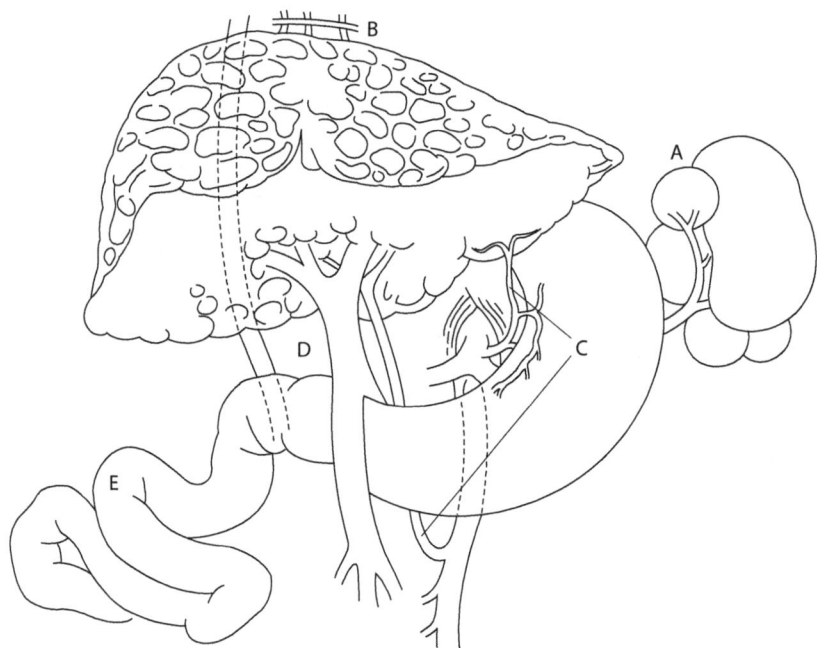

**Figure 10.7.** Commonly associated anatomic findings in patients who have situs inversus and billary atresia. A, polysplenia; B, interrupted inferior vena cava with azygous discontinuation; C, aberrant arterial supply with left hepatic artery from either left gastric artery or from superior mesenteric artery; D, preduodenal portal vein; E, gut malrotation.

## Hypersplenism

Hypersplenism can be considered as a state in which the spleen is more harmful than beneficial and splenectomy will improve the patient's state. Hypersplenism is usually associated with anaemia, neutropenia or thrombocytopema. The neutropenia may be so severe as to cause recurrent infections and the thrombocytopenia may be associated with purpura. It is vitally important to obtain a good bone marrow sample as a part of the routine work-up of patients with suspected hypersplenism. Table 10.2 lists conditions that may be associated with hypersplenism.

In assessing whether the removal of an enlarged spleen will benefit the patient there are two main factors to be considered: the cause of splenomegaly and whether there is a significant degree of hypersplenism.

There are some conditions in which splenectomy is almost always associated with an improvement in the patient's clinical condition. However, there are many disorders including haemolytic anaemia, the myeloproliferative states, Felty's syndrome and some malignancies in which there may be a significant degree of splenomegaly and hypersplenism, but it is not clear to what degree the spleen is contributing to the clinical disability.

In malaria, alterations in the white blood picture are rather marked and stable and hence are used by clinicians as one of the differential diagnostic symptoms. These changes are largely characterized by leucopenia, neutropenia with a shift in the direction of staff neutrophils and eosinopenia with relative lymphocytosis [4].

## Focal Disease of the Spleen

### Cysts

Cystic lesions of the spleen have a varied aetiology, and include the "true" cyst containing an epithelial lining and believed to be congenital in origin, the "false" cyst, which is probably post-traumatic, and other less common lesions

# BENIGN DISEASE OF THE SPLEEN

**Table 10.2.** Conditions associated with hypersplenism

|  | Syndrome | Specific diseases of clinical importance |
|---|---|---|
| Primary | Idiopathic non-tropical splenomegaly | Dacie's syndrome |
|  | Cysts and tumours | Haemangioma |
|  |  | Haemangiosarcoma |
| Secondary | Acute and chronic infections | Tuberculosis |
|  |  | Subacute bacterial endocarditis |
|  |  | Kala-azar |
|  | Tropical splenomegaly | Malaria |
|  | Hodgkin's disease |  |
|  | Non-Hodgkin's lymphoma |  |
|  | Infiltrative disorder |  |
|  | (a) Hereditary | Gaucher's disease |
|  | (b) Acquired | Sarcoidosis |
|  |  | Arnyloidosis |
|  | Autoinimune disorders | Felty's syndrome |
|  |  | Systemic lupus erythematosus |
|  | Haematological "big spleen" syndromes | Primary myeloid metaplasia |
|  |  | Chronic leukaemia |
| Portal hypertension | Presinusoidal | Schistosomiasis |
|  | Sinusoidal | Cirrhosis |
|  | Postsinusoidal | Budd–Chiari syndrome |
|  | *Other presinusoidal:* |  |
|  | Portal vein occlusion |  |
|  | Cavernomatous transformation as in cases of neonatal umbilical sepsis |  |
|  | Splenic vein obstruction |  |
|  | ("Left-sided portal hypertension") |  |

such as cystic neoplasms and parasitic cysts (hydatid cyst).

On radiographic examination, a large, usually solitary splenic mass is identified in the left upper quadrant of the abdomen. While these are most commonly found in patients in the second or third decade, they may also be discovered in children.

On $^{99m}$technetium-sulphur colloid scintigraphy, a splenic cyst will be seen as a large photopenic zone representing the mass, often partially surrounded by a crescent of normal but compressed spleen.

On CT a splenic cyst appears as a large, well-defined, non-enhancing, near-water density lesion having a smooth wall. It is usually found in subscapular locations, but approximately one-third are located deep within the spleen. Although approximately 80% are solitary and unilocular, 20% are multiple or multilocular.

Ultrasound is also useful for identifying the splenic origin of the cyst, as well as in distinguishing cystic from solid complex lesions.

## Splenic Abscess

This condition is most often secondary to disease elsewhere. Many cases of left-sided subphrenic abscess originate as abscesses of the spleen, and as a rule result from contiguous or from metastatic infection; the latter is more frequent and begins with clotting or from emboli. Contiguous infection spreads from the lung sometimes after injury; from the colon; rarely from the stomach. The appendix and fallopian tube are distant sources of infection, and splenic abscess can follow typhoid fever, dysentery, relapsing fever and influenza. The abscess following typhoid fever is said to have the best prognosis. Chronic tuberculosis may occur.

Splenic abscess may be multiple in haematogenous spread (75%) or solitary due to infarction, haematoma and direct extension. Complications of splenic abscess include fistula formation, rupture (43% mortality) and sepsis.

Ultrasonography reveals the appearance of splenic abscess as focal or multifocal lesions,

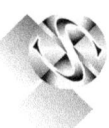

simple cysts or complex mass and bright echoes, if there is a gas. CT scan reveals a hypodense area, fluid ± gas density or portal venous gas (rare).

### Candidal Abscess

- Occurs most frequently in immunocompromised patients.
- Hasa microabscess pattern.
- May mimic *Pneumocystis carinii*, MAC, *Bordetella*, Gaucher's disease, sarcoid.

Ultrasonography reveals:

- wheel within wheel
- bulls-eye
- hypoechoic
- echogenic, shadowing.

### Hamartoma

Splenic hamartomas are usually solitary but may be multiple. White pulp or red pulp tissue, or a mixture thereof, may predominate. Plain films are either normal or show some degree of splenomegaly.

Calcifications found in splenic hamartomas range from punctate to stellate in configuration, and have been found in the fibrotic portions of the lesions rather than within the vascular channels. The solid lesion may appear nearly isodense with the spleen on contrast-enhanced CT. Cystic hamartomas demonstrate both solid and cystic components on CT and ultrasound.

### Lymphoma

Lymphomatous involvement of the spleen as a manifestation of systemic lymphonia is common. whereas primary splenic lymphoma is relatively uncommon. Lymphoma in the spleen characteristically involves the white pulp, frequently appearing as nodules. In advanced disease, the entire spleen may be replaced by tumour. Splenomegaly in splenic lymphoma is not a reliable sign.

On ultrasonography, lymphomatous involvement of the spleen is usually seen as single or multiple inhomogeneous, hypoechoic, nodular lesions of variable size.

### Haemangioma

Although rare, the haemangioma is the most common benign tumour of the spleen, it is usually asymptomatic and frequently presents as splenomegaly or as a mass in the left upper quadrant

#### Radiology

- Plain film: splenomegaly, rare calcification.
- Anglography: hypovascular or predominantly hypervascular.
- Ultrasonography: echogenic or complex.
- CT: calcification, homogeneous solid or multicystic and rim enhancement; may fill in.

### Lymphangioma

- Usually diffuse but may be focal.
- May be part of systemic angiomatosis (lung, liver, kidney, bone, etc.).
- Patients complain of pain, rarely coagulaopathy; there may be other symptoms and signs if other organs are involved.
- Simple (capillary), cavernous, and cystic types.
- Plain films: splenomegaly- calcification rare.
- Angiography: "Swiss cheese" pattern.
- Ultrasonography/CT/MRI: multilocular cysts or multiple cysts – rarely, one (abdominal) cyst.
- Internal echoes or higher density if blood, debris or proteinaceous fluid present – MR characteristics of lymph.

### Treatment

Treatment of proven splenic abscesses has previously been splenectomy and antibiotics. However, over the last 20 years there has been a definite trend towards splenic conservation in relation to trauma, with clear evidence of predisposition to fatal sepsis and haematological disturbance after splenectomy. This can be achieved by percutaneous drainage of splenic abscesses (ultrasound-guided drainage) if there is no improvement in the condition after antibiotic chemotherapy.

# BENIGN DISEASE OF THE SPLEEN

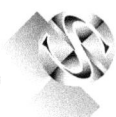

## Diffuse Disease

### Splenomegaly

Splenomegaly is probably the most common finding in the presence of diffuse splenic disease. The differential diagnosis of splenomegaly and associated findings may help in differentiating the various causes. However, many diseases causing splenomegaly without specific characteristics can be diagnosed on the basis of clinical or laboratory data.

### Splenomegaly due to Increased Demand for Splenic Function

1. *Reticuloendothelial system hyperplasia (for removal of defective erythrocytes).* Spherocytosis – early sickle cell anaemia – ovalocytosis – thalassaemia major – haemoglobinopathies – paroxysmal nocturnal haemoglobinuria – nutritional anaemia.
2. *Immune hyperplasia: (response to infection).* Infectious mononucleosis – AIDS – viral hepatitis – cytomegalovirus – SBE – bacterial septicaemia – congenital syphilis – splenic abscess – tuberculosis – histoplasmosis – malaria – leishmaniasis – trypanosomiasis.
3. *Disordered immuno regulation.* Rheumatoid arthritis (Felty's syndrome) – systemic lupus erythematosus – collagen vascular diseases – serum sickness – immune haemolytic anaemias – immune thrombocytopenia – immune neutropenias – drug reactions – angioimmunoblastic lymphadenopathy – sarcoldosis – thyrotoxicosis – (benign lymphoid hypertrophy).
4. *Extramedullary haematopoiesis.* Myelofibrosis – marrow damage by toxins, radiation, strontium – marrow infiltration by tumours, leukaemias, Gaucher's disease.

### Splenomegaly due to Abnormal Pplenic or Portal Blood Flow

Cirrhosis – hepatic vein obstruction – portal vein obstruction (intrahepatic or extrahepatic) – cavernous transformation of portal vein – splenic vein obstruction – splenic artery aneurysm – hepatic schistosomiasis – congestive heart failure – hepatic echinococcosis – portal hypertension (due to any of the previous causes): Bantl's disease.

### Infiltration of the Spleen (Intracellular or Extracellular)

Amyloidosis – Gaucher's disease – Niemann–Pick disease – Tangier disease – Hurler's syndrome and other mucopolysaccharidoses – hyperlipidaemias.

### Benign and Malignant Cellular Infiltrations

Letikaemias (acute, chronic, lymphoid, myeloid, monocytic) – lymphomas – Hodgkin's disease – myeloproliferative syndromes (e.g. polycythamia vera) – angiosarconias – metastatic tumours (melanoma is most coininon) – eosinophilic granuloina – histiocytosis X – hamartomas – haemangiomas, fibromas, lymphangiomas – splenic cysts.

### Unknown Aetiology

Idiopathic splenomegaly – berylliosis – iron deficiency anaemia.

## Spleen and Haematological Diseases

### The Spleen and Sickle Cell Disease

Sickle cell disease is due to homozygous inheritance of the HbS variant. It is one of the commonly inherited haemoglobinopathies worldwide, with a variable spectrum of severity. In the eastern province of Saudi Arabia, sickle cell disease (SCD) is common and has been reported to be more benign than in other parts of the world. This has been attributed to high levels of HbF and the frequently associated alpha thalassaemia.

The standard treatment of SCD has remained largely unchanged. It involves general preventive measures, as well as therapy for specific complications. One of the main organs to be

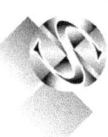

affected early in SCD is the spleen, which is commonly enlarged during the first decade of life, but then undergoes progressive atrophy, due to repeated attacks of vaso-occlusion and infarction, leading to siderofibrotic nodules (autosplenectomy).

## Indications for Splenectomy in SCD

As a general rule, splenectomy should be avoided in patients with SCD, as these patients are already susceptible to infection, especially during the first 3 years of life. This is attributed to several factors, which include early splenic dysfunction. Other contributory factors include defective opsonisation due to abnormality of the alternative pathway for complement activation, neutrophil dysfunction, deficiency in heat-labile serum opsonising activity and lack of circulating specific antibodies characteristic of early infancy.

To obviate the risks of splenectomy, and especially of overwhelming post-splenectomy infection (OPSI), splenic preservation is being increasingly advocated. The main indications for splenectomy in SCD are (1) acute splenic sequestration crisis, (2) hypersplenism, and (3) splenic abscess.

## Splenic Sequestration

Much of the severe morbidity and mortality of sickle cell anaemia in the first few years of life is a consequence of the so-called acute splenic sequestration crisis. These catastrophic events are characterised by severe anaemia, splenomegaly, hypovolaemic shock and sudden death, and it was suggested that patients had literally "bled into their spleen". Infants and young children with sickle cell anaemia whose spleens have not yet undergone multiple infarctions and subsequent fibrosis, and those individuals with other forms of sickle cell disease, whose spleens remain enlarged into adult life, can suddenly have intrasplenic pooling of vast amount of blood.

During severe splenic sequestration, the spleen becomes enormous, filling the abdomen and even reaching into the pelvis. The usual clinical manifestations of this complication are sudden weakness, pallor of the lips and mucous membranes, tachycardia, tachypnoea, and abdominal fullness. Splenic sequestration is one of the most dangerous events in the life of a patient with sickle cell anaemia and must be promptly treated. Treatment of the acute splenic sequestration is directed toward the prompt correction of hypovolaemia with plasma expanders followed by red cell transfusion. A dramatic regression of splenomegaly and rise in haemoglobin level can occur in a short time after transfusion.

## Spleen and Idiopathic Thrombocytopenic Purpura (ITP)

Idiopathic thrombocytopenic purpura mainly affects females between the ages of 15 and 50 years. It presents with bruising, usually after trauma or pressure, and examination reveals variable numbers of petechial haemorrhages in the skin. The clinical course is often intermittent and chronic. The platelets of affected patients become sensitised by antiplatelet IgG autoantibodies and are then removed from the circulation. Many patients need no treatment if their platelet count remains over $50 \times 10^9/l$ and no spontaneous bleeding occurs. If the count falls below $20 \times 10^9/l$, the risk of bleeding increases. Splenectomy is indicated, the spleen being the initial and major site of antibody production and also the major site of platelet destruction. Good results are usually obtained, with approximately 80% of patients having a satisfactory outcome, no longer requiring steroids to maintain an adequate number of platelets. However, in more heavily sensitised patients, platelets can continue to be destroyed elsewhere in the reticuloendothelial system, including the liver, and after an initial good response a relapse may also occur secondarily to an acute bacterial or viral illness. A good response is most likely in patients under 45 years, in those in whom the thrombocytopenia is less severe, and in those who have shown at least an initial response to steroid therapy. At operation, the spleen is usually of normal size and no special technique is needed for its removal, although a careful search must be made to ensure that no splenunculi remain. Although the preoperative platelet count may be very low, platelet transfusion is not begun until the splenic vessels have been ligated, when 6 to 10 units of platelet may be transfused. In addition, some patients may benefit from high doses of intravenous gammaglobulin preoperatively

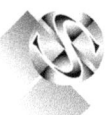

to raise the platelet count to an acceptable level (greater than $20 \times 10^9/l$).

## Spleen and Spherocytosis

The disorders of the red cell membrane are a very heterogeneous group. They fall into two main categories – inherited and acquired. Inherited red cell membrane disorders are mainly caused by a decrease in the expression of one or more specific proteins on the membrane of the cell. This causes the membrane to become unstable by splenic pitting, causing spherocytosis of the cell. Spherocytes, being less deformable than discocytes, become trapped in the microcirculation of the spleen and are destroyed by the spleen and the reticuloendothelial (RE) system, resulting in haemolytic anaemia.

The most common of the hereditary membrane defects is hereditary spherocytosis (HS). This is a very clinically heterogeneous disorder in which the whole spectrum of gravity may be covered, from no clinical expression to death in utero. Most patients experience haemolytic anaemia, with or without the need for regular blood transfusion, but the disease may be complicated by aplastic or haemolytic crises and biliary tract disease.

The diagnosis of HS has always been based on clinical symptoms and laboratory data, the most common clinical signs being jaundice, anaemia, splenomegaly and biliary stones together with the presence of spherocytes in the peripheral blood film. The traditional methods of diagnosing spherocytosis are the osmotic fragility test, autohaemolysis, acid glycerol lysis, Pink test and cryohaemolysis test. These tests are insensitive because the results are subjective as they rely on human judgement to decide whether the test is positive or negative. A new technique has been developed, the dye-binding flow cytometric method for detection of red cell membrane abnormalities.

Pyruvate kinase deficient reticulocytes are able to circumvent their defect by using the oxidative phosphorylation pathway to produce ATP. This ability is diminished when the reticulocytes are exposed to hypoxia or when they mature to adult red cells. This explains why most of the haemolysis occurs when the reticulocytes are trapped in the hypoxic environment of the spleen and why a paradoxical rise in reticulocyte number occurs after splenectomy.

### Treatment

1. *Medical care.* Simple blood transfusion for anaemia or exchange transfusion for severe hyperbilirubinaemia may be needed for symptomatic newborns.
2. *Surgical care.* For surgical care, consider splenectomy and partial splenectomy. Preoperative vaccination (Pneumovax) and preoperative antibiotics should be given to avoid OPSI.

*Splenectomy*

- This surgical procedure is frequently performed to eliminate or minimise the need for blood transfusion.
- Splenectomy is not curative but may eliminate or decrease the need for blood transfusions in transfusion-dependent patients.
- In an attempt at splenic conservation, partial splenectomy has been tried but results are not satisfactory and total splenectomy may be resorted to.

*Gallstones*

Pigment stones are a common complication of congenital spherocytosis and are found most often in young adults in the third decade of life. The presence of stones is usually considered an indication for cholecystectomy at the same time as splenectomy. If not done simultaneously, we prefer splenectomy first. Bile duct stones should be classically treated.

## Spleen and Thalassaemia

The pathogenesis of the anaemia of thalassaemia is multifactorial. Inclusion bodies are rarely found in the peripheral blood of thalassaemic patients with a normally functioning spleen. However, splenectomised patients with thalassaemia major show inclusion bodies within their red cells, indicating that the spleen is important for the clearance of globin chain precipitates. $^{51}$Cr-labelled red cell studies show increased uptake of the thalassaemic cells by the spleen.

Light microscopic examination of splenic tissue from patients with thalassaemia major shows an accumulation of red cells within the splenic cords. The interendothelial slits are the most important barrier to red cell passage: electron microscopic studies demonstrate marked distortion of the thalassaemic cells as they pass through these apertures, and red cells containing inclusion bodies are disrupted during their passage through them.

Splenomegaly is a common sequela of thalassaemia major. This can result in hypersplenism and increased red cell transfusion requirements. Hypertransfusion programmes designed to maintain the patient's haemoglobin within the normal range have decreased the spleen size in some patients, which may be due to diminished red cell pooling, or possibly a reduction in extramedullary haematopoiesis within the spleen.

Some thalassaemia patients benefit from splenectomy performed to alleviate the hypersplenism and decrease red cell transfusion requirements. Several studies have attempted to define factors capable of predicting the optimal time for splenectomy in these patients. Some would recommend splenectomy when transfusion requirements progressively rise above their previous baseline.

# Spleen and Tropical Diseases

## Tropical Splenomegaly Syndrome (Hyper-reactive Malarial Splenomegaly, Big Spleen Disease)

### Definition

Tropical splenomegaly syndrome or big spleen disease is massive enlargement of the spleen resulting from an abnormal immune response to repeated attacks of malaria. It is seen among residents of areas for endemic malaria and it is not species specific. It occurs mainly in tropical Africa, but also in parts of Vietnam, New Guinea, India, Sri Lanka, Thailand, Indonesia, South America and the Middle East. It must be differentiated from splenomegaly associated with acquisition of immunity in endemic and hyperendemic areas.

Tropical splenomegaly syndrome is characterized by massive splenomegaly, hepatomegaly, marked elevations in levels of serum IgM and malaria antibody. Hepatic sinusoidal lymphocytosis is also seen. In about 10% of African patients, it may be associated with peripheral lymphocytosis (B cells).

The peripheral smear shows manifestations of hypersplenism. Malarial parasites are not found in the peripheral blood. There is an increase ill the serum levels of polyclonal IgM with cryoglobulinaemla.

### Differential Diagnosis

The condition should be differentiated from other causes of splenomegaly in the tropics, i.e. kala-azar, schistosomasis, post-necrotic cirrhosis, thalassaemia, leukaemia, lymphoma, myelofibrosis, non-tropical idiopathic splenomegaly and Felty's syndrome.

### Surgery in Hyper-reactive Malarial Splenomegaly

In patients with uncomplicated hyper-reactive malarial splenomegaly, splenectomy seems to produce initial symptomatic improvement, with correction of anaemia, IgM and hypersplenism, and with an acceptable operative mortality. However, subsequent mortality rates, apparently due to overwhelming sepsis or malaria. Splenectomy seems indicated in the minority of patients who do not respond to prolonged antimalarial medication.

## Spleen and Kala-azar (Visceral Leishmaniasis)

*Leishmania donovani* parasites invade the reticuloendothelial cells of the spleen (liver and lymph nodes) and multiply. Patients with progressive disease develop marked splenomegaly due to hyperplasia of reticuloendothelial cells that are filled with parasites, and splenic infarcts are common. In acute cases, the spleen is smooth and friable, but it is firm in the more usual chronic cases.

*Splenectomy* is occasionally employed in patients with visceral leishmaniasis who are resistant to other forms of treatment. There is usually a rise in haemoglobin levels and white blood cell and platelet counts after splenectomy, but additional chemotherapy is necessary, because cure is unlikely otherwise.

## Spleen and Schistosomiasis

Splenomegaly and hypersplenism result from chronic *Schistosoma mansoni* infection and are frequent indications for splenectomy in endemic areas of the world. Partial splenectomy (segmental splenectomy) has been described for this disorder [5,6]. Fifty-one patients who underwent segmental splenectomy and 44 patients treated by total splenectomy for schistosomiasis were followed: the percentage of T lymphocytes increased after segmental splenectomy, and there was also an increased T-helper:T-suppressor cell ratio after segmental splenectomy. Only two patients required conversion from partial to total splenectomy for technical reasons, and no increase in size of the splenic remnant was noted during the subsequent 2 to 4 years. To our knowledge, this is the largest series of randomized elective partial (segmental) splenectomies reported and provides encouraging data in favour of the concept of partial splenectomy for hypersplenism.

Massive splenomegaly may suggest the presence of a splenic follicular lymphoma. This rare tumour occurred in 1% of patients with hepatic schistosomiasis who underwent splenectomy. It is the only malignancy whose incidence is definitely increased in hepatic schistosomiasis. Although no definite relation between the size of the spleen and other data could be detected, it can be said that a shrunken liver, varices, haematemesis and ascites were fairly common with huge enlargement of the spleen. Ascites, in particular, was commoner with huge enlargement of the spleen than otherwise.

*Classification of portal hypertension* as suggested by [7] is outlined below.

Group 1. Bilharzial splenomegaly without other clinical evidence of portal obstruction or ascites.

(a) With normal or critical portal vein pressure.
(b) With high portal vein pressure.

Group 2. Bilharzial splenomegaly with varices but no ascites.

(a) With no history of haematemesis, either with normal or critical portal vein pressure or with high portal vein pressure.
(b) With history of haematemesis, either with normal or critical portal vein pressure or with high portal vein pressure.

Group 3. Bilharzial splenomegaly with ascites but no varices, either controllable by medical treatment or not.

Group 4. Bilhazial splenomegaly combined with varices and ascites.

## Complications of Splenectomy in the Tropics

Although complications of splenectomy are the same as elsewhere, some tropical diseases can have an impact on the spleen. In addition, acute malaria is common immediately after splenectomy, especially when blood transfusion is used. Infestation of donated blood is common in endemic areas and the infective dose of parasites is small. The risk of acute and chronic malaria after splenectomy in patients with hyper-reactive malarial splenomegaly is probably increased by the genetic defect these patients have in their immune response to the parasite. A therapeutic course of an antimalarial such as chloroquine is indicated perioperatively in all patients undergoing splenectomy; prophylaxis is then necessary for life in malarious regions to reduce the risk of fatal malaria. Asplenic patients from malaria-free countries should be warned against travel to malarious areas, even with appropriate chemoprophylaxis.

Overwhelming babesiosis has been reported as a rare long-term complication of splenectomy. The incidence of overwhelming bacterial sepsis after splenectomy may be greater in the tropics than temperate zones, and the mortality rate also seems higher, perhaps due to delays and deficiencies in treatment. Pneumococcal and other antibacterial vaccines may offer protection, but are no substitute for preservation of at least a portion of normally perfused spleen whenever technically possible.

## Spleen and Brucellosis

Human brucellosis is a multisystem disease with a broad spectrum of clinical manifestations. After haematogenous dissemination, circulating *Brucella* organisms are removed by reticuloendothelial cells in the liver, spleen and bone marrow. Suppurative disease of the liver and/or spleen is a rare and serious complication of human brucellosis. In the English language literature, only nine cases have been reported, all involving adults with chronic infection. [8] reported the case of a young child in whom abscesses of the liver and spleen developed during acute brucellosis. *Brucella melitenesis* was cultured from an aspirate of the liver and from bone marrow. After percutaneous drainage of the liver abscess, the patient responded to a 56-day course of antimicrobial therapy.

With the advent of non-invasive imaging techniques such as ultrasonography and CT, diagnosis and localisation of abscesses are now relatively easy, which allows for the timely initiation of appropriate therapy. Clinicians should be aware of this unusual complication of brucellosis in children and should include *Brucella* on the list of pathogens causing pyogenic liver and splenic abscesses.

## Tuberculous Splenomegaly

Splenic tuberculosis is rare and may present as a splenic abscess or with hypersplenism. The presence of multiple hypoechoic lesions on ultrasonography of the spleen in an HIV-positive patient is highly suggestive of disseminated tuberculosis. The diagnosis is usually made following surgical resection of the diseased spleen. The size of the spleen in tuberculosis varies from normal to very large. In acute miliary tuberculosis, the spleen is commonly involved and the cut surface shows numerous tubercles 1 to 2 mm in diameter. The miliary tubercles are similar in size to the lymphoid follicles, but are more numerous. They are pale yellow, unlike the lymph. follicles, which are grey. In the less acute forms the tubercles are large and fuse together. In chronic non-miliary tuberculosis involvement of the spleen is much less frequent and the number of tubercles may be small. Tuberculous splenomegaly may complicate tuberculous pneumonia. A therapeutic test with antituberculous drugs brings about some improvement, and there is less danger of dissemination of the tubercle bacilli if splenectomy is undertaken.

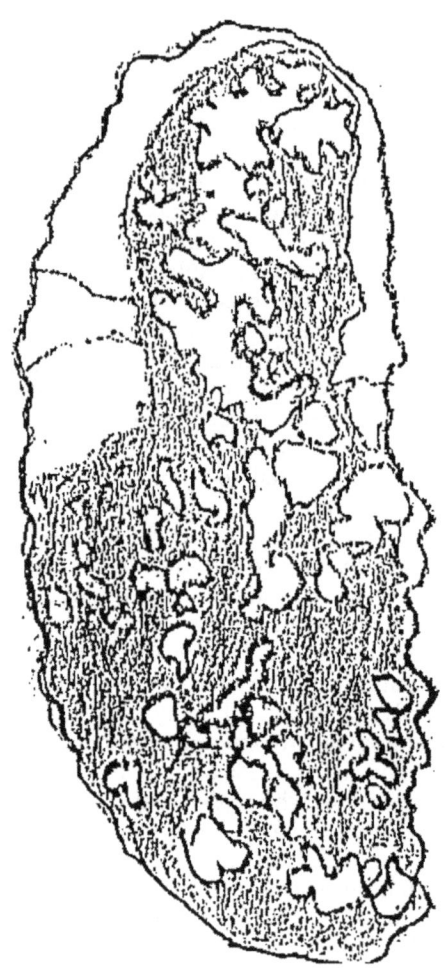

Diagram showing tuberculosis of the spleen. The cut surface is studded with caseous foci varying in size from about $1\frac{1}{2}$ cm downwards and in parts coalescing into larger areas.

## Spleen and HIV Infection

The important role of the spleen in maintaining immune competence is clear, prompting numerous researchers and clinicians to ask whether removing the spleen might place individuals with compromised immune status (people with HIV or AIDS), and those receiving chemotherapy, at an increased risk for sepsis or opportunistic infections.

Lymphoreticular tissues such as lymph nodes and spleen are thought to be major sites for HIV viral replication throughout the natural history of HIV infection and AIDS, The spleen, while integral to the maintenance of immune competence, also represents a "reservoir" where HIV virions pool, accumulate and replicate during the disease's asymptomatic phase. Up to 20% of individuals with asymptomatic HIV disease experience ITP (idiopathic thrombocytopenic purpura), which is often successfully treated via splenectomy, yielding long-lasting platelet increases in more than 80% of patients. Splenectomy has been associated with a relative leucocytosis and lymphocytosis. Increased lymphocyte counts, as well as changes in the cytokine environment after splenectomy, may also play a role in moderating the course of HIV infection, but it is not known whether (or how) such immunomodulatory changes relate to the surgical removal of the HIV reservoir, the spleen. Randomised clinical trials are required to evaluate more fully the role of splenectomy in HIV and to elucidate the complex role of immunomodulatory agents in this clinical setting.

## Gaucher's Disease (GD)

GD is the most prevalent lysosomal sphingolipid storage disorder. It is an autosomal recessive disorder that results from a deficiency in β-glucocerebrosidase with accumulation of the substrate glucosylceramide in monocytes and macrophages. Type 1 GD usually starts in childhood with most patients presenting before the age of 10. GD causes growth retardation, hepatosplenomegaly, hypersplenism, bone involvement (avascular necrosis) and central nervous system involvement. Intravenous enzyme replacement is the therapy of choice and has changed life expectancy, reduced organomegaly and improved haematological disorder. Partial splenectomy (removal of 85–90%) may improve severe hypersplenism and mechanical problems, but the remaining spleen enlarges and the preoperative condition recurs in most patients. Total splenectomy is postponed as far as possible in life due to the risk of post-splenectomy sepsis, accelerated hepatic and bone lipid deposition with earlier appearance of osteolytic changes (painful crisis).

## Niemann–Pick Disease

This is caused by specific genetic mutations; the four forms of Niemann–Pick disease are all characterised by an accumulation of sphingomyelin and cholesterol in cells, particularly in the cells of major organs, such as the liver and the spleen. The three most commonly recognised forms of the disease are types A, B and C. Types A and B Niemann–Pick are both caused by the deficiency of a specific enzyme activity, acid sphingomyelinase (ASM). If ASM is absent or not functioning properly, sphingomyelin cannot be metabolised properly and is accumulated within the cell, eventually causing cell death and the malfunction of major organ systems. The mutations for types A and B have been extensively studied, particularly among the Ashkenazi Jewish population, and DNA tests for these forms of Niemann–Pick are available.

## Amyloidosis of the Spleen

*Sago spleen* is a morbid condition of the spleen, produced by amyloid degeneration of the organ, in which a cross-section shows scattered grey translucent bodies looking like grains of sago (dry granulated starch, much used for making puddings and also, as starch, for stiffening textile fabrics).

Sago spleen has two different anatomical patterns. Most commonly, the amyloid deposition is limited to the splenic follicles, resulting in the gross appearance of a moderately enlarged spleen dotted with grey nodules (so-called "sago" spleen). Alternatively, the amyloid deposits may spare the follicles and mainly infiltrate the red pulp sinuses, producing a large, firm spleen mottled with waxy discolorations ("lardaceotis "spleen).

## Myelofibrosis

Myelofibrosis is a disorder in which fibrous tissue may replace the precursor cells that produce normal blood cells in the bone marrow, resulting in abnormally shaped red blood cells, anaemia, and an enlarged spleen. Eventually, fibrous tissue replaces so much of the bone marrow that production of all blood cells is reduced. When this happens, the anaemia becomes severe, the reduced number of white blood cells cannot fight infections, and the reduced number of platelets cannot prevent bleeding. The body produces blood cells outside the bone marrow, mainly in the liver and spleen, which may enlarge; this condition is called idiopathic myeloid metaplasia.

Often, myelofibrosis produces no symptoms for years. Eventually, the anaemia makes people weak and tired, they feel unwell and lose weight. The enlarged spleen and liver may cause pain in the abdomen.

## Treatment

No available treatment can effectively reverse or permanently slow the progression of this disorder, although the anticancer drug hydroxyurea may decrease the size of the liver or spleen. Rarely, the spleen becomes extremely large and painful and may have to be removed. Infections are treated with antibiotics.

# Vascular Diseases

## Splenic Artery Aneurysm

Splenic artery aneurysms and pseudoaneurysms are rare, but clinically important vascular lesions with a high risk of rupture. Splenic artery aneurysms are the most frequent visceral arterial aneurysms, accounting for 60% of all splanchnic artery aneurysms.

The most common aetiologies include medial degeneration with superimposed atherosclerosis, congenital, mycotic, portal hypertension, fibromuscular dysplasia, and pseudoaneurysms from trauma and pancreatitis. Pseudoaneurysms of the splenic artery occur secondary to injury from released pancreatitis enzymes.

Splenic artery aneurysm and pseudoaneurysm are diagnosed by CT scan, the common finding is high central density surrounded by a peripancreatic collection (clot within a pseudoaneurysm), although it is common to mistake a pancreatic pseudocyst for a splenic pseudoaneurysm and vice versa.

Dissecting aneurysm of the splenic artery may occasionally occur, producing acute severe pain in the left hypochondrium and loin. It is diagnosed by CT, MRI and subtraction digital angiography.

## Treatment

Splenectomy is an easier approach to the management of splenic artery aneurysm in cases of emergency management of ruptured aneurysm. Other options are either operative repair or percutaneous transcatheter embolisation. The latter is performed via selective arterial catheterisation with initial deployment of a coil in the neck extending proximally.

## Splenic Vein Thrombosis

The pathophysiology of splenic vein thrombosis includes compression, encasement and inflammation around the splenic vein. In most cases thrombosis is related to pancreatic carcinoma or chronic pancreatitis; however, the list of causes is long and includes trauma and large masses causing compression.

Radiological findings may demonstrate evidence of the underlying cause of the splenic vein thrombosis; for example, pancreatic calcifications on plain films in a patient with chronic pancreatitis, or a large pancreatic mass seen on CT.

## Splenic Infarct

Splenic infarct is a rare form of pathology. The infarct may be segmental or global, involving the entire organ. It is the result of arterial or venous compromise, and is associated with a heterogeneous group of diseases. Surgery is indicated only in the presence of complications such as haemorrhage, rupture, abscess or pseudocyst.

### Frequency

Splenic infarct is most commonly associated with haematological disorders. The propensity for splenic infarction in sickle haemoglobinopathies is well known.

The mechanism of splenic infarction in sickle cell disease is attributed to crystallisation of the abnormal haemoglobin during periods of hypoxia or acidosis. The rigid erythrocyte leads to rouleaux formation and occlusion of the splenic circulation.

Systemic embolisation can also result in splenic infarct. It occurs most commonly in the setting of a left atrial or ventricular mural thrombus formed as the result of acute myocardial infarction. While autopsy series report a 9%

## BENIGN DISEASE OF THE SPLEEN

incidence of splenic infarction in early deaths following an acute myocardial infarction, clinical series report a much lower incidence of splenic embolisation, probably reflecting the silent clinical course of many splenic infarcts.

Iatrogenic splenic embolisation as in the management of hypersplenism and portal hypertension may produce localised infarction or massive infarction following splenic artery ligation in the treatment of the portal hypertension.

Splenic infarct can be diagnosed by imaging procedures.

### Treatment

*Medical Therapy*

Surgery is indicated only in the presence of complications. Otherwise, the infarcted spleen can be left in situ and the patient observed. The principal mainstay of medical therapy is analgesia with either narcotics or non-steroidal anti-inflammatory agents.

*Surgical Therapy*

- Splenectomy is indicated in splenic abscess when aspiration or catheter drainage fails to treat the patients. In view of the small but real risk of fatal overwhelming post-splenectomy sepsis, splenic preservation is preferable whenever possible.
- In cases of torsion of a wandering spleen, splenopexy with splenic salvage is the procedure of choice in the well-perfused, non-infarcted spleen.
- Complications such as bleeding or pseudocyst formation may also be amenable to splenic salvage using techniques of conservative splenectomy.
- If there is perisplenic inflammation and dense adhesions that make splenectomy difficult, preoperative splenic artery embolisation, which purposely infarcts the remaining spleen, may minimise blood loss, which can otherwise be quite profuse in these difficult dissections. Intraoperative ligation of the splenic artery at the superior margin of the pancreas in the lesser sac is another alternative to minimise blood loss if the spleen is enlarged.

## Splenic Arteriovenous Fistula

Blunt or penetrating injury to the abdomen leading to splenic arteriovenous fistula (AVF) is well known and described in the literature. The other notable causes of splenic AVF are high intra-abdominal pressure such as in pregnancy and childbirth, post-splenectomy and following rupture of a splenic artery aneurysm into the splenic vein. The development of portal hypertension in patients with AVF could be related to an increase in intravenous pressure resulting from increased blood flow or arterialisation of the portal venous system. This is a potentially treatable entity and splenectomy with resection of fistula resulted in resolution of signs and symptoms in all reported cases. The AVF evolved over a long time after initial trauma or surgery. Increased venous pressure of the splenic vein and portal vein may lead to formation of gastric varices and dilation of the inferior mesenteric vein, which drains into the splenic vein.

It was also believed that normal liver function or biopsy in patients with portal hypertension should be followed up by Doppler sonography and angiography to visualise any splanchnic AVF. A history of abdominal trauma, splenectomy, multiple pregnancies and presence of splenic artery aneurysm are strong indicators. Suggestive clinical features include a pulsatile or soft mass in the upper abdomen with palpable thrill and machinery murmur on auscultation. The ideal treatment in selected patients would be to embolise the AVF.

*Splenosis* refers to autotransplantation of individual fragments of splenic tissue left behind after either operative or traumatic removal of the spleen. Although rarely symptomatic, splenosis may cause intestinal obstruction since the splenules link adjacent loops of bowels to each other, kinking and obstructing them. Tomographic selective splenic scintigraphy with sulphur colloid and heat-damaged red cells is the most sensitive method to detect splenosis. Patients who undergo emergency splenectomy for trauma are at a much higher risk of developing splenosis than those splenectomised due to haematological conditions. Spilled splenic tissue seeds the peritoneum, takes root and grows into vascularised splenules. Experimental evidence (Folkman) suggests that the presence of a large amount of vascularised spleen inhibits the growth of other splenic tissue in mice, providing a theory why patients who undergo partial splenectomy, splenography or are merely observed after splenic rupture have almost no splenosis. Management of splenosis is expectant.

## Investigations of the Cause of Splenomegaly

Clinical examination must include a very careful study of the superficial lymph nodes and the tonsillar and adenoid tissues, a search for stigmas of liver disease, a full examination of the skin for evidence of purpura or bruising, and a complete survey of all the systems.

A few simple laboratory investigations will provide the cause for most cases of splenomegaly. Almost all the splenomegalies associated with haematological disorders can be diagnosed by a complete blood examination together with a bone marrow aspiration. Liver disease is often associated with abnormal liver function tests or oesophageal varices on barium swallow examination. Liver biopsy may be necessary to determine the type of liver pathology. The diagnosis of lymphoma or other reticuloendothelial malignancies may be accomplished by biopsy of a suitable node, the liver or another involved organ, lymphangiography or bone marrow biopsy, in some cases diagnostic splenectomy may be necessary.

The various infections that produce splenomegaly may be identified from appropriate haematological or serological studies. Infectious mononucleosis is diagnosed by the finding of atypical lymphocytes in the blood, a positive Paul–Bunnell test (or related screening procedures) and a rising anti-Epstein–Barr virus titre. In those who have travelled to the tropics, malarial parasites should be looked for and the marrow examined for Leishman–Donovan bodies in cases of leishmaniasis (kala-azar).

Special investigations in splenic disorders include radiography, ultrasonography, computed tomography (CT), magnetic resonance imaging (MRI), angiography, splenoportography, measurement of portal venous pressure (percutaneous intrasplenic pressure and wedged hepatic venous pressure) and scintigraphy.

## Splenic Index

Bleeding from oesophageal varices with its high mortality rate is a known complication in patients with cirrhosis. The clinical course in these cirrhotic patients shows progressive splenomegaly. A study by Watanabe et al [9] tried to determine if the splenic size in cirrhotic patients correlated with the severity of oesophageal varices, gastric varices and liver function.

The splenic index is also used in malaria surveys to estimate the size of the spleen among people in areas endemic for malaria during epidemiological studies.

## Rupture of the Spleen: Aetiology

### Traumatic Rupture

A splenic injury can be closed, open or iatrogenic. Minor trauma such as a fall from a bicycle, donkey or a camel may lead to rupture of the spleen in childhood as the ribs are more flexible and the spleen is relatively large and less protected. At any age, splenic enlargement produced by malaria, vascular malformation, haematological causes, infectious mononueleosis and splenic fixity by perisplenic adhesion may predispose to easy rupture after minor injuries and that is why corporal punishment is prohibited in areas endemic for malaria.

The importance of preserving splenic function for both children and adults is now well recognised.

The early complications of the non-operative management of a ruptured spleen include failure to detect continuing splenic haemorrhage and associated injury requiring laparotomy. In the longer term, delayed rupture of a subcapsular haematoma or post-traumatic cysts may occasionally follow splenic preservation and should be managed by capsular repair, partial splenectomy, or unroofing and drainage of cysts, whenever possible. Intraperitoneal implantation of splenic fragments (splenosis) does not seem to provide asplenic patients with protection from severe infection and is no substitute for appropriate lifetime prophylaxis.

# BENIGN DISEASE OF THE SPLEEN

## Non-traumatic Rupture

Non-traumatic rupture of an entirely normal spleen arguably does not occur in the absence of a coagulopathy, and even the diseased spleen rarely ruptures spontaneously. Subcapsular haemorrhage in an acutely inflamed, enlarged and congested spleen is probably the most common mechanism of pathological rupture. Trivial trauma may have been forgotten or disregarded.

Acute malaria is the most common cause of non-traumatic splenic rupture in the tropics. The incidence is highest during initial attacks of malaria, but even then it is rare. The chronically enlarged spleen may undergo a degree of capsular fibrosis, which protects it somewhat from rupture.

Infectious causes of spontaneous rupture, such as *Salmonella*, Epstein–Barr virus and hepatitis virus, probably occur more commonly in the tropics, while haematological and neoplastic causes have a similar incidence in tropical and temperate areas.

## Staging of Splenic Trauma

*Staging classification*:

Grade 1: capsule tear or minor parenchymal laceration.

Grade 2: capsular avulsion.

Grade 3: major parenchymal fracture or laceration or penetrating gunshot or stab wound.

Grade 4: severe parenchymal stellate fracture, crush, bisection or hilar injury.

Grade 5: shattered spleen (or multiply injured patient).

## Management

*Non-operative management*:

1. Selectively stable patients with grade 2 or less injuries (controversial)
2. In children higher levels of splenic injury tend to be accepted for observation (follow with CT, serial haematocrits, close observation).

*Operative management* (after failure of non-operative management):

1. Trend now toward saving the spleen (splenorrhaphy) with the use of intraoperative packing, pledged sutures, polyglycolic mesh wrap, hemisplenectomy, omental wrap.
2. Splenectomy (total or partial) for grade 4–5 injuries.
3. Conservative therapy should be critically evaluated the patient has multiple injuries (i.e. head injuries).
4. Operative trauma results in injury to the spleen in roughly 2% of operations and most of these can be repaired if the injury is noted at the time.
5. Other concerns: autotransplantation of splenic mass does not protect against infection.

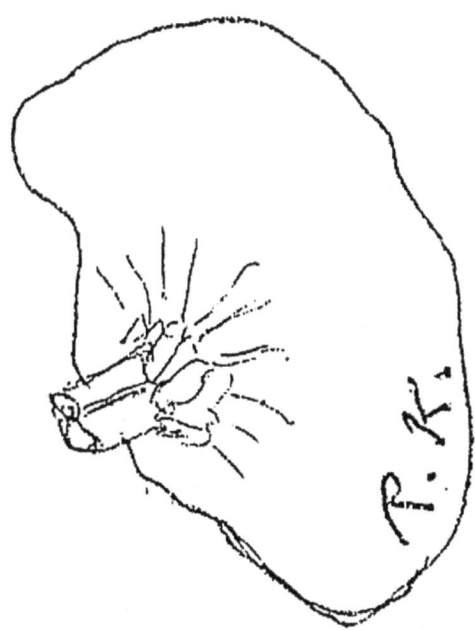

Diagram showing that when the spleen has been severely damaged, but the hilar vessesls are intact, a synthetic absorbable mesh wrap may be used to provide haemostasis by gentle compression.

## Splenectomy

### Indications

The accepted indications for splenectomy have changed dramatically over time. Splenic trauma is the most common surgical indication for splenectomy, although attempts at splenic preservation are increasingly important. Splenic cysts, tumours, and vascular lesions may also require surgical removal. Whenever possible, splenic tissue is preserved to decrease the risk of septicaemia, but total splenectomy occasionally is necessary.

Early reports of splenectomy for trauma exist, but the first documented splenectomy occurred in 1849 for splenomegaly. By the 1950s, splenomegaly with hypersplenism was the most common indication for splenectomy, whereas staging of Hodgkin's disease predominated in the 1970s.

Indications for splenectomy were determined on the basis of the patient's primary diagnosis. Trauma included all splenectomies performed for blunt or penetrating injury to the spleen. Incidental splenectomies included all spleens removed as a planned portion of another procedure (e.g., distal pancreatectomy). Iatrogenic cases were defined as removal of the spleen secondary to intraoperative injury. Any splenectomy performed for treatment or staging of leukaemias or Hodgkin's or non-Hodgkin's lymphomas was included under haematological malignancies. Cytopenia included anaemia, leukopenia, or thrombocytopenia not secondary to a haematological malignancy and was subcategorised into thrombocytopenia (Idiopathic and thrombotic thrombocytopenic purpura (ITP and TTP)) and haemolytic anaemia. All splenectomies for causes or complications of left-sided portal hypertension or during decompressive shunt procedures were included in the category of portal disorders. Diagnostic splenectomies were performed to clarify preoperative uncertainty, including cases of splenic tumours, splenomegaly of unclear aetiology, and fevers of unknown origin. All miscellaneous conditions not assignable to the above categories were included I "other", including pyruvate kinase deficiency, infarctions secondary to septic emboli, and Felty's syndrome.

## Medical Indication

Some causes of haemolytic anaemia are successfully treated by splenectomy, including congenital spherocytosis, elliptocytosis, pyruvate deficiency (membrane damage of the red cells and distortion with premature culling by the spleen), thalassaemia and acquired immune haemolytic anaemia.

## Surgical Indications

1. Rupture of spleen.
2. Removal of tumours, cysts or vascular anomalies.
3. Need for adequate exposure of left upper quadrant (LUQ).
4. Certain shunting procedures.
5. For staging of Hodgkin's disease and other lymphoreticular malignancies.

# Complications of Splenectomy

## Overwheiming Post-splenectomy Infection (OPSI)

There is overwhelming sepsis, fatal within 12–24 hours. Sixty per cent of cases are due to pneumococci, the rest to meningococcal, *Haemophilus influenzae*, staphylococci, etc.

- Risk of sepsis is 200 greater than in normal children.
- Risk of overwhelming sepsis is low (0.5–1%) when splenectomy is done for rupture of spleen, spherocytosis or ITP.
- Risk is higher for alpha-thalassaemia (24.8%), histiocytosis or lipidosis.
- Risk is highest in conditions that predispose to infection such as Wiskott–Aldrich syndrome.

*Pneumococcus* vaccine and vaccine against *H. influenzae* should be given as a prophylaxis; these are best given 10 days before elective splenectomy and preoperatively in anticipation of splenic trauma.

Booster doses of Pneumovax 23 are not recommended due to possible reactions, except maybe for those who are vaccinated before 2 years of age. Surgery should be deferred until 5–6 years of age due to the higher risk of sepsis for infants and young children and also the poor response to vaccines before 18–24 months of age. Accessory spleen (present in 10–18%) should be looked for in surgery. Penicillin prophylaxis (for life?) or intermittent penicillin with illness should be given. Immediate medical

## BENIGN DISEASES OF THE SPLEEN

evaluation for any febrile illness should always be undertaken.

Pneumovax 23 only covers 85% of serotypes and meningococcal vaccine only cover serotypes A, C, Y and W-135. Conjugated pneumococcal vaccine (seven serotypes) for those < 2 years of age is currently being tested.

Although post-splenectomy sepsis is uncommon in the immediate postoperative period, patients who undergo incidental splenectomy as part of another procedure or secondary to an iatrogenic injury do appear to have an increased rate of morbidity and mortality compared with their counterparts without splenectomy. Traditionally, splenectomy was a common part of operations for cancer in the left upper quadrant. Recent studies have failed to show a survival advantage for splenectomy as a routine part of resection for gastric carcinomas unless the distal pancreas is directly involved. Furthermore, an increased mortality has been shown for the additional unnecessary procedure. Animal studies have also shown an increased risk for hepatic metastases for colon cancer in splenectomized mice, possibly related to the impact on the host immune system. Because of the increased morbidity and mortality from splenectomy, more attempts are being made at splenic conservation after iatrogenic injury.

The rise in diagnostic splenectomies is possibly a result of improvement in radiographic techniques. Asymptomatic splenic masses accounted for a large portion of the splenectomies for diagnostic purposes in the second 5-year period after CT scanning developed its current prevalence. These lesions may have gone undetected and unnoticed had a CT scan not been performed on these patients for other indications.

There has been a decrease in overall incidence of splenectomy in cytopenic patients over the past 20 years, with that decrease secondary to the thrombocytopenic population. Patients with haemolytic anaemia had a clear increase in incidence of splenectomy. The reason for the decline in the thrombocytopenic group is unclear. Several studies have shown an ongoing role for splenectomy in the treatment of patients with ITP and TTP, particularly patients refractory to plasmaphoresis and steroids.

Parasitic infections are liable to recur after splenectomy in patients from endemic areas and may appear in unusual forms. There is increased risk of cerebral malaria, and of febrile illness in which the classical intermittent pattern is not present and the parasites are demonstrated only with difficulty in the blood, but which responds promptly to antimalarial drugs.

### Other Complications of Splenectomy

- Haemorrhage (postoperative haemorrhage)
- Pulmonary atelectasis
- Subphrenic abscess
- Pancreatic fistula
- Gastric fistula
- Thrombocytosis

## Alternatives to Splenectomy

### Partial Splenectomy

With the recognition of post-splenectomy sepsis and infections and the availability of improved radiographic imaging, efforts have increased over the past two decades to avoid unnecessary splenectomy. The initial efforts were made within the field of trauma, clearly showing non-operative splenic salvage as a viable alternative in appropriately selected patients.

Although the risk of post-splenectomy sepsis was originally thought to be restricted to the first 2 to 3 years following splenectomy, it is now clear that the asplenic adult may be vulnerable for many years after the event and perhaps indefinitely. The critical task is to achieve a balance between ablation and conservation of the spleen. A possible solution was suggested by Maddison [10] who first used the technique of embolisation of the spleen with autologus blood clots. Unfortunately, there was a high risk of complications, and in particular abscess formation, which precluded this from being used as an alternative to surgical splenectomy. Subsequently Witte et al [11] showed that hypersplenism could be treated by partial ablation of the splenic mass by segmental embolisation of parenchyinal arteries with gel foam. Although this method was also associated with complications including pleural effusion, sepsis and splenic abscess, the preservation of a degree of prograde arterial flow does appear to protect

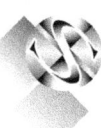

10 · UPPER GASTROINTESTINAL SURGERY

against the serious and frequent complication of total splenic infarction. Partial embolisation has also been used successfully to treat myelofibrosis, spherocytosis and thalassaemia, while others have used it to treat hypersplenism in portal hypertension.

## Segmental Splenectomy

Increasing recognition of unique and significant functions of the spleen has stimulated interest in the development of therapeutic alternatives to total splenectomy. Techniques for partial splenic resection and splenic salvage, initially developed for the management of splenic trauma, are being applied to an increasing number of conditions in which reduction, rather than total ablation, of splenic tissue is desired. In a study by *Kamel and Dunn* [5] segmental splenectomy was evaluated in 51 patients who required splenectomy to relieve the symptoms of schistosomal splenomegaly, and their course was compared with that of 44 patients who underwent total splenectomy in an unrandormised study (Figures 10.8 and 10.9).

### Surgical Technique [5]

Segmental splenectomy involves removal of a part of the spleen, based on its segmental blood supply. This procedure is a compromise between the need to remove the great bulk of splenic tissue responsible for hypersplenism and discomfort, and the desirability of preserving normal splenic function. The opinion of the authors is to leave splenic tissue nearly equal to the weight of normal spleen, i.e. 150 g of spleen. The authors applied segmental splenectomy on five patients with hepatosplenic schistosomiasis and they concluded that this procedure is safe and well tolerated in such patients.

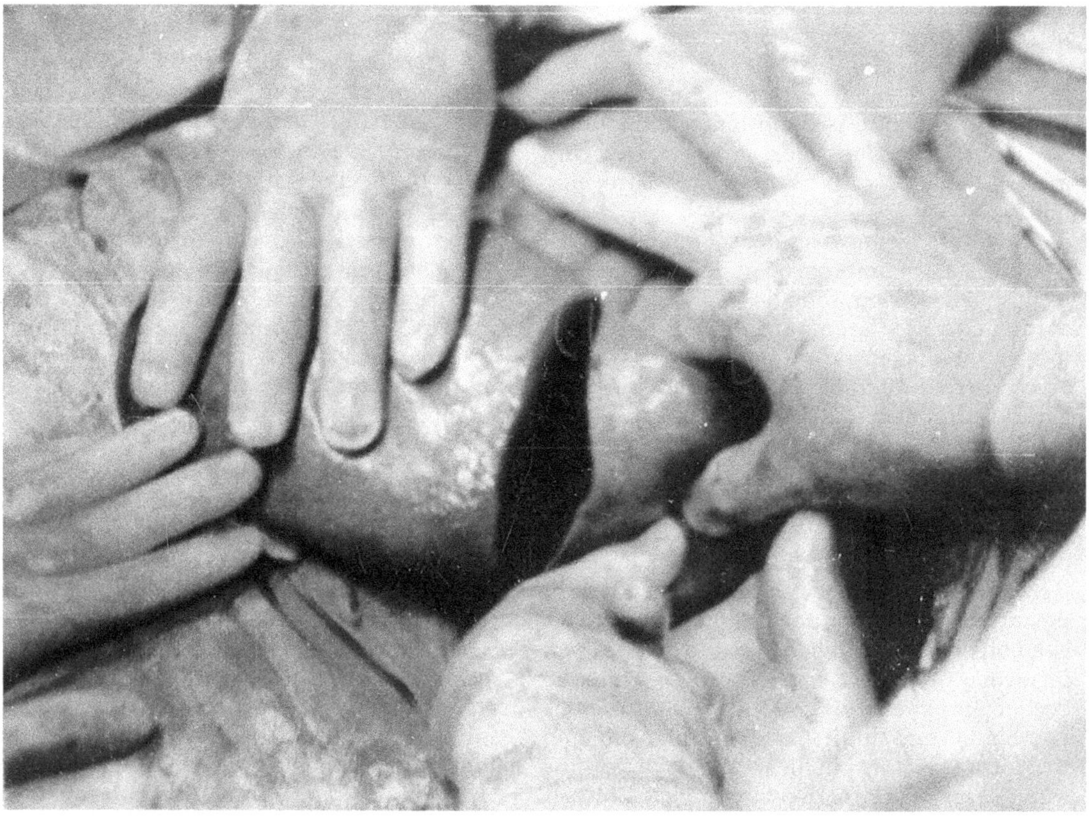

**Figure 10.8.** Haemostatic compression of the spleen using manual pressure by the thumbs and forefingers of the second assistant. The cut on the diaphragmatic surface of the spleen is shown as done in segmental splenectomy.

# BENIGN DISEASES OF THE SPLEEN

## Splenorrhaphy

### Indications

Spleens that have been injured and are bleeding require splenorrhaphy (repair of the spleen) or if this is not successful a splenectomy is indicated. Most commonly these injuries are from car or bike accidents, falls, kicks, etc.

### Preoperative Evaluation

All patients require blood tests to verify that they are bleeding internally despite blood transfusions and medications. Frequently a CT scan is used to locate the spleen as a cause of internal bleeding.

### Procedure

The cracks in the spleen, which cause the bleeding, are repaired using sutures. Frequently this does not completely stop the bleeding and additional techniques must be used including blood-clotting agents applied to the bleeding areas, mesh wrapped around the spleen to hold it together or removal of small fragments of the spleen.

## Laparoscopic Splenectomy

Laparoscopic splenectomy (LS) was first described by Delaitre et al [12], but unlike laparoscopic cholecystectomy, did not gain immediate widespread adoption. As laparoscopic techniques have expanded, the frequency of LS has increased rapidly since 1995.

The location and size of the spleen make its exposure relatively difficult. The spleen's proximity to the pancreatic tail and its ample blood supply require tedious operative dissection and advanced laparoscopic skills. ITP is the most common non-traumatic indication for splenectomy, and the small size of the spleen in this disease renders it amenable to the

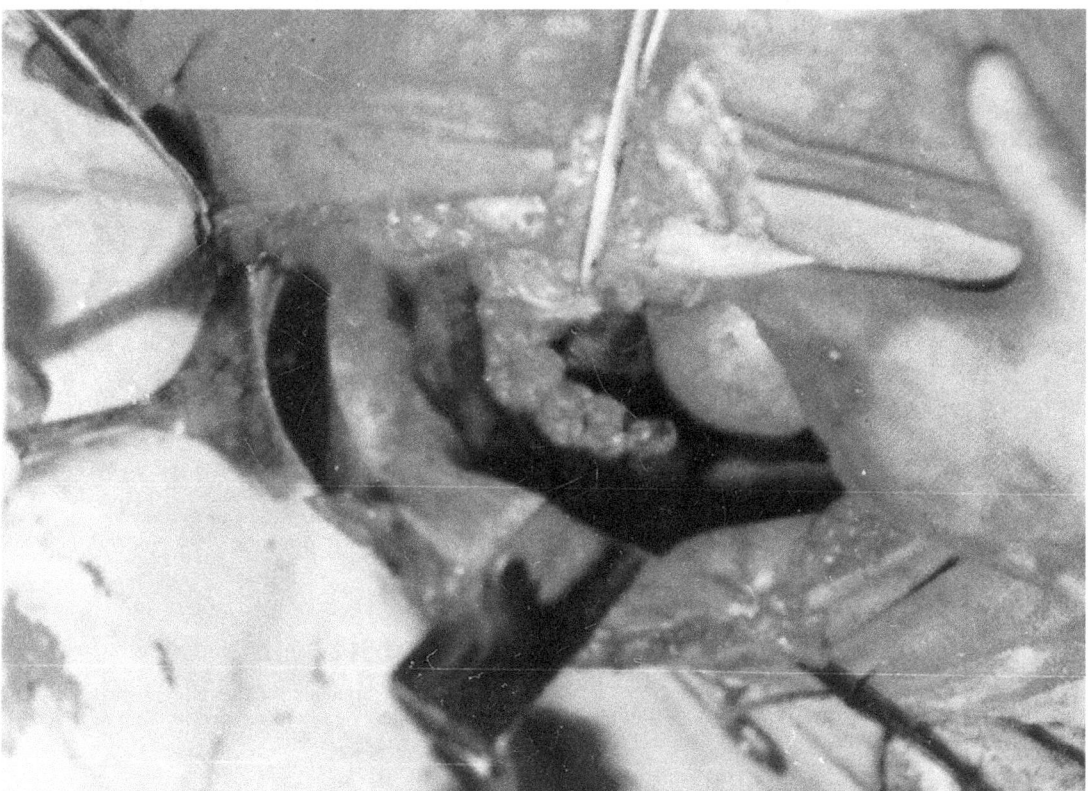

**Figure 10.9.** The splenic remnant with an omental patch in place. The final appearance after segmental splenectomy.

laparoscopic approach. Although controversial, a maximum splenic size of approximately 20 cm in diameter has been recommended. However, with increasing experience, LS is being applied successfully to patients with larger spleens. Indications such as hereditary spherocytosis, haemolytic anaemia, Hodgkin's disease, lymphoma, idiopathic neutropenia, sarcoidosis and thrombotic thrombocytopenic purpura are now considered for LS.

LS is feasible, safe and effective. With increasing surgical experience, shorter operative time, the postoperative advantages of laparoscopic versus open surgery, and lower costs, LS is emerging as the procedure of choice and soon may be the standard method of elective splenectomy.

## Hepatisation of the Spleen

Allogeneic human hepatocyte transplantation has been used in both acute and chronic liver failure. Both transplantation into the liver via the portal vein and ectopic transplantation into the spleen have been also used. In pilot studies, liver and splenic hepatocyte transplantation has been shown to be both safe and potentially effective in humans as a bridge to orthotopic transplantation.

Immunosuppression is required in all patients receiving allogeneic human hepatocyte transplantation.

The spleen appears to be the preferred site due to fibrosis and loss of blood supply to the liver. In animal models, hepatisation of the spleen is a well-described phenomenon and results in replacement of the splenic pulp with cords of functioning hepatocytes that perform hepatic functions including synthesis of albumin and clotting factors, detoxification of ammonia and oxidative metabolism.

## Acknowledgement

I would like to acknowledge Professor Manar El-Tonsy (Professor of Parasitology, Faculty of Medicine, Ain-Shams University) for her assistance during preparation of this chapter.

## Questions

1. List congenital abnormalities of the spleen.
2. What are the indications for splenectomy?
3. What are the complications of splenectomy?
4. List tropical diseases affecting the spleen.

## References

1. Kyber E. Über die Mitz des Menchen und effiliger Säugetiere. *Arch mikroskop Anat Entwicklungsmechanik* 1870;6:540–70.
2. Gupta CD, Gupta SC, Arora AK, Heya Singh P. Vascular segments in the human spleen. J Anat 1976;121: 613–6.
3. Mikhail Y, Kamel R, Nawar NNY, Rafla MFM. Observations on the mode of termination and parenchymal distribution of the splenic artery with evidence of splenic lobation and segmentation. J Anat 1979;128(2): 253–8.
4. Kassirsky, IA, Demiana NA, Lysenko AY. Malaria. In: A *Handbook on tropical diseases.* Moscow, 1974; 38 (111 Russian).
5. Kamel R, Dunn MA. Segmental splenectomy in schistosomiasis. Br J Surg 1982;69:311–13.
6. Kamel R, Dunn MA,; Skelly RR et al. Clinical and immunological results of segmental splenectomy in schistosomiasis. Br J Surg 1986;73:544–7.
7. Kamel R et al. 1966
8. Vallejo JG, Stevens AM, Dutton RV, Kapla SL. Hepatosplenic abscesses due to *Brucella melitensis*: report of a case involving a child and review of the literature. Clin Infect Dis 1996;22:485–9.
9. Watanabe S, Hosomi N, Kitade Y et al. Assessment of the presence and severity of oesophagogastric varices by splenic index in patients with liver cirrhosis. J. Comput Assist Tomogr 2001; 24:788–94.
10. Maddison, FE. Embolic therapy of hypersplenism. Invest Radiol 1973;8:280–1.
11. Witte CL, Van Wyck DB, Witte MH et al. Ischemia and partial resection for control of splenic hyperfunction. Br J Surg (1982);69:531–5.
12. Delaitre B, Maignien B. Splenectomy by the laparoscopic approach. A report of a case (letter). Press Med 1991;20(44):2263.

## Further Reading

Bowdler A,J. A Textbook on: The spleen, structure, function and clinical significance. London: Chapman and Hall Medical, (1990).

# 11

# Epithelial Neoplasms of the Oesophagus

Derek Alderson and Jonathan H. Vickers

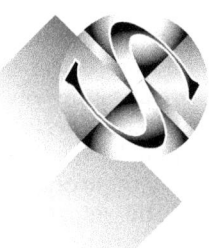

## Aims

- To describe the incidence of oesophageal cancer worldwide.
- To outline common management of the condition.
- To describe standards methods of pre-operative assessment.
- To put treatment options in context.

## Introduction

Both benign and malignant epithelial tumours occur in the human oesophagus. The former, however, are all extremely rare. True papillomas, adenomas and hyperplastic polyps do occur but the majority of "benign" tumours are not epithelial in origin and arise from other layers of the oesophageal wall. They are collectively referred to as gastrointestinal stromal tumours (GIST) and while the majority are truly benign, malignant counterparts are well described.

Most benign oesophageal tumours are small and asymptomatic and the most important point in their management is usually to carry out an adequate number of biopsies to prove beyond reasonable doubt that the lesion is not malignant. The remainder of this chapter will focus on primary malignant epithelial oesophageal neoplasms. Although again well described in many case reports, the oesophagus is an unusual site for the occurrence of secondary carcinomas, with the exception of bronchogenic carcinoma involving the oesophagus by direct invasion of the primary and/or contiguous lymph nodes.

## Oesophageal Cancer

Oesophageal carcinoma is an aggressive tumour which is difficult to cure. Worldwide, it is the sixth most common cancer although there is wide geographical variation. Its incidence in the Western world is relatively modest (United Kingdom male: 14.0, female: 9.2 per 100 000 population) [1], although there is reliable evidence that this has been rising steadily in recent years due to a dramatic rise in the incidence of adenocarcinomas which now account for 75% of cases. It is the ninth highest cause of death due to malignant disease in males in the United Kingdom [1] and has an overall 5-year survival from the time of diagnosis of only 5–10%. Early lesions tend to be asymptomatic. The majority of patients present with advanced disease, when the chances of cure are small.

Radical but potentially curative surgery, either alone or in combination with other modalities, also carries significant risk to the patient. The average United Kingdom 30-day operative mortality for oesophagectomy is 11% [2,3]. This reflects not only the magnitude of the procedure but also other patient-related factors

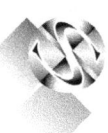

such as advanced age and co-morbid cardiorespiratory disease. This has implications for the organisation of oesophageal cancer services. Surgeons performing ten or more resections annually tend to have significantly lower mortality figures than those who do fewer than six.

The appropriate selection of patients for either potentially curative radical treatment, or for less invasive palliative therapies is therefore of great importance. The principal determinant of long-term survival in patients with oesophageal cancer is tumour stage (TNM) at the time of diagnosis. Historically, due to the limitations of some imaging techniques and the relative inaccessibility of the oesophagus, such information has proved difficult to obtain. Technological advances and use of imaging modalities in combination (e.g. spiral computed tomography, endoscopic ultrasound, laparoscopy) have helped improve the collection of reliable staging information, which is vital for planning therapeutic strategies and using resources appropriately.

## Demographics and Aetiology

Most oesophageal malignancies are either adenocarcinomas or squamous cell carcinomas. Adenocarcinoma arises either in columnar lined epithelium (Barrett's oesophagus) or rarely in glands within the oesophageal wall. There has been a steady increase in the proportion of adenocarcinomas compared with squamous carcinomas in the last 10 to 20 years in Western series thought to be due to a rising incidence of gastro-oesophageal reflux disease (GORD) and consequently of Barrett's oesophagus. Despite this, however, worldwide 85% of all oesophageal cancers are squamous.

Squamous cell carcinoma (SCC) occurs mainly in the elderly and affects predominantly males. Its aetiology is not fully understood, but certain nutritional and mineral deficiencies (vitamin C, retinol, fresh fruit and vegetables, zinc, selenium, molybdenum) are implicated, as is exposure to known carcinogens, including nitrosamines, petroleum oil derivatives, aflatoxin and tobacco. Certain pathological conditions of the oesophagus have also been implicated such as achalasia, chronic oesophagitis, caustic injuries and Plummer–Vinson syndrome, all of which are associated with an increased risk of developing squamous cell carcinoma [4]. Chronic alcohol ingestion and a positive family history are further contributing factors. There are huge geographical variations in incidence of SCC, with over 60% of the total world cases occurring in parts of China. Other high incidence areas include Central Asia, Transkei, parts of India, and the Caribbean.

Adenocarcinoma also predominantly affects males. Some gastric tumours, arising in the cardia can spread upwards into the distal oesophagus, and may make nomenclature confusing. Up to 80% of oesophageal adenocarcinomas contain associated columnar lined epithelium, suggesting an origin in areas of Barrett's mucosa. Recent studies of tumour-related genes, such as p53, also support the view that most oesophageal adenocarcinomas arise on a background of this type of metaplasia. As a consequence, adenocarcinoma occurs most frequently (90%) in the distal oesophagus. Factors implicated in the development of squamous cell carcinoma are less apparent in the development of adenocarcinoma. The most important factor is long-standing reflux disease, and the associated development of Barrett's oesophagus, although recent evidence suggests that obesity (independent of reflux disease) is also a risk factor [5].

## Methods of Spread

Both adenocarcinomas and squamous cell carcinomas tend to disseminate early. Sadly, the classical presenting symptoms of dysphagia, regurgitation and weight loss are often absent until the primary tumour has become advanced and so the tumour is often well established before the diagnosis is made. Tumours can spread in three ways: invasion directly through the oesophageal wall, via lymphatics or via the bloodstream. Direct spread occurs both laterally through the component layers of the oesophageal wall and longitudinally within the oesophageal wall. Sakata showed that longitudinal spread is mainly via the submucosal lymphatic channels of the oesophagus [6]. The pattern of lymphatic drainage is therefore not segmental, as in other parts of the gastrointestinal tract. Consequently the length of oesophagus involved by tumour is frequently much longer than the macroscopic length of the malignancy at the epithelial surface. Lymph node spread occurs commonly. Akiyama demonstrated that although the direction of spread to regional lymphatics is predominantly caudal, the involvement of lymph nodes is potentially widespread, and can also occur in a cranial direction [7]. Any regional lymph node from the superior mediastinum to the coeliac axis and lesser curve of the stomach may be involved regardless of the location of the primary lesion within the oesophagus. Haematogenous spread may involve a variety of different organs including the liver, lungs, brain and bones. Tumours arising from the intra-abdominal portion of the oesophagus may also disseminate transperitoneally.

## Investigations

### History and Clinical Examination

These are as important as for any other clinical condition. Most oesophageal neoplasms present with mechanical symptoms, principally dysphagia, but sometimes also regurgitation, vomiting, odynophagia (painful swallowing) and weight loss. Clinical findings suggestive of advanced malignancy include recurrent laryngeal nerve palsy, Horner's syndrome, chronic spinal pain and diaphragmatic paralysis. Other factors making surgical cure unlikely include weight loss of more than 20%, and loss of appetite. Cutaneous tumour metastases or enlarged supraclavicular lymph nodes may be seen on clinical examination and indicate disseminated disease. Specialised investigations are usually needed to obtain diagnostic tissue samples (all neoplasms) or provide more detailed staging data (malignant neoplasms).

### Diagnostic Tests

#### Endoscopy

This is the first line investigation for most oeosphageal disorders, and for follow-up of patients after treatment. It also has an important therapeutic role. Early fibreoptic instruments utilising the principle of total internal reflection to transmit images to the eye have now been largely superseded by video-endoscopes in which the fibreoptic bundle is replaced by an electronic chip which transmits its the image to an external TV monitor. Endoscopy provides an unrivalled direct view of the oesophageal mucosa and any lesion, allowing its site and size to be documented. Cytology and/or histology specimens taken via the endoscope are crucial for accurate diagnosis. The combination of histology and cytology increases the diagnostic accuracy to more than 95%. The chief limitation of conventional endoscopy is that only the mucosal surface can be studied and biopsied. Other investigations are therefore usually required to define the extent of local or distant spread. Early lesions may be missed despite enhancing techniques such as staining the oesophageal wall with Lugol's iodine because they cause no demonstrable mucosal abnormality and there are usually no symptoms to alert the clinician.

#### Barium Swallow

Radiological techniques are limited in their use because they show only mucosal detail and provide no means of obtaining tissue samples. Although contrast studies can yield useful information about the extent of an oesophageal lesion, its exact location and the degree of luminal narrowing, all of these can nearly always be assessed equally well by endoscopy. Diagnostic endoscopy with biopsy should be undertaken whenever possible in patients with progressive dysphagia regardless of the radiological findings. Barium swallow may, however, be a useful alternative investigation where endoscopic examination is not possible or may be dangerous (e.g. in tightly stenotic tumours, achalasia or pharyngeal pouch), although it is more likely to miss small neoplasms than endoscopy. Large lesions causing axis deviation of the oesophagus on barium swallow are invariably advanced (T4) and incurable.

### Staging Investigations

#### Background

The most widely used pathological staging system is the World Health Organisation TNM (Tumour, Node, Metastasis) classification [8].

Table 11.1 shows the TNM system for oesophageal cancer in its most recently updated

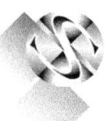

**Table 11.1.** TNM staging scheme for oesophageal cancer

| | |
|---|---|
| Tis | High grade dysplasia |
| T1 | Tumour invading lamina propria or submucosa |
| T2 | Tumour invading muscularis propria |
| T3 | Tumour invading beyond muscularis propria |
| T4 | Tumour invading adjacent structures |
| Tx | Primary tumour cannot be assessed |
| N0 | No regional lymph node metastases |
| N1 | Regional lymph node metastases |
| Nx | Lymph nodes cannot be assessed |
| M0 | No distant metastases |
| M1(a) | Coeliac node involved (for distal oesophageal tumours) |
| | Supraclavicular node involved (for proximal tumours) |
| M1(b) | Coeliac or supraclavicular node involved if not remote from tumour site (i.e. not 1a) |
| | All other distant metastases |
| Mx | Distant metastases cannot be assessed |

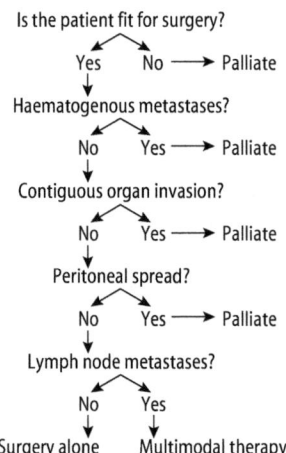

**Figure 11.1.** How to deal with oesophageal cancer.

form. Like all pathological systems, it is reliant on the nature and extent of the surgery performed. For example, performing more extensive radical surgical lymphadenectomy provides a more accurate assessment of the "N" stage. There is accumulating evidence that many patients described as N0 in the past were probably N1, a phenomenon described as stage migration.

Staging information may be gathered before the commencement of therapy, during therapy, (e.g. at open operation), or following treatment (histology or post mortem). The techniques commonly used to provide preoperative staging data are described below, along with a suggested algorithm (Figure 11.1).

## Blood Tests

These are of limited value. Blood tests reveal nothing about local invasion or regional lymph node spread, and to date, no reliable tumour marker for oesophageal cancer has been isolated from peripheral blood. The presence of abnormal liver function tests (LFTs) may suggest the presence of liver metastases, but this is generally too insensitive to be diagnostic. Many patients with known liver metastases have normal LFTs. At best, abnormal LFTs only reinforce clinical suspicion of spread to the liver, and further imaging is usually required to confirm the diagnosis.

## Transcutaneous Ultrasound

It is difficult to visualise mediastinal structures with transcutaneous ultrasound. With the relatively low frequency sound waves used, good depth of tissue penetration is achieved at the expense of poor image resolution. In addition, the mediastinal organs are surrounded by bone and air which renders them largely inaccessible to external ultrasound. The technique is used therefore mainly to assess spread to the liver, the whole of which can be clearly visualised by standard transcutaneous ultrasound. Haematogenous spread can be more fully assessed by combining ultrasound with chest radiography.

## Bronchoscopy

Many middle and upper third oesophageal carcinomas (and therefore usually squamous carcinomas) are sufficiently advanced at the time of diagnosis that the trachea or bronchi are already involved. Bronchoscopy may reveal of either impingement or invasion of the main airways in over 30% of new patients. In some cases, therefore, bronchoscopy alone can confirm that the tumour is locally unresectable.

## Laparoscopy

This is a useful technique for the diagnosis of intra-abdominal and hepatic metastases [9]. It has the advantage of enabling tissue samples or peritoneal cytology to be obtained and is the only modality reliably able to detect peritoneal tumour seedlings. This may be particularly important for tumours arising from the intra-abdominal portion of the oesophagus and oesophagogastric junction. Laparoscopic ultrasonography is useful for assessing spread to coeliac and other posterior wall nodal groups, which are normally not seen using conventional optical laparoscopes.

## Computed Tomography (CT)

The normal thoracic oesophagus is easily demonstrated by CT scanning. The mediastinal fat planes are usually clearly imaged in healthy individuals and any blurring or distortion of these images is a fairly reliable indicator of abnormality. Spiral and thin slice CT permit structures such as lymph nodes to be adequately imaged, down to a minimum diameter of about 5 mm. Distant organs such as the liver, lung, adrenal and kidney are easily seen and metastases within them visualised with high accuracy (94-100%). However, CT cannot reliably define the depth of invasion through the oesophageal wall, a structure normally less than 5 mm thick. In cachectic patients with dysphagia and malnutrition, the mediastinal fat plane may be virtually absent, making local invasion more difficult to assess. CT scanning is also of limited value for assessing lymph node involvement. The principal CT criterion for detecting lymph node metastasis is node size; greater than 5 mm in diameter in the mediastinum or 10 mm in the abdomen is usually considered indicative of malignancy. Smaller nodes cannot reliably be visualised and it is not possible to distinguish between enlarged lymph nodes which have reactive changes only and metastatic nodes. Similarly, micrometastases within normal-sized nodes cannot be detected.

The accuracy of correctly predicting lymph node status by CT scanning is in the range of 70-90%. Understaging of malignant nodal disease is the more common error – whilst the specificity of nodal staging using CT may be acceptable (80-90%), the sensitivity is usually low (20-40%). On this basis it is not usually possible to confidently base therapeutic strategies on CT assessment of lymph nodes.

## MRI Scanning

MRI does not expose the patient to ionising radiation and needs no intravascular contrast medium, although intra-oesophageal air or contrast medium may help to assess wall thickness. MRI can differentiate between soft tissue masses and vascular structures within the mediastinum, and just as for CT, distant metastases to organs such as the liver are usually reliably identified.

Current literature indicates no significant additional benefits of MRI scanning over CT [10]. Perhaps the advent of new MRI technologies (real-time or cine MRI) and the development of small coils that can be placed endoluminally may lead to substantial improvements

## Endoscopic Ultrasound (EUS)

The two principal prognostic factors for oesophageal cancer are the depth of tumour penetration through the oesophageal wall and regional lymph node spread. Although CT will detect distant metastasis, its limited axial resolution precludes reliable assessment of both the depth of wall penetration and lymph node involvement. EUS can determine the depth of spread of a malignant tumour through the oesophageal wall (T1-3), invasion of adjacent organs (T4), and metastasis to lymph nodes (N0 or N1). It can also detect contiguous spread downward into the cardia and more distant metastases to the left lobe of the liver (M1).

EUS technology combines flexible endoscopy and high frequency ultrasound delivered endoluminally via miniature probes mounted at the tip of an endoscope. For oesophageal lesions the combination of high frequency ultrasound (7.5-20 MHz) and the ability to position the probe directly adjacent to the target organ provides images of unparalleled resolution (less than 1 mm). The image range with EUS is inversely proportional to the ultrasound frequency used. There is no intervening gas between the echo probe and the target lesion, thus avoiding air artefact

EUS visualises the oesophageal wall as a multilayered structure. The layers represent ultrasound interfaces rather than true anatomical layers, but there is close enough correlation to allow accurate assessment of the depth of invasion through the oesophageal wall. Structures smaller than 5 mm can be clearly seen, enabling very small nodes to be imaged. The EUS image morphology of such structures provides an additional means of distinguishing malignant from reactive or benign lymph nodes. For submucosal lesions, EUS can demonstrate the wall layer of origin of a lesion, suggesting the likely histological type.

Two different EUS systems have been developed. One uses a mechanically driven rotating radial scanner, the other uses a solid-state electronic linear array ultrasound probe. Radial scanners produce circular images at right angles to the long axis of the endoscope, essential as transverse sections of the mediastinum. Linear images are in the sagittal plane, which makes orientation and interpretation more difficult, but these sector scans enable tissue samples to be obtained via EUS-guided fine needle aspiration biopsy using a metal biopsy needle directed within the scanning plane and a steerable bridge system as for endoscopic retrograde cholangiopancreatography (ERCP).

In the mediastinum the aorta and other great vessels, the aortic wall, the heart valves and chambers, regional mediastinal lymph node groups and the wall of the oesophagus can all be imaged in detail by scanning from within the oesophagus (Figure 11.2).

Classically, the wall of the upper alimentary tract is visualised by EUS as a five-layered structure of alternating high and low echogenicity (Figure 11.3). Sometimes the five layers are condensed into three. The anatomical layers represented are shown in Figures 11.4 and 11.5. These intramural layers are significant in terms of assessing "T" stage. The extent of local tumour infiltration is determined by noting

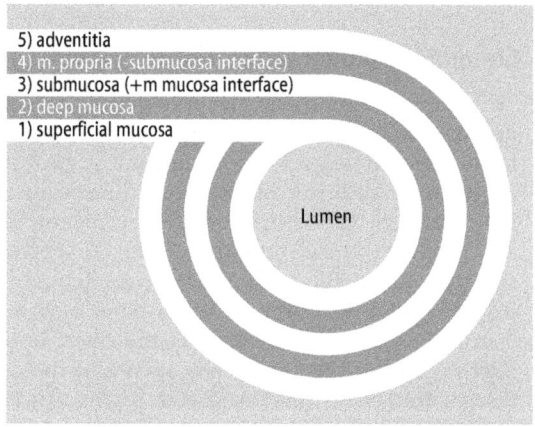

**Figure 11.3.** Five-layered EUS wall structure.

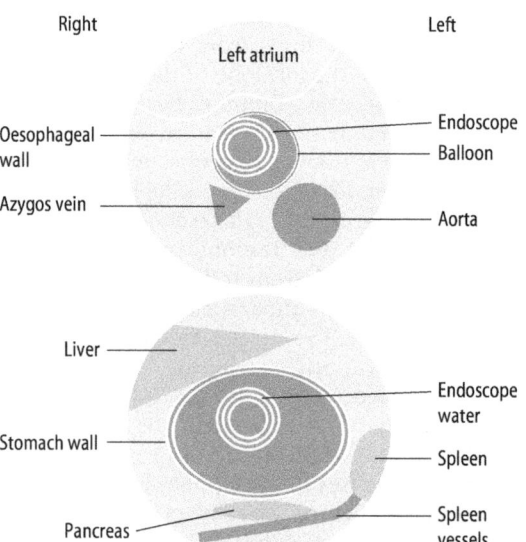

**Figure 11.2.** EUS views through chest and abdomen using a radial scanner.

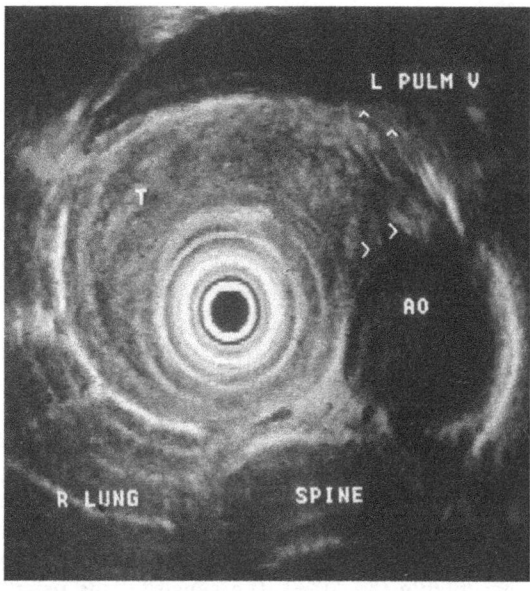

**Figure 11.4.** A locally advanced tumour involving the aortic wall and left pulmonary vein. Note the marginal irregularity and loss of bright interface (T4).

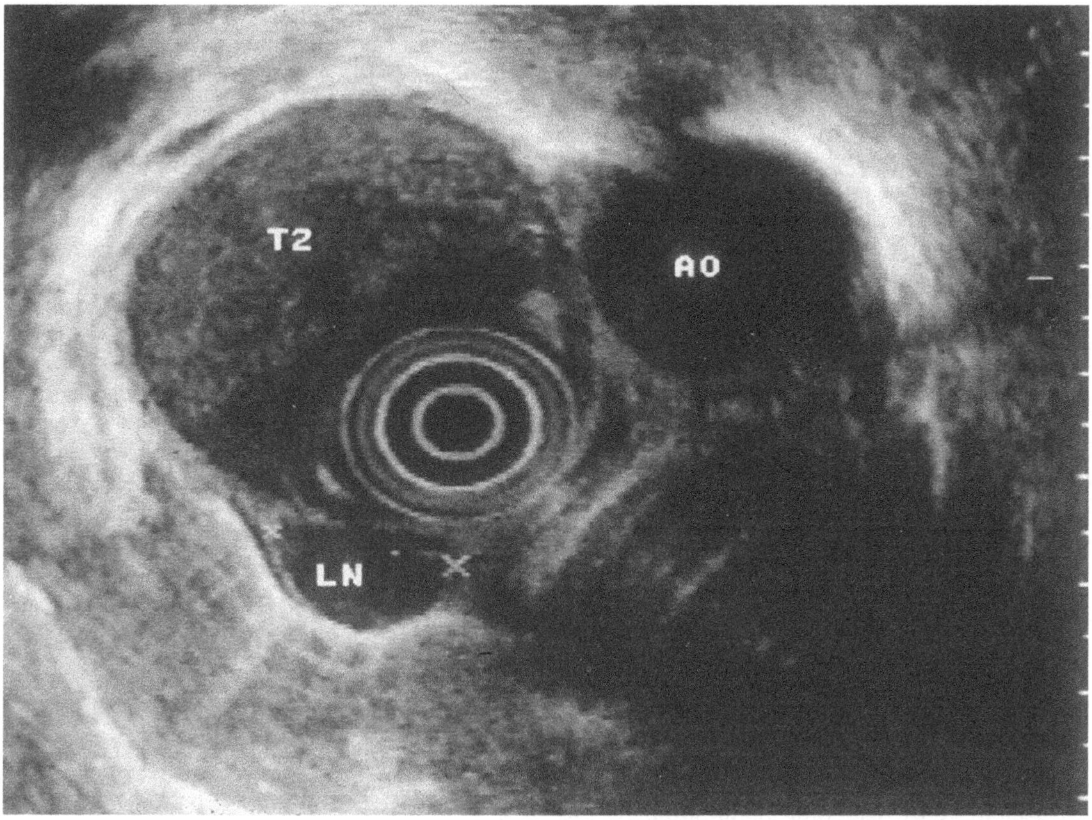

# EPITHELIAL NEOPLASMS OF THE OESOPHAGUS

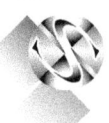

**Figure 11.5.** A tumour of similar overall size to Fig. 11.4, but note the clear margin with bright interface (T2).

which layers remain intact and which are replaced by tumour.

The real-time nature of EUS images confers additional benefits, notably the ability to distinguish blood vessels from other objects of similar size, such as lymph nodes. Colour Doppler, available on some EUS systems, can also help.

The exceptionally high image resolution of EUS reveals the internal architecture of lymph nodes. This information is useful for distinguishing between malignant and benign lymph nodes (Table 11.2). With EUS, image morphology and node size in combination help to determine nodal involvement, rather than node size alone as in CT and MRI.

## The Role of Staging

Once the initial diagnosis of a malignant oesophageal neoplasm has been made, patients should be assessed first in terms of their general

**Table 11.2.** Lymph node evaluation criteria using EUS

| Criterion | Malignant | Benign |
|---|---|---|
| Size | Large (<5 mm) | Small |
| Shape | Round | Elliptical/flat |
| Echo density | Echo poor | Echo dense |
| Heterogeneity | Homogeneous | Heterogeneous |
| Grouping | Solitary | Clusters |
| Borders | Regular | Irregular |

health and fitness for potential therapies. Their preferences should also be considered. Most potentially curative therapies include radical surgery although chemoradiotherapy is an alternative in squamous cell carcinoma. Patients who are unfit for, or who do not wish to contemplate, radical treatments should not be investigated further but should be diverted to appropriate palliative therapies, depending on symptoms and current quality of life. Only those patients suitable for potentially curative therapies should proceed to staging investigations to rule out haematogenous spread and then to assess locoregional stage (EUS ± laparoscopy). This will distinguish between early (T1/ T2, N0) and advanced lesions (T3/T4, N1) and indicate whether surgery alone or multimodal therapy is most appropriate. Where attempted cure is deemed possible, the aim should be to provide the best chance of cure while minimising perioperative risks. In general, surgery alone should be reserved for patients with early disease, and multimodal therapy used in patients with locally advanced disease, in whom the chance of cure by surgery alone is small (generally less than 20%).

# Treatment of Oesophageal Cancer

## Treatments with Palliative Intent

At the time of diagnosis, around two-thirds of all patients with oesophageal cancer will already have incurable disease. The aim of palliative treatment is to overcome debilitating or distressing symptoms while maintaining the best quality of life possible for the patient. Some patients do not require specific therapeutic interventions but do need supportive care and appropriate liaison with community nursing and hospice care services. Close communication between primary and secondary care is therefore of great importance in optimising quality of life for them.

As dysphagia is the predominant symptom in advanced oesophageal cancer, the principal aim of palliation is to restore adequate swallowing. A variety of methods are available and given the short life expectancy of most patients, it is important that the choice of treatment should be tailored to each individual. Tumour location and endoscopic appearance are important in this regard, as is the general condition of the patient.

## Chemotherapy and/or Radiotherapy

Careful patient selection is important. Good performance status and the absence of co-morbid disease are particularly desirable in patients considered for palliative chemotherapy alone or in combination with radiotherapy. A number of studies have reported good clinical responses in around two-thirds of patients, using a variety of regimens but generally including cisplatin and 5-fluorouracil. Most studies demonstrate modest improvements in survival, with an average life expectancy of around 9 months. There is no great difference between adenocarcinomas and squamous cell carcinomas [11,12]. Radiotherapy alone will improve dysphagia also in about two-thirds of patients. It is important to realise that improvement is slow and therefore this treatment is best suited to patients with milder degrees of dysphagia. The addition of brachytherapy to external beam radiotherapy does lead to faster relief of dysphagia but at the expense of an increased risk of fistula formation. In randomised trials, combination chemoradiotherapy produces higher response rates than radiotherapy alone, with a further modest prolongation in survival to around one year [13].

## Endoscopic Treatment

### Oesophageal Dilatation

This is only appropriate for patients with a very short life expectancy, as recurrent dysphagia is inevitable, usually within 2 to 4 weeks. Serious complications, including haemorrhage and perforation, will occur in up to 10% of patients.

### Injection Therapy

Intratumoral injection of absolute alcohol is useful in soft polypoid tumours and those situated immediately below the cricopharyngeus, where intubation is inappropriate. Injection therapy can also be useful to control bleeding. In well-selected cases, this method does improve dysphagia but usually needs to be repeated on a monthly basis.

### Thermal Ablation

This can be achieved using lasers, photodynamic therapy or argon plasma coagulation. Whichever thermal method is used, it is contraindicated in patients with aerodigestive fistulas but like ethanol injection it may be particularly useful in tumours close to the cricopharyngeus. All three techniques produce a marked improvement in dysphagia but require repetition, usually at about monthly intervals as tumour regrowth occurs. Complications, including perforation, have been reported in up to 5% of patients and photosensitivity may be a problem with photodynamic therapy. All thermal methods can be used in conjunction with other palliative modalities including radiotherapy and stenting. In addition, thermal methods can be useful as a means of recanalising stents if tumour ingrowth should occur.

*Oesophageal Intubation*

This is an effective method of relieving dysphagia in a single procedure. Semi-rigid plastic tubes have gradually been replaced in the last 10 years by self-expanding metal stents because the latter seem easier to insert as they do not require preliminary dilatation for tube placement. There is little evidence to suggest that the improvement in dysphagia is different between semi-rigid and self-expanding stents, although case series would indicate that the ability to take solid food is more widely achieved with self-expanding than rigid stents. Procedure-related morbidity occurs in around 10% of patients and by eliminating the preliminary dilatation step, this may be slightly lower for self-expanding stents. In both cases, prior radiotherapy or chemotherapy seems to lead to a higher rate of complications [14]. Covered self-expanding metal stents are particularly useful as a means of occluding areodigestive fistulas.

A variety of self-expanding stent configurations are available. Those that are widest in diameter may cause significant tracheal compression when placed in the upper half of the oesophagus, while placement at the oesophagogastric junction with an intragastric component to the stent will result in gastro-oesophageal reflux and a significant risk of aspiration, particularly in the elderly and frail.

## Treatments with Curative Intent

Once oesophageal neoplasms reach the submucosal layer of the oesophagus, the tumour has access to the lymphatic system, meaning that even at this early local stage, there is an incidence of nodal positivity for both squamous cell and adenocarcinomas of between 10% and 50%. The rarity of intramucosal cancer in symptomatic patients means that there are no randomised studies to compare different approaches to this type of very early disease.

Even in Barrett's oesophagus, where high grade dysplasia and early cancer coexist, most centres favour oesophageal surgery and many centres exclude elderly or unfit patients from surveillance programmes, so there is considerable selection bias in most case series that have examined local therapies for these very early tumours. All forms of local ablation have been used successfully. Endoscopic ultrasound should be used to try and establish the intramucosal nature of such a malignancy and exclude nodal metastasis.

## Non-surgical Treatments

Radiotherapy alone was widely used as a single modality treatment for squamous cell carcinoma of the oesophagus until the late 1970s. The 5-year survival overall was 6%. As a result, multimodal approaches were adopted throughout the 1980s, initial trials indicating that similar long-term survival rates could be obtained to surgery. Subsequent randomised studies, essentially confined to patients with squamous cell carcinoma, have indicated significant survival advantages with chemoradiotherapy over radiotherapy alone [15,16]. While it is clear that chemoradiotherapy does offer a prospect of cure for patients who may not be fit for surgery, particularly in squamous cell carcinoma, the high rate of loco-regional failure has meant that surgery remains the mainstay of attempted curative treatments for both adenocarcinoma and squamous cell carcinoma in patients who have potentially resectable disease and are fit for oesophagectomy. In most Western series, this represents about one-third of patients with adenocarcinoma and a slightly lower percentage of patients with squamous cell carcinoma.

There is considerable current debate regarding the selection of patients in whom surgery should be considered, along with the identification of those who would be most appropriately treated by surgery alone and those requiring a multimodal approach. In terms of the latter, both neoadjuvant and adjuvant approaches have been adopted using chemotherapy and/or radiotherapy. There is no evidence that postoperative chemotherapy or radiotherapy has any significant effect on survival.

It is essential that oesophagectomy should be performed with a low hospital mortality and complication rate. Case selection, case volume and experience of the surgical team are all important. Preoperative risk analysis has shown that this can play a major part in reducing hospital mortality [17].

There are really no circumstances in the Western world where surgery should be undertaken if it is not part of an overall treatment plan aimed at cure. The principle of oesophagectomy is to deal adequately with the local tumour in order to minimise the risk of local recurrence and achieve an adequate lymphadenectomy to reduce the risk of staging error. Although studies in Japan would indicate that more extensive lymphadenectomy is associated with better survival, this may simply reflect more accurate staging. A number of studies support the view that the proximal extent of resection should ideally be 10 cm above the macroscopic tumour and 5 cm distal. When such a margin cannot be achieved proximally, particularly with squamous cell carcinoma, there is evidence that postoperative radiotherapy can minimise local recurrence, though it does not improve survival [18].

Adenocarcinoma commonly involves the gastric cardia and may therefore extend into the fundus or down the lesser curve. Some degree of gastric excision is essential in order to achieve adequate local clearance and accomplish an appropriate lymphadenectomy. Excision of contiguous structures such as crura, diaphragm and mediastinal pleura all need to be considered as methods of creating negative resection margins.

It follows that surgery alone is best suited to patients with disease confined to the oesophagus (T1, T2) without nodal metastasis (N0). As a result of careful preoperative investigation, most of these patients are now identifiable and can be offered surgery alone, with a prospect of cure of between 50% and 80% [19,20]. Patients with more advanced stages of disease require either multimodal approaches or entry into appropriately designed trials.

## Oesophagectomy

Histological tumour type, its location and the extent of the proposed lymphadenectomy all influence the operative approach. This is largely an issue of surgical preference, although it should be recognised that a left thoracoabdominal approach is limited proximally by the aortic arch and should be avoided when the primary tumour is at or above this level. Similarly, trans-hiatal oesophagectomy is unsuitable for most patients with squamous cell carcinoma because a complete mediastinal lymphadectomy is not easily achieved by this approach in most centres. The most widely practised approach is the two-phase Lewis–Tanner operation, with an initial laparotomy and construction of a gastric tube, followed by a right thoracotomy to excise the tumour and create an oesophagogastric anastomosis. The closer this is placed to the apex of the thoracic cavity, the fewer problems there are with reflux disease. Three-phase oesophagectomy (McKeown) may be more appropriate for more proximal tumours in order to achieve better longitudinal clearance, although the additional distance gained is less than many surgeons believe. A third cervical incision also permits lymphadenectomy in this region.

The extent of lymphadenectomy is highly controversial. For squamous cell carcinoma, because a higher proportion of patients will have middle and upper third tumours in the thoracic oesophagus, the rationale behind a three-phase operation with three-field lymphadenectomy is more understandable, even though this approach has not been adopted widely in the West. For adenocarcincoma, the incidence of metastases in the neck is relatively low in the context of patients who would be otherwise curable. For this reason, two-phase operations with two-field lymphadenectomy seem the most logical operations. While two-field lymphadenectomy does not substantially increase operative morbidity or mortality, the same cannot be said for more extended operations.

While many centres have reduced hospital mortality to single figures following oesophagectomy, the complication rate remains high. At least one-third of all patients will develop some significant complication after surgery. The most common of these is respiratory, followed by anastomotic leakage, chylothorax and injury to the recurrent laryngeal nerves. The most common late problem is benign anastomotic stricture, which seems to be more likely, with cervical rather than intrathoracic anastomoses, although the problem is usually easily dealt with by endoscopic dilatation.

## Neoadjuvant Treatments with Surgery

Apart from the earliest stages of disease, surgery alone produces relatively few cures in either

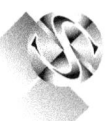

## EPITHELIAL NEOPLASMS OF THE OESOPHAGUS

squamous cell or adenocarcinoma patients. This led to a number of trials throughout the 1980s and 1990s to investigate the value of chemotherapy and surgery or chemoradiotherapy and surgery compared with surgery alone. The results of these are shown in Table 11.3.

Many of these studies are open to criticism on the grounds of trial design or patient numbers. Nevertheless, positive results in favour of neoadjuvant therapy for adenocarcinoma in both the Walsh and MRC studies indicate that it is no longer appropriate to consider surgery alone as the gold standard treatment for most patients who are surgical candidates with adenocarcinoma. The exact role of surgery in a multimodal approach to squamous cell carcinoma is an unresolved issue and the results of ongoing trials must be awaited.

## Conclusion

The management of malignant oesophageal neoplasms remains challenging. Late presentation with advanced disease is still a common scenario. The ability to reliably detect patients with potentially curable lesions remains crucial.

With the advent of more reliable pretreatment staging investigations and the continuing development of novel therapies, there is now a better opportunity to select patients on an individual basis for the treatment modality most appropriate to their situation. The variety of available therapies continues to broaden and highlights the need for a multidisciplinary approach to patient care. While the debate around radical surgery versus multimodal treatments is likely to develop further in the future,

**Table 11.3.** Randomised trials of neoadjuvant chemotherapy ± radiotherapy with surgery

| | No | Histology SCC | Adeno | RT (Gy) | Chemotherapy | pCR (%) | Overall survival Median | 3 years (%) | p |
|---|---|---|---|---|---|---|---|---|---|
| Nygaard et al 1992 [21] | | | | | | | | | |
| CRT + surgery | 47 | 47 | 0 | 35 | Cisplatin, bleomycin | N/S | 7 m | 17 | 0.3 |
| Chemotherapy + surgery | 50 | 50 | 0 | | Cisplatin, bleomycin | N/S | 6 m | 3 | |
| Radiotherapy + surgery | 48 | 48 | 0 | 35 | | N/S | 8 m | 21 | |
| Surgery only | 41 | 41 | 0 | | | | 6 m | 9 | |
| Apinop et al 1994 [22] | | | | | | | | | |
| CRT + surgery | 35 | 35 | 0 | 40 | 5FU, cisplatin | 20 | 10 m | 26 | 0.4 |
| Surgery only | 34 | 34 | 0 | | | | 7 m | 20 | |
| Le Prise et al 1994 [23] | | | | | | | | | |
| CRT + surgery | 41 | 41 | 0 | 20 | 5FU, cisplatin | 10 | 10 m | 19 | 0.6 |
| Surgery only | 45 | 45 | 0 | | | | 11 m | 14 | |
| Walsh et al 1996 [24] | | | | | | | | | |
| CRT + surgery | 58 | 0 | 58 | 40 | 5FU, cisplatin | 22 | 16 m | 32 | 0.01 |
| Surgery only | 55 | 0 | 55 | | | | 11 m | 6 | |
| Bosset et al 1997 [25] | | | | | | | | | |
| CRT + surgery | 143 | 143 | 0 | 37 | Cisplatin | 20 | 19 m | 36 | 0.8 |
| Surgery only | 139 | 139 | 0 | | | | 18 m | 34 | |
| Kelsen et al 1998 [26] | | | | | | | | | |
| Chemotherapy + Surgery | 213 | 98 | 115 | | 5FU, cisplatin | 2.5 | 14.9 m | 23 | 0.53 |
| Surgery only | 227 | 106 | 121 | | | | 16.1 m | 26 | |
| Urba et al 2001 [27] | | | | | | | | | |
| CRT + Surgery | 50 | N/S | N/S | 45 | 5FU, cisplatin, vinblastine | 28 | 17 m | 30 | 0.15 |
| Surgery only | 50 | N/S | N/S | | | | 18 m | 16 | |
| MRC 2002 [28] | | | | | | | | | |
| Chemotherapy + Surgery | 400 | 123 | 265 | | 5FU, cisplatin | 4 | 17 m | 24 | 0.0014 |
| Surgery only | 402 | 124 | 268 | | | | 13 m | 17 | |

SCC, squamous cell carcinoma; Adeno, adenocarcinoma; RT, radiotherapy m, months.

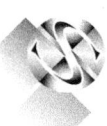

the present role of radical resection as the mainstay of treatment aimed at cure should be acknowledged. Clinicians must, however, remember that all available potentially curative therapies carry the risk of significant morbidity and as such these should only be offered in large centres where there is a wide experience in management of patients with oesophageal cancer.

## Questions

1. Outline the differences in oesophageal cancer incidence internationally.
2. List the key factors in determining appropriate treatment.
3. Compare and contrast operative approaches to oesophageal cancer treatment.
4. Discuss the role of neoadjuvant and adjuvant treatment in oesophageal cancer.

## References

1. HMSO. Cancer statistics registrations: Cases of diagnosed cancer in England and Wales. OPCS, 1986.
2. Gilleson E, Powell J, McConkey C et al. Surgical workload and outcome after resection for carcinoma of the oesophagus and cardia. Br J Surg 2002;89(3):344–8.
3. Rahamim J, Cham CW et al. Oesophagogastrectomy for carcinoma of the oesophagus and cardia. Br J Surg 1993;80(10):1305–9.
4. Ribeiro U, Posner M, Safatle-Ribeiro A et al. Risk factors for squamous cell carcinoma of the oesophagus. Br J Surg 1996;83(9):1174–85.
5. Lagergren J, Bergstrom, R Nyren O et al. Association between body mass and adenocarcinoma of the esophagus and gastric cardia. Ann Intern Med 1999;130:883–90.
6. Sakata K. Uber die Lymphgefassedes Oesophagus und Uber Siene Regionaren Lymphrusen Mit Berucksichtigung der Verbreitung des Carcinomas Mitt Grenzgebeit. Med Chir 1903;11:634.
7. Akiyama H, Tsurumaru M, Kawamura T, Ono Y. Principles of surgical treatment for carcinoma of the oesophagus. Ann Surg 1981;194(4):438–46.
8. Sobin L, Wittekind C (eds) TNM classification of malignant tumours, 5th edn. New York: John Wiley, 1997.
9. Molloy R, McCourtney J, Anderson J et al. Laparoscopy in the management of patients with cancer of the gastric cardia or oesophagus. Br J Surg 1995;82(3):352–4.
10. Quint L, Glazer G, Orringer M. Oesophageal Imaging by MR and CT: Study of normal anatomy and neoplasms. Radiology 1985;156:727–31.
11. Webb A, Cunningham D, Scarffe JH et al. Randomized trial comparing epirubicin, cisplatin, and fluorouracil versus fluorouracil, doxorubicin, and methotrexate in advanced esophagogastric cancer. J Clin Oncol 1997;15:261–7.
12. van der Gaast A, Kok TC, Kerkhofs L et al. Phase I study of a biweekly schedule of a fixed dose of cisplatin with increasing doses of paclitaxel in patients with advanced oesophageal cancer. Br J Cancer 1999;80:1052–7.
13. Herskovic A, Martz K, Al Sarraf M et al. Combined chemotherapy and radiotherapy compared with radiotherapy alone in patients with cancer of the esophagus. N Engl J Med 1992;326:1593–8.
14. Siersema PD, Hop WC, Dees J et al. Coated self-expanding metal stents versus latex prostheses for esophagogastric cancer with special reference to prior radiation and chemotherapy: a controlled, prospective study. Gastrointest Endosc 1998;47:113–20.
15. Smith TJ, Ryan LM, Douglass HO Jr et al. Combined chemoradiotherapy vs. radiotherapy alone for early stage squamous cell carcinoma of the esophagus: a study of the Eastern Cooperative Oncology Group. Int J Radiat Oncol Biol Phys 1998;42(2):269–76.
16. Al-Sarraf M, Martz K, Herskovic A et al. Progress report of combined chemoradiotherapy versus radiotherapy alone in patients with esophageal cancer: an intergroup study. J Clin Oncol 1997;15:277–84.
17. Bartels H, Stein HJ, Siewert JR. Preoperative risk analysis and postoperative mortality of oesophagectomy for resectable oesophageal cancer. Br J Surg 1998;85:840–4.
18. Tam PC, Sui KF, Cheung HC et al. Local recurrences after sub-total oesophagectomy for squamous cell carcinoma. Ann Surg 1987;205:189–94.
19. Bonavina L. Early oesophageal cancer: results of a European multicentre survey. Group Européen pour L'Etude des Maladies de L'Oesophage. Br J Surg 1995;82:98–101.
20. Hölscher AH, Bollschweiler E, Schneider PM et al. Early adenocarcinoma in Barrett's oesophagus. Br J Surg 1997;84:1470–3.
21. Nygaard K, Hagen S, Hansen HS et al. Pre-operative radiotherapy prolongs survival in operable esophageal carcinoma: A randomized, multicentre study of pre-operative radiotherapy and chemotherapy. The second Scandinavian trial in esophageal cancer. World J Surg 1992;16:1104–10.
22. Apinop C, Puttisak P, Preecha N. A prospective study of combined therapy in esophageal cancer. Hepatogastroenterology 1994;41:391–3.
23. Le Prise E, Etienne PL, Meunier B et al. A randomized study of chemotherapy, radiation therapy, and surgery versus surgery for localized squamous cell carcinoma of the esophagus. Cancer 1994;73:1779–84.
24. Walsh TN, Noonan N, Hollywood D, et al. A comparison of multimodal therapy and surgery for esophageal adenocarcinoma. N Engl J Med 1996;335:462–7.
25. Bosset JF, Gignoux M, Triboulet JP et al. Chemoradiotherapy followed by surgery compared with surgery alone in squamous-cell cancer of the esophagus. N Engl J Med 1997;337:161–7.
26. Kelsen DP, Ginsberg R, Pajak TF et al. Chemotherapy followed by surgery compared with surgery alone for localized esophageal cancer. N Engl J Med 1998;339:1979–84.
27. Urba SG, Orringer MB, Turrisi A et al. Randomized trial of preoperative chemoradiation versus surgery alone in patients with locoregional esophageal carcinoma. J Clin Oncol 2001;19:305–13.
28. Medical Research Council Oesophageal Cancer Working Group. Surgical resection with or without preoperative chemotherapy in oesophageal cancer: a randomised controlled trial. Lancet 2002;359:1727–33.

# 12

# Epithelial Neoplasms of the Stomach

Peter McCulloch

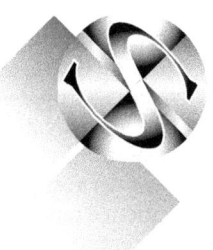

## Aims

- To discuss the causes of changing patterns of gastric cancer.
- To evaluate methods of improving early detection.
- To summarise current staging techniques.
- To explain current controversies about gastrectomy for cancer.
- To define the place of non-surgical treatments.

Properly speaking there are very few epithelial neoplasms of the stomach. Benign adenomas of gastric epithelium exist, and gastrinomas and gastric carcinoids are both well recognised, although whether these latter two qualify as epithelial tumours is a matter of how liberally the term is defined. The most important epithelial neoplasm is gastric carcinoma, and consequently the bulk of this chapter will be concerned with this subject.

Although the focus of Western efforts against cancer has shifted to other areas, gastric carcinoma remains one of the largest causes of cancer mortality worldwide. Its poor prognosis globally is related to the difficulty of early diagnosis, the need for major surgery in an elderly, unfit population and the limited efficacy of non-surgical treatments.

## Pathology

### Degree of Differentiation and Site

Gastric cancer seems to be divisible into two subtypes whose natural history and aetiology are quite distinct. The type of gastric cancer which remains endemic in the Far East, parts of South America and Eastern Europe is principally a disease of the distal stomach, associated with chronic gastritis, intestinal metaplasia and atrophy of the mucosa. The type which is increasing rapidly in incidence in Western countries is commonly found near the oesophagogastric junction, and is not associated with significant gastritis. The histological appearances of gastric cancer have been classified on completely different bases by a number of authorities. The classification of Lauren, which describes tumours as intestinal or diffuse, remains influential, partly because it has been found to correspond to a dichotomy in the molecular biology of gastric tumours. The system has serious problems, however, principally a degree of subjectivity in the definitions of the two classes which leads to very considerable inter-interpreter variation. The classifications of Ming and of Goseki have found favour in different degrees, but neither is universally used. The Japanese Research Society for Gastric Cancer (JRSGC) has its own system, which recognises signet cell cancers and few others as exceptions which cannot be fitted into a spectrum of degrees of differentiation. All of the systems struggle with the common finding of great heterogeneity in histological appearance between different areas of the same tumour. In broad terms, cancers in areas of high endemic incidence tend to be distal and intestinal, or well differentiated, whereas those in lower incidence areas have a greater probability of being diffuse and proximal.

## Mode of Spread

Gastric cancer shares with colorectal cancer an origin in the luminal epithelium of the gut, a position within the peritoneal cavity and a portal venous drainage arrangement, but their metastatic behaviour is strikingly different. Gastric cancer has a very marked propensity towards loco-regional nodal spread, rarely if ever metastasising via the bloodstream before spreading to numerous local nodes. Autopsy series show that many patients dying from gastric cancer still had no evidence of disease outwith the affected organ and the regional lymph nodes. Gastric cancer also has a greater propensity, once it has breached the serosa, to spread via the peritoneal surfaces, shedding miliary metastatic nodules in a fashion which renders the patient essentially incurable. In contrast to colorectal cancer, in which isolated liver metastases suitable for surgical resection occur quite frequently, only 30 of about 5000 gastric cancers in one very large series were eligible for this kind of treatment. There is some evidence from studies of early gastric cancer in Japan that well-differentiated cancers may metastasise rather more frequently to the liver and poorly differentiated tumours to the nodes. Limited evidence on the natural history of early (mucosal and submucosal) cancer also suggests that there is a major acceleration in the growth rate and metastatic potential of the tumour once the mucosa is breached. Mucosal cancers have an incidence of positive nodes of around 2% in Japanese series, whereas this increases about tenfold when the lamina propria has been breached. The transition from early cancer to advanced cancer in the Japanese classification (T2+ disease in Union Internacional Contra la Cancrum (UICC) staging terms) appears to take an average of 4–7 years, whereas the progression of T2+ from diagnosis to inoperability or death is measurable in months.

## Staging

### Staging Systems

Staging is performed differently in North America, Japan and Europe, a fact which contributes significantly to international misunderstanding about treatment and outcome. An attempt to unify the staging systems in 1987 has not, unfortunately, been repeated following revisions of the Japanese and UICC classifications in subsequent years. All staging systems concentrate on wall invasion and nodal metastasis, but the Japanese system retains the definition of "early gastric cancer" for T1 n(any) cancers. The 5th edition of the UICC system changed the basis of nodal classification from an anatomical one (n1 nodes defined as within 3 cm of the primary tumour) to a numerical one (n1 now means 1–6 positive nodes). Several studies have shown this approach to be superior to the 4th edition, and at least equal to the more complex anatomical system used in Japan in terms of prognostic value.

### Stage Migration and Associated Problems

Since nodal metastasis plays such a dominant role in the prediction of prognosis in gastric cancer, more radical lymphadenectomy and more diligent pathological examination lead inevitably to a "stage migration" phenomenon [1]. This means that more radically operated patients are more likely to be allocated a more advanced stage, because more nodes are found and examined. It can be predicted that this will lead to an apparent survival improvement in each stage group, even if radical surgery is completely ineffective. This is because each stage group will contain a proportion of patients that would have been in a lower stage category if the extent of surgery had been less radical, and the overall survival of the group will therefore be bought up. This phenomenon is one of the major difficulties which have prevented a clear answer to the question which still remains over the benefits of radical nodal clearance. Various authors have attempted to estimate the effects of stage migration in different subgroups. Most have concluded that the groups whose apparent survival is changed most are the intermediate stages II, IIIA and IIIB. These are also the stages for which the predicted survival benefits of radical gastrectomy are greatest. Although ingenious attempts have been made to circumvent the problem, only an overall population survival benefit from more radical nodal dissection within a randomised trial would be scientifically valid, and this has not yet been reported.

# Aetiology

## Genetic Influences

The genetic basis of gastric cancer is less well understood than that of colorectal or breast cancer, but progress has been made in identifying come common mutations and deletions. As with most carcinomas, loss of normal p53 function and over-expression or gain-of-function mutation of growth factor receptors such as EGF, c-erbB2 and c-Met are common findings, as are mutations in the "second messenger" chain of protein kinases which mediate growth factor effects, such as k-Ras. There is an important association of diffuse type gastric cancer with loss of function of the E-cadherin molecule, which normally acts as one of the main adhesion molecules anchoring cells to each other in the epithelial sheet. The proteins which interact with E-cadherin in this role also have other roles to play, and one in particular, β catenin, is an important player in the so-called Wnt signalling pathway, which also involves the APC molecule associated with familial polyposis coli and colorectal cancer. Over-expression of β catenin in the cytoplasm or reduction of expression on the membrane of the cell is associated with poor outcome in gastric as well as colorectal cancer. Attempts have been made to develop a schema of genetic changes associated with the stages in gastric carcinogenesis. These have been complicated by the apparently different nature of diffuse and intestinal cancers. The existence of a recognisable progression of premalignant changes in the former has allowed recognition of early and later changes. In diffuse cancer, the lack of any recognisable premalignant mucosal abnormality hinders these studies, but it does seem quite clear that the commonly found mutations and deletions are quite different in the two forms. E-cadherin loss is strongly associated with diffuse cancer, and a number of families have now been described in whom inherited loss of one E-cadherin allele predisposes to diffuse gastric cancer at an early age when the other allele is mutated or lost [2]. C-erbB2 over-expression, on the other hand, is associated with intestinal cancer. Correa has described a gastritis–atrophy–metaplasia–dysplasia–cancer sequence which applies to typical cases of intestinal cancer in endemic areas, and Tahara has developed a putative sequence of associated genetic abnormalities. The number of such abnormalities associated with diffuse cancer is at least as large, but the lack of an observable progression histopathologically has prevented identification of the order in which these tend to occur.

## Helicobacter pylori

The importance of *Helicobacter* infection in the causation of gastric cancer is universally accepted, and the organism has been classified as a grade 1 carcinogen by the World Health Organisation. A large multinational study of *H. pylori* infection and gastric cancer incidence showed a predicted fivefold variation between populations with zero and 100% infection rates [3]. Another convincing strand of evidence is the development of cancer in an animal model in which Mongolian gerbils were infected with a closely related *Helicobacter*. The *H. pylori* organism usually infects the gastric mucosa during the first 3 years of life, and there is evidence that it causes an acute vomiting illness which may assist its further spread by oral–oral contamination. The response to colonisation depends partly on genetic and partly on environmental factors. There is evidence that the interleukin 1 genotype of the individual may help to determine whether infection is more likely to result in cancer or a benign ulcer, and other genes related to immune and inflammatory responses may be implicated [4]. The strain of the organism may also play a role: the strain of the organism and the type of toxins it produces, particularly the CAG antigen, is reported by some workers to affect the chance of cancer. The fact that *Helicobacter* acts over several decades to produce a state of chronic inflammation and atrophy with reduction in acid production explains why the organisms are often absent at the time of cancer diagnosis: the higher pH of the atrophic stomach leads to greater competition from other organisms which are able to survive in the less hostile conditions. It is important to note that H. pylori is NOT implicated in cancer of the cardia, which is the only type of gastric cancer which is on the increase worldwide. There is some evidence that CAG-positive H. pylori infection of the distal stomach may actually be protective against cancers at the oesophagogastric junction, perhaps because the infection promotes gastric atrophy and therefore reduces acid reflux.

## Diet

Dietary influences which increase the risk of chronic gastritis appear to synergise with infection to increase further the chance of cancer developing. The strongest association is with a diet high in salt and poor in vitamins C and E. Some evidence from supplementations studies supports a role for these antioxidant vitamins in cancer prevention. The role of salt is thought to be both direct and indirect, causing osmotic damage as well as encouraging the conversion of dietary nitrates to nitrites. In the achlorhydric conditions of chronic atrophic gastritis the latter are readily converted to carcinogenic nitrosamines through fermentation by bacteria.

## Alcohol and Tobacco

The evidence from studies of alcohol intake in the causation of gastric cancer and cancer of the gastro-oesophageal junction suggests that it is not a significant risk factor – indeed wine may be slightly protective in the latter. Smoking, on the other hand, is clearly implicated in cardia cancer, with evidence of a dose–response effect and a risk ratio for smokers compared with non-smokers.

## Reflux

The cause of the rapid increase in proximal gastric and junctional cancer is not yet clear, but there is persuasive evidence that one essential factor is gastro-oesophageal reflux. Epidemiological studies have linked the condition strongly with symptomatic reflux, and with both obesity and a high fat diet, both of which increase the risk of reflux disease. One influential study shows a risk ratio of over 3 for cardia cancer in people with a long history of reflux disease, with evidence of a dose–response effect; it should be noted that there is an even stronger association with cancer of the distal oesophagus [5]. There is experimental evidence to indicate that the combined effects of bile and acid are significantly more genotoxic than either substance alone. The rise in the incidence of the condition correlates temporally with diet and lifestyle changes which have led to increases in obesity and reflux disease in many populations, and it is interesting to note that this rise has not been seen in populations where reflux and obesity are still uncommon, such as the Japanese. Reflux alone is not a sufficient explanation for the rise in the incidence, as brief reflection makes clear. It does not explain the very strong male predominance seen in most studies, and some degree of synergism with another factor such as smoking may be needed for carcinogenesis.

# Epidemiology and Incidence

## Pandemic Distal Cancer

The dramatic decline in distal gastric cancer in the West is well documented, and has been described as an accidental public health triumph. Figures for the incidence of the disease worldwide show the variable nature of the decline, which has been sharpest in affluent countries with a predominantly Caucasian population and a low population density, such as the USA, Canada, Australia and New Zealand. In these countries the disease has declined by as much as eightfold over the last 50 years. In Western Europe the decline, whilst highly significant, has been considerably less steep, and this is even more so for the countries in the Far East and South America where the populations are still affected by high incidence rates. Continuing high rates of H. pylori infection, adverse dietary factors and genetic predisposition may all play a role in determining these population differences.

## Junctional Cancer

Cancer of the gastro-oesophageal junction is said to be the fastest-increasing solid malignancy of adult life in the Western world, increasing in incidence by about 3–4% per

# EPITHELIAL NEOPLASMS OF THE STOMACH

annum over the last 30 years. Some recent data suggest there may be an element of misclassification bias, but most authorities agree that the increase is real. The associations with male sex, obesity, smoking and reflux noted in epidemiological studies suggest possible aetiological factors, but the work of establishing the pathogenetic pathways by which these work is in its early stages. Most workers have reported no association of this type of cancer with *H. pylori* infection, whilst some have provided suggestive evidence of an inverse relationship between infection and incidence – that is to say that infection may actually be protective.

# Diagnosis and Screening

## The Problem of Early Detection

Gastric cancer begins as an epithelial proliferation and disorganisation which has no features which either stimulate pain receptors or influence function significantly. It is therefore inherently difficult to diagnose at an early stage. Breakdown of the mucosa with ulceration, pain and bleeding can occur at an early stage, but more commonly not until the tumour is well established, and the same applies to functional disturbance, which occurs either when the lumen begins to be obstructed or when the infiltration of the gastric wall and its intrinsic nervous system is widespread enough to cause problems with normal motility and emptying.

Japanese clinicians, for whom gastric cancer is high on the list of public health problems, have paid greater attention than any others to the possibility of screening for the disease. They estimate that up to 40% of early gastric cancers are associated with symptoms, and therefore many of their so-called screening services are focused on investigation of symptomatic or concerned patients. The evidence that the symptoms these patients suffer from are due to the cancer rather than to the almost invariable background of chronic gastritis is scanty. The combination of a high incidence and meticulous investigation has led to a high pick-up rate of early lesions in Japanese programmes, and both Japanese and Western authors commonly attribute the very high incidence of early cancer in Japan to screening. If we define screening in the strict sense of testing the asymptomatic population by invitation, however, it quickly becomes clear that this alone cannot be responsible for the Japanese success. The screening programme in Japan appears to be rather fragmented, and the proportion of the population at risk which is reached by any one programme is very small. Even when all programmes are taken together, it is clear from the detection rates compared with the overall incidence rate for early gastric cancer that the majority of early cancer cases are detected outside the screening programme. The key feature would appear to be the high level of awareness and concern in the Japanese population, which leads over 40% of men over 40 to seek investigation every year, according to a recent opportunistic study. There is evidence from observational studies of patients who refused or missed treatment that the progression of intramucosal malignancy in the stomach is slow, and this gives greater opportunities for detection at an easily treatable stage if the at-risk population can be identified and can be persuaded to have an accurate test. Japanese authors have shown that serum measurement of pepsinogen I and II ratios is specific and sensitive enough to be considered as a screening tool in their population, but the approach is dependent on detecting severe gastric atrophy, and would therefore be less useful in the West. There have been few Western attempts to improve early detection, despite the obvious benefits which would accrue. There has been a gradual shift in the direction of earlier detection over the last 20 years, which has correlated with the more widespread use of gastroscopy for the investigation of dyspepsia. There is no good evidence to support the assertion that open access endoscopy improves early detection rates, but by increasing population access to gastroscopy it is likely to act in this direction.

An approach which has been shown to have a positive effect in a well-designed study is close liaison between specialists and GPs in the screening of dyspeptic patients and referral of those most at risk for early gastroscopy [6]. This approach led to a 25% incidence of early gastric cancer in the study group, although most of these lesions were in fact detected at yearly follow-up gastroscopy organised after severe gastritis, severe metaplasia or dysplasia was found on initial examination. A case-control study of symptom characteristics showed that patients with symptoms of less than 6 months' duration, continuous symptoms, and symptoms which include either anorexia with weight loss or dysphagia are over 20 times more likely to have cancer than the average dyspeptic patient. A recent study of health education by letter, however, showed that, although the information initially increased the operation rate, it had no effect on overall survival.

## Investigations

The definitive investigation when gastric cancer is part of the differential diagnosis is a careful gastroscopy under good conditions. These should include good sedation, smooth muscle relaxant such as hyoscine, and good quality video-endoscopy with facilities for applying anti-foaming agents and dye-spray with indigo-carmine to show up details of mucosal topography. An experienced endoscopist with these facilities should be able to detect even very small mucosal lesions with a high degree of accuracy. There are a number of well-recognised pitfalls and difficulties in the endoscopic diagnosis of gastric cancer:

1. Gastric ulcer. The controversy over whether cancer develops in benign ulcers is over 100 years old, but largely irrelevant to the management of the situation. The patient is usually an elderly female, and the ulcer is resistant to normal drug therapy. Biopsies are often repeatedly negative until eventually a diagnosis of cancer is made.
2. Linitis plastica. The diagnostic clue in this type of cancer is usually the inability to perform a gastroscopy due to a non-distensible stomach.
3. Gastric outlet obstruction. The build-up of food residue and fluid in the obstructed stomach can make endoscopy impossible.
4. Blind spots. Small tumours high on the lesser curve, or hidden amongst the rugae of the mid-body can be difficult to detect.

Repeated lavage of the stomach via a nasogastric tube is the unpleasant but essential preliminary to gastroscopy in the obstructed stomach. The routine use of dye-spray with indigo-carmine to delineate the surface topography of the mucosa is stressed as an important tool for the detection of subtle early cancers by Japanese endoscopists, but there is no good evidence from well-designed comparisons to demonstrate its value over care and experience.

Histology is usually diagnostic, but where no evidence of invasion is found in the biopsy, Western pathologists tend to diagnose dysplasia when mitoses are frequent, cells are pleiomorphic and the normal palisade structure of the epithelium is disturbed. An elegant blind comparison between pathologists from Japan and Western countries demonstrated that Japanese pathologists are far more likely to rely on morphology alone than their Western colleagues [7], which may go some way to explaining the extremely high incidence of early cancer in Japan. Interestingly, after strip biopsy, invasive cancer was found in most of the specimens the Japanese pathologists diagnosed as malignant purely on morphology, a situation closely akin to that of severe dysplasia in Barrett's oesophagus.

Barium meal is useful in linitis plastica, as it confirms the non-distensibility of the stomach, usually with a distinctive pattern. It can also give an indication of the likely nature of gastric outlet obstruction when endoscopy is made difficult by accumulated debris. It is less accurate than gastroscopy in most other situations, and is not recommended as a first line investigation for gastric cancer. Multiple biopsies (more than 12) from the edge of the ulcer are recommended in non-healing ulcers. Histological proof of malignancy can be hard to obtain on endoscopy in large chronic ulcers in the elderly, even where subsequent surgery proves malignancy. Biopsies are commonly negative or inconclusive in linitis, because the malignant cells infiltrate the submucosal layer and excite an enormous fibrotic reaction. Occasionally where there is genuine doubt about the diagnosis of linitis, cytology using an injection needle via the endoscope may provide confirmation. In this situation endoscopic ultrasound is valuable, as it provides a very characteristic picture.

## Staging

### Purposes of Staging

Staging is important because it allows prediction of outcome, and can therefore be used as a marker for the quality of treatment, but more importantly because it determines treatment choices. Proof that disease is very early may allow minimally invasive surgical treatment, whereas proof of dissemination may preclude surgery or change its nature and intent. Great advances in staging accuracy have been made during the last 10 years, and these have permitted a great reduction in "open and shut" cases where irresectable disease is only discovered at laparotomy. Avoiding the pain, debility and hastened demise associated with such operations should be a major goal of staging investigations.

## Staging Modalities

CT scanning remains important in staging gastric cancer, mainly because of its ability to detect liver metastases. Modern spiral CT can have sensitivity and specificity values as high as 96% and 86% for liver secondaries. Its accuracy is less good, but still useful in relation to direct invasion of other structures and organs by the tumour. In this context CT has a high positive predictive value but is relatively non-specific. Ultrasound is less sensitive than CT for the detection of distant metastases, but endoscopic ultrasound probes have proved very useful for determining the thickness of wall invasion (T stage), where their accuracy exceeds that of any other modality. Staging laparoscopy has by far the highest sensitivity for the detection of peritoneal deposits of any known modality, and may detect liver metastases missed by CT. Several authors have reported that treatment decisions were changed in up to 25% of cases after laparoscopy. Attempts to extend its value by taking washings for cytology have shown a low yield of positives with conventional techniques, but this increases several fold if immunohistochemical techniques are used to detect specific tumour-associated antigens such as cytokeratins. A positive result using conventional cytology indicates an extremely poor prognosis, and is used by some authors to exclude patients from curative surgery, but the prognostic implications of a positive result using the more sensitive immunohistochemical approach is still not entirely clear, and may be compatible with long-term survival. Laparoscopic ultrasound is reported to make a difference to treatment decisions in an additional 8% of cases.

## Importance of Fitness Assessment

Although tumour staging and fitness assessment are usually regarded as separate processes, they are in practice two complementary halves of a process of decision-making by which the surgeon determines the risks and benefits associated with operative and other treatment options and thereby selects between them. The population who suffer from oesophagogastric cancer in Western countries is elderly and unhealthy: a lifelong smoking habit is the rule, and overt evidence of chronic heart or lung disease is extremely common. It is therefore very common to encounter patients in whom staging shows an eminently operable tumour, but fitness assessment suggests that curative resection is likely to prove fatal. Where surgery is clearly out of the question, judgement is not troubled, but a common dilemma is the patient whose tumour is apparently advanced but technically resectable with a small but measurable chance of long-term survival – say T3n2 – but whose fitness, whilst not hopeless, is a cause for serious concern. One problem for surgeons is the absence of any reliable prognostic fitness test which can be applied before the operation. Most experienced surgeons use a subjective global judgement based on their experience, commonly referred to by facetious titles such as the "end of the bedogram". The patent impossibility of standardising or defining this makes a comparative assessment of selection criteria very difficult, and this in turn makes evaluation of surgical mortality rates highly debatable, in view of the very clear inverse correlation between selectivity and operative mortality. In a recent survey of recognised specialist authorities, only about 40% used the ASA grade as a criterion for case selection, and the only objective tests which were used more commonly than this were spirometry results. Neither these nor objective tests of cardiac function have thus far been shown to outperform subjective judgement in predicting death or complications after surgery. The lack of a simple objective means of predicting risk from fitness is a problem for upper gastrointestinal (GI) surgeons which requires urgent attention.

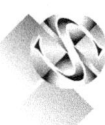

## Recommendations

Staging should include good quality CT scanning of the abdomen and chest for all patients in whom open surgery is being considered. Endoscopic ultrasound adds further information especially about T stage, and should be employed if available. Patients in whom there is a significant risk of peritoneal metastasis (all patients with T2+ gastric, junctional or lower oesophageal adenocarcinomas) should undergo staging laparoscopy unless symptoms or other factors have predestined their treatment, but cytology and laparoscopic ultrasound remain investigational in terms of their staging value. Fitness assessment should include basic spirometry and some form of objective assessment of exercise tolerance.

## Surgical Treatment

### Endoscopic Mucosal Resection

The method of endoscopic mucosal resection (EMR) has been pioneered by the Japanese, who have a unique experience of large numbers of very early carcinomas. The method consists of injection of fluid under the mucosa and submucosa to separate them from the muscle wall, followed by demarcation, grasping and excision of the lesion with a suitable margin of unaffected tissue. Randomised trials have not been performed, but large well-documented prospective series have confirmed that the method can be safely carried out for some early tumours. The criteria used by most Japanese units have included (a) size less than 2 cm, (b) morphological type I or II, (c) no associated ulceration, (d) no definite invasion of the submucosa. Using these conservative criteria, zero recurrence rates at 5 years have been achieved. Bolder attempts have been made particularly in the frail elderly, where open surgery seemed fraught with danger. These have shown that large lesions can be safely excised, and that perforation of the muscle, which can occur, can usually be repaired endoscopically using clips. Most non-Japanese endoscopists will have limited experience of the technique, and its likely place in most settings will be for patients whose lesion is early enough to give reason for optimism that the tumour can be completely excised and whose fitness precludes an open resection.

### Laparoscopic Resection Methods

Several ingenious methods for resecting gastric lesions from the inside of the stomach using laparoscopic instruments has been described. One approach has been to fix the stomach to the abdominal wall and introduce a Buess-type operating sigmoidoscope allowing minimally invasive procedures on the back wall of the organ and near the gastro-oesophageal junction, where EMR is difficult. More conventional laparoscopic approaches to wedge resection of tumours have been described, but are only applicable when the tumour is suitably placed, usually near the greater curvature. Several cases of laparoscopically assisted gastrectomy have been described, but the technique has not been widely adopted. It seems unlikely that it will become feasible except for early cancer in thin individuals. The concerns about possible port-site metastasis which have affected other types of minimally invasive cancer surgery apply equally to gastric cancer.

## Curative Resection (Open)

### General Principles

The principles of all attempts at curative surgery for gastric cancer are: First, to ensure complete resection of the primary tumour with adequate resection margins; second, to perform en-bloc nodal dissection of lymph nodes which are likely to be involved, and whose inclusion in the resection is likely to improve survival; third, to reconstruct the GI tract in a fashion which minimizes bile reflux across the anastomosis; fourth, to resect adjacent organs and tissues only where necessary to ensure a complete removal of all macroscopic tumour.

### Total Versus Subtotal

The Italian trial by Bozzetti and colleagues [8] has essentially answered the question of whether a total gastrectomy has any advantages over a subtotal operation for tumours where both are technically feasible: it does not. This finding is supported by a mass of weaker evidence, showing consistently higher mortality and postoperative malnutrition rates with the total resection, and failing to report any evidence of improved long-term survival. The original concept of a total gastrectomy for diffuse cancers and a subtotal operation for intestinal lesions has therefore been refuted.

## D1 Versus D2 Dissection

The extent of lymph node dissection has been the major controversy in gastric cancer surgery for several decades, and remains a subject of lively debate. It was noted in the early twentieth century that gastric cancer commonly remained localised to the stomach and adjacent nodes even in the terminal stages. Nodal mapping studies using injected dyes showed that lymph drainage from the stomach proceeded centrifugally in an orderly and predictable fashion and direction, the nodes affected and the order in which they stained being dependent on the part of the stomach injected with dye. These observations led surgeons to propose radical operations to remove the stomach and surrounding nodal chains en-bloc. Initial reports on this approach from the USA in the 1950s were alarming, with high mortality rates and no survival benefit.

Subsequent development of the technique in Japan, however, was associated with reports of spectacularly improved survival compared to historical controls. The Japanese approach involved identification of concentric tiers of nodes spreading outward from the stomach, and called for the resection of the entire tier likely to contain metastases on the basis of previous database information, plus an extra tier outside this to ensure a safety margin. The nodal tiers were numbered 1, 2, 3 and 4 outward from the stomach, and the resections labelled D1–D4 according to the outer limit of the nodal clearance. The majority of tumours fell into a category requiring D2 resection, which involved en-bloc clearance of the perigastric nodes and of all the nodes along the main branches of the coeliac axis. The initial Japanese doctrine also recommended routine resection of the spleen and distal pancreas during total gastrectomy, in order to ensure full nodal clearance along the splenic artery.

The presence or absence of real benefit from the nodal clearance has been the subject of fierce debate. Two very small and two large randomised trials have been performed, none of which have found a survival advantage for extended nodal dissection, and all of which have either found or suggested increased risks of complications and death following the procedure [9,10]. On the other hand, numerous impressive case series record the excellent results from specialist centres employing this technique, whilst there are no similar impressive reports from advocates of D1 surgery. The trials were clearly influenced by the fact that most surgeons spent a substantial part of their trial participation time on a steep learning curve, and by the difficulty of ensuring that patients received the assigned surgery. Subsequent subgroup analysis has found a possible benefit for D2 surgery in some of the groups where this might be predicted – for example patients with T3 tumours [11]. Direct comparison between D1 and D2 results on a stage for stage basis has been confounded by the "stage migration effect". Sensible analysis of the data has been hampered by the fact that all surgeons with a special interest have a view on this issue, and the views tend to be strongly held. In attempting a near objective analysis, the literature provides no good evidence of a survival benefit for D2 gastrectomy, but plenty of hints that this may exist, particularly for fit patients with intermediate stages of disease. The figures show results of a recent meta-analysis of randomised studies, plus a systematic review of the other evidence. Despite all that has been written on this subject, the large degree of uncertainty that still remains suggest the need for yet further trial work, whilst highlighting the need for better quality control and monitoring of the surgery actually delivered.

## Operation for Junctional Tumours

Examination of the mortality and survival results for cancer surgery in the upper GI tract shows that in both regards the worst location for tumours is at the oesophagogastric junction. The reasons for this are not entirely clear, but the adverse anatomical features of the area probably play a role. Access for the surgeon is particularly awkward here, and the lymphatic drainage of the area is diverse, draining to nodes in the lower mediastinum, upper abdomen, and also via the bare area of the stomach to the deeper layers of para-aortic nodes around the left renal vein. The diaphragmatic hiatus, pericardium and pleura are all adjacent to the oesophagus in this area, so direct invasion is a common problem. The controversy over the

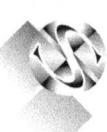

## 12 · UPPER GASTROINTESTINAL SURGERY

origin of tumours in this area and the different perspectives of the specialists who operate on them have led to a situation where tumours only different in position by 2 or 3 cm may be dealt with by completely different operations. The options can be divided into different means of exposure, different choices as to which part of the gut tube to resect and different views on the extent of lymph node dissection. This history means that there are very few good quality comparative studies of the different surgical approaches.

The following summary is therefore largely based on a personal interpretation of numerous case series, and cannot be regarded as evidence based. Thoracic surgeons traditionally approach the area through the left chest and divide the diaphragm to expose the abdominal organs. This allows good exposure of the tumour and in most reports has a low mortality, but limits the extent of oesophageal resection and makes extensive nodal dissection in the abdomen and middle mediastinum difficult. Some GI surgeons approach junctional tumours from below via a purely abdominal incision, opening or excising the hiatus to reach the posterior mediastinum. This allows easy nodal dissection in the abdomen and avoids the respiratory problems associated with a thoracotomy, but limits the extent of oesophagus which can be comfortably resected and the upper extent of mediastinal lymphadenectomy. This can result in a poorer symptomatic result because of excessive bile reflux and taking the literature overall, the lower mediastinal gastro-oesophageal anastomosis has an apparently inferior leak rate. The Ivor Lewis approach of an abdominal plus a right thoracic incision allows the widest exposure of the structures, allowing both subtotal oesophagectomy and full thoracic and abdominal lymph node dissection. It pays for this with the morbidity from two large incisions, and many series using this approach report high mortality rates. The option of a blind trans-hiatal removal of the whole thoracic oesophagus is favoured by some because it allows a high oesophageal anastomosis without requiring a thoracotomy. A recent meta-analysis suggests that it does achieve its original aim of reducing cardiorespiratory morbidity and mortality compared to the Ivor Lewis procedure, but it does not allow controlled nodal clearance in the mediastinum. Where tumours involve the stomach to a significant extent many surgeons perform a total gastrectomy, whilst some perform a proximal resection only. Where the tumour is a type I or II lesion, most surgeons spare the stomach for use as a tube to reconstitute the GI tract, but the extent of oesophageal resection varies. Surgeons who opt for an extensive gut tube resection need to use an interposed segment of colon or jejunum for reconstitution, adding to the duration and potential morbidity of the operation. Finally, the selection of extensive or limited nodal dissection in the abdomen depends on the surgeons' evaluation of the benefits or otherwise of extended lymphadenectomy, based on the limited and difficult literature alluded to above.

All that can safely be said is that the ideal operation for tumours at the oesophagogastric junction should produce adequate proximal and distal resection margins, a high rate of clear circumferential margins, a low operative mortality and a good functional result. It is unfortunately improbable that trials will ever be conducted to determine which of the options achieves these desiderata most consistently.

## Complications and their Management

Gastrectomy for cancer has historically been a high risk operation, and it remains so in many settings. There is a striking difference in mortality rates between series from specialist units and studies of general surgical experience, and between different countries. The main causes of mortality are respiratory and cardiac complications, anastomotic leaks and local sepsis. The prevalence of underlying cardiac and respiratory problems is probably an important determinant of whether patients survive their complications. Preoperative preparation can reduce chest infections, but is not widely practised. Postoperatively, excellent analgesia, intensive physiotherapy and appropriate hydration are important in reducing chest infection: there is evidence that excessive hydration and cooling intraoperatively can both increase infection risks. Patients undergoing D2 surgery are more prone to develop pancreatic fistulas because the anterior capsule of the organ is removed. These are not dangerous complications as long as infection does not supervene. Prompt radiologically guided drainage of abscess is usually effective. Patients with complications often have significant delay in establishing oral feeding, so many surgeons insert a feeding jejunostomy.

Long-term complications of gastrectomy have been well described for many years. Malnutrition is the commonest problem, and is more severe for total gastrectomy patients. There is some evidence that creating a pouch of jejunum may reduce the impact of this problem in the first 2 to 3 years, when it tends to be a at its worst. Vitamin $B_{12}$, vitamin C, iron and calcium are the specific micronutrients likely to be poorly absorbed after gastrectomy, and most surgeons give supplements to prevent this. Bile reflux can cause nausea, anorexia, abdominal pain in some patients. It tends to be more symptomatic in total gastrectomy patients; most patients with a Billroth II reconstruction have significant but asymptomatic bile reflux gastritis. Where reflux and inflammation are clearly associated with major symptoms, revision surgery is likely to be successful. A much more difficult group are patients with persistent abdominal pain and nausea without evidence of a specific cause. Some patients with dumping have pain as part of the syndrome, but most do not. Conservative measures and time usually help dumping, but a variety of revision operations have been proposed. Finally, after partial gastrectomy the need for continued surveillance of the stomach remnant for second cancers should be remembered.

## Outcomes: Morbidity, Mortality and Survival

Reports on the outcome of surgery for gastric cancer vary enormously in the impression they give of the success rate of surgery. There are a number of important reasons for this, and it is worth considering these to avoid being confused or misled.

Population studies use cancer registry or other population records to identify all people in a region with gastric cancer, and to follow their survival from diagnosis. This approach includes many frail elderly patients who are clearly unsuitable for surgery, and gives a depressingly low figure for 5-year survival, usually around 5% in Western studies. There are wide variations between countries in the figures produced using this kind of approach, but it is likely that many of these are due to incomplete verification of the diagnosis, or differences in death certification procedures.

The figures reported in hospital-based retrospective cohort studies or case series, which are by far the most common type of study in gastric cancer therapy, are much more encouraging. This is because two forms of selection have "weeded out" the cases with the worst prognosis. Patients referred to hospital in whom a definite diagnosis is made are, as a group, younger and fitter than those who are deemed too ill and frail to benefit from such referral. Once diagnosed, a further selection is usually made by the physician caring for the patient, who decides whether it is sensible to consult a surgeon. Once again, the patients denied referral will, as a group, be older, sicker, and have more advanced cancer than those who are referred. Surgeons then undertake their own fitness assessment and staging procedures before deciding whether to attempt resection of the tumour, and once again exclude a poorer-risk population. Finally, many series report only on the outcome of patients who underwent a potentially curative or R0 resection. In the majority of reports this represents only about 70% of those who underwent gastrectomy, the remainder being shown to have unresectable residual disease either by observations made during the operation or by the pathologist's report on the resected specimen. Given this series of selection steps it is easy to understand the contrast between the figures given by population studies and those given by hospital series. These have improved in most parts of the world both in terms of 5-year survival and in terms of postoperative mortality. A recent systematic review found that specialist centres reported mortality rates averaging less than 4% and 5-year survival rates averaging 53% [11].

Contemporary figures from Western Europe, the USA and the Far East reveal another source of confusion. Japanese figures are consistently superior to those from any other nation, and Far Eastern results in general show a trend towards better operative mortality and longer survival than those from Europe, with the USA trailing behind. Analysis of the stage distribution in the various series reveals major differences which go some way towards explaining this consistent pattern, with the best results occurring where the diagnosis is made earliest. In the same way, mortality results may reflect differences in the

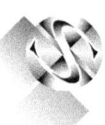

population burden of other diseases, particularly cardiovascular and respiratory disease, as well as differences in the average age of the patients operated on (nearly 10 years when Europe and Japan are compared). There is increasing interest in risk-adjusted analysis of short-term results, as these still vary enormously within national populations, for reasons which are not clear. Complete and accurate recording of mortality and survival results on a common basis which allows for adjustment by the most important risk factors is desirable but expensive, and has not yet been achieved nationally in any country.

There is considerable evidence that very large specialist centres with a very high throughput have the best results in a number of cancer surgery situations. The evidence in relation to gastric cancer is conflicting and relatively weak in both quantity and quality, and comparisons are generally available only for mortality results. Recent British data do show a trend towards decreased mortality with increasing case volume [12], but some studies contradict this. High case volume tends to be strongly correlated to other positive factors such as long experience, special clinical and research interests and being in a major institution with good facilities for preoperative assessment and postoperative care. Large units are also better able than small ones to provide specialist technical training within a limited programme and to conduct meaningful audits of their results. The best mortality results worldwide continue to come from Japan, where one leading centre recently recorded 1000 consecutive gastrectomies without a death. There are European and American centres with mortality rates as low as 2%, but the median UK rate was 13% in a recent survey of practice in about 30 hospitals. Comparison of published overall 5-year survival figures is confounded by the very different stage distributions in different populations, and stage-specific data are confounded by the stage migration effect of different nodal dissection policies. One way of partly circumventing this difficulty is to look at survival rates for T3+ disease without considering nodal status. A 5-year survival rate of 30% amongst T3 tumours or for node-positive tumours would be considered excellent, and figures of this kind were reported as long ago as the early 1970s.

## Palliative Resection

Palliative resection has a limited role to play in the modern management of gastric cancer. As with all palliative surgery, there must be a careful weighing of the risks and benefits. The benefits include prolonging survival, and there is little doubt that this occurs in many cases, although no trial could ethically be conducted. The average survival range after palliative resection (R2 in UICC terms) is 6–24 months, so the amount of time bought is not huge, but may be considered very valuable by patients and their families. The other expected benefit is relief of symptoms, and here there is often a problem. Vomiting and dysphagia caused by obstruction of the lumen can be reliably improved by surgery, but if these are not part of the clinical pattern, little other worthwhile benefit can be predicted. Persistent nausea and early satiety are often warning signs of widespread peritoneal or retroperitoneal perineural infiltration, and surgery will not help either of these problems. Pain is not commonly a serious problem in this condition: anorexia is, but is not commonly helped by gastric resection. Bleeding may warrant resection if it is torrential and life-threatening, but anaemia without overt bleeding can often be treated by repeated transfusion without ever needing to resort to operation, and without major haemorrhage ever developing. Where palliative gastrectomy is warranted, partial distal operation is more likely to give a good quality of postoperative life. Palliative total gastrectomy should only be considered in otherwise fit individuals who consent understanding the limited benefits to them. Preoperative nutritional support is very important in the majority of cases, and needs to be given for at least 2 weeks to be of any benefit in reducing morbidity and mortality.

## Other Palliative Surgery

The conventional palliative option for gastric cancers which cannot be resected has been gastroenterostomy, but the outcomes reported are extremely poor. Median survival after this procedure is only 3 to 6 months, but more importantly, only about half of the patients ever leave hospital after the operation, and the mortality rate is as high as 25%. Gastroenterostomy can only help a patient with gastric cancer by

# EPITHELIAL NEOPLASMS OF THE STOMACH

allowing them to eat and preventing vomiting. If these are not prominent symptomatic problems, bypass will not help. Even if they are, many advanced cases have widespread invasion of the autonomic nerves in the coeliac axis and small bowel mesentery, or widespread peritoneal invasion, and in these cases functional obstruction often persists even after gastroenterostomy. Modern minimally invasive options for specific problems include endoscopic self-expanding stenting of the pylorus or duodenum, laser treatment or arterial embolisation for bleeding and alcohol injections of the coeliac axis for pain. These can all be very useful in selected patients but all have potential for making matters worse. Tumours at the gastro-oesophageal junction behave symptomatically like oesophageal cancers, and stenting or laser therapy are the commonest endoscopic options. Open surgical bypass is rarely feasible, although palliative oesophagojejunal bypass has been described.

## Non-surgical Treatment

### Adjuvant and Neoadjuvant Chemotherapy

Chemotherapy as an adjunct to potentially curative surgery has been subjected to numerous randomised controlled trials (RCTs) over a 30-year period, but remains controversial. Five meta-analyses of the trial data have varied only slightly in their conclusions depending on which trials they have excluded. Overall, trials suggest a modest but significant survival benefit for chemotherapy with a risk ratio for death of between 0.7 and 0.9 compared to surgery alone [13]. The picture is complicated by the fact that a large number of trials have been conducted in Japan, where the context, trial design and populations studied have been unique and distinct. The results of the Japanese trials analysed separately are much more positive than those of the other studies, but there is concern about whether this is due to faults in the design of many earlier Japanese RCTs. Amongst the Western trials, two early trials with positive results contribute strongly to the overall outcome. Neither trial used a regimen which would be considered acceptable in modern practice, and their applicability is therefore minimal. The results of a large British trial of neoadjuvant therapy with ECF (epirubicin, cisplatin and infusional 5-fluorouracil) are likely to prove very influential. At present sceptical surgeons are able to justify withholding chemotherapy on the basis of the above analysis. Enthusiasts generally advocate pre- rather than postoperative therapy. The main argument for this is the pragmatic one that many patients are unfit to receive postoperative chemotherapy after a gastrectomy. Surgical concerns about the potential for an increased mortality risk after chemotherapy have not so far been borne out, but the trials conducted have not been powered to test this hypothesis.

Intraperitoneal chemotherapy has had some strong advocates and has been the subject of at least eight randomised trials. The rationale is to prevent the peritoneal recurrence which often causes death after apparently curative resection in cases where the tumour has breached the serosa. Two approaches can be defined: one group of workers advocate hyperthermic perfusion of the abdomen with cisplatin either alone or with other drugs, at the time of surgery. The other school have tried insertion of a Tenckhoff or other catheter for repeated postoperative dosing with milder regimens. Some reports suggest significant dangers with the perioperative approach, which clearly requires a much higher level of intensive monitoring and experience to administer it safely. Half of the trials have reported a survival benefit, and the approach clearly remains experimental.

### Adjuvant and Neoadjuvant Radiotherapy

Radiotherapy has had limited attention in gastric cancer because of early experience showing that it caused severe toxicity. As well as the problems of nausea, vomiting and bleeding associated with irradiating the stomach, the incidental dose to the liver was reported to be potentially dangerous. Intraoperative radiotherapy to the stomach has been used in a few small series, but the infrastructure required is formidably cumbersome and expensive, and the results thus far have not justified expanded trials. Combined chemoradiation as an adjuvant to surgery was tried by the British Stomach

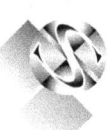

Cancer group in the 1980s, and showed no benefits. In 2001, a large US study reported impressive survival benefits from chemoradiation in association with gastrectomy [14]. This result is currently regarded with considerable scepticism because of the documented poor quality of the surgery performed. Further studies with quality control of the surgery are needed to determine whether the neoadjuvant therapy did more than compensate for inadequate surgery in this study.

## Biological Response Modifiers

Japanese and Chinese surgeons have included a number of unconventional treatments together with chemotherapy in randomised trials. A recent meta-analysis suggested an overall benefit from the use of these substances, most of which are bacteria and fungus-derived antigenic preparations designed to stimulate the immune system. Further well-designed studies of these substances are needed. Non-chemotherapy approaches to therapy which have been tried in Western countries in recent years have included the matrix metalloproteinase inhibitor marimastat and the gastrin peptide vaccine G17dt (Gastrimmune). Marimastat showed a near-significant survival benefit in a placebo-controlled trial in advanced inoperable disease, but significant problems with musculoskeletal stiffness and contractures occurred. No therapeutic data on Gastrimmune have yet been published.

## Palliative Chemotherapy

There is evidence that palliative chemotherapy prolongs life compared to best supportive therapy in gastric cancer patients of good performance status. Bearing in mind the side effects of anorexia, nausea and vomiting, tiredness and weakness which can occur, the likely effect on quality of life needs to be carefully assessed and discussed with the patient before embarking on treatment. Several groups have attempted to use chemotherapy to downstage inoperable disease and then proceed to operation in those in whom the treatments appeared successful. Results to date have been relatively disappointing, with a high percentage of early relapses, but a few patients have achieved long-term survival which could not have been expected with conventional treatment.

## Questions

1. Outline the staging systems for gastric cancer.
2. What relevance have genes?
3. What are the common sites for gastric cancer?
4. Discuss the arguments in the surgical approaches to gastric cancer.

## References

1. Feinstein AR, Sosin DM, Wells CK. The Will Rogers phenomenon: Stage migration and new diagnostic techniques are a source of misleading statistics for survival in cancer. N Engl J Med 1985;312:1604–8.
2. Guilford P, Hopkins J, Harraway J et al. E-cadherin germline mutations in familial gastric cancer. Nature 1998;392(6674):402–5.
3. EUROGAST Study Group. An international association between *H. pylori* infection and gastric cancer. Lancet 1993;34:1359–62.
4. El-Omar EM, Carrington M, Chow WH et al. Interleukin-1 polymorphisms associated with increased risk of gastric cancer. Nature 2000;404(6776):398–402.
5. Lagergren J, Bergstromn R, Lindgren A, Nyren O. Symptomatic gastro-oesophageal reflux as risk factors for oesophageal adenocarcinoma. N Engl J Med 1999;340:825–31.
6. Hallissey MT, Allum WH, Jewkes AJ et al. Early detection of gastric cancer. BMJ 1990;301:513–15.
7. Schlemper RJ, Itabashi M, Kato Y et al. Differences in diagnostic criteria for gastric carcinoma between Japanese and western pathologists. Lancet 1997;349(9067):1725–9.
8. Bozzetti F, Marubini E, Guilano B et al. Total versus subtotal gastrectomy: surgical morbidity and mortality rates in a multicentre Italian randomised study. Ann Surg 1997;226:613–20.
9. Bonenkamp JJ, Hermans J, Sasako M, van de Velde CJH. Extended lymph-node dissection for gastric cancer. N Engl J Med 1999;340:908–58.
10. Cuschieri A, Weeden S, Fielding J et al. Patients survival after $D_1$ and $D_2$ resections for gastric cancer: long-term results of the MRC randomised surgical trial. Br J Cancer 1999;79:1522–30.
11. McCulloch P, Niita ME, Kazi H et al. Gastrectomy with extended lymphadenectomy for the primary treatment of gastric cancer. Systematic review submitted to Cochrane collaboration.
12. Bachmann MO, Alderson D, Edwards D et al. Cohort study in South and West England of the influence of specialization on the management and outcome of patients with oesophageal and gastric cancers Br J Surg 2002;89(7):914–22.
13. Earle CC, Maroun JA. Adjuvant chemotherapy after curative resection for gastric cancer in non-Asian patients: revisiting a meta-analysis of randomised trials. Eur J Cancer 1999;35:1059–64.
14. MacDonald JS, Smalley SR, Benedetti J et al. Chemoradiotherapy after surgery compared with surgery alone for adenocarcinoma of the stomach or gastro-oesophageal junction. N Engl J Med 2001;345:725–30.

# 13

# Cancer at the Gastro-oesophageal Junction (Epidemiology)

Gill M. Lawrence

## Aims

To identify change patterns of gastro-oesophageal cancer.

## Introduction

Cancers of the stomach and the oesophagus are amongst the ten most common cancers in the world. In 1985 there were estimated to be 755 000 new stomach cancers and 304 000 new oesophageal cancers diagnosed worldwide [1]. At that time, as now, there were marked differences in the incidence of stomach cancer between countries with this cancer being the most common cancer in developing countries and the fourth most common cancer in developed countries. In 1985 the lowest incidence of stomach cancer was recorded in India (age-standardised incidence rate 2.1 per 100 000 population) and the highest in Japan (age-standardised incidence rate 93.3 per 100 000 population) where stomach cancer accounted for one-third of all male cancers and almost one-quarter of female cancers. Because of these high incidence rates, the Japanese have introduced a screening programme for stomach cancer which has led to the diagnosis of 30–40% of tumours at an early stage. Coupled with aggressive treatment, this has resulted in much improved survival rates [2].

Stomach cancer incidence and mortality have been linked with dietary risk factors such as high intake of salt, fat, starches and carbohydrates (from grains and starchy foods), and dietary nitrate (from water or via the pickling and smoking of food) [3]. A high intake of preserved foods is believed to increase the risk of stomach cancer due to the presence of nitrites which form carcinogenic N-nitroso compounds when mixed with gastric juices. Chronically high levels of infection with *Helicobacter pylori* have also been positively correlated with a high incidence of stomach cancer [4], with carriers of the bacteria having 3–6 times the risk. This link with *H. pylori* infection has been suggested as an explanation for the higher levels of stomach cancer in the more deprived sections of the UK population [5]. Other risk factors for stomach cancer include occupational exposure to dust (pottery industry), medical conditions such as atrophic gastritis, intestinal metaplasia and pernicious anaemia. Stomach cancer rates are also higher in people with blood group A and with hereditary non-polyposis colon cancer.

In 1985 the lowest rates of oesophageal cancer were recorded in Israeli Jews (age-standardised incidence rate 1.4 per 100 000 population) and the highest in Calvados in France (age-standardised incidence rate 26.5 per 100 000 population) [1]. There is also a high risk "Asian oesophageal cancer belt" extending from the Caspian Sea in northern Iran, through the former southern Republics of the USSR to western and northern China [6]. Almost half of the world's oesophageal cancers occur in China [1]. In China and Iran, poor nutrition (in particular zinc deficiency) and ingestion of opium pyrolysates and preserved food high in nitrosamines and mycotoxins is thought to be responsible for the high incidence rates. Human papilloma virus (subtypes 16 and 18) has also been implicated in areas of particularly high prevalence in China. Squamous cell carcinoma is the most common histology in the upper two thirds of the oesophagus and adenocarcinoma in the lower third.

Alcohol and tobacco consumption are major risk factors associated with squamous cell carcinoma of the oesophagus in Europe and the Americas and the two compounds act synergistically. Thus, in a French control study, the relative risks for heavy drinkers and heavy smokers were 5.1 and 18 respectively, while the relative risk for those who smoked and drank heavily was 44.4 [7]. Furthermore, in Calvados where the incidence of oesophageal cancer in men is particularly high, the trend in risk amongst successive birth cohorts has a pattern characteristic of other alcohol-related cancers such as those of the tongue, mouth, pharynx and larynx. Gastro-oesophageal reflux and body mass index have been identified as factors strongly associated with increased risk of adenocarcinoma of the oesophagus [8].

## Temporal Trends in Stomach Cancer Incidence and Mortality

The incidence of stomach cancer is decreasing by 2–4% worldwide each year, mainly because of a decrease in the "intestinal" type of adenocarcinoma. These changes have been correlated with the introduction of refrigeration as a means of food preservation, which has reduced the need for salting, pickling and smoking. The increased consumption of fresh fruits, raw vegetables and salads is also believed to have played an important role in the reduction of stomach cancer worldwide [9]. This is thought to be due to the presence in these foods of antioxidants such as vitamins C and E which inhibit nitrosation. This interpretation is further supported by migrant studies which consistently demonstrate that immigrants and their offspring assume the stomach cancer lifetime risk of their host country.

Overall stomach cancer incidence and mortality rates are approximately 2.5 times as high in men, but there is some variation in these ratios with age (see Figure 13.1). In people aged 45 to 74 incidence rates are around three times higher in men than in women but the incidence

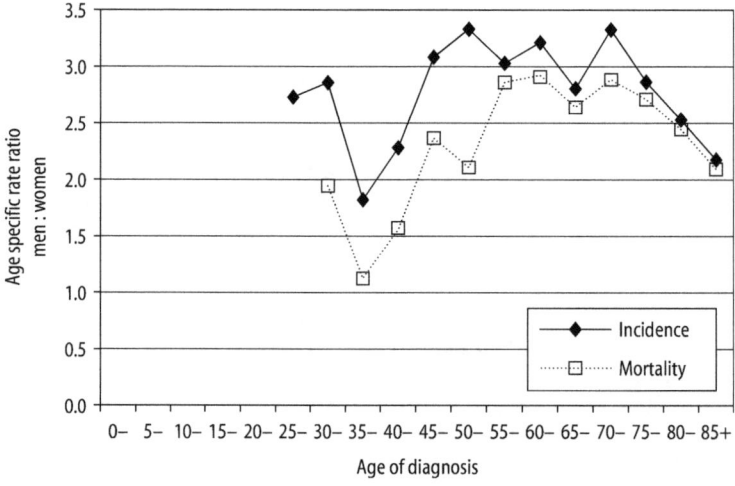

**Figure 13.1.** Age-specific rate incidence and mortality rate ratios for men and women in the West Midlands diagnosed with or dying from stomach cancer in the period 1996 to 2000.

# CANCER AT THE GASTRO-OESOPHAGEAL JUNCTION (EPIDEMIOLOGY)

rate ratio is lower in younger and older people. Mortality rates are also approximately three times higher in men aged 55 to 75 but the mortality rate ratio declines with age in men and women aged less than 55 and over 75.

Figure 13.2 shows the decreases in stomach cancer incidence and mortality that occurred in men and women in England and Wales between 1971 and 1999. Age-standardised incidence rates fell in men by 41% (from 31.8 to 18.9 per 100 000) and in women by 51% (from 15.1 to 7.3 per 100 000). At the same time, age-standardised mortality rates decreased in men by 60% (from 31.7 to 12.6 per 100 000) and in women by 66% (from 14.9 to 5.0 per 100 000). Stomach cancer mortality fell at a faster rate than incidence in both sexes, although this effect is slightly greater in men.

## Temporal Trends in Oesophageal Cancer Incidence and Mortality

Improvements in oesophageal cancer incidence and mortality in some countries have been correlated with increases in the consumption of fresh fruit and vegetables. However, in many European countries the benefits of these nutritional improvements have been largely offset by increasing alcohol and tobacco consumption with the result that oesophageal cancer incidence and mortality rates are rising. Figure 13.3 shows the increases in oesophageal cancer incidence and mortality that occurred in men and women in England and Wales between 1971 and 1999. Age-standardised incidence rates rose in men by 67% (from 7.6 to 12.8 per 100 000) and in women by 34% (from 4.2 to 5.7 per 100 000). At the same time, age-standardised mortality rates increased in men by 66% (from 7.6 to 12.7 per 100 000) and in women by 28% (from 4.0 to 5.2 per 100 000).

Figure 13.4 shows how age-specific incidence rate ratios for oesophageal cancers diagnosed in men and women in the West Midlands changed between 1980 and 2000. Incidence rates increased by 50% in men and women aged 60 and over during this time period. However, in men there was also a marked increase in the 45–59 age band which was not apparent in women.

## Variation in Stomach and Oesophageal Cancer Incidence with Deprivation

Similar decreases in stomach cancer incidence to those seen in England and Wales have

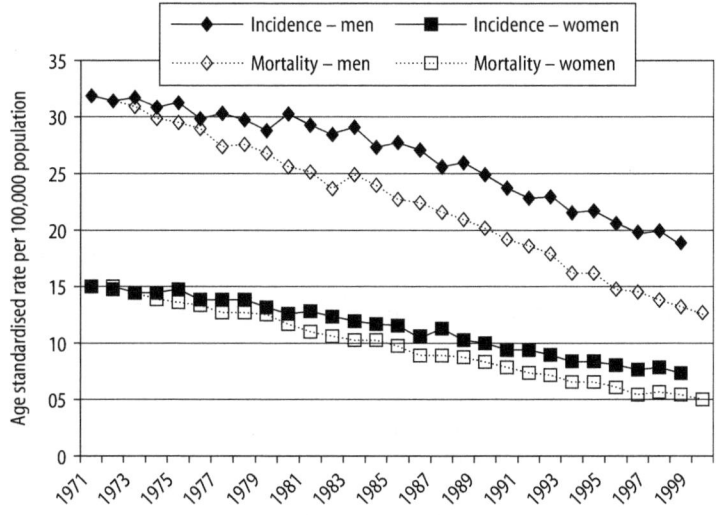

**Figure 13.2.** Temporal changes in stomach cancer incidence and mortality in England and Wales during the period 1971 to 1999.

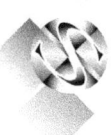

13 · UPPER GASTROINTESTINAL SURGERY

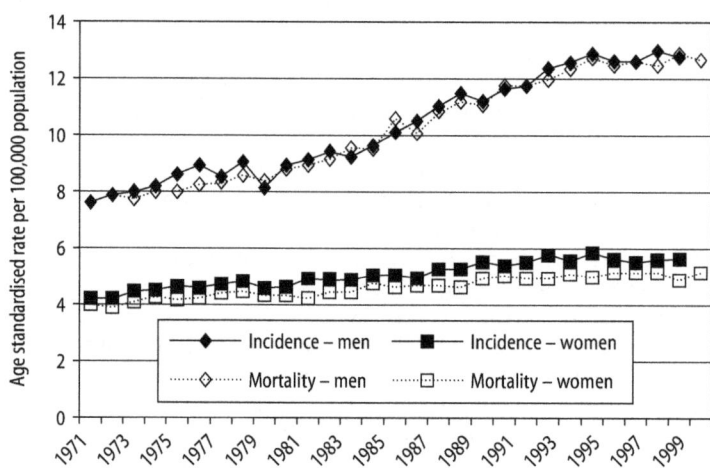

**Figure 13.3.** Temporal changes in oesophageal cancer incidence and mortality in England and Wales during the period 1971 to 1999.

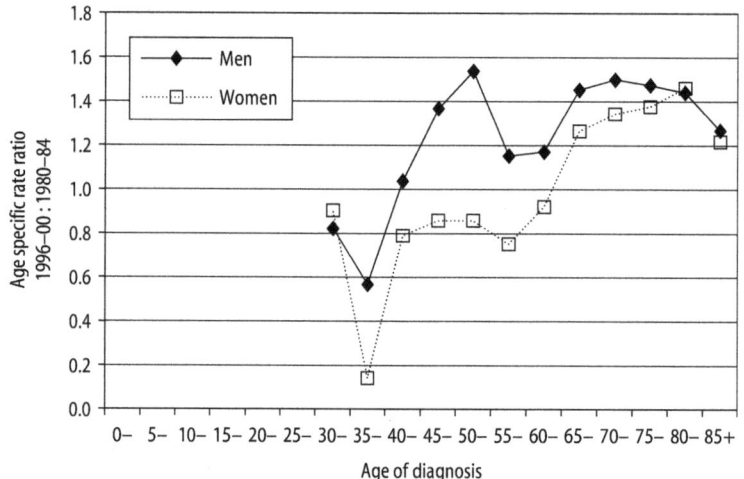

**Figure 13.4.** Changes in age-specific oesophageal cancer incidence rate ratios for men and women in the West Midlands diagnosed in 1980–84 and 1996–2000.

occurred in the West Midlands. However, in this region the rate of change has varied markedly with deprivation status [10], consistent with the suggestion that early infection with *Helicobacter pylori* prior to the widespread introduction of refrigeration is a major risk factor for stomach cancer. Figure 13.5a shows how stomach cancer incidence in men and women varied in the most affluent and most deprived sections of the West Midlands population between 1984 and 1998. These data clearly demonstrate that the overall decrease in male stomach cancer that was apparent in the West Midlands during this time was mainly due to a 31% decrease in incidence in the most deprived men (from 40.4 per 100 000 in 1984–86 to 27.9 per 100 000 in 1996–98). The majority of this change took place in the period from 1985–87 to 1992–94 when a 34% fall in incidence was seen. The situation was very different in the most affluent men. In this group stomach cancer incidence remained reasonably stable at around 19 per 100 000 between 1984–86 and 1994–96 and then increased by 15% to reach 21.9 per 100 000 in 1996–98. Similar effects were

# CANCER AT THE GASTRO-OESOPHAGEAL JUNCTION (EPIDEMIOLOGY)

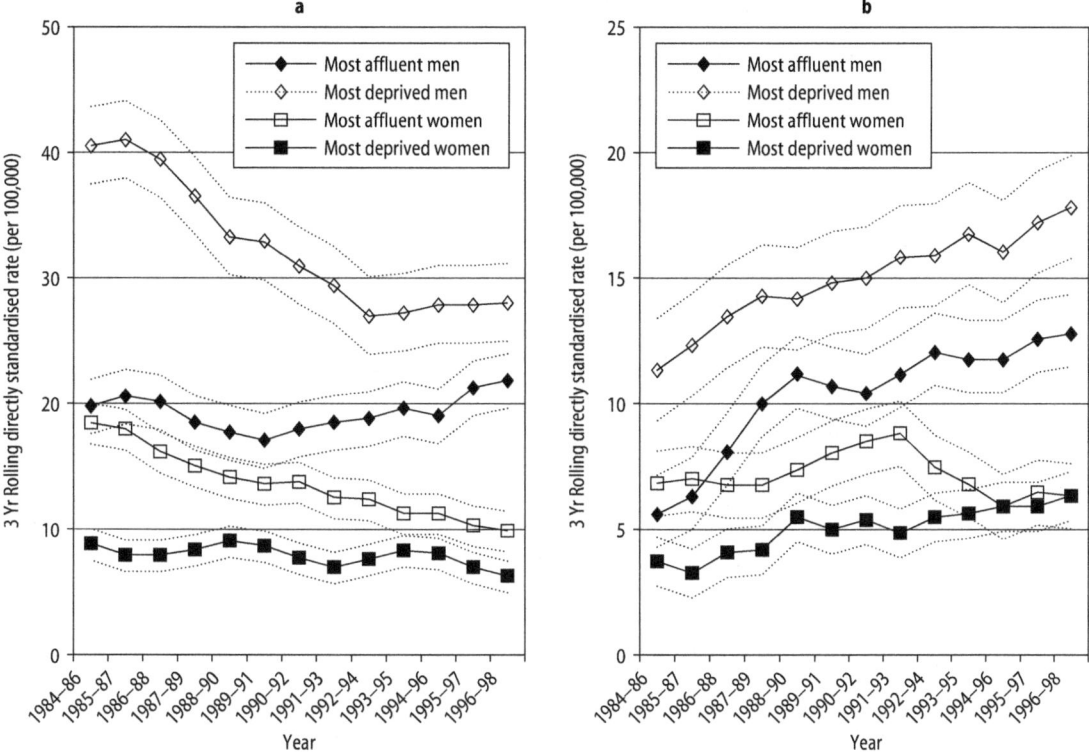

**Figure 13.5.** Variation in stomach and oesophageal cancer incidence rates with deprivation in men and women diagnosed in the 15-year period 1984–98; 95% confidence intervals are indicated by dotted lines. **a** Three-year rolling directly age-standardised stomach cancer incidence rates in men and women from Townsend bands 1 (most affluent) and 5 (most deprived). **b** Three-year rolling directly age-standardised oesophageal cancer incidence rates in men and women from Townsend bands 1 (most affluent) and 5 (most deprived).

seen in women where stomach cancer incidence in the most deprived group fell by 47% from 18.5 per 100 000 in 1984–86 to 9.9 per 100 000 in 1996–98 while that in the most affluent women remained fairly constant at around 8 per 100 000 until 1994–96 when it decreased by 21% to reach 6.3 per 100 000 in 1996–98.

Table 13.1 shows that these temporal changes in stomach cancer incidence in men and women caused the rates in the most affluent and most deprived categories to converge. In 1984–86 the incidence rates in the most affluent men and women were less than half the rates in the most deprived men and women (rate ratios 0.49 and 0.48 for men and women respectively). By 1996–98, the differences in the stomach cancer incidence in the two groups of men and women were much smaller, with the rates in the most affluent men and women being only 22% and 36% lower than those experienced by their most deprived counterparts (rate ratios 0.78 and 0.64 in men and women respectively).

The overall increase in male oesophageal cancer seen in England and Wales over the last 28 years is also apparent in the West Midlands. Figure 13.5b shows that this increase occurred in the most affluent and the most deprived men, but that the effect was much greater in the former (127% compared with 57%). In both groups, incidence increased most rapidly between 1984–86 and 1988–90 (from 5.7 per 100 000 to 11.2 per 100 000 in the most affluent men and from 11.4 per 100 000 to 14.2 per 100 000 in the most deprived men). After this time there was a steady and sustained increase in both groups, with incidence rising an additional 14% in the most affluent men and by an additional 25% in the most deprived men.

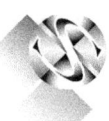

**Table 13.1.** Variation in 3-year rolling directly age-standardised stomach and oesophageal cancer incidence rates in the West Midlands in men and women in the most affluent (Townsend band 1) and most deprived (Townsend band 5) categories with cancers diagnosed in the 15-year period 1984–98 (95% confidence intervals are shown in brackets)

| | Men | | | Women | | |
|---|---|---|---|---|---|---|
| Diagnosis years | Most affluent incidence rate | Most deprived incidence rate | Most affluent: Most deprived Incidence rate ratio | Most affluent incidence rate | Most deprived incidence rate | Most affluent: Most deprived Incidence rate ratio |
| *Stomach cancer* | | | | | | |
| 1984–86 | 19.86 (17.65–22.07) | 40.43 (37.04–43.82) | 0.49 | 8.80 (7.50–10.09) | 18.45 (16.47–20.42) | 0.48 |
| 1990–92 | 18.05 (15.89–20.21) | 30.90 (27.93–33.88) | 0.58 | 7.70 (6.50–8.89) | 13.79 (12.08–15.51) | 0.56 |
| 1996–98 | 21.91 (19.51–24.30) | 27.92 (25.03–30.81) | 0.78 | 6.34 (5.26–7.42) | 9.85 (8.41–11.29) | 0.64 |
| *Oesophageal cancer* | | | | | | |
| 1984–86 | 5.65 (4.47–6.82) | 11.36 (9.53–13.19) | 0.50 | 3.75 (2.91–4.60) | 6.84 (5.54–8.14) | 0.55 |
| 1990–92 | 10.46 (8.84–12.07) | 15.02 (12.91–17.14) | 0.70 | 5.40 (4.37–6.43) | 8.53 (7.13–9.92) | 0.63 |
| 1996–98 | 12.81 (10.99–14.63) | 17.84 (15.48–20.20) | 0.72 | 6.37 (5.25–7.50) | 6.29 (5.12–7.47) | 1.01 |

Similar but smaller increases in oesophageal cancer incidence were recorded in the most affluent women, with a 46% rise between 1984–86 and 1988–90 (from 3.8 per 100 000 to 5.5 per 100 000) and a further 16% increase from 1988–90 onwards. The picture in the most deprived women is, however, more complex. In this group, there was no significant change in oesophageal cancer incidence between 1984–86 and 1996–98, but this overall picture masks a 29% increase in incidence to 8.8 per 100 000 in 1991–93 followed by a similar decrease over the following 7 years.

As with stomach cancer, these temporal changes in oesophageal cancer incidence with time in women caused the rates in the most affluent and most deprived categories to converge (Table 13.1). Thus, in 1984–86 the incidence rate in the most affluent women was only half the rate in the most deprived women (rate ratio 0.55) but, by 1996–98, the incidence rates in the two groups of women are almost the same (rate ratio 1.01). A similar but less marked reduction in the difference in incidence between the most affluent and the most deprived groups was seen in men. Here, whereas in 1984–86 oesophageal cancer incidence in the most affluent men was only half the rate of that in the most deprived men, by 1996–98 the rate in the most affluent men was only 28% lower (rate ratios 0.50 and 0.72 for 1984–86 and 1996–98 respectively).

## Survival from Stomach and Oesophageal Cancer

Survival from stomach and oesophageal cancer is generally poor. Survival varies markedly with stage at diagnosis, with 5-year survival rates for stage I, II, III, IVA and IVB tumours diagnosed in the West Midlands region in 1972–91 being 76.9%, 33.5%, 10.7%, 2.1% and 0.2% respectively [11]. Overall survival rates in England and Scotland are lower than the European average, with only 11–12% of stomach cancer patients and 7–9% of oesophageal cancer patients diagnosed in 1985–89 alive after 5 years; the European weighted averages being 21% and 10% respectively [12]. It is likely that variation in stage at diagnosis is the main factor accounting for the differences in survival between England and other European countries. However, after subsite and stage are taken into consideration, the low proportion of stomach

## CANCER AT THE GASTRO-OESOPHAGEAL JUNCTION (EPIDEMIOLOGY)

cancer patients undergoing surgery has also been identified as a factor contributing to the relatively poor survival recorded in England. Five-year survival rates for these cancers diagnosed in whites in the USA in 1983–88 at 18% and 9% are similar to the European average [13]. Much higher 5-year survival rates (47% and 15% respectively for stomach and oesophageal cancers diagnosed in 1975–89) have been reported in Japan. Although more widespread use of endoscopy in Japan and the introduction of a mass screening programme are probably responsible in part for these variations, the use of different criteria for the histological diagnosis of early gastric carcinoma in Japan and Western countries may also be a contributory factor [14].

Although survival from stomach and oesophageal cancer is poor, relative survival rates have improved in both men and women in England and Wales over the last 25 years (Figure 13.6). Thus, for stomach cancer 5-year relative survival rates increased in men from 3.9% to 9.7% and in women from 4.9% to 11.6% for cancers diagnosed in 1992–94 compared with 1971–75. For oesophageal cancer 5-year relative survival rates increased in men from 2.9% to 5.7% and in women from 5.1% to 8.8% for cancers diagnosed in the two time periods.

Stomach cancer survival varies with age at diagnosis in both men and women, with between 15 and 20% of men and women aged 15–49 diagnosed in England and Wales in 1992–94 surviving for 5 years compared with only 5–10% of those aged 70 or older (Figure 13.7a). Five-year relative survival rates from oesophageal cancers diagnosed in the same time period were generally lower than for stomach cancer in men, ranging from 0.9% in men aged 80–99 to 8.8% in men aged 40–49. Five-year relative survival was significantly higher in women in all but the oldest age group studied, varying between 2.5% in women aged 80–99 and 29.1% in woman aged 15–39 (Figure 13.7b). The reason for these large variations in survival between men and women is not clear but it may be related to the relatively higher incidence of adenocarcinoma in men compared with women.

## Cancer at the Gastro-oesophageal Junction

It is generally accepted that intestinal metaplasia both in the oesophagus (Barrett's oesophagus) and at the gastro-oesophageal junction has premalignant potential and that these metaplastic changes can progress through dysplasia to adenocarcinoma [15]. The mucosal changes characteristic of Barrett's oesophagus are believed to occur as a consequence of extended gastro-oesophageal reflux during which contents of the stomach or duodenum pass into the oesophagus. Gastro-oesophageal reflux occurs

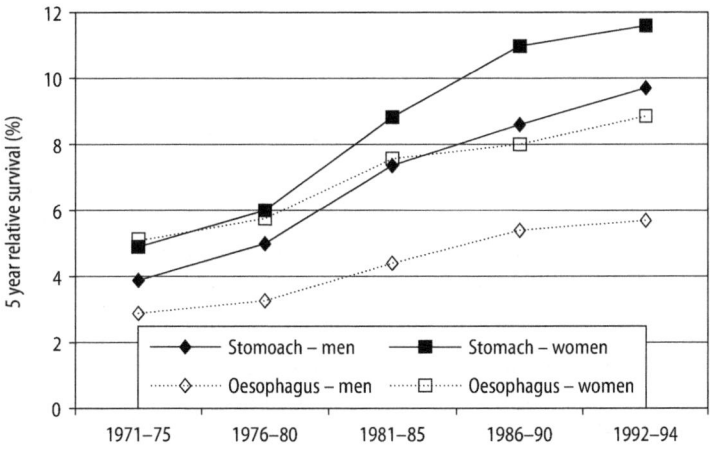

**Figure 13.6.** Temporal changes in 5-year relative survival from stomach and oesophageal cancers diagnosed in men and women in England and Wales between 1971 and 1994.

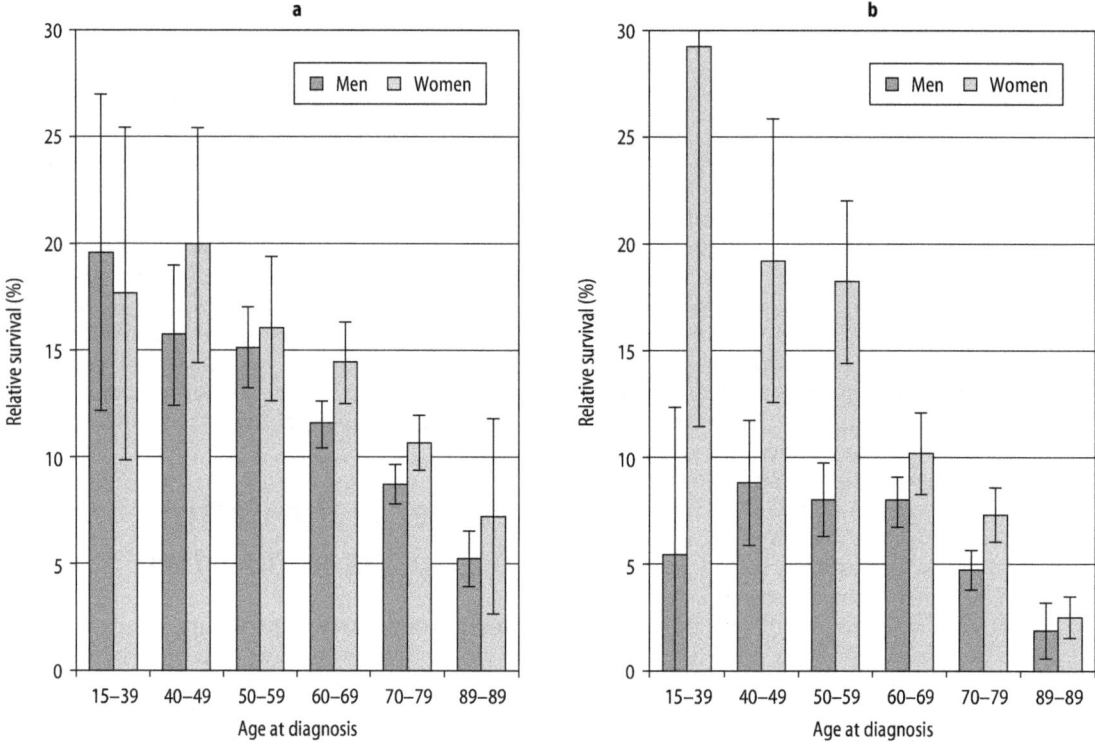

**Figure 13.7.** Five-year relative survival rates for (a) stomach cancer and (b) oesophageal cancer diagnosed in men and women in England and Wales in the period 1992 to 1994.

more frequently in overweight individuals, particularly those with excess abdominal fat. This may be in part due to a reduction of pressure in the lower oesophageal sphincter related to high fat consumption. It has also been suggested that drugs such as proton pump inhibitors and $H_2$-receptor blockers might potentiate adenocarcinoma of the gastro-oesophageal junction by reducing the acidity of the gastric juice and decreasing its bile-neutralising capability. More recently, dietary nitrate has been implicated in the development of cancers at the gastro-oesophageal junction through conversion in the gastric juice in the presence of vitamin C into the highly reactive and potentially toxic NO free radical.

Annual increases in the incidence of adenocarcinoma of the oesophagus in men of between 9% and 20% have been reported in the UK and other parts of Europe, the USA and Australia [16]. Figure 13.8 illustrates the increase in age-standardised incidence of adenocarcinoma in the oesophagus that occurred in men and women in England and Wales between 1971 and 1998. Over this time period there was a 3.68-fold increase in the incidence of adenocarcinoma in men and a 2.65-fold increase in women while the incidence of cancers with other or non-specific morphology remained relatively constant in both sexes. This suggests that the increases in adenocarcinoma did not arise because of improvements in the coding and classification of oesophageal tumours.

Further evidence to support this interpretation comes from an examination of the relationship between oesophageal cancer subsite and morphology. Figure 13.9 shows the subsite distribution in the oesophagus of adenocarcinomas and cancers with other morphology (including squamous cell carcinomas and cancers with non-specific morphology) in men and women in England and Wales diagnosed in 1971 and 1998. Over this time period in men there was a 8.17-fold increase in the number of adencarcinomas diagnosed in the lower third of the oesophagus and a 3.36-fold increase in the

# CANCER AT THE GASTRO-OESOPHAGEAL JUNCTION (EPIDEMIOLOGY)

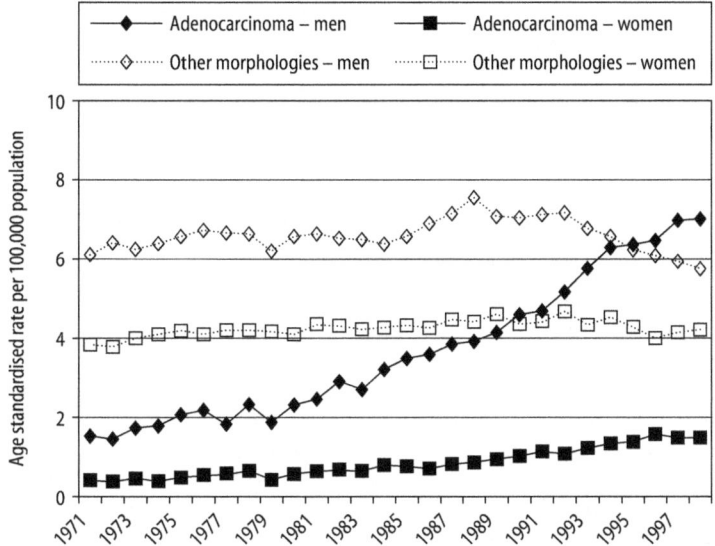

**Figure 13.8.** Age-standardised incidence rates of adenocarcinoma and other morphologies (including non-specific morphologies) in the oesophagus in men and women in England and Wales from 1971 to 1998.

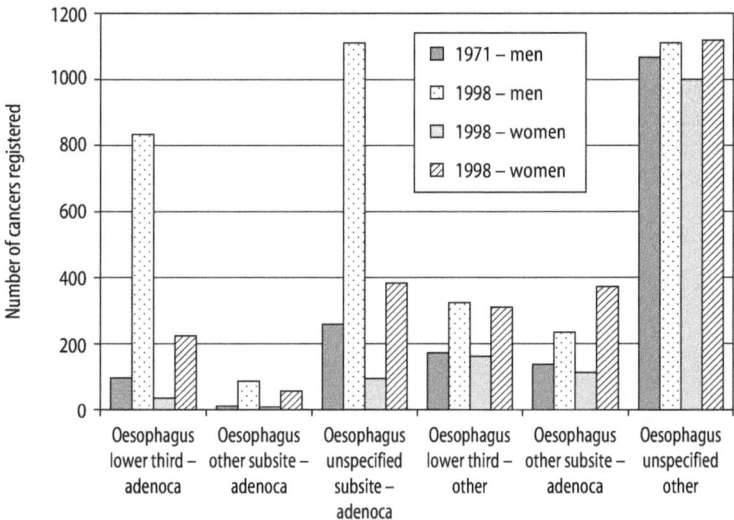

**Figure 13.9.** Temporal changes in subsite and morphology recorded in oesophageal cancers diagnosed in men and women in England and Wales in 1971 and 1998.

number of adenocarcinomas diagnosed in unspecified subsites within the oesophagus. Smaller increases were also apparent in women, with an 85% increase in adenocarcinomas in the lower third of the oesophagus and a 75% increase in unspecified subsites. These changes were, however, not accompanied by equivalent decreases in the incidence of oesophageal cancers with unspecified subsite and morphology. Therefore data indicate that increases in adenocarcinomas of the oesophagus are not spurious and that they have not arisen because of improvements in the collection of information relating to subsite and morphology.

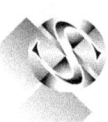

## 13 · UPPER GASTROINTESTINAL SURGERY

On the other hand, comparable data for stomach cancer shown in Figure 13.10 cannot be used to refute the suggestion that overall increases in the incidence of adenocarcinoma between 1971 and 1998 are due mainly to improvements in the quality of the data relating to subsite and morphology. Thus, although the number of adenocarcinomas registered in the stomach during this time period increased by 77% in men and 35% in women, these changes were accompanied in both sexes by 3-fold decreases in the numbers of cancers with other or unspecified morphology. It is, however, possible that the 4.31-fold increase in adenocarcinoma of the gastric cardia is real because the male to female incidence rate ratio at this site (3.6–4.0) is much higher than for other sites (2.0–2.4). If the increase in adenocarcinoma in the cardia was due to improved subsite recording, the male to female rate ratio for gastric cancer with an unspecified subsite should have decreased as the sex rate ratio in the cardia increased. In fact, the male to female incidence rate ratios increased at both sites between 1971 and 1998 (from 3.6 to 4.4 in the cardia and from 2.0 to 2.2 in the unspecified subsites).

Adenocarcinoma is the most common type of cancer in the stomach. Increases in the incidence of adenocarcinoma in the lower oesophagus could therefore occur if more tumours at or near the gastro-oesophageal junction were identified as being of oesophageal rather than gastric origin. It has been suggested that only centres with a special interest in oesophageal and gastric surgery can accurately classify whether a tumour of the gastro-oesophageal junction is in the distal oesophagus, the true gastric cardia or the gastro-oesophageal junction. It may thus be reasonable from an epidemiological standpoint, to consider adenocarcinoma of the oesophagus and the gastric cardia to be the same disease and to combine the incidences of adenocarcinomas at the two locations [17]. Such an approach is consistent with the two cancers having a similar phenotype and a similar prevalence of the p53 gene mutation.

Figure 13.11 shows the increases in age-standardised incidence rates that occurred between 1980 and 1998 in cancers diagnosed in the oesophagus and gastric cardia in men and women in the West Midlands. During this time the incidence rate of adenocarcinoma in men increased 1.8-fold (from 6.8 per 100 000 to 12.1 per 100 000) and that in women more than doubled (from 1.3 per 100 000 to 2.8 per 100 000). During the same time period the incidence of squamous cell carcinoma remained constant at around 3.7 per 100 000 in both sexes and the incidence of cancers with other non-specific morphologies decreased slightly.

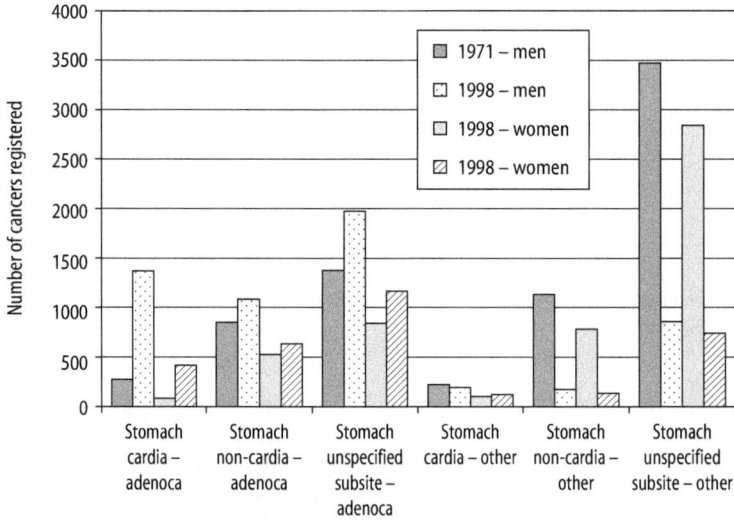

**Figure 13.10.** Temporal changes in subsite and morphology recorded in stomach cancers diagnosed in men and women in England and Wales in 1971 and 1998.

# CANCER AT THE GASTRO-OESOPHAGEAL JUNCTION (EPIDEMIOLOGY)

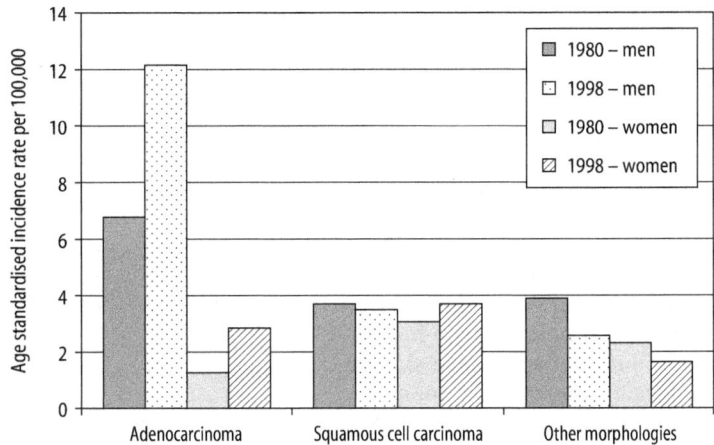

**Figure 13.11.** Variation in age-standardised incidence rates with morphology for cancers in the oesophagus and gastric cardia diagnosed in men and women in the West Midlands in 1980 and 1998.

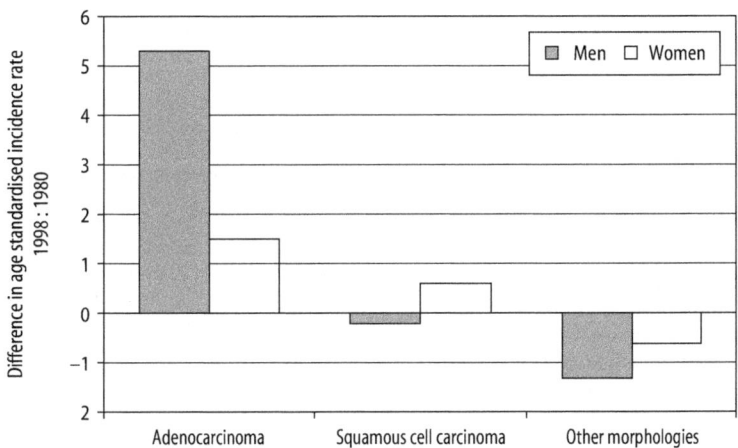

**Figure 13.12.** Differences between the age-standardised incidence rates for adenocarcinomas, squamous cell carcinomas and cancers with other and non-specific morphologies for cancers in the oesophagus and gastric cardia diagnosed in men and women in the West Midlands in 1980 and 1998.

Details of the subsite specific changes in incidence rate that took place in cancers of the oesophagus and gastric cardia in men and women in the West Midlands between 1980 and 1998 are provided in Figure 13.12. This shows that in both sexes, the increases in the incidence of adenocarcinoma could not be accounted for by decreases in squamous cell carcinomas or cancers with other non-specific morphology. It is therefore likely that these cancers arose because of new factors affecting the aetiology of the disease.

## Conclusions

While stomach cancer incidence and mortality are generally declining, increases in oesophageal cancer incidence and mortality have occurred in many countries over the last 20–30 years. In the West Midlands, decreases in stomach cancer incidence are much greater in the most deprived men and women. Improvements in food preservation with the introduction of refrigeration resulting in reduced levels of infection with *Helicobacter pylori* are probably the most likely

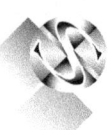

explanation for this finding. Although, as with stomach cancer, the incidence of oesophageal cancer is generally higher in the most deprived men and women, the rate of increase of oesophageal cancer incidence in the West Midlands is considerably greater in the most affluent men and women. Oesophageal cancer incidence and mortality are approximately twice as high in men and in recent years there has been a marked increase in incidence in the 45–59 age band which is not apparent in women. Epidemiological studies combining data for the gastric cardia and the oesophagus have shown that adenocarcinomas account for the majority of this rise in incidence. Increased gastro-oesophageal reflux linked to high fat consumption and the expanding use of proton pump inhibitors and $H_2$-receptor blockers may be responsible for these changes.

## Acknowledgements

I am grateful to Dr Mike Quinn, Director of the National Cancer Intelligence Centre at the Office for National Statistics, for providing the incidence and mortality data for England and Wales that have been included in this chapter. I would also like to thank the staff in the West Midlands Cancer Intelligence Unit who diligently abstract, code and quality assure the cancer registration data collected for the West Midlands region and Dr Cheryl Livings and Miss Sarah Baggott for their assistance with data analysis. Finally, my thanks go to the NHS Trusts and Private Hospitals which provide cancer registration data and without whose continued cooperation valuable epidemiological studies such as those I have described would not be possible.

## Questions

1. Where is cancer of the stomach common?
2. Where is cancer of the oesophagus common?
3. What has happened to the incidence of these two cancers?

## References

1. Parkin DM, Muir CS, Whelan S (eds) Cancer incidence in five continents, Vol VI. IARC Scientific Publications No. 120. Lyon: International Agency for Research on Cancer, 1992.
2. Hisamichi S, Sugawara N. Mass screening for gastric cancer by x-ray examination. Jpn J Clin Oncol 1984;14:211–23.
3. Judd PA. Diet and pre-cancerous lesions of the stomach. Eur J Can Prev 1993;2 (Suppl 2):65–71.
4. Eurogast Study Group. An international association between *Helicobacter pylori* infection and gastric cancer. Lancet 1993;341:1359–62.
5. Brewster DH, Fraser LA, McKinney PA. Socioeconomic status and risk of adenocarcinoma of the oesophagus and cancer of the gastric cardia in Scotland. Br J Cancer 2000;83(3):387–90.
6. Coleman MP, Esteve J, Damiecki P, Arslan A, Renard H. Trends in cancer incidence and mortality, Chapter 11. IARC Publications No.121. Lyon: International Agency for Research on Cancer, 1993.
7. Tuyns A, Pequignot G, Jensen O. Le cancer de l'oesophage en Ille-et-Vilaine en fonction des niveaux de consommation de l'alcool et de tabac. Bull Cancer (Paris) 1977;64:45–60.
8. Lagergren J, Bergstrom R, Lindgren A, Nyren O. Symptomatic gastro-oesophageal reflux as a risk factor for esophageal adenocarcinoma. N Engl J Med 1999;340:825–31.
9. World Cancer Research Fund. Food, nutrition and the prevention of cancer: a global perspective. Washington DC: American Institute for Cancer Research, 1997.
10. West Midlands Cancer Intelligence Unit. Cancer and Deprivation Report 2002.
11. Fielding JWL, Powell J, Allum W et al. Cancer of the stomach. Clinical Cancer Monographs, Volume 3. Basingstoke: Palgrave Macmillan 1989.
12. Faivre J, Forman D, Esteve J, Gatta G, Eurocare Working Group. Survival of patients with oesophageal and gastric cancers in Europe. Eur J Cancer 1998;34:2167–75.
13. Kosary CL, Ries LAG, Miller BA et al. SEER Cancer statistics review 1973–1992. NIH Pub No. 96:2789; 1995.
14. Schlemper R J, Itabashi M, Kato Y Differences in diagnostic criteria for gastric carcinoma between Japanese and Western Pathologists. Lancet 1997;349:1725–29.
15. Li H, Walsh TN, Hennessy TPJ. Carcinoma arising in Barrett's oesophagus. Surg Gynaecol Obstet 1992:175:167–72.
16. Bollschweiler E, Wolfgarten E, Gutschow C, Holscher A. Demographic variations in the rising incidence of esophageal adenocarcinoma in white males. Cancer 2001;92:549–55.
17. Sihvo EIT, Salminen JT, Ramo OJ, Salo JA. The epidemiology of oesophageal adenocarcinoma: has the cancer of the gastric cardia an influence on the rising incidence of oesophageal adenocarcinoma? Scand J Gastroenterol 2000;10:1082–86.

# 14

## Neoplasms of the Small Bowel

Aviram Nissan and Martin S. Karpeh

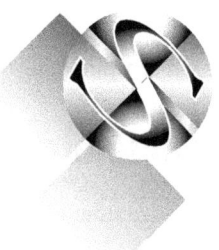

## Aims

To identify neoplasms of the small bowel, and their epidemiology, aetiology and treatment.

## Introduction

Tumors of the small bowel are rare, accounting for only 1–3% of gastrointestinal neoplasms [1]. The low incidence of tumors in the small bowel is intriguing given the fact that it comprises 75% of the length of the alimentary tract and 90% of its surface area. Furthermore, the small intestine is located between the stomach and the colon, which both have a high incidence of neoplastic diseases. The diagnosis is relatively difficult because of the rare incidence of the disease and because of the non-specific presentation of small bowel tumors.

The limited ability to obtain good imaging of the small bowel further increases the interval between onset of symptoms and diagnosis [2]. Novel diagnostic techniques such as enteroclysis, magnetic resonance imaging (MRI), and enteroscopy provide better imaging and can provide the clinician with valuable information [3]. However, most of these diagnostic modalities require special expertise and are rarely applied for the diagnosis of non-specific gastrointestinal symptoms typical to small bowel tumors. Local excision or segmental resection is the treatment of choice for benign lesions located distal to the ligament of Treitz. Benign lesions arising in the duodenum, especially periampullary lesions, require more complex surgical intervention in the form of limited resection or pancreaticoduodenctomy (Whipple's procedure).

The treatment of malignant lesions depends mainly on the histologic type and the stage of disease. Due to the lack of large retrospective or prospective randomized clinical trials, the treatment of small bowel malignancies, such as adenocarcinoma, is based mainly on the extrapolation of data obtained from studies of malignancies with similar biological features. Because the natural history of adenocarcinoma of the duodenum has many similarities with adenocarcinoma of the stomach, similar treatment guidelines are recommended.

Tumors of the jejunum and ileum, meanwhile, resemble adenocarcinoma of the colon and therefore should be treated accordingly. Surgery remains the mainstay of treatment in all adenocarcinomas of the small bowel regardless of their location. Selection of adjuvant chemotherapy should be done according to the location and stage of disease [4]. Chemoradiation might be beneficial for adenocarcinoma of the duodenum, because of its positive effect on gastric cancer and the fixed location of the duodenum. The role of radiation therapy in adenocarcinomas arising in the other portions of the small intestine is limited because of its mobility

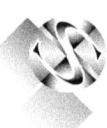

## Epidemiology

The incidence of both benign and malignant small bowel neoplasms is low, and the incidence of neoplasms per surface area is even lower. The majority (two-thirds) of small bowel lesions are malignant with a crude incidence of 0.4 to 1 cases per 100 000 population per year [5]. The incidence varies according to the method of diagnosis: surgery or autopsy. In a comprehensive analysis [6], data from cancer registries participating in the Surveillance, Epidemiology, and End-Results (SEER) Program from 1973 to 1990 were analyzed to determine the incidence of small bowel tumors. An average annual incidence rate of 9.9 per million people was reported, with carcinoid and adenocarcinoma being the most common histological subtypes, followed by lymphomas and sarcomas. Over 90% of cases occurred in people over the age of 40. During the 18-year study period, the incidence of small bowel tumors has risen slowly.

In a review of the American National Cancer Database, maintained by the American College of Surgeons and the American Cancer Society, 14 253 cases of small bowel cancer diagnosed between 1985 and 1995 were found [7]. Adenocarcinoma was the most common histologic subtype with 4995 (35%) cases followed by 3934 (28%) cases of carcinoid, 2967 (21%) cases of lymphoma, and 1441 (10%) of sarcoma; 55% of the adenocarcinomas arising in the duodenum, 18% in the jejunum, 13% in the ileum, and the remaining 14% in non-specified sites.

Incidence reports of small bowel neoplasms vary from region to region (Table 14.1). The variance in incidence and breakdown to histologic subtypes reflects not only true variability but also the small number of cases in each report.

## Aetiology

The low incidence of small bowel neoplasms compared with the neighboring organs, stomach, and colon is intriguing. Both adenomatous polyps and adenocarcinoma are distributed unevenly, with the vast majority of these neoplasms located in the 25 cm long duodenum. By contrast, the minority of tumors are located in the remaining 300 cm of jejunum and ileum. Despite its length and relatively large surface area and its exposure to a variety of ingested carcinogens, the small bowel is resistant to carcinogenesis. The relative resistance of the small intestine was studied by many investigators [8,9], but neither animal models nor clinical studies provided solid evidence to support one hypothesis or another. Cooper et al [10] compared the Bristol Royal Infirmary experience of treating primary adenoma and adenocarcinoma of the small bowel with the effects of treating 88 rats with intravenous azoxymethane (a known colonic carcinogen). In the patients 40% of the neoplasms were located in the duodenum, 24% in the jejunum, and 36% in the ileum, whereas in the azoxymethane-treated rats 65% of the neoplasms were located in the duodenum, 32% in the jejunum, and 3% in the ileum. The ratio of small to large bowel neoplasms in their experiment was 1 to 4,

**Table 14.1.** Histologic breakdown of small bowel neoplasms in selected series from different populations

| Author | Period (years) | Region | N | Adenocarcinoma (%) | Carcinoid (%) | Lymphoma (%) | Sarcoma (%) | Other (%) |
|---|---|---|---|---|---|---|---|---|
| Garcia Marcilla | 15 | Spain | 69 | 38 | 10 | 42 | 10 | 0 |
| Frost | 30 | California | | 63 | 6 | 15 | 13 | 3 |
| DiSario | 25 | Utah | 328 | 24 | 41 | 22 | 11 | 2 |
| Serour | 26 | Israel | 61 | 30 | 10 | 37 | 23 | 0 |
| Ciccarelli | – | Connecticut | 51 | 33 | 39 | 16 | 12 | 0 |
| Laws | 16 | Alabama | 45 | 36 | 29 | 11 | 24 | 0 |
| Barclay | 30 | Canada | 209 | 35 | 45 | 10* | 9 | 1* |
| Howe | 10 | USA (NCDB) | 14 253 | 35 | 28 | 21 | 10 | 6 |

*Lymphomas and other tumors are reported together.
NCDB, National Cancer DataBase.

# NEOPLASMS OF THE SMALL BOWEL

compared with 1 to 50 in reported series in humans.

This observation might imply a connection between bile and carcinogenesis, but the results were the same when the experiment was repeated in rats whose bile was surgically diverted.

## Predisposing Factors

The predisposing conditions for small bowel neoplasms can be divided into three groups (Table 14.2): (a) inflammatory disorders such as Crohn's disease, (b) disorders of the immune system such as AIDS, congenital immunodeficiency disorders, or patients receiving immunosuppressive therapy, and (c) genetic disorders such as familial adenomatous polyposis (FAP) or hereditary non-polyposis colon cancer (HNPCC).

Other factors including occupational hazards and lifestyle factors such as smoking or alcohol intake were investigated in two European multicenter case-control studies [11,12]. A cohort of 70 patients diagnosed with small bowel adenocarcinoma (SBA) during the study period (1995–1997) were compared with 2070 matched controls. Beer and spirits intake were associated with small bowel adenocarcinoma, with an odds ratio (OR) of 3.5 and 95% confidence intervals (CI) of 1.5–8.0. However, there was no association between smoking or total alcohol intake and adenocarcinoma of the small bowel. In a second study of the same group, investigators identified occupational clustering of SBA. The strongest industrial risk factors for SBA were dry cleaning, manufacture of workwear, mixed farming (women), and manufacture of motor vehicles (men). A significantly increased risk of SBA was found among men employed as building caretakers (OR 6.7; CI 1.7 to 26.0) and women employed as housekeepers (OR 2.2; CI 1.1 to 4.9); general farm laborers (OR 4.7; CI 1.8 to 12.2); dockers (OR 2.9; CI 1.0 to 8.2); dry cleaners or launderers (OR 4.1; CI 1.2 to 13.6); and textile workers (OR 2.6; CI 1.0 to 6.8).

## Regional Enteritis (Crohn's Disease)

Regional enteritis or Crohn's disease is an inflammatory bowel disease that affects mainly people in their 3rd and 4th decades of life. It has long been associated with a high incidence of adenocarcinoma of the small bowel and colon. The first case of small bowel malignancy identified in a patient with Crohn's disease was reported by the same group that originally described the disease in 1932. Interestingly, when the surgical approach to the treatment of Crohn's disease was changed from radical resection to bypass surgery, the same group described a high incidence of adenocarcinoma in the bypassed loop of small bowel. Since then, numerous reports of small bowel neoplasms arising in patients with Crohn's disease have been published.

**Table 14.2.** Predisposing factors for small bowel neoplasms

| | |
|---|---|
| *Inflammatory conditions* | |
| Regional enteritis (Crohn's disease) | Adenocarcinoma |
| | Lymphoma |
| Celiac sprue | Lymphoma |
| | Carcinoid |
| | Adenocarcinoma |
| Tuberculosis | Lymphoma |
| *Immune deficiencies* | |
| Acquired immune deficiency syndrome | Kaposi's sarcoma, lymphoma |
| Common variable hypogammaglobulinemia | Lymphoma |
| *Genetic syndromes* | |
| Familial adenomatous polyposis | Adenoma, adenocarcinoma |
| HNPCC | Adenoma, adenocarcinoma |
| Peutz–Jeger | Adenocarcinoma |
| Neurofibromatosis | Adenocarcinoma |

## Coeliac Disease (Non-tropical Sprue)

Celiac disease is associated with an increased risk of certain gastrointestinal malignancies, especially of the small bowel. In addition to lymphoma, there is an increased incidence of gastrointestinal adenocarcinoma in patients with malabsorption due to celiac disease. This is frequently manifested by a loss of response to gluten withdrawal. Metachronous malignancies are well established in the colon, where adenocarcinoma is common, but are exceptional in the small intestine. It was suggested that the subgroup of celiac patients unresponsive to gluten-free diet are more prone to develop small bowel malignancies, but this hypothesis was never proven. Cases of carcinoid tumors of the small intestine have been reported in patients with celiac disease. Small bowel lymphoma, both B cell and T cell, is the most common malignancy reported in association with celiac disease, with higher incidences of T-cell lymphomas reported.

## Tuberculosis

Intestinal tuberculosis is a rare disease in industrial countries and is often mistaken for Crohn's disease. However, in Asia where intestinal tuberculosis is more frequently encountered, there are several reports of lymphoma complicating intestinal tuberculosis.

## Acquired Immunodeficiency Syndrome (AIDS)

Patients with the acquired immunodeficiency syndrome (AIDS) are known to be at increased risk for developing a small bowel malignancy. The rising incidence of small bowel lymphoma over the past two decades has occurred mainly in patients with immunodeficiency disorders such as AIDS or chronic immunosupression following organ transplantation. Balthazar et al [13] reported finding small bowel lymphoma in 52% of AIDS patients in their study of patients with intestinal lymphomas. Other authors also emphasized the association between AIDS and small bowel lymphoma. Most of the reported cases were diagnosed by laparotomy, presenting with intussusception, perforation, biliary obstruction, or small bowel obstruction.

Kaposi's sarcoma is a neoplasm arising mainly in immunodeficient patients, The association between Kaposi's sarcoma and AIDS is well known. In fact, about one-third of all patients with AIDS have Kaposi's sarcoma. Gastrointestinal involvement has been noted in 50% of homosexual men with cutaneous Kaposi's sarcoma and AIDS [14]. Numerous reports of Kaposi's sarcoma of the gastrointestinal tract in AIDS patients have been published in the medical literature. Diagnosis is made by small bowel imaging, either by computed tomography (CT) scan, MRI or enteroclysis. Recommended treatment depends on the individual patient's general condition and the symptoms related to the lesion. Surgical resection, if feasible, is the treatment of choice for Kaposi's sarcoma of the small intestine. Others have suggested using radiation therapy as a single mode therapy or in the adjuvant setting.

## Immunosuppression

Patients are at an increased risk for developing malignancies following organ transplantation. Lymphomas, skin malignancies, Kaposi's sarcomas, and cervical/vulvar neoplasms are the most common, but visceral malignancies are also well documented, with a reported frequency ranging from 1% to 6% [15]. These visceral tumors represent a mix of neoplasms that were clinically occult at the time of transplantation and those that arise de novo after transplantation. There are several reports in the literature of small bowel neoplasms, mainly lymphomas, in patients receiving immunosuppressive therapy following solid organ transplant.

## Hypogammaglobulinemia

Common variable hypogammaglobulinemia or adult-onset hypogammaglobulinemia are genetic disorders of the immune system. There are several reports describing an association between these rare disorders and lymphoma of the small intestine.

## Familial Adenomatous Polyposis (FAP)

FAP is an autosomal dominant syndrome manifested by hundreds of adenomas that arise in

# NEOPLASMS OF THE SMALL BOWEL

the colon and rectum. It accounts for 0.5% of these cancers and the lifetime incidence of colorectal cancer is nearly 100%. The adenomatous polyposis coli (APC) gene is located on chromosome 5q and well-described germline mutations are associated with the different FAP phenotypes.

Patients with FAP are at considerable risk of developing extracolonic manifestations of the disease. Desmoid tumors of the abdominal cavity, and duodenal adenomas and carcinomas are the most serious ones. It is estimated that some 10% of all FAP patients will develop desmoids, whereas 50–90% of FAP patients will suffer from duodenal adenomas predominantly concentrated on or around the major papilla.

Desmoid tumors and duodenal carcinomas are major causes of death in those patients in whom a prophylactic proctocolectomy has been performed. Although some investigators suggest that the adenoma–carcinoma sequence, which is generally accepted for colorectal adenomas, also applies for the duodenal adenomas in FAP patients, it is not clear whether these patients should be screened for upper gastrointestinal adenomas. As these polyps are usually small, multiple, and difficult to remove, the benefit of endoscopic surveillance would be the early detection of cancer. In addition, evidence that screening and early treatment leads to an improvement of the prognosis is not available. Although the role of (procto)colectomy in the treatment of large-bowel polyps is well established in FAP patients, the treatment of their duodenal counterparts is still open to debate. The risk of the development of periampullary cancer is not high enough to warrant an aggressive prophylactic surgical approach after the discovery of duodenal adenomas. Some authors suggest intraoperative enteroscopy at the time of proctocolectomy and describe small bowel adenomas in 59% of the patients investigated.

## Hereditary Non-polyposis Colorectal Cancer (HNPCC)

HNPCC is an autosomal dominant syndrome first described by Lynch. In HNPCC families colorectal cancers not associated with extensive polyposis are the hallmark of the disease. Extracolonic neoplasms are also common and include endometrial, ovarian, gastric, hepatobiliary, and urinary tract cancers. Mutations in DNA mismatch repair genes are found in 30–35% of HNPCC patients. DNA microsatellite instability with replication error-positive phenotype are present in all HNPCC patients as well as in 15% of sporadic colorectal cancers.

The incidence of small bowel cancer in HNPCC patients was studied by Rodriguez-Bigas et al 16]. Forty-two individuals from 40 HNPCC families developed 42 primary and 7 metachronous small bowel tumors, including 46 adenocarcinomas and 3 carcinoid tumors. Mismatch repair gene mutations were present in 15 of 42 patients (36%). The small bowel was the first site of carcinoma in 24 patients (57%). Aarnio et al calculated the lifetime risk of developing various HNPCC-related cancers in a cohort of 414 patients, and found that the lifetime risk for small bowel cancer was only 1%, compared with 78% for colorectal cancer.

## Peutz–Jeghers Syndrome

Peutz–Jeghers syndrome is an autosomal dominant disorder characterized by gastrointestinal hamartomatous polyps and cutaneous pigmentation. Although the hamartomas typical of Peutz–Jeghers syndrome are benign in nature, it is has been recognized that Peutz–Jeghers patients are at increased risk for the development of malignant neoplasms of the small bowel. A molecular locus associated with this syndrome has recently been assigned to chromosomal region19p13.3. The LKB1 gene (GenBank accession number U63333), also referred to as STK11, had previously been identified and is located at that site. This gene, which encodes for a serine threonine kinase, is present as a somatic mutation in most patients with Peutz–Jeghers syndrome. Patients with this mutation can also develop cancers at sites outside of the gastrointestinal tract such as in the cervix and ovaries.

## Neurofibromatosis (von Recklinghausen's Disease)

Neurofibromatosis type 1 (von Recklinghausen's disease) is an autosomal dominant genetic disorder characterized by café au lait spots, pigmented hamartomas (Lich nodules) of the iris, and cutaneous neurofibromas. While the association between neurofibromatosis and neuroendocrine tumors is well described, there are several reports of adenocarcinoma of the small bowel arising in patients with von Recklinghausen's disease.

## Clinical Presentation

In general, small bowel tumors, either benign or malignant, present with non-specific gastrointestinal symptoms. Symptoms are related to the underlying histology, location of the tumor, and the extent of disease. The main groups of symptoms include pain, obstructive symptoms, symptoms related to bleeding, and symptoms related to effects on adjacent organs such obstructive jaundice secondary to periampullary tumors. Other symptoms such as palpable mass, perforation, or weight loss are present less frequently, although in a single report of 58 small bowel tumors, the most frequent symptoms were weight loss and abdominal lump [17]. A large proportion of patients are asymptomatic at diagnosis.

Pain is non-specific, can be related to partial obstruction, stretching of the serosa, or neural invasion of the tumor. Usually it is a dull, intermittent pain related to food intake, and it is poorly localized. The non-specific pain that is characterized as varying in location and quality is usually interpreted as a functional disorder and many of the patients are diagnosed with "irritable bowel syndrome" or their symptoms are attributed to other incidental findings such as gallstones or diverticulosis.

Bleeding is rarely acute; more commonly patients have chronic iron-deficiency anemia with related symptoms of weakness and fatigue. Intermittent acute bleeding is the exception.

Small bowel obstruction as the presenting symptom of a small bowel tumor may occur as a result of a luminal obstruction related to concentric adenocarcinoma. Intratumoral hemorrhage in a large leiomyosarcoma or lymphoma can cause obstruction. A less common reason for small bowel obstruction is intussusception (Figure 14.1). In a retrospective series, Eisen et al reported 22 cases of small bowel intussusception. The majority were secondary to benign conditions and in the eight patients with malignant underlying lesions these were all metastatic lesions. Begos et al reported 11 cases of small bowel or ileocolic intussusception; only one case was secondary to primary leiomyosarcoma of the small bowel. Azar et al reported that 48% of 44 enteric intussusceptions studied were associated with malignant underlying lesions. Only one patient had primary adenocarcinoma of the small bowel and another patient presented with an undifferentiated carcinoma. Overall it is estimated that the underlying etiology in 20–50% of adult small bowel intussusception is malignant and the vast majority of the cases will be metastatic. A summary of the findings of these three studies is outlined in Table 14.3.

## Diagnosis

The non-specific nature of symptoms related to small bowel tumors results in a long interval between the onset of symptoms and diagnosis. A lag period of up to 3 years for the diagnosis of benign tumors and 18 months for malignant tumors was reported. The diagnostic work-up is usually long, expensive, and involves at least one invasive procedure. The diagnostic work-up of the individual patient depends on the presenting symptoms. Patients presenting with pain or mild obstructive symptoms such as cramps, occasional vomiting, or distension are best approached radiologically, whereas patients presenting with bleeding symptoms will benefit from an endoscopic approach.

Table 14.3. Underlying pathology of small bowel intussusception

| Author | N | Benign tumors | Malignant tumors | | Other benign conditions |
|---|---|---|---|---|---|
| | | | Primary | Metastatic | |
| Eisen | 22 | 5 | 0 | 8 | 9 |
| Begos | 11 | 1 | 1 | 2* | 7 |
| Azar | 44 | 6 | 2 | 19 | 17 |

* One patient with carcinomatosis.

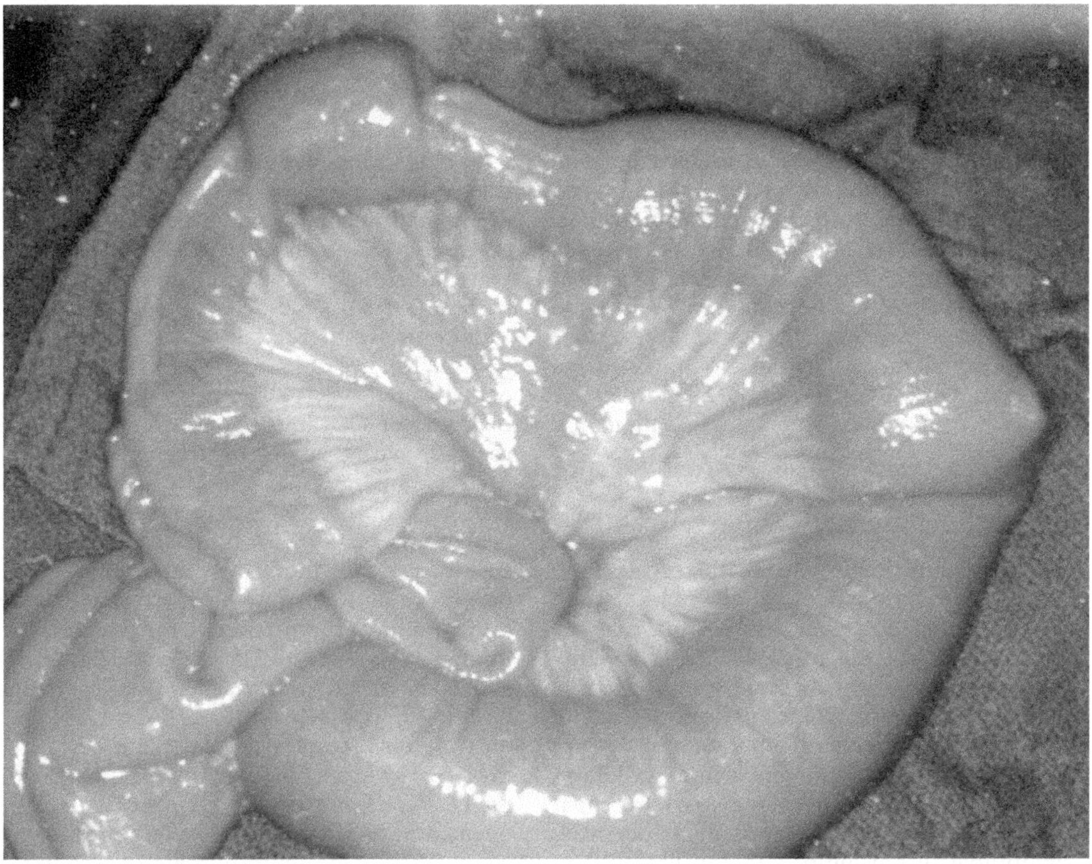

## NEOPLASMS OF THE SMALL BOWEL

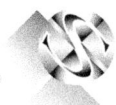

**Figure 14.1.** Intraoperative photograph of a small bowel intussusception secondary to a primary small bowel gastrointetinal stromal tumor. The patient presented with classic symptoms of a small bowel obstruction.

## Plain Abdominal X-Rays

The work-up of non-specific abdominal pain includes using plain abdominal films as an initial screening tool. The value of plain abdominal films in the diagnosis of small bowel tumors is limited to identifying complete or partial obstruction. In most cases, a CT scan of the abdomen and pelvis should be performed.

## Computed Tomography of the Abdomen

A CT scan performed with both intravenous and oral contrast material can detect benign and malignant tumors of the small bowel and in many cases differentiate between the two entities. Leiomyoma, the most common benign lesion of the small bowel, will appear as a round, smoothly outlined, homogeneous soft tissue mass, showing marked contrast enhancement. In the absence of distant metastasis or clear invasion to adjacent organs, there is not a clear radiologic distinction between leiomyomas and leiomyosarcomas. However, lesions greater than 6 cm tend to carry higher malignant potential. Large adenomatous polyps can be detected by CT scan. The image typically appears as an ill-defined intraluminal soft tissue mass, surrounded by oral contrast. Lipomas show up on the CT scan as a smooth, homogeneous, ovoid mass, with a density comparable to fat. Intussusception is clearly seen on CT scan as a classic "target" lesion.

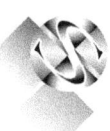

The value of a CT scan is not only in the diagnosis of malignant small bowel tumors, but also in the evaluation of the extent of disease and staging. The appearance of adenocarcinoma of the small bowel on CT scan is similar to the appearance of adenocarcinoma of the colon and includes the following radiological appearances: annular stricture formation, polypoid mass, or other filling defect. Ulceration is frequently seen, either in the form of an ulcerated mass or an ulcer. However, duodenal ulcers are common and the presence of malignancy in these lesions is exceedingly rare. Ulcers located in the distal duodenum or other parts of the small intestine should be viewed as suspicious for malignancy.

## Barium Radiology

Most of the small bowel tumor patients presenting with pain or partial obstruction will require further radiologic studies to establish the diagnosis. Upper gastrointestinal barium radiology is still the most frequent modality used in the work-ups of these symptoms. The correct diagnosis in symptomatic patients with small bowel tumors is obtained only in 50% of the cases by conventional barium radiology. The low yield of conventional barium upper gastrointestinal studies results primarily from suboptimal distensibility and the presence of overlapping segments. Strictures, small masses or mural lesions such as leiomyomas may be easily overlooked, especially in the presence of an underlying disease such as Crohn's disease.

Enteroclysis has an important role in the diagnosis of small bowel tumors. Briefly, a transnasal intubation of an 8F catheter is performed and manipulated beyond the ligament of Treitz. Methylcellulose-barium solution is used to distend the small bowel and obtain optimal imaging of the small bowel. Enteroclysis was shown to be effective in the detection of small bowel tumors and other diseases [18].

## Magnetic Resonance (MR) Enteroclysis

Enteroclysis provides only indirect information about the small bowel wall and the surrounding tissues. MR enteroclysis, although still investigational, shows great promise in providing accurate information about intraluminal, mural, and extraluminal lesions of the small bowel. The small bowel is distended with 1500–3000 ml of methylcellulose-water solution. The transit of the water in the small bowel is documented by MR fluoroscopy; the examination is completed when the water reaches the colon in cross-sectional MR images. Luminal distension by methylcellulose provides the ability to distinguish even small lesions. Umschaden et al [19] compared conventional barium with MR enteroclysis in 30 patients with symptoms of either inflammatory bowel disease or small bowel obstruction. In 24% of the patients, the MR enteroclysis showed abnormalities not seen in conventional barium enteroclysis. Furthermore, extraluminal lesions, such as superior mesenteric vein thrombosis, were seen on the MR enteroclysis. The advantage of water as a contrast material is clear. It is well tolerated by the patients and unlike after a barium swallow, a subsequent CT scan or other radiographic examinations can be performed immediately after the MR without delay, and it avoids the problems associated with inspissated barium in patients with partial small bowel obstructions. However, since MRI is performed in a closed space not easily accessible to the medical staff, the risk of vomiting and subsequent aspiration should be taken into account when MRI of partially obstructed patients is performed.

## Small Bowel Endoscopy

The major advances in fiberoptic technology enabled the development of flexible endoscopic instruments for the diagnosis and treatment of gastrointestinal diseases. While esophagogastroduodenoscopy and colonoscopy became the main diagnostic tools for esophageal, gastric, and duodenal tumors and tumors of the colon and rectum (colonoscopy), small bowel endoscopy (enteroscopy) is limited to very few specialty centers around the world. The main reason for the slow development of enteroscopy is the lack of a driving force. Small bowel pathology, excluding Crohn's disease, which can be diagnosed and followed by small bowel barium studies and CT scan, is rare. The length of the small bowel and the technical complexity of passing an endoscopic instrument beyond the ligament of Treitz or retrogradely through the ileocecal valve necessitate the development of complex instruments and a long learning curve. Therefore, developing complex and expensive instruments that require significant expertise and training for an infrequent use is not in the interest of most clinical investigators and industrial researchers.

Despite that, major progress in small bowel endoscopy has been made over the past few years. The development of a wireless capsule endoscopy was a major breakthrough in small bowel imaging. Preliminary reports show accuracy and great promise for this imaging method [20]. Push enteroscopy is practiced in several specialty centers mainly to identify occult gastrointestinal bleeding. Descamps et al reported that out of 233 such patients, the enteroscope was passed successfully, under sedation, beyond the ligament of Treitz in 229 patients. Pathology was identified in 53% of the patients examined. Other groups also reported a high yield with minimal complications of enteroscopy. Lewis et al examined 258 patients with obscure gastrointestinal bleeding using small bowel enteroscopy. A small bowel tumor was found in 5% of patients. In 50% of patients no diagnosis could be made, but when the cause of obscure bleeding was discovered, small bowel tumors were the single most common lesion in patients younger than 50 years. Intraoperative enteroscopy is a more invasive technique with a high yield of occult bleeding detection.

# Management

## Benign Epithelial Tumors

### Adenomatous Polyps (Adenomas)

Adenomatous polyps are the second most common symptomatic benign tumor of the small bowel, and the most common benign tumors in autopsy studies. The majority of adenomas are found in the duodenum, with a decreasing incidence toward the distal ileum. Villous adenomas of the duodenum usually present with obstructive jaundice, and the diagnosis is easily made by endoscopic biopsy. The propensity for malignant transformation varies with age, location in the duodenum, and size. Villous adenomas diagnosed over the age of 50 years, larger than 5 cm, and located distally in the duodenum carry the highest risk of malignant transformation. Although some authors recommend transduodenal excision, the high recurrence rate and the risk of missed diagnosis of adenocarcinoma drive many surgeons toward pancreaticoduodenectomy (Whipple's procedure). Lesions located distal to the ampulla of Vater can be managed by transduodenal excision. The vast majority of patients with FAP have multiple duodenal polyps. Surgical excision of multiple villous adenomas in the duodenum is not recommended. Endoscopic follow-up with multiple biopsies is recommended in most cases. If high-grade dysplasia or malignant transformation identified, radical surgery is the treatment of choice.

### Brunner's Gland Adenoma (Hamartoma)

Brunner's gland enlargement is sometimes called Brunner's gland adenoma or hamartoma. There is controversy as to whether these lesions should be classified as hyperplasias, neoplasia, or hamartoma. Whatever the classification, this type of adenoma rarely undergoes malignant degeneration. Symptoms at presentation depend on the size of the tumor and range from a lack of symptoms to chronic upper gastrointestinal bleeding and duodenal or biliary obstruction. Treatment involves either endoscopic removal of pedunculated lesions or surgical resection of larger lesions.

## Malignant Epithelial Tumors

### Adenocarcinoma

Adenocarcinoma is the most common malignant tumor of the small bowel. However, because it is an uncommon disease, knowledge of its natural history and prognosis is limited. Management of gastrointestinal neoplasms such as adenocarcinoma of the colon or gastric adenocarcinoma is based mainly on data obtained from prospective randomized trials. Since adenocarcinoma of the small bowel is relatively uncommon, its management is based on extrapolation of data from gastric and colon cancer trials and retrospective studies that show great variability in the management of duodenal adenocarcinoma.

Joesting et al [16] reviewed the records of 104 patients with adenocarcinoma of the duodenum. They found that 50% of the lesions were resectable, and the 5-year survival rate for patients with resectable lesions was 46%. Eight patients treated with segmental resections for lesions in the third and fourth portions of the duodenum were alive for at least 5 years. Survival was directly related to nodal status, the grade of the lesion, and the ability of the surgeon to minimize or eliminate operative mortality. Rotman et al studied factors influencing survival of 46 patients with adenocarcinoma of the duodenum resected with curative intent. They concluded that resection of adenocarcinoma of the duodenum should be performed whenever possible, even in the presence of lymph node metastasis and pancreatic spread. Barnes et al [22] retrospectively reviewed the hospital records of 67 patients with non-ampullary adenocarcinoma of the duodenum treated at the University of Texas M.D. Anderson Cancer Center. A curative resection was performed in 36 of the 59 (61%) patients who underwent surgery. The 5-year survival difference between resected and unresected patients was 54% versus 0%, respectively ($p < 0.0001$). No survival difference was noted between patients who underwent pancreaticoduodenectomy rather than wide local excision. Other authors showed that resectability was the single most important factor influencing survival of patients with adenocarcinoma of the duodenum.

The role of preoperative chemoradiation in the treatment of adenocarcinoma of the duodenum and pancreas was studied by Coia et al in a prospective non-randomized trial. Radiation was given at a total dose of 50.4 Gy with two cycles of chemotherapy given concurrently (5-fluorouracil and mitomycin-C) with radiation. Surgery was performed 4–6 weeks after completion of chemoradiation. Thirty-one patients with a median follow-up of 4.5 years were studied. Twenty-seven patients had pancreatic cancer and four patients had adenocarcinoma of the duodenum. Twenty-one patients were initially judged to be unresectable and ten potentially resectable prior to chemoradiation. All four patients with adenocarcinoma of the duodenum underwent complete resection. A complete pathologic response was seen in all four patients and all were alive at the time of analysis.

In summary, based on these small studies, the treatment recommendations for adenocarcinoma of the duodenum include surgical resection for early lesions and preoperative chemoradiation for locally advanced lesions.

Adenocarcinoma of the jejunum and ileum should be managed by surgical resection of the tumor-bearing segment with its lymphatic drainage. Adjuvant chemotherapy utilizing 5-fluorouracil and leucovorin should be added for node-positive patients. A comprehensive analysis of the National Cancer Database was performed by Howe et al [7]. Of the 4995 cases of adenocarcinoma of the small intestine they reviewed, surgery as a single therapy was performed in 48%, surgery combined with radiotherapy in 2%, surgery with chemotherapy in 13%, and a combination of all three therapeutic modalities was delivered in 4% of the patients. Radiation alone was delivered in 2% of the cases, chemotherapy alone in 5%, and chemoradiation in 3%. In 3% of the patients treatment modality was unknown, and the remaining 20% did not receive any treatment. Median survival was 19.7 months and the 5-year survival was 30.5%. In a multivariate analysis of this group of patients, disease-specific survival was adversely affected by age >75, presence of tumor in the duodenum versus jejunum or ileum, tumor stage, tumor grade, and the noncancer directed surgery.

Prognosis can be reliably predicted by the American Joint Committee on Cancer (AJCC) TNM staging system [23] as shown in Table 14.4.

# Lymphoproliferative Disorders

## Lymphoid Hyperplasia

Primary hyperplasia of the intestinal lymphoid tissue is a non-neoplastic change that produces visible lesions. Focal lymphoid hyperplasia typically affects the terminal ileum of children and young adults. It may present as a polypoid lesion up to a size of 5 cm. Diffuse nodular lymphoid hyperplasia is a rare disorder that may involve the entire small intestine or colon. It might be associated with late onset hypogammaglobulinemia. Management includes careful follow-up to detect additional lymphomas that can arise in these patients.

**Table 14.4.** TNM staging

*Primary tumor (T)*
- TX: Primary tumor cannot be assessed
- T0: No evidence of primary tumor
- Tis: Carcinoma in situ
- T1: Tumor invades lamina propria or submucosa
- T2: Tumor invades muscularis propria
- T3: Tumor invades through the muscularis propria into the subserosa or into the non-peritonealized perimuscular tissue (mesentery or retroperitoneum) with extension 2 cm or less
- T4: Tumor perforates the visceral peritoneum or directly invades other organs or structures (includes other loops of the small intestine, mesentery, or retroperitoneum more than 2 cm, and the abdominal wall by way of the serosa; for the duodenum only, includes invasion of the pancreas)

*Regional lymph nodes (N)*
- NX: Regional lymph nodes cannot be assessed
- N0: No regional lymph node metastasis
- N1: Regional lymph node metastasis

*Distant metastasis (M)*
- MX: Distant metastasis cannot be assessed
- M0: No distant metastasis
- M1: Distant metastasis

*AJCC stage groupings*
- Stage 0: Tis, N0, M0
- Stage I: T1, N0, M0
  T2, N0, M0
- Stage II: T3, N0, M0
  T4, N0, M0
- Stage III: Any T, N1, M0
- Stage IV: Any T, Any N, M1

## Malignant Lymphomas

Half of non-Hodgkin's lymphomas (NHL) of the gastrointestinal tract arise in the stomach, 40% in the small intestine and 10% in the colon. The diagnosis of primary gastrointestinal lymphoma requires the absence of superficial palpable lymph nodes or radiologically detectable mediastinal lymph nodes, normal white cell count, predominance of the gastrointestinal lesion, and tumor-free liver and spleen. There are several classification systems for lymphomas: the most popular one is the Revised European-American Lymphoma (REAL) classification.

Immunoproliferative small intestinal disease (IPSID), α-heavy chain disease, Mediterranean lymphoma, or mucosa-associated lymphoid tissue (MALT) lymphoma are all synonyms of the same proliferative disorder of IgA-producing B lymphocytes. It affects children and young adults, primarily in Mediterranean countries. These lesions commonly affect the duodenum and proximal jejunal mucus or the etiology remains unclear. Diarrhea and weight loss are the main presenting symptoms. Treatment with broad-spectrum antibiotics to prevent its transformation into a high-grade lymphoma has been theorized, but chemotherapy is the treatment of choice.

Primary T-cell gastrointestinal lymphomas are rare. Enteropathy-associated T-cell lymphoma (EATL) accounts for about one-third of small intestinal lymphomas and usually affects adults over the age of 60. The disease progress rapidly and might cause small bowel perforation. The prognosis is poor, with an overall 5-year survival of 10%. A number of small intestinal T-cell lymphomas may develop in the absence of celiac disease. Some cases are identical to EATL, but some differ in their molecular or cytologic markers. Several cases of primary Hodgkin's disease of the gastrointestinal tract have been reported in the literature.

Treatment options for localized small intestinal lymphomas include surgical resection, which may suffice for disease localized to the bowel wall if 12 or more lymph nodes are removed and prove negative. However, the addition of combination chemotherapy should be considered as well. For extension of disease to the regional lymph nodes, surgical resection at the time of diagnosis followed by combination chemotherapy is the treatment of choice. For unresectable and extensive disease, combination chemotherapy is the treatment of choice. In addition, radiation therapy is often used to reduce the risk of recurrence in the tumor bed.

## Carcinoid Tumour

The majority of carcinoid tumors arise in the gastrointestinal tract, most frequently in the appendix, followed by the small intestine, rectum, colon, and stomach. In several studies, carcinoid tumors of the small intestine accounted for 18–25% of all carcinoids. Patients with small intestinal carcinoids present in the sixth or seventh decade of life, most commonly with abdominal pain or partial small bowel obstruction. The majority present with lymph node or distant metastasis and 5–7% present with carcinoid syndrome. In general tumor size correlates directly with the presence of lymph node metastasis and survival. The risk of metastases begins to increase significantly for tumors 2 cm or greater. Five-year survival is estimated to be 65% in patients with locoregional disease and 36% in patients with distant disease. Segmental resection of the small bowel with draining mesenteric lymph nodes is the treatment of choice for locoregional disease. The role of surgery is limited in advanced disease.

## Mesenchymal Small Bowel Neoplasms

Gastrointestinal mesenchymal tumors can be divided into two categories: those with distinct histologic features such as lipomas or hemangioma, and those that do not have clear-cut histologic features and cannot be classified into any specific cell lineage. Tumors in the second category are called gastrointestinal stromal tumors (GIST).

The classification of GIST is difficult because these tumors lack differentiated cellular characteristics, they might be heterogeneous, and they can share overlapping features of several entities. Assessment of the malignant potential of GIST tumors is done by size (>5 cm) and mitotic count (>10/10 high power field). These parameters are not always accurate in predicting the malignant potential of a certain tumor.

## Gastrointestinal Stromal Tumors (see Chapter 15)

The cellular *morphology* of GIST ranges from predominantly spindle-shaped to epithelioid. Moreover the differentiation *pathways* can vary from indeterminate to myoid or neural. Recent studies have indicated that the interstitial cells of Cajal, postulated to act as pacemaker cells of the gastrointestinal tract, could be candidates for GIST origin. The c-*kit* proto-oncogene, which encodes a growth factor receptor with tyrosine kinase activity, has been postulated to play an important role in tumorigenesis. Monoclonal and polyclonal antibodies directed at the c-*kit* gene product expressed on the cell surface (CD117/c-kit) are essential in resolving the histopathological differential diagnosis between GIST and true gastrointestinal smooth muscle neoplasms, schwannomas, and other gastrointestinal mesenchymal tumors. Increasing tumor size and mitotic activity favor aggressive tumor behavior, whereas the prognostic value of germline and somatic mutations within the c-*kit* proto-oncogene remains to be further elucidated. In a retrospective review, Clary et al [24] studied the clinical differences between leiomyosarcomas occurring within the abdomen and retroperitoneum and GIST. A total of 561 patients, 239 with GIST and 322 with leiomyosarcoma, were studied. Patients with GIST were older, with a median age of 58 years. The 5-year disease-specific survival for GIST and leiomyosarcoma were 28% and 29%, respectively. Another study from the same group looked at the clinical patterns of recurrence of GIST. Of the 200 patients studied, 46% had primary disease without metastasis, 47% had metastasis, and 7% had isolated local recurrence. In patients who underwent complete resection, the 5-year actuarial survival was 54%. Recurrence of disease after resection was mainly intra-abdominal, affecting the original tumor site, the peritoneum, and the liver.

Treatment of localized disease is by surgical resection. A major development in the treatment of metastatic c-*kit*-positive GIST is the introduction of the selective tyrosine kinase inhibitor STI571. STI-571 has already shown clinical value in BCR-ABL-positive leukemias. Preliminary results from clinical trials show good response of c-*kit*-positive GIST to STI-571[25].

## Leiomyomas

Leiomyomas of the small bowel are the most common symptomatic small bowel benign tumors. Leiomyomas account for 20–40% of benign small bowel tumors. In autopsy series, the incidence of small bowel leiomyomas is second only to adenomatous polyps.

Since clinical distinction of benign and malignant lesions is extremely difficult, size is an important predictor of malignancy. Histologic criteria for malignancy include mitotic activity, necrosis, and nuclear pleomorphism. Treatment includes segmental resection of the small bowel loop containing the tumor. Enucleation or local excision can be performed in cases of small leiomyomas of the duodenum.

## Leiomyosarcomas

Well-differentiated leiomyosarcomas are hard to distinguish from leiomyomas because both appear as firm, rubbery masses. Some of the leiomyosarcomas are large with areas of hemorrhage or necrosis and these are obviously malignant. Tumor diameter of more than 5 cm is considered a predictive factor of low-grade malignancy. Factors associated with better outcome are complete surgical resection without violation of the tumor pseudocapsule, a localized growth pattern, low histologic grade, and size <5 cm. Lymphatic invasion and nodal metastases are distinctly uncommon.

## Other Benign Tumors

Lipomas of the small bowel are rare tumors presenting with symptoms of abdominal pain consistent with partial small bowel obstruction. In the case of a single lesion, segmental resection is the proper surgical treatment choice. However, in the case of multiple lipomas, more complex surgical decision-making is required.

Angiomas of the small bowel are less common, may be multifocal, and usually present as occult gastrointestinal bleeding. Treatment includes segmental resection of the small bowel after the lesion has been localized either preoperatively or intraoperatively.

Neurofibromas can occur as a single lesion or as part of diffuse neurofibromatosis. Upper digestive tract involvement has been estimated to occur in 2% to 25% of patients with systemic neurofibromatosis. Typically, the involvement is characterized by submucosal neurofibromas originating in the submucosal nerve plexus.

# Secondary (Metastatic) Neoplasms of the Small Bowel

Several malignant neoplasms show predilection to metastasize to the small intestine. Metastatic malignant melanoma is the most common, followed by bronchiogenic carcinoma and breast cancer. A report of 103 cases of malignant melanoma of the small bowel from the Armed Forces Institute of Pathology [26] showed that primary lesions preceded intestinal disease by an average of 5.6 years for cases diagnosed in surgery and 2.1 years if diagnosed by autopsy. They concluded that small bowel involvement by melanoma, even without a known primary, is probably metastatic. Bender et al reported on 32 patients with malignant melanoma metastasis involving the small bowel. The sensitivity of small bowel barium follow-through and CT scan in detection of small bowel metastasis was 58% and 66%, respectively. Krige et al reported 18 patients with small bowel metastasis of malignant melanoma who underwent complete resection with a median survival of 4.5 years. They concluded that surgical resection is indicated both for symptoms relief and for prolongation of life. Other authors reported similar results supporting segmental resection of small bowel involved with metastatic malignant melanoma.

Berger et al reviewed 1544 patients with lung cancer and found 7 patients with small intestinal metastasis. In all but one case, patients were diagnosed following resection of lung cancer. Mosier et al reviewed 37 cases in the literature and 3 cases from their own experience of lung cancer small bowel metastasis.

In summary, metastatic lesions are rarely found in the small intestine, with malignant melanoma being the most common followed by bronchiogenic carcinoma.

## Questions

1. What are the most common types of small bowel tumors?
2. What are the methods used for diagnosis of neoplasms?
3. What are the small bowel features of FAP and what tumors commonly develop in the small bowel after panproctocolectomy?
4. What are the conditions that can progress to the development of small bowel neoplasms?
5. Outline the staging system for small bowel neoplasms.

# References

1. Coit DG. Cancer of the small intestine. In: DeVita VT (ed.) Cancer: Principles and practice of oncology. Philadelphia: Lippincott Williams & Wilkins, 2001;1204–13.
2. Maglinte DD, Chernish SM, Bessette J et al. Factors in the diagnostic delays of small bowel malignancy. Indiana Med 1991;84:392–6.
3. Dixon PM, Roulston ME, Nolan DJ. The small bowel enema: a ten year review. Clin Radiol 1993;47:46–8.
4. Jigyasu D, Bedikian AY, Stroehlein JR. Chemotherapy for primary adenocarcinoma of the small bowel. Cancer 1984;53:23–5.
5. Barclay TH, Schapira DV. Malignant tumors of the small intestine. Cancer 1983;51:878–81.
6. Chow JS, Chen CC, Ahsan H, Neugut AI. A population-based study of the incidence of malignant small bowel tumours: SEER, 1973–1990. Int J Epidemiol 1996;25:722–8.
7. Howe JR, Karnell LH, Menck HR, Scott-Conner C. The American College of Surgeons Commission on Cancer and the American Cancer Society. Adenocarcinoma of the small bowel: review of the National Cancer Data Base, 1985–1995. Cancer 1999;86:2693–706.
8. Coop KL, Sharp JG, Osborne JW, Zimmerman GR. An animal model for the study of small-bowel tumors. Cancer Res 1974;34:1487–94.
9. Calman KC. Why are small bowel tumours rare? An experimental model. Gut 1974;15:552–4.
10. Cooper MJ, Williamson RC. Enteric adenoma and adenocarcinoma. World J Surg 1985;9:914–20.
11. Kaerlev L, Teglbjaerg PS, Sabroe S et al. Occupation and small bowel adenocarcinoma: a European case-control study. Occup Environ Med 2000;57:760–6.
12. Kaerlev L, Teglbjaerg PS, Sabroe S et al. Is there an association between alcohol intake or smoking and small bowel adenocarcinoma? Results from a European multicenter case-control study. Cancer Causes Control 2000;11:791–7.
13. Balthazar EJ, Noordhoorn M, Megibow AJ, Gordon RB. CT of small-bowel lymphoma in immunocompetent patients and patients with AIDS: comparison of findings. AJR Am J Roentgenol 1997;168:675–80.
14. Wall SD, Friedman SL, Margulis AR. Gastrointestinal Kaposi's sarcoma in AIDS: radiographic manifestations. J Clin Gastroenterol 1984;6:165–71.
15. Torbenson MS, Wang J, Nichols L et al. Occult non-hematopoietic malignancies present at autopsy in solid organ transplant patients who died within 100 days. Transplantation 2001;71:64–9.
16. Rodriguez-Bigas MA, Vasen HF, Lynch HT et al. Characteristics of small bowel carcinoma in hereditary nonpolyposis colorectal carcinoma. International Collaborative Group on HNPCC. Cancer 1998;83:240–4.
17. Gupta S, Gupta S. Primary tumors of the small bowel: a clinicopathological study of 58 cases. J Surg Oncol 1982;20:161–7.
18. Gourtsoyiannis N, Mako E. Imaging of primary small intestinal tumours by enteroclysis and CT with pathological correlation. Eur Radiol 1997;7:625–42.
19. Umschaden HW, Szolar D, Gasser J et al. Small-bowel disease: comparison of MR enteroclysis images with conventional enteroclysis and surgical findings. Radiology 2000;215:717–25.
20. Appleyard M, Glukhovsky A, Swain P. Wireless-capsule diagnostic endoscopy for recurrent small-bowel bleeding. N Engl J Med 2001;344:232–3.
21. Joesting DR, Beart RW Jr, van Heerden JA, Weiland LH. Improving survival in adenocarcinoma of the duodenum. Am J Surg 1981;141:228–31.
22. Barnes G, Jr., Romero L, Hess KR, Curley SA. Primary adenocarcinoma of the duodenum: management and survival in 67 patients. Ann Surg Oncol 1994;1:73–8.
23. AJCC. Small intestine. American Joint Committee on Cancer: AJCC cancer staging manual. Philadelphia: Lippincott-Raven, 1997; 77–81.
24. Clary BM, DeMatteo RP, Lewis JJ, Leung D, Brennan MF. Gastrointestinal stromal tumors and leiomyosarcoma of the abdomen and retroperitoneum: a clinical comparison. Ann Surg Oncol 2001;8:290–9.
25. Joensuu H, Roberts PJ, Sarlomo-Rikala M et al. Effect of the tyrosine kinase inhibitor STI571 in a patient with a metastatic gastrointestinal stromal tumor. N Engl J Med 2001;344:1052–6.
26. Elsayed AM, Albahra M, Nzeako UC, Sobin LH. Malignant melanomas in the small intestine: a study of 103 patients. Am J Gastroenterol 1996;91:1001–6.

# 15

# Stromal Upper GI Tract Neoplasms

Stephan T. Samel and Stefan Post

## Aims

- Definition and differential diagnosis of gastrointestinal stromal tumors.
- Epidemiology and common clinical features of GIST.
- Diagnostic characteristics and pathological confirmation of diagnosis.
- Surgical approach and options for non-surgical treatment.

## Introduction

The term *sarcoma* for malignant tumors arising from mesenchymal cells is old and has its origin in the Greek term *sarx* for flesh. This term referred to the fleshy appearance of certain tumors on cross-sections. Modern pathologists believed that sarcomas consist of different types of mesenchymal cells. But there was disagreement over their cellular origin. The pathologist Franz Schuh from Vienna in the late nineteenth century proposed reserving the term for tumors of muscle cell origin but found little support for this. Precursors of various mesenchymal cell types had already been identified in sarcomas and a subsequent definition by T. Billroth found broad acceptance: a sarcoma was a tumor, "which consists of a tissue derived from precursors of connective substances (connective tissue, cartilage, bone), muscle and nerve" *Lectures on general surgical pathology and therapy*, 8th edn, Berlin, 1876). We will see, that such a stem cell concept still applies in the case of gastrointestinal stromal tumor (GIST). In the early twentieth century the smooth muscle cell origin of mesenchymal neoplasm's was favored and tumors were called leiomyomas and leiomyosarcomas or epithelioid leiomyomas/-sarcomas and leiomyoblastomas respectively [1]. The British pathologist Arthur Purdy Stout and his coworkers never questioned the smooth muscle origin of stromal tumors and they found a good correlation between the number of mitoses and malignancy. But they noticed that some stromal tumors do metastasize despite a low mitotic count and these tumors did not always fit into the general histomorphology of smooth muscle neoplasms. Such tumors of uncertain biological behavior have since been known as *Stout's bizarre smooth muscle tumors* or *stromal tumors of uncertain malignant potential* (STUMP). More elaborate understanding of the nature of mesenchymal neoplasms arising in the stomach and intestines took some more decades of research. Looking at leiomyomas of the stomach through the electron microscope in the late 1960s, Welsh discovered that some of these tumors lacked smooth muscle cell differentiation [2]. Mazur and Clarke in 1983 confirmed that some leiomyomas/leiomyosarcomas of the stomach lacked smooth muscle cell differentiation. Others were positive for S100 and showed immunohistochemical characteristics of Schwann cells [3]. It was believed then that stromal tumors basically consisted of undifferentiated cells [4]. In view of the histomorphological heterogeneity of these tumors the general term *gastrointestinal stromal tumors* was introduced.

Today we understand that stromal tumors of the gastrointestinal tract are specific c-KIT positive gastrointestinal neoplasms of differing histomorphological and ultrastructural phenotype and biological behavior. The common feature of GISTs is their expression of the c-KIT, a growth factor receptor with tyrosine kinase activity. They predominately occur in the stomach, are less frequent in the small bowel and rarely arise in the colorectum, esophagus or in the omentum or mesentery. The variety of synonymous denominations for GIST in literature, e.g. STUMP (smooth muscle cell tumor of uncertain malignant potential) or GIPACT (gastrointestinal pacemaker cell tumor) [5], reflects the state of consent and disconsent regarding this group of neoplasms [6]. When looking through the literature of the past four decades concerned with stromal tumors of the digestive tract, the reader will find different classifications and an inconsistent use of terminology. Many authors used the term sarcoma in the former understanding of Stout, referring to both stromal tumors and true smooth muscle neoplasms, until the late 1980s and many conclusions drawn from such patient series ought to be considered with care. This chapter will summarize the current understanding of the pathology of GISTs and its implications for surgical and non-surgical therapy.

## Classification of GISTs and their Differentiation from Other Mesenchymal Tumors of the GI Tract

### GIST

Gastrointestinal stromal tumors (GISTs) are defined as mesenchymal neoplasms of the digestive tract with spindle cell, epithelioid or pleomorphic differentiation. On immunohistochemistry and by ultrastructural examination myogenic, neural, bi-directional and dedifferentiated subclasses have been classified [7]. The tumor cells express the c-KIT, a growth factor receptor with tyrosine kinase activity (CD 117). The c-KIT is expressed in normal interstitial cells in the digestive tract too, called interstitial cells of Cajal (ICC). During embryogenesis the tyrosine kinase receptor seems to be essential for the development of Cajal cells. Santiago Ramon Cajal, a Spanish anatomist, had discovered this type of primitive nerve cells in the early twentieth century. These cells are located around the myenteric plexus in adults and are currently believed to play a pivotal rote in gastrointestinal motility [8]. In the fetal intestines ICCs can be found in the outer smooth muscle cell layer [9]. Because GISTs share immunohistochemical and ultrastructural features with Cajal cells, an origin of GIST from these Cajal cells or a common stem cell origin of both has been suggested [5]. Cajal cells are capable of differentiating into smooth muscle cells suggesting some stem cell like potential [10]. These recent findings further support the concept of a Cajal cell origin of GIST. In this respect GISTs are "true" stromal tumors.

Activating mutations in the exon 11 of the c-KIT gene are believed to be a central pathogenic factor in the development of GIST [11]. These mutations cause a pathological signal transduction activation by ligand-independet phosphorylization of the c-KIT tyrosine kinase. Because approximately half of GIST in larger series lack mutations in the exon 11, relevant mutations are suspected on other loci as well. In a minority of GIST lacking the exon 11 mutation, for example, mutations are localized on exon 9 and 13 [12]. Identification of relevant mutations may have implications for therapy. It has been shown that inhibition of the pathological activation of tyrosine kinase is a possible treatment strategy in other tumors, in which treatment with specific tyrosine kinase inhibitors has shown promising results. Since both malignant GIST and sarcoma demonstrate a rigorous resistance against conventional chemotherapy the pathological tyrosine kinase activity is as yet the only potential target of non-surgical treatment of GIST. For patients with advanced or metastatic stromal tumors, therefore, the detection of c-KIT expression is crucial for treatment.

The group of c-KIT-positive GISTs represent the majority of gastrointestinal tumors of mesenchymal origin. Omental stromal tumors too are positive for c-KIT and like GIST show mutations of the c-KIT oncogene. Omental GISTs may originate from recently identified omental Cajal-like c-KIT-positive cells [13]. Metastatic melanoma, a frequent metastatic tumor of the GI tract, and intestinal angiosarcoma may express c-KIT in half of the cases too.

## GANT

Gastrointestinal autonomic nerve tumors (GANT), originally called "plexosarcomas" [14,15] most probably represent a subset of GIST. GANTs are positive for c-KIT and share the histological and immunohistochemical characteristics of GIST and ICC. The even more obvious similarities of GANT with ICC have led to the hypothesis that GANT is probably the most differentiated form of GIST. GANTs differ by having a specific ultrastructure similar to that of neural tissue of the plexus myentericus. These specific features, dendritic processes with dense neuroendocrine granules, become evident on electron microscopy only. Clinically GANTs present like GISTs and prognosis is probably the same.

## Other Gastrointestinal Tumors of Mesenchymal Origin

A small proportion of mesenchymal GI neoplasms, e.g. leiomyomas and leiomyosarcomas and schwannomas, share histogenetic and pathogenic features of GIST, but are c-KIT negative. In addition, other mesenchymal tumors unrelated to GIST and negative for c-KIT can be found along the digestive tract and may clinically simulate GIST. These include desmoid tumors, inflammatory fibroid tumors, myofibroblastic tumors and invasive retroperitoneal dedifferentiated liposarcoma.

### True Leiomyomas

Benign leiomyomas consist of well-differentiated smooth muscle cells. They represent the majority of mesenchymal tumors of the esophagus and the colorectum. Leiomyomas of the stomach or the small bowel are less frequent. Esophageal leiomyoma usually occurs in male patients younger than those with GIST. These intramural and often calcified tumors only a few millimeters in size remain asymptomatic in most cases and may be found incidentally on chest X-rays. Some esophageal leiomyomas, however, may develop to larger tumors and may cause dysphagia and bleeding. Some families have been reported to show a frequent incidence of multiple esophageal and upper gastrointestinal lesions (familial esophageal and upper gastrointestinal leiomyomatosis) [16]. Colorectal leiomyomas form intraluminal polyps. They usually remain small and asymptomatic as well and are incidentally found on colonoscopy on elder patients. Some surgeons prefer to perform resection rather than local excision in patients with leiomyomas because differentiation from leiomyosarcoma may be difficult at first sight. If the resected tumor is benign, surgery is curative and there is no recurrence.

### True Leiomyosarcomas

Malignant gastrointestinal leiomyosarcomas (LMS) share the histological pattern of well-differentiated smooth muscle cells with other sarcomas of vascular or retroperitoneal origin. Like GIST they occur in older patients and share a similar clinical course and prognosis. In a retrospective study of 561 patients with mesenchymal gastrointestinal neoplasms from Memorial Sloan Kettering Cancer Center [17] 43% of patients had had GIST and 57% had had LMS. The latter were predominately female (67%) and younger than patients with GIST. Hepatic recurrence was more frequent in GIST, whereas pulmonary spread predominated in LMS. Five-year-survival was 28 and 29% respectively.

### Schwannomas

Little is known about gastrointestinal schwannomas. They are rare benign or malignant solitary or multiple intramural tumors arising from Schwann cells of Auerbach's plexus. They occur incidentally or in association with von Recklinghausen's disease. Clinically and grossly they resemble GIST in many features. Electron microscopy often is necessary to confirm diagnosis. Like GIST, they occur in older patients and predominate in the stomach. Less frequently they occur in the small and large bowel. Gastrointestinal bleeding is the most commonly observed clinical feature and early recurrence of malignant schwannoma after surgery has been reported [18].

## Epidemiology of GIST

Mesenchymal tumors account for less than 1% of gastric malignomas but for more than 10% of malignant tumors of the small bowel. In Western countries the incidence of mesenchymal malignomas of stomach and small bowel has been estimated as 1.2–1.8 per million [19] and 1.3 per million respectively [20]. These data represent both stromal and smooth muscle cell neoplasms. In a recent epidemiological study from Sweden the incidence of GIST was estimated as 10–20 per million. The proportion of malignant GIST was 20–30% in this study [18]. It is still unclear whether GISTs are more likely to occur in males but many studies show a male predominance among patients. GISTs are neoplasms of the sixth and seventh decade, rarely occurring in patients younger than 40 years of age, and they are very rare among children. In children inflammatory myofibroblastic tumor, a benign neoplasm, is far more frequent and may clinically and grossly simulate GIST [21].

More than two-thirds of patients with GIST have stromal tumors of the stomach and in a quarter of cases GIST is located in the small bowel. GIST of the esophagus (< 5%) and the colorectum (5%) are sporadic findings. GIST-like tumors have occasionally been found in the omentum and mesentery [18].

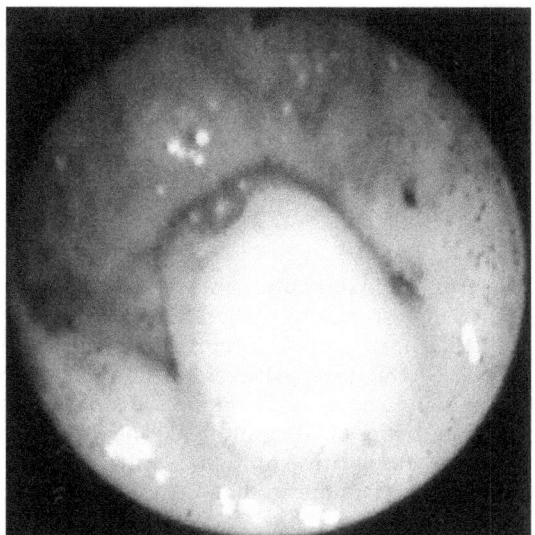

**Figure 15.1.** Submucosal polypoid GIST of the stomach on endoscopy.

## Clinical Presentation and Typical Findings

The clinical presentation of GIST lacks characteristic features. Many cases are discovered incidentally on endoscopy, laparotomy or radiological studies. Endoscopically GISTs may present as submucosal nodules or pedicles covered by mucosa (Figure 15.1) or they may present as a mediastinal mass or extraluminal pedicular tumors on imaging studies (Figure 15.2). GIST and LMS may look alike on ultrasound examination (US), computed tomography (CT), magnetic resonance imaging (MRI) and on laparotomy (Figure 15.3). Symptoms are associated with increasing tumor size. Larger GISTs of the esophagus may cause dysphagia or dyspepsia and mediastinal pain. However, leiomyoma is more common in this localization

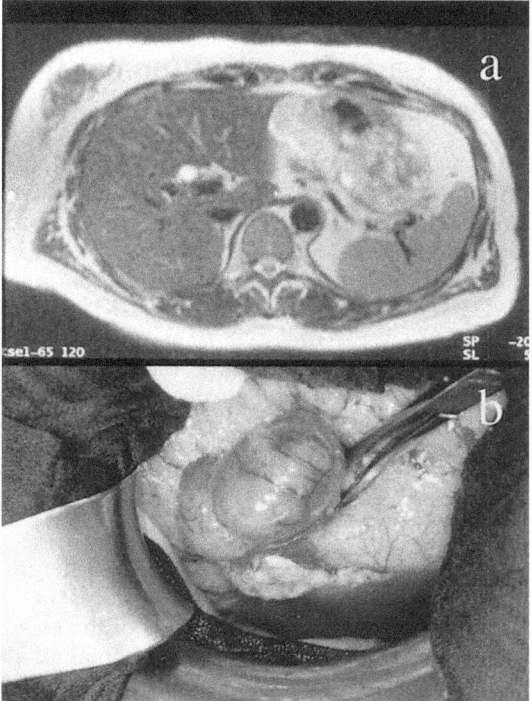

**Figure 15.2.** Transversal computed tomography **a** and intraoperative macrophotograph **b** demonstrating an extraluminal pediculate malignant GIST of the stomach in a male patient.

## STROMAL UPPER GI TRACT NEOPLASMS

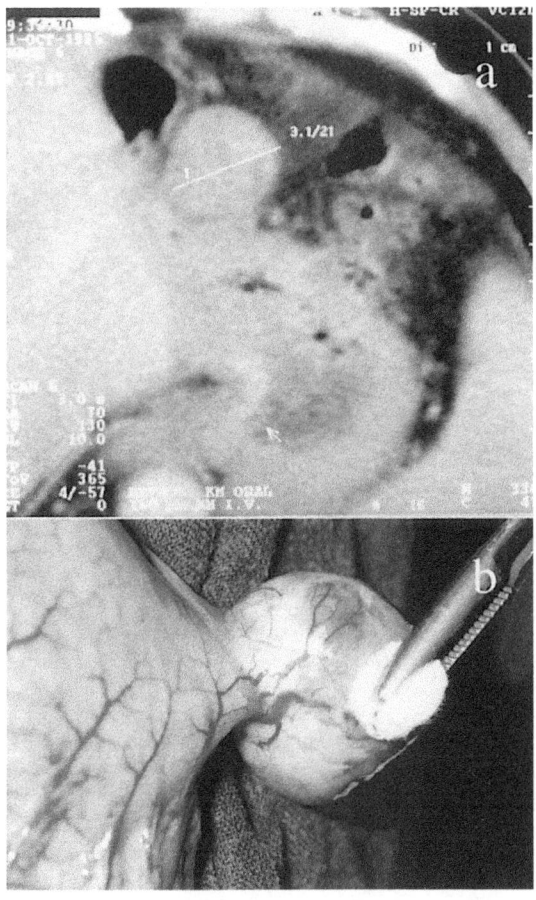

**Figure 15.3.** Transversal computed tomography **a** and intraoperative macrophotograph **b** demonstrating an extraluminal pediculate leiomyosarcoma of the stomach in a male patient.

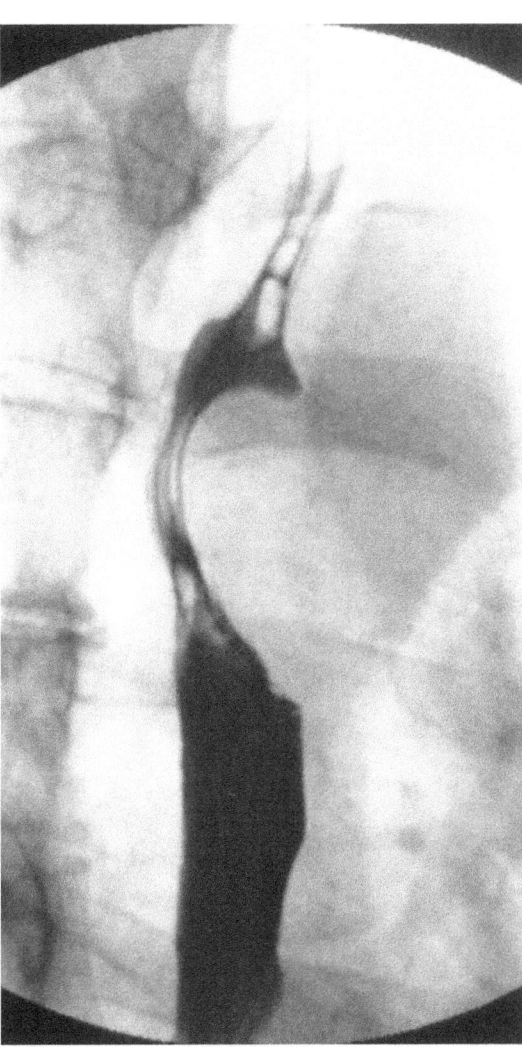

**Figure 15.4.** Esophageal enema demonstrating leiomyoma, 3 cm in diameter, in a 60-year-old female patient. GIST is uncommon in this localization.

(Figure 14.4). Larger GISTs of the stomach usually present with upper abdominal discomfort or hemorrhage. Upper gastrointestinal bleeding may lead to the diagnosis of upper intestinal tumor in most patients with GIST [22] (Figure 15.5). The clinical presentation of GIST past the stomach is likely to be determined by obstructive tumor growth. Patients may present with recurrent abdominal pain, acute bowel obstruction, intussusseption or perforation. GIST of the rectum may form a large submucosal mass causing perineal or pelvic pain or obstruction. Small and large bowel enema may demonstrate and localize intramural tumor or obstruction of the digestive tract. US and CT can determine tumor site and extent of tumor growth. Confinement to the gastrointestinal muscular layer can be demonstrated by endoscopic ultrasound (EUS). MRI may help to characterize GIST, demonstrating a homogeneous isointense mass on T2-weighted images [23,24].

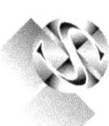

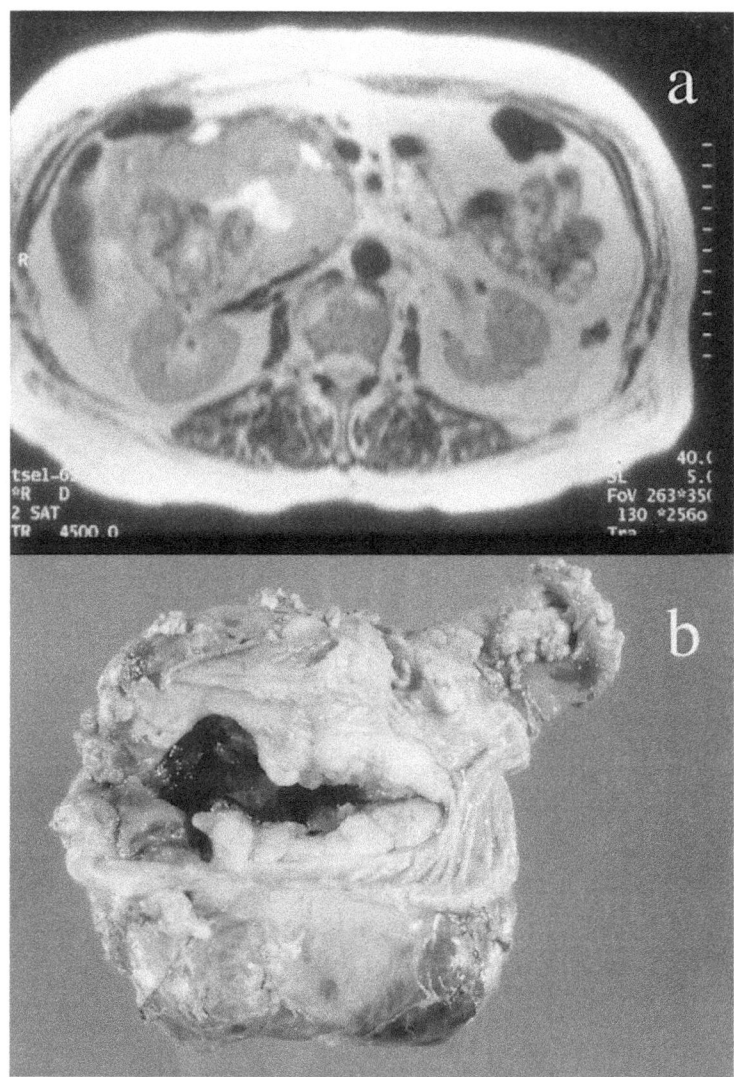

**Figure 15.5.** Transversal magnetic resonance image **a** of advanced malignant duodenal GIST with hepatic metastases in a 66-year-old female. The excavated tumors had caused severe acute intestinal bleeding. Pylorus preserving partial duodenopancreatectomy was performed for palliation **b**.

## Diagnosis of GIST on Histology and Immunohistochemistry

GIST present with a regular pattern of spindle or epithelioid-like sometimes pleomorphic stromal cells on cross-sections (Figure 15.6a). In order to confirm the diagnosis of GIST immunohistochemistry should be performed (Table 15.1). Vimentin, an unspecific marker of mesenchymal tissue generally shows a positive reaction in GIST. The majority of GISTs are positive for CD34 (Figure 15.6b). c-KIT-positive tumor cells are found in 100% of GISTs and confirm the diagnosis (Figure 15.6c). c-KIT-positive gastrointestinal tumors other than GIST are usually of metastatic origin. Reactivity for sm-actin, ms-actin and desmin antibodies is

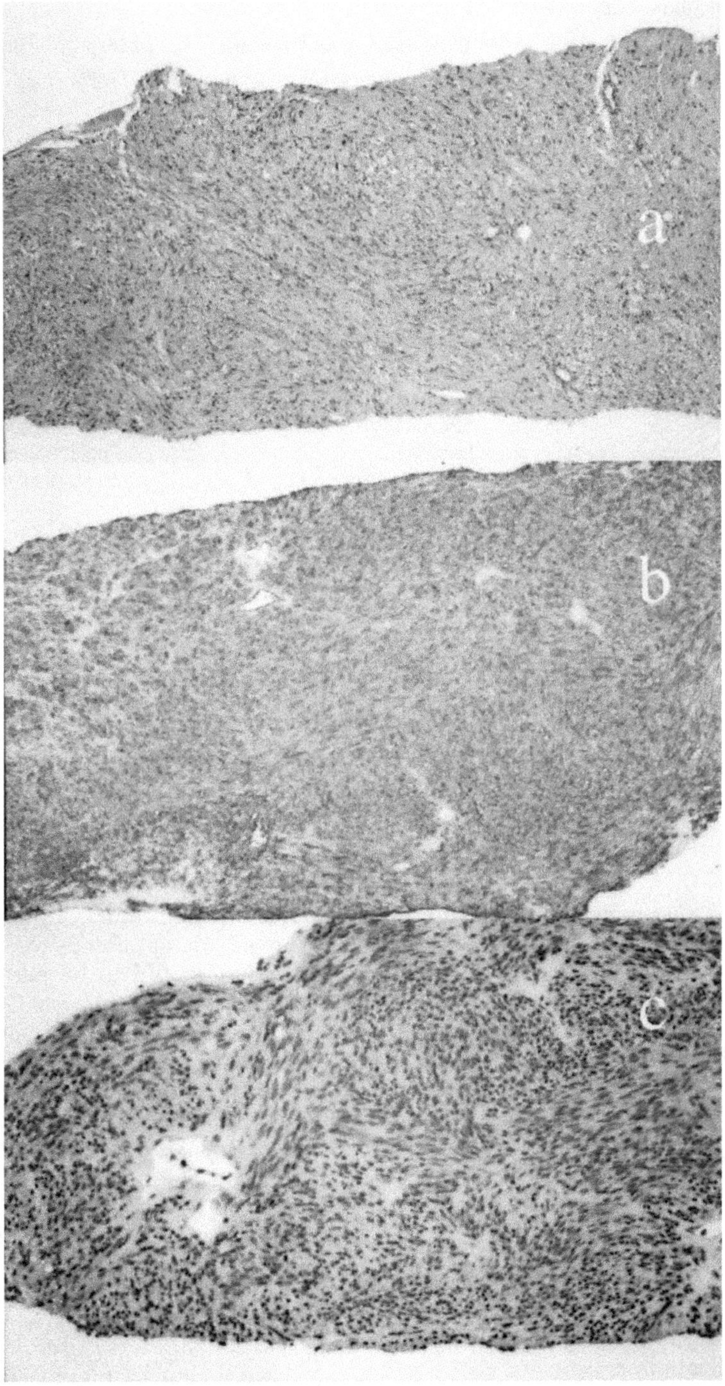

## STROMAL UPPER GI TRACT NEOPLASMS

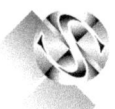

**Figure 15.6.** Typical histological and immunohistochemical pattern of malignant spindle cell GIST of the stomach. **a** Hematoxylin–eosin staining (10×) demonstrating a typical spindle cell pattern. **b** Positive immunostaining for CD34 (10×) **c** Positive c-KIT-immunostaining (10×) confirming diagnosis of GIST.

**Table 15.1.** Immunohistochemical markers of GIST

| Antibody | Reactivity in GIST (%) | Differential tumor diagnosis | Expression in normal tissue |
|---|---|---|---|
| CD117 | 100 | Gastrointestinal metastases from:<br>Melanoma<br>Clear cell sarcoma<br>Endometrial cancer<br>Small cell lung cancer<br>Ewing's sarcoma<br>Large cell lymphoma<br>Reed Sternberg cell in Hodgkin's lymphoma<br>Mastocytosis<br>AML<br>Glioma<br>Germinoma | Cells of Cajal<br>Mast cell<br>Hematopoietic stem cells<br>Basal cells and immature Langerhans cells of the epidermis<br>Epithelial cells<br>Glial cell<br>Osteoblasts |
| Vimentin | 100 | Stromal tissue | Stromal tissue |
| CD34 | 75 | Leiomyoma<br>Leiomyosarcoma<br>Solitary fibrous tumor<br>Dermatofibrosarcoma protuberans<br>Karposi's sarcoma<br>Lipoma<br>Neurofibroma<br>Vascular tumors<br>Epithelioid sarcoma | Endothelial cells<br>Mesenchymal stem cells |
| Smooth muscle actin | 50 | Leiomyoma<br>Leiomyosarcoma | Muscle cells |
| Desmin | 30 | Leiomyoma<br>Leiomyosarcoma | Muscle cells |
| S100 | 15 | Schwannoma | Schwann cells |

frequent but not always present. Schwann cells can be detected on immunohistochemistry (S100 protein) in less than 20% of GISTs [18].

## Treatment

### Surgery

Patients with GIST should to be referred for surgury particularly because no therapeutic alternatives are yet at hand. Radical curative resection is the most important prognostic factor in patients with GIST. However, some peculiarities of tumor biology may allow a modified treatment strategy with regard to tumor status and localization.

### Esophagus and Stomach

Leiomyoma is the most common non-epithelial tumor of the esophagus whereas GIST is more frequent in the stomach. Small and benign mesenchymal tumors of the esophagus may be removed on endoscopy or by local excision. Resection should to be performed in patients with malignant esophageal GIST or leiomyosarcoma. The difference between esophageal leiomyoma and leiomyosarcoma may be difficult to recognize at first sight and some surgeons prefer oncological esophageal resection in benign cases too. In the stomach very small GIST and leiomyoma may be removed on endoscopy. Like leiomyoma small GISTs are benign in most cases. In patients with borderline or malignant GIST of the stomach, on the other hand, surgical tumor removal is mandatory. In contrast to gastric adenocarcinoma, however, malignant GISTs of the stomach prefer a vertical rather than a lateral submucosal growth pattern. In small gastric GIST a safety margin of 2–3 cm may therefore be oncologically sufficient and subtotal resection or atypical local tumor removal (wedge resection) may be employed. Lymphadenectomy can be limited to suspected mediastinal or perigastric lymph nodes. A rationale for systematic lymphadenectomy does not exist either for esophageal or for gastric GIST.

## Duodenum

In GIST of the duodenum the choice of procedure is extremely difficult. Although, unlike cholangiocarcinoma or pancreatic cancer, duodenal GIST usually causes upper intestinal bleeding rather than cholestasis, these tumors will require partial duodenopancreatectomy if their status is in question. Only small and supposedly benign tumor nodules can be removed, like adenomas, on endoscopy, by pancreas-preserving procedures or via a transduodenal approach.

## Bowel

Surgery should aim at radical, complete, and if necessary multivisceral, removal of small bowel GIST because only complete tumor removal can provide cure. Since lymphatic spread is rare, radical systematic lymphadenectomy may not be necessary [25].

Surgery for malignant colorectal GIST should also be performed in accordance with the principles of oncological surgery. Experience and evidence regarding local transanal resection of malignant GIST has not yet been gathered. Surgery of GIST in the lower rectum should therefore be limited to small low grade tumors.

## Additive Therapy

For locally irresectable or metastatic GIST no effective chemo- or radiotherapy was available during the 1990s, since GIST like LMS is unresponsive to conventional chemotherapy. Early experience with systemic treatment using the tyrosine kinase inhibitor STI-571 (imatinib mesylate) directed against the c-KIT receptor tyrosine kinase protein, however, has been encouraging [26]. Heikki Joensuu and coworkers reported the case of a 50-year-old woman who had initially presented with metastatic GIST of the stomach. The patient returned a little more than a year after curative surgery with local, peritoneal and hepatic tumor. After failure of initial chemotherapy with thalidomide and interferon α the patient was recruited for receiving a study protocol of 100 mg oral STI-571 four times daily. Within a month of treatment the patient had complete tumor remission on positron emission tomography (PET) and a marked decrease of tumor volume on MRI. The evident tumor remission had lasted for 11 months at the time of publication. Most recently Demitri, von Mehren, Blanke, Joensuu and coworkers have reported on a randomized multicenter trial evaluating the response of patients with advanced irresectable GIST to treatment with imatinib mesylate. A total of 147 patients were randomized for this study. Response to a protocol of either 400 mg or 600 mg of imatinib daily was recorded in 53.7% of these patients; 27.9% of patients had stable disease. These responses have been durable during a median follow-up of 24 weeks. On the other hand, there was a considerable rate of non-responders (13.6%) as well. The drug, a non-toxic chemotherapeutical agent, previously evaluated in the treatment of BCR-ABL-positive leukemia, had only mild side effects such as dyspepsia and diarrhea, fatigue and, less frequently, gastrointestinal bleeding. Yet this phase II study was not sufficiently powered to detect significant differences between both study groups regarding tumor response and toxicity of treatment and to decide on the optimal dosage of imatinib [27]. In summery and conclusion, however, imatinib mesylate is the first and at the time only effective and well-tolerated systemic treatment for patients with advanced irresectable GIST.

# Assessment of Tumor Status and Prognosis

The biological and clinical behavior of GIST demonstrates a broad variability at all gastrointestinal locations. Whereas small gastric GISTs regularly take a benign clinical course, gastric GISTs larger than 5 or 10 cm demonstrate malignant features and have a poor prognosis [28]. Small tumors usually have a low mitotic count of less than 2 per 10 high power field (HPF). More mitoses per HPF usually suggest an uncertain tumor status or malignancy. Grading of GIST has been correlated to the number of mitosis for this reason (Table 15.2). Yet a third group of GISTs with low mitotic count nevertheless has been noted to display an uncertain malignant potential. Despite a low mitotic count

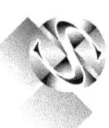

**Table 15.2.** Grading of GIST of the stomach with reference to the mitotic count [30]

| Cell type | Number of mitoses/10 HPF | Status |
|---|---|---|
| Spindle cell | 0–4 | Benign |
| | 5–9 | Borderline |
| | >10 | Malignant |
| Epithelioid cell | 0–1 | Benign |
| | 2–9 | Borderline |
| | >10 | Malignant |

**Table 15.4.** Risk assessment of gastric GIST using a simple triple pattern [30]

| | High risk | Low risk |
|---|---|---|
| Size (cm) | >5 | <5 |
| Mitotic count (n/10 HPF) | >2 | <2 |
| PCNA index (%) | >10 | <10 |

large GISTs may metastasize. Taking both size and number of mitoses into consideration probably allows a more accurate projection of prognosis. GISTs with a mitotic count of >10 per 10 HPF are regarded as high grade malignancies being frequently associated with a diffuse hepatic and peritoneal spread. These observations have been made for GIST of the stomach only. In intestinal GIST no mitotic count of prognostic significance has yet been determined [29].

The relevance of many other macroscopic, histological, molecular and genetic aspects of these tumors for determining the risk of invasive or metastatic tumor growth has been investigated. So far only a few factors have been confirmed to be indicative of a poor prognosis by different authors (Table 15.3). A pattern of risk assessment still applying in the clinical setting using tumor size, mitotic count and the proliferating cell nuclear antigen (PCNA) index was proposed by Franquemont and Frierson in 1995 (Table 15.4) [30].

Local tumor recurrence or peritoneal or hepatic (bone and lung are rare) spread occurs in up to half of the patients with malignant gastric stromal tumors. Leiomyosarcoma predominately spreads to the lung.

Recent survival data are derived from few and in part retrospective patient series. Many of the older studies may not have clearly differentiated between sarcoma and malignant GIST. A retrospective study from Memorial Sloan Kettering Cancer Center [17] found less than 30% of patients alive 5 years after R0 resection of GIST or LMS. From a more recent analysis of 200 cases of GIST the authors report a 5-year survival rate of 54% [28].

Most authors have found a survival advantage in favor of gastric GIST and a female gender. Hansson et al report a 5-year survival rate of 39.4% in men and 62.4% in women, in a study of 313 patients with LMS and GIST of the stomach [19]. A Japanese study reports a 10-year survival rate of 74% for malignant gastric GIST and 17% for malignant intestinal GIST [31]. Resection status on microscopy is regarded as a crucial factor influencing prognosis [17].

**Table 15.3.** Assessment of status and prognosis in GIST

| | Risk factors | Discussion/references |
|---|---|---|
| Macroscopy | Diameter < 5 cm | Gastric GIST seems to be less malignant than extragastric GIST of same size and mitotic count [32] |
| | Extragastric localization | Extragastric GIST seems to have a poorer prognosis than gastric GIST of same size and mitotic count [32] |
| Histology | Mitotic frequency >10 per 10 HPF | A proportion of GISTs may metasta-size despite a low mitotic count [30] |
| Immunohistochemistry | Ki-67/MIB-1 proliferation index >4% | Predictive for distant spread [33] |
| | Bcl-2 protein | Correlation with poor prognosis [34] |
| | Cellular apoptosis | Correlation with better survival [34] |
| | PCNA index | Correlation with prognosis in some studies [30] |
| Molecular biology | c-KIT mutations | c-KIT mutations are more frequent in malignant GIST [35]. Different c-KIT oncogenes possibly form distinct subgroups of GIST [18] |
| DNA analysis | DNA aneuploidy | May differentiate benign from malignant GIST [33] |

## Conclusion

Mesenchymal tumors account for less than 1% of malignancies in the stomach but for more than 10% in the small bowel. Their incidence in Western countries has been estimated as 1.2–1.8 per million and 1.3 per million respectively. A major proportion of these neoplasms, historically called sarcomas, because they were believed to be of smooth muscle cell origin, have been recognized as different from tumors which indeed arise from smooth muscle cells (true leiomyoma/sarcoma) and other mesenchymal cells of the gastrointestinal tract. These specific neoplasms have been termed as "gastrointestinal stromal tumors" (GIST). GISTs are genetically characterized by mutations of the c-KIT gene causing a pathologic activation of the tyrosine kinase signal pathway. Yet it is increasingly evident that the GIST group, despite common genetic features, is made up of a heterogeneous and poorly understood variety of gastrointestinal neoplasms of spindle cell, epithelioid and pleomorphic histomorphology and uncertain biological behavior. Currently, GISTs are thought to arise from the distinctive interstitial c-KIT-positive cells of Cajal found in the gastrointestinal tract. An explanation of the histomorphological, ultrastructural and prognostic peculiarities of GIST may lie in the stem cell potential of Cajal cells.

More than half of GISTs are found in the stomach as incidental submucosal tumors on endoscopy, usually benign, or larger intramural tumors of borderline or malignant behavior. GISTs of the stomach seem to have a better prognosis than GISTs of the esophagus and the small and large bowel with respect to size and mitotic count. Yet various other aspects of histomorphology, immunohistochemistry, molecular and genetic biology are suspected to determine the clinical course of GIST. Like true sarcomas GISTs show a remarkable resistance to radiotherapy and conventional chemotherapy. Radical curative surgery therefore is regarded as the main independent prognostic factor for patients with GIST. Systematic lymphadenectomy, on the other hand, does not seem to be crucial for prognosis because GISTs rarely show lymphatic spread. Metastases from GIST usually are confined to the liver and less frequently to the peritoneum. A considerable proportion of patients present with primarily metastatic disease. In these patients and those with recurrent disease systemic treatment with imatinib mesylate has been recognized to cause a durable tumor response in about 50%. Imatinib, a non-toxic inhibitor of tyrosine kinase, pathologically activated in GIST, represents the first and at the present time only effective therapeutic approach for patients with irresectable GIST.

## Acknowledgement

Radiological images have been kindly provided by Prof. Dr Christoph Dueber MD, Dept of Clinical Radiology, microphotographs by PD Dr Walter Back, MD, Dept of Pathology, University Hospital Mannheim, University of Heidelberg.

## Questions

1. How do GISTs differ from other mesenchymal neoplasms of the GI tract?
2. What is the supposed cellular origin of GIST?
3. How do you confirm the diagnosis of GIST?
4. Characterize the biological behavior of GIST.
5. How would you try to assess the malignant potential of GIST?
6. GIST and true leiomyosarcoma are both regularly unresponsive to chemotherapy. Which feature of GIST provides a novel therapeutic approach in advanced irresectable disease?

## References

1. Goulden T, Stout AP. Smooth muscle tumors of the gastrointestinal tract and retroperitoneal tissues. Surg Gynecol Obstet 1941;73:784–8.
2. Welsh RA, Meyer AT. Ultrastructure of gastric leiomyoma. Arch Pathol Lab Med 1969;87:71–81.
3. Mazur MT, Clark HB. Gastric stromal tumors. Reappraisal of histogenesis. Am J Surg Pathol 1983; 7:507–19.
4. Appelman HD. Smooth muscle tumors of the gastrointestinal tract. What we know now that Stout didn't know. Am J Surg Pathol 1986;10 (Suppl 1):83–99.

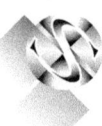

5. Kindblom LG, Remotti HE, Aldenborg F, Meis-Kindblom JM. Gastrointestinal pacemaker cell tumor (GIPACT): gastrointestinal stromal tumors show phenotypic characteristics of the interstitial cells of Cajal. Am J Pathol 1998;152:1259-69.
6. Chan JK. Mesenchymal tumors of the gastrointestinal tract: a paradise for acronyms (STUMP, GIST, GANT, and now GIPACT), implication of c-KIT in genesis, and yet another of the many emerging roles of the interstitial cell of Cajal in the pathogenesis of gastrointestinal diseases? Adv Anat Pathol 1999; 6:19-40.
7. Erlandson RA, Klimstra DS, Woodruff JM. Subclassification of gastrointestinal stromal tumors based on evaluation by electron microscopy and immunohistochemistry. Ultrastruct Pathol 1996;20:373-93.
8. Rumessen JJ, Thuneberg L. Pacemaker cells in the gastrointestinal tract: interstitial cells of Cajal. Scand J Gastroenterol Suppl 1996;216:82-94.
9. Wester T, Eriksson L, Olsson Y, Olsen L. Interstitial cells of Cajal in the human fetal small bowel as shown by c-KIT immunohistochemistry. Gut 1999;44:65-71.
10. Torihashi S, Nishi K, Tokutomi Y et al. Blockade of kit signaling induces transdifferentiation of interstitial cells of Cajal to a smooth muscle phenotype. Gastroenterology 1999;117:140-8.
11. Kitamura Y, Hirota S, Nishida T. Molecular pathology of c-KIT proto-oncogene and development of gastrointestinal stromal tumors. Ann Chir Gynaecol 1998;87:282-6.
12. Lasota J, Wozniak A, Sarlomo-Rikala M et al. Mutations in exons 9 and 13 of KIT gene are rare events in gastrointestinal stromal tumors. A study of 200 cases. Am J Pathol 2000;157:1091-5.
13. Sakurai S, Hishima T, Takazawa Y et al. Gastrointestinal stromal tumors and KIT-positive mesenchymal cells in the omentum. Pathol Int 2001; 51:524-31.
14. Walker P, Dvorak AM. Gastrointestinal autonomic nerve (GAN) tumor. Ultrastructural evidence for a newly recognized entity. Arch Pathol Lab Med 1986; 110:309-16.
15. Herrera GA, Cerezo L, Jones JE et al. Gastrointestinal autonomic nerve tumors. 'Plexosarcomas'. Arch Pathol Lab Med 1989;113:846-53.
16. Rosen RM. Familial multiple upper gastrointestinal leiomyoma. Am J Gastroenterol 1990;85:303-5.
17. Clary BM, DeMatteo RP, Lewis JJ et al. Gastrointestinal stromal tumors and leiomyosarcoma of the abdomen and retroperitoneum: a clinical comparison. Ann Surg Oncol 2001;8:290-9.
18. Miettinen M, Lasota J. Gastrointestinal stromal tumors – definition, clinical, histological, immunohistochemical, and molecular genetic features and differential diagnosis. Virchows Arch 2001;438:1-12.
19. Hansson LE, Sparen P, Nyren O. Stomach leiomyosarcoma: secular trends in incidence and survival in Sweden, 1960-1989. Scand J Gastroenterol 1998;33:540-3.
20. Chow JS, Chen CC, Ahsan H, Neugut AI. A population-based study of the incidence of malignant small bowel tumours: SEER, 1973-1990. Int J Epidemiol 1996;25:722-8.
21. Karnak I, Senocak ME, Ciftci AO et al. Inflammatory myofibroblastic tumor in children: diagnosis and treatment. J Pediatr Surg 2001;36:908-12.
22. Kim IH, Kim PS, Lee DH et al. Gastric malignant stromal tumor with long stalk impacted into duodenum. Yonsei Med J 1999;40:510-3.
23. Shojaku H, Futatsuya R, Seto H et al. Malignant gastrointestinal stromal tumor of the small intestine: radiologic–pathologic correlation. Radiat Med 1997;15:189-92.
24. Hama Y, Okizuka H, Odajima K et al. Gastrointestinal stromal tumor of the rectum. Eur Radiol 2001;11:216-9.
25. Tworek JA, Appelman HD, Singleton TP, Greenson JK. Stromal tumors of the jejunum and ileum. Mod Pathol 1997;10:200-9.
26. Joensuu H, Roberts PJ, Sarlomo-Rikala M et al. Effect of the tyrosine kinase inhibitor STI571 in a patient with a metastatic gastrointestinal stromal tumor. N Engl J Med 2001;344:1052-6.
27. Demetri GD, von Mehren M, Blanke CD et al. Efficacy and safety of imatinib mesylate in advanced gastrointestinal stromal tumors. N Engl J Med 2002;347:472-80.
28. DeMatteo RP, Lewis JJ, Leung D et al. Two hundred gastrointestinal stromal tumors: recurrence patterns and prognostic factors for survival. Ann Surg 2000;231:51-8.
29. Emory TS, O'Leary TJ. Prognosis and surveillance of gastrointestinal stromal/smooth muscle tumors. Ann Chir Gynaecol 1998;87:306-10.
30. Franquemont DW, Frierson HF Jr. Proliferating cell nuclear antigen immunoreactivity and prognosis of gastrointestinal stromal tumors. Mod Pathol 1995;8:473-7.
31. Ueyama T, Guo KJ, Hashimoto H et al. A clinicopathologic and immunohistochemical study of gastrointestinal stromal tumors. Cancer 1992;69:947-55.
32. Emory TS, Sobin LH, Lukes L et al. Prognosis of gastrointestinal smooth-muscle (stromal) tumors: dependence on anatomic site. Am J Surg Pathol 1999;23:82-7.
33. Carrillo R, Candia A, Rodriguez-Peralto JL, Caz V. Prognostic significance of DNA ploidy and proliferative index (MIB-1 index) in gastrointestinal stromal tumors. Hum Pathol 1997;28:160-5.
34. Cunningham RE, Abbondanzo SL, Chu WS et al. Apoptosis, bcl-2 expression, and p53 expression in gastrointestinal stromal/smooth muscle tumors. Appl Immunohistochem Mol Morphol 2001;9:19-23.
35. Ernst SI, Hubbs AE, Przygodzki RM et al. KIT mutation portends poor prognosis in gastrointestinal stromal/smooth muscle tumors. Lab Invest 1998;78:1633-6.

# Further Reading

(The following list of selected recent articles includes papers by pathologists and surgical and medical oncologists.)

Berman J, O'Leary TJ. Gastrointestinal stromal tumor workshop. Hum Pathol 2001;32:578-82.

DeMatteo RP, Lewis JJ, Leung D et al. Two hundred gastrointestinal stromal tumors: recurrence patterns and prognostic factors for survival. Ann Surg 2000;231:51-8.

Franquemont DW. Differentiation and risk assessment of gastrointestinal stromal tumors. Am J Clin Pathol 1995;103:41-7.

Graadt van Roggen JF, van Velthuysen ML, Hogendoorn PC. The histopathological differential diagnosis of gastrointestinal stromal tumours. J Clin Pathol 2001;54:96-102.

Joensuu H, Fletcher C, Dimitrijevic S et al. Management of malignant gastrointestinal stromal tumours. Lancet Oncol 2002;3:655-64.

Miettinen M, Lasota J. Gastrointestinal stromal tumors – definition, clinical, histological, immunohistochemical, and molecular genetic features and differential diagnosis. Virchows Arch 2001;438:1-12.

Savage DG, Antman KH. Imatinib mesylate – a new oral targeted therapy. N Engl J Med 2002;346:683-93.

Tworek JA, Appelman HD, Singleton TP, Greenson JK. Stromal tumors of the jejunum and ileum. Mod Pathol 1997;10:200-9.

# 16

## Neoplasms of the Spleen

Mark G. Coleman and Michael R. Thompson

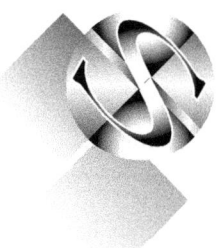

### Aims

- To identify the origin of splenic neoplasms.
- To discuss the most efficient modes of investigation and diagnosis.
- To give the indications for splenectomy.
- To explain how to manage the complications and sequelae of splenectomy.

*The spleen is an organ full of mystery*
(Galen, Greek physician AD 129–200)

## Introduction

The spleen is the largest lymphoid organ in the body, and is situated in the left hypochondrium. The size and shape of a spleen varies, but is described as being solid, measuring around 3 × 8 × 13 cms in dimension, weighing 75–100 g and lying between the ninth and eleventh ribs [1]. There are two anatomical components: the red pulp, consisting of sinuses lined by endothelial macrophages and cords (spaces), and the white pulp, which has a structure similar to lymphoid follicles. The marginal zone separates them. Its arterial blood supply, the splenic artery, is a branch of the coeliac axis, and its venous drainage, via the splenic vein, is through the portal venous system. Between 14 and 30% of individuals have accessory splenic tissue, usually found within the gastrocolic or greater omenta. Splenic enlargement, splenomegaly, is first clinically detectable by an increase in percussion dullness before it is palpable in the abdomen below the left costal margin on inspiration.

The spleen is part of the reticuloendothelial system and has many roles as part of immune and haematological processing. These include filtering bloodborne bacteria and debris, removing fragmented, damaged or senescent red cells, red cell remodelling, and in certain circumstances, haemopoiesis. There is also a red cell, platelet and lymphocyte storage capacity, which is limited in humans. Like lymph nodes, the spleen also has immune functions including antibody production, cell-mediated responses and phagocytosis.

Not surprisingly, therefore, most neoplastic processes that involve the spleen are a manifestation of a wider haematological disorder, most often lymphoma. Primary neoplasms of the spleen are rare. The majority of non-haematogenous malignancies are a result of direct spread from adjacent organs, e.g. carcinomas of the stomach, pancreas, kidney or colon. The diagnosis is usually made by cross-sectional imaging such as ultrasound (US), computed tomography (CT) or magnetic resonance scan (MR).

## Differential Diagnosis

Space-occupying lesions in the spleen may be classified as cystic, cystic/solid or solid (Table 16.1). Solid lesions may be diffuse or discrete lesions, and discrete lesions may be solitary or multiple. In each case there will be a differential diagnosis.

## Causes of Splenic Enlargement

### Primary

- Primary non-haematopoietic neoplasms of the spleen are rare. There are two types depending on the cell of origin. The commonest are of vascular origin, the sinus endothelium giving rise to angiosarcomas and endotheliomas. The connective tissue elements give rise to spindle cell tumours and fibrosarcomas.
- Primary splenic neoplasms may be classified into benign lesions, which include haemangiomas, lymphangiomas or hamartomas, intermediate lesions such as haemangioendotheiomas, and malignant lesions such as angiosarcomas.

Non-neoplastic splenic enlargement is covered in Chapter 10.

### Angiosarcoma

Angiosarcomas are the most common primary malignancy found in the spleen [2]. Most often, a solitary well-defined haemorrhagic nodule is found, though the spleen may be diffusely involved. Presentation clinically in 75% of patients is with abdominal pain, the remainder through spontaneous rupture, or through symptoms of hypersplenism such as anaemia, thrombocytopenia or a consumption coagulopathy. There are characteristic contrast enhancement features on CT and MR that can aid the diagnosis. The spleen is palpable in 85% of patients. The prognosis is poor, with a rapidly fatal course. Pathogenesis is unknown although arsenicals, vinyl chloride (used in the manufacture of plastics) and thorium oxide (Thorotrast, a contrast medium used in radiology in the first half of the twentieth century) have been implicated. Treatment is by prompt splenectomy and chemotherapy, although response is poor.

### Haemangioma

Haemangiomas are the most frequently occurring benign neoplasm found in the spleen. In autopsy series they are found in 0.03 to 14% of patients [3,4]. They are believed to be congenital in origin and arise from sinusoidal epithelium. They may be single or multiple and occur as part of a widespread angiomatosis. Infarction, thrombosis, haemorrhage or fibrosis may occur (Figure 16.1). They are slow growing and tend to be asymptomatic, though they may present with pain, rupture and features of hypersplenism such as anaemia or consumption coagulopathy. Rarely, they undergo malignant transformation.

### Littoral Cell Angiomas

Littoral cell angiomas are a form of angioma that occur exclusively in the spleen and display distinct immunohistochemical properties [5]. They contain vascular and histiocytic elements and most often form multiple nodules within the spleen although a focal form is described.

Table 16.1. The differential diagnosis and category of space occupying lesions of the spleen

| Cystic | Cystic/Solid | Solid – diffuse | Solid – discrete |
|---|---|---|---|
| Epidermoid cysts | Abscess | Lymphoma | Hamartoma |
| Haemangiomas | Metastasis | Leukaemia | Metastasis |
| Lymphangiomas | Epidermoid cysts | | Infarct |
| | Haemangiomas | | Angiosarcoma |
| | Lymphangiomas | | Lymphoma |
| | Haematoma | | |
| | Lymphoma | | |

# NEOPLASMS OF THE SPLEEN

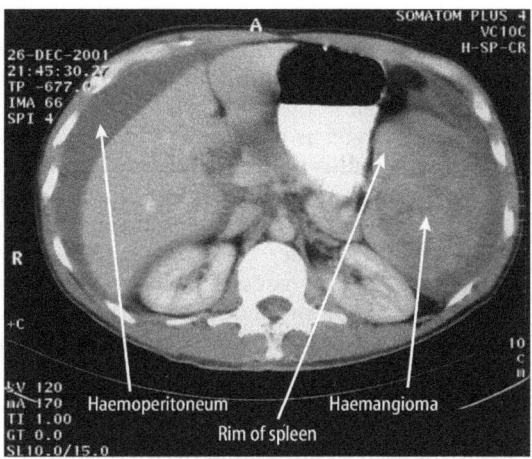

**Figure 16.1.** A computer tomogram (oral and intravenous contrast) of the abdomen in a 42-year-old man with an acute abdomen. There is a large central splenic haemangioma, which has ruptured into the peritoneal cavity. Spontaneous rupture is an uncommon mode of presentation of splenic neoplasm, which requires prompt recognition and treatment by emergency splenectomy.

There is also a malignant variant described. Littoral cell angiomas usually present with features of hypersplenism such as splenomegaly, thrombocythaemia and anaemia. On contrast-enhanced CT there are multiple small low attenuation areas in the portal venous phase.

## Lymphangioma

Lymphangiomas are rare benign congenital neoplasms that are most commonly found in the neck or axillae [6]. They rarely occur in the spleen and are usually asymptomatic. They may be visualised on US as single or multiple hypoechoic lesions, or on CT, which will demonstrate splenomegaly with multiple discrete low attenuation lesions, which are non-enhancing on injection of intravenous contrast.

## Haemangioendotheliomas

Haemangioendotheliomas of the spleen are rare, and are considered to be of intermediate/borderline malignancy. Microscopically, they are composed of vascular and stromal elements [7]. Both types of elements show moderate atypia and rare mitoses.

## Haematological Malignancy

### Leukaemia

Most leukaemias are associated with infiltration of the spleen, which may result in functional hypersplenism. Although the overall risk of spontaneous rupture in leukaemic patients is 1%, this is the single commonest cause of spontaneous splenic rupture, especially in acute leukaemias. Rupture is particularly associated with acute myeloid, acute lymphoblastic and hairy cell leukaemias. The pattern of splenic involvement follows the migratory pathway of the normal benign cellular counterparts.

### Chronic lymphocytic leukaemia (CLL)

Fifty per cent of patients with CLL have splenomegaly, though it is usually a late feature. In 5% of CLL patients, splenomegaly is progressive. Splenic infiltration may be diffuse or miliary and affects both the red and white pulp. The density of the infiltrate reflects the peripheral lymphocyte count.

### Chronic Myeloid Leukaemia (CML)

Splenomegaly is a characteristic feature of CML and is found in 90% of cases [8]. The red pulp is preferentially affected and the spleen becomes large, red and diffusely involved. Marked splenomegaly is an adverse prognostic factor due to impairment of the response to platelet transfusion and other effects of hypersplenism.

### Hairy Cell Leukaemia

This is a low grade B-cell malignancy that mainly affects middle-aged men and results in splenomegaly in about two-thirds of cases [9]. Most commonly the spleen is diffusely enlarged and massive splenomegaly may occur. Microscopically, only the red pulp is infiltrated in contrast to other B-cell malignancies, and there is an absence of nodules. The splenic hilar nodes are often involved.

### Lymphomas

Lymphomas are malignant tumours of the lymphoreticular system that are classified in Hodgkin's and various subtypes of non-Hodgkin's according to the histological appearance. Most lymphomas present with fever, malaise and weight loss, often associated with painless lymphadenopathy.

Various patterns of involvement of the spleen are noted in lymphoma from reactive enlargement to lymphomatous replacement of its substance (Figure 16.2). Prior to the advent of CT, abdominal lymphoma staging was carried out by laparotomy. At laparotomy, the para-aortic and coeliac lymph nodes were biopsied, wedge and needle liver biopsy was carried out, a splenectomy performed, and an iliac crest bone marrow biopsy done. Staging laparotomy, against CT has not been shown to improve survival and has important negative effects such as delay in commencement of chemotherapy, infection risk following splenectomy and the potential for serious complications. Splenomegaly in all lymphoma cases has a 36% sensitivity and 61% specificity for splenic involvement [10].

## Hodgkin's Disease

In Hodgkin's disease, the earliest involvement is by recognisable Reed–Sternberg cells at the periphery of the Malphigian body. Typically later involvement is with scattered foci and architectural destruction. A spleen over 400 g in weight is always histologically infiltrated and many below this weight. Splenic infiltration is a manifestation of bloodborne dissemination of the disease, and occurs in one-third of patients with Hodgkin's disease. Splenomegaly may also be observed as a secondary effect without malignant infiltration. Malignant infiltration occurs initially in the white pulp, in the T-cell-dependent peri-arteriolar lymphoid sheath, and the red pulp becomes enlarged secondarily by extension. As the process of splenic infiltration continues, single or multiple discrete tumour nodules form which become confluent with progression. There is adverse prognosis associated with nodular splenic involvement.

## Non-Hodgkin's Lymphoma (NHL)

NHL is the most common malignant process to affect the spleen, with 40–50% of NHL patients having splenic involvement, but the spleen is usually only mildly or moderately enlarged. In about 1% the spleen is the only detectably involved organ. NHL is characterised by diffuse homogeneous, or miliary infiltration, or by masses that are either solitary or multiple with varying histological patterns according to the type and grade of the disease. The commonest form is the low grade type, in which miliary infiltration usually occurs, and the second commonest, the large cell type, in which solitary or multiple masses are usually found. Expansion by infiltration occurs in the white pulp, particularly with low grade lymphoma. Discrete tumour-like masses are characteristic of the more aggressive intermediate or high grade lymphoma. Microscopically, B-cell lymphomas initially involve the B-cell-dependent germinal centres and mantle zones. T-cell lymphoma infiltration occurs in the peri-arteriolar sheaths and less frequently in the marginal zones.

## Secondary Malignancy

Isolated metastasis to the spleen is relatively rare compared with metastases to other organs such as liver, lungs and bone [11]. Theoretically, this is thought to be because the microenvironment of the spleen is not favourable to the growth of tumour cells, or because of the lack of afferent lymphatics to the spleen, or the sharp origin of the splenic artery from the coeliac trunk. Most often it occurs in the presence of widespread disseminated malignant disease. The incidence of splenic metastases ranges from

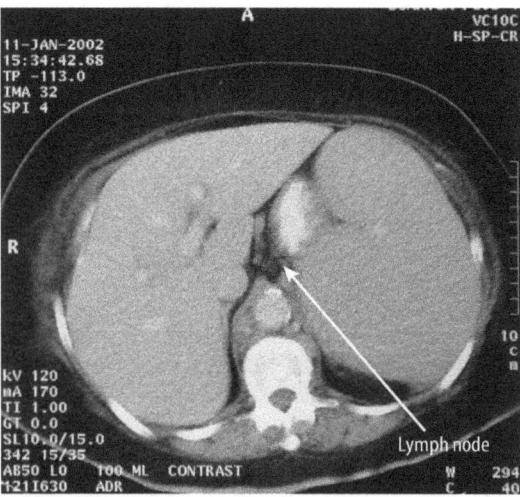

Figure 16.2. A computer tomogram (oral and intravenous contrast) of the abdomen in a patient with diffuse lymphomatous infiltration of the spleen and para-aortic lyphadenopathy. CT has superseded laparotomy in the staging of lymphoma.

0.3 to 7% of patients with disseminated malignancy at post-mortem [12]. The majority are asymptomatic and discovered either during staging investigations, at surgery or at autopsy. The common causes in large autopsy series are breast, lung, colorectal and ovarian carcinomas, and melanomas, which probably reflects the incidence of the primary disease.

## Direct Spread

The location of the spleen results in direct spread of tumours of the pancreas, colon and stomach.

### Gastric Cancer

Direct spread to the spleen may occur from a cancer of the greater curve or fundus of the stomach. The practice in general from gastric cancer is to avoid splenectomy unless specifically indicated because of direct invasion and the need for total macroscopic clearance. Splenectomy is only indicated if a curative result can be achieved by en-bloc splenectomy or pancreaticosplenectomy. In such cases a node dissection of the splenic artery or hilum may be required, but this is now often accomplished without splenectomy in most cases (station 10 node dissection) [13]. The addition of splenectomy to resection of the stomach, pancreas or colon may result in increased rate of septic and thromboembolic complications. Theoretically there may be a long-standing adverse effect on the immune system in these cancer patients.

### Colon Cancer

In colon carcinoma, as with other organs directly invaded by a colonic primary, the spleen is often ressected in continuity with the bowel to achieve a curative margin. There is no evidence that this is to the detriment of long-term survival in such patients [14]. Several cases of isolated splenic metastasis have been described, also treated by splenectomy [15].

## Diagnosis

## Plain Radiology

On a plain abdominal radiograph, the spleen may leave an impression on the gastric air bubble or an indentation on the splenic flexure. It is invisible on straight X-ray if it is of normal size.

## Isotope Scanning

Technetium-99m radio-isotope labelled colloid injected intravenously is preferentially taken up by reticuloendothelial cells in the spleen [16]. When scanned using a gamma camera, splenic size may be assessed and perfusion defects noted. This technique has fallen from general use since the advent of CT but would differentiate between avascular and vascular neoplasms.

## Ultrasound Scanning

Ultrasonography is often used as a preliminary diagnostic tool and can help to differentiate between benign and malignant lesions in the spleen [17]. Solitary lesions, anechoic mass or lesions with hyperechoic foci suggesting calcification are predictive for benign lesions, whereas multifocal or diffuse lesions, mixed echoic lesions and the presence of extrasplenic abdominal masses are predictive of a malignant process.

Lymphomatous infiltration may be nodular or diffuse; in Hodgkin's lymphoma, the lesions are uniformly hypodense. Due to its superiority in the detection and evaluation of intra-abdominal lymphadenopathy, CT has largely superseded US in the staging of lymphoma.

## Computed Tomography

CT has superseded operative staging for abdominal lymphoma [18]. Its advantages are that it is non-invasive. However, it cannot detect disease in normal size nodes (micronodular involvement) or differentiate reactive from infiltrated nodes.

Hamartomas have equal attenuation to normal splenic tissue and can be difficult to detect.

## Magnetic Resonance Imaging

Since the magnetic tissue characteristics of the normal spleen are indistinguishable from the average tissue characteristics of metastatic cancer, there is a limit to the use of MR in the detection and evaluation of solid splenic neoplasms [19].

Hamartomas may be hyper- or hypointense relative to normal spleen on a T2-weighted image, and all demonstrate heterogeneous enhancement on administration of contrast (gadolinium) [20].

## Indications for Splenectomy (Table 16.2)

Before the advent of accurate cross-sectional imaging, splenectomy was used in neoplasms of the spleen for accurate diagnosis and staging, often in conjunction with node sampling. However, this is uncommon since the advent of CT [21]. Occasionally, for lymphoma or leukaemia, where the spleen involvement is predominant, splenectomy may be indicated to downstage disease prior to conventional chemotherapy. Contiguous spread or local node involvement from a gastric, pancreatic, colonic, renal or adrenal primary may necessitate splenectomy en-bloc to achieve a curative resection (see above). Symptomatic enlargement producing abdominal pain and fullness, and hypersplenism (anaemia, thrombocytopenia or consumptive coagulopathy) may also be indications for splenectomy [22]. Occasionally, spontaneous rupture may require emergency splenectomy.

## Preoperative Preparation

The patient should be immunised against pneumococcal, *Haemophilus* and meningococcal infections as soon as the decision to operate is made [23]. Splenectomy results in reduced antibody responsiveness, especially in young or immunosuppressed patients. Vaccination results in a twofold increase in the antibody titres within 2 weeks. The resulting protection lasts at least 5 years though the exact duration is unknown. Immunisation should be carried out as soon as the decision to operate is made.

In the presence of coagulopathy due to thrombocytopenia, perioperative platelet transfusion may be required. In cases where the platelet count is very low ($<20 \times 10^9$/l), such transfusion may only be effective once the vascular pedicle is secured and divided due to rapid platelet consumption by the spleen [24].

## Technique

The operative approach depends upon the indication and the degree of splenomegaly and associated conditions such as portal hypertension.

### Open Splenectomy

The spleen is usually approached through an upper midline or left paramedian incision. The paramedian incision may give better access to the spleen, but it is less useful if the spleen is massive or other procedures such as cholecystectomy are contemplated. Initial ligation of the splenic artery through the lesser sac may reduce bleeding during removal of the spleen. This is best approached through the gastrocolic omentum. Thereafter the spleen can be safely immobilised by division of the splenorenal ligament. Alternatively the hilar structures may be approached, dissected and divided directly without resort to the lesser sac. The chosen approach is the preference of the operating surgeon.

### Laparoscopic Splenectomy

The safety and efficacy of laparoscopic splenectomy is well established for benign conditions such as idiopathic thrombocytopenia purpura or hereditary spherocytosis [25]. The potential risks of this approach for malignant neoplasms are dissemination of malignant cells in the peritoneum or the trocar sites, and architectural disruption during the process of maceration required to remove the specimen through a small incision. Thorough preoperative staging investigations, careful operative technique and the use of wound protectors during maceration and removal should mitigate these problems.

**Table 16.2.** The indications for splenectomy

| |
|---|
| Diagnosis – lymphomas, now largely superseded by CT |
| Staging – lymphomas, now largely superseded by CT |
| Downstaging – isolated splenic lymphomas |
| Metastasis – isolated or direct spread |
| Symptoms – pain, fullness or early satiety |
| Hypersplenism – anaemia, thrombocytopenia, consumptive coagulopathy |

Conditions that increase the vascularity and friability of the spleen such as lymphoma, as well as massive splenomegaly (>1.5 kg), may be relative contraindications to laparoscopic splenectomy. The operating time for laparoscopic splenectomy is greater than for open splenectomy, although the newer technique is in its relative infancy. There is a comparable incidence of the numbers of accessory spleens found during the procedure. The morbidity of the open and laparoscopic procedures is similar. Postoperative hospital stay is reduced for the laparoscopic approach [26].

## Postoperative Complications

### General

After splenectomy, pulmonary atelectasis commonly affects the left lower lobe, which is reduced by preoperative physiotherapy. Gastric ileus is also common and a nasogastric tube is usually required for 2–3 days postoperatively.

Significant per- and postoperative haemorrhage may occur with splenectomy (Table 16.3), especially after removal of a large spleen (> 1500 g) [27]. Reoperation may be required, or a subphrenic haematoma may develop. A tube drain is often placed at the time of splenectomy, though there is no evidence that this reduces the possibility of reoperation. Patients with myelofibrosis are particularly at high risk.

### Specific Complications

#### Thrombocytosis

In up to 75% of patients there is an increase in the platelet count immediately after splenectomy, which peaks at 7–12 days and lasts for 2–3 weeks (usually $600–1000 \times 10^9/l$) [28]. If the platelet count is over $750 \times 10^9$, oral aspirin should be administered (150 mg/dl). This does not seem to be associated with an elevated risk of deep vein thrombosis and specific antithromboembolic prophylaxis is not indicated in patients undergoing splenectomy [29].

Portal vein thrombosis may occur, particularly after splenectomy for massive splenomegaly and where the platelet count is high. The consequences may be serious with intractable ascites, hepatic failure and, often, death.

### Overwhelming Post-splenectomy Infection (OPSI)

This is a fulminant bacteraemia that may occur after splenectomy. Clinically it presents with shock, coma, coagulopathy and adrenal haemorrhage. The common organisms isolated are *Streptococcus pneumoniae*, *Escherichia coli*, *Neisseria meningitides* and *Haemophilus influenzae* [30].

It occurs for two reasons: first, due to the lack of red pulp, which results in a deficiency of phagocytosis to clear exogenous organisms, and second, due to the lack of white pulp, which leads to a failure of bacterial opsonisation with antibodies. The incidence of OPSI is 1–5% in large series, and it is more common in children and adolescents [31]. It usually occurs within 3 years after splenectomy, but has been described up to 30 years later. There is a very high mortality, up to 75% [31]. There is also an increased susceptibility to parasitic infections such as malaria [31].

## Long-term Management

All splenectomised patients should receive postoperative prophylactic penicillin for at least 2 years; thereafter they should also be covered

Table 16.3. The specific complications of splenectomy

| Peroperative | Early postoperative | Late postoperative |
|---|---|---|
| Bleeding | Bleeding | Overwhelming post-splenectomy infection (OPSI) |
| Gastrotomy | Gastroparesis or perforation | |
| Pancreatic damage | Pancreatic abscess, fistula or pancreatitis | |
| Missed splenunculus | Thrombocytosis | |
| | Portal vein thrombosis | |
| | Pulmonary; lobar collapse or effusion | |

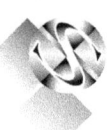

## 16 · UPPER GASTROINTESTINAL SURGERY

with penicillin during any infectious illness [32]. Guidelines may vary in different centres. The hazard of overwhelming infection is greatest in:

- children under the age of 16
- the first 2 years after splenectomy
- patients with underlying impairment of immune function.

Pneumococci are susceptible to a range of antibiotics. An increasing proportion of pneumococci, however, have become resistant to antibiotics, although the proportion in the UK is much lower than in many other European countries. Data collected by the Public Health Laboratory Service (PHLS) have shown that the proportion of pneumococci resistant to penicillin has risen from 0.3% in 1989 to 7.5% in 1997, and the proportion resistant to erythromycin has risen from 3.3% in 1989 to 11.8% in 1997 [33].

### Antibiotics

A typical regimen for antibiotics is 250–500 mg phenoxymethylpenicillin or amoxicillin once a day (adults), or in the case of allergy to penicillin, erythromycin (250 mg once a day in adults). Amoxicillin is better absorbed than phenoxymethylpenicillin and has a longer shelf life. A therapeutic dose should be taken in the event of any illness with shivering, fever or malaise. Doctors attending any asplenic patients with severe infection should give parenteral benzylpenicillin and arrange hospital admission.

### Patient Identification (Figure 16.3)

It is recommended that patients after splenectomy carry a card or wear a medical alert bracelet to identify their asplenic status in case of subsequent illness or injury. Cards are available from the Department of Health (PO Box 410, Wetherby, LS23 7LL, UK). This is of particular importance after laparoscopic splenectomy where no major incision will be visible.

### Immunisation

A single dose of polyvalent polysaccharide pneumococcal vaccine is recommended for all patients aged 2 years or above for whom it is not contraindicated. This should be done as soon as possible after splenectomy or ideally 4–6 weeks before surgery. There is a conjugated vaccine available for children between 2 months and 2 years. Reimmunisation is recommended every 5–10 years.

Immunisation against *Haemophilus* B should be given in a single dose at the same time as pneumococcal vaccination. The recommendations for reimmunisation are under review.

Annual immunisation for influenza may be beneficial.

All patients should be offered meningococcal C conjugate vaccine. There is no information on the need for further doses.

## Conclusions

Surgery for the spleen is currently changing since the development of advanced laparoscopic surgery over the last decade. In most instances surgeons well trained in complex minimal access techniques carry out such procedures. Whilst laparoscopic surgery has much to offer in terms of the reduction of postoperative pain and hospital stay, it is vital that this is not at the expense of increased morbidity when compared to open surgery.

There remains no general consensus as to the long-term prevention of infective illness in asplenic patients. It is therefore the responsibility of the individual clinician to take appropriate advice in this regard.

## Areas of Controversy

- Laparoscopic splenectomy
- Long-term antibiotics
- Immunisation

## Questions

1. Give the differential diagnosis of space-occupying lesions of the spleen.
2. What is the most common malignant process to affect the spleen?
3. What immunisations are recommended prior to surgery and how long is this effective for?
4. Detail postoperative risks of splenectomy.

## NEOPLASMS OF THE SPLEEN

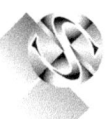

### INFORMATION ABOUT SPLENECTOMY FOR PATIENTS

Splenectomy is an operation to remove the spleen. Doctors may perform a splenectomy because the spleen has been damaged, or is diseased, or contains a growth or tumour, or because it is the site of extensive breakdown of red blood cells.

Some people are born without a spleen or their spleen does not work properly. They will have the same problems as someone whose spleen has been removed.

**WHAT DOES THE SPLEEN DO?**

The spleen helps the body's defence against bacterial infections. If you do not have a spleen you will be able to cope with most infections, but in some cases serious infection may develop very quickly. The risk of serious infection is higher in children than in adults, although the risk is still very small.

**WHAT YOU SHOULD DO**

- Make sure that your doctors and dentists know that you do not have a spleen. Carry a card or wear an identifying bracelet or necklace to alert other people in an emergency.

- Vaccinations are available which will prevent infection. If you have not already been given an injection of pneumococcal vaccine, ask your doctor for one. This will help protect you against some infections and should be repeated every five to ten years. You should also have a Haemophilus influenzae type b (Hib) vaccine if you have not already been immunised. Meningococcal vaccine may be required if you travel to certain countries abroad (ask your doctor for advice).

### I HAVE NO FUNCTIONING SPLEEN

I am susceptible to overwhelming infection, particularly pneumococcal
Please show this card to the nurse or doctor if I am taken ill

ALWAYS CARRY THIS CARD WITH YOU

**Figure 16.3.** A card issued by the Department of Health for patients to carry after splenectomy. These are available with an information leaflet for patients from the Department of Health, PO Box 777, London SE1 6XH.

# References

1. Moossa AR, Shackford SR. The spleen and lymph nodes. Essential Surgical Practice, 2nd edn. Wright, 1988; 1114–35.
2. McGinley K, Googe P, Hanna W, Bell J. Primary angiosarcoma of the Spleen: A case report and review of the literature. South Med J 1995;88(8):873–75.
3. Pines B, Rabinovitch J. Hemangioma of the spleen. Arch Pathol 1942;33:487–503.
4. Husni EA. The clinical course of splenic hemangioma. Arch Surg 1961;83:681–8.
5. Ziske C, Meybehm M, Sauerbruch T, Schmidt-Wolf IG. Littoral cell angioma as a rare cause of splenomegaly. Ann Hematol 2001;80(1):45–8.
6. de Perrot M, Rostan O, Morel P, Le Coultre C. Abdominal lymphangioma in adults and children. Br J Surg 1998;85(3):395–7.
7. Katz JA, Mahoney DH, Shukla LW et al. Endovascular papillary angioendothelioma in the spleen. Pediatr Pathol 1988;8(2):185–93.
8. Bourgeois E, Caulier MT, Rose C et al. Role of splenectomy in the treatment of myelodysplastic syndromes with peripheral thrombocytopenia: a report of six cases. Leukemia 2001;15(6):950–3.
9. Jaiyesimi IA, Kantarjian HM, Estey EH. Advances in therapy for hairy cell leukemia. A review. Cancer 1993;72(1):5–16.
10. Coon WW. Surgical aspects of splenic disease and lymphoma. Curr Probl Surg 1998;35(7):543–646.
11. Lee S, Morgenstern L, Phillips EH et al. Splenectomy for isolated splenic metastases: a changing clinical spectrum. Am Surg 2000;66(9):837–40.
12. Lam KY. Metastatic tumours to the spleen. Arch Pathol Lab Med 2000; 124:526–30.
13. Sugimachi K, Kodama Y, Kuimashiro R Critical evaluation of prophylactic splenectomy in total gastrectomy for stomach cancer. Gann 1985;71:704–9.
14. Varty PP, Linehan IP, Boulos PB. Does concurrent splenectomy at colorectal cancer resection influence survival? Dis Colon Rectum 1993;36(6):602–6.
15. Weathers BK, Modesto VL, Gordon D. Isolated splenic metastases from colorectal carcinoma: report of a case and review of the literature. Dis Colon Rectum 1999;42(10):1354–48.
16. Armas R, Thakur ML, Gottschalk A. A simple method of spleen imaging with 99mTc-labelled erythrocytes. Radiology 1979;132(1):215–16.
17. Wan YL, Cheung YC, Lui KW et al. Ultrasonographic findings and differentiation of benign and malignant focal spenic lesions. Postgrad Med J 2000;76(898): 488–93.
18. Urban BA, Fishman EK. Helical CT of the spleen. Am J Roentgenol 1998;170(4):997–1003.
19. Torres GM, Terry NL, Mergo PJ, Ros PR. MR imaging of the spleen. Magn Reson Imaging Clin N Am 1995; 3(1):39–50.
20. Ramani M, Reinhold C, Semelka RC et al. Splenic hemangiomas and hamartomas: MR imaging characteristics of 28 lesions. Radiology 1997;202(1):166–72.
21. Munker M, Stengel A, Stabler A et al. Diagnostic accuracy of ultrasound and computed tomography in the staging of Hodgkin's disease. Cancer 1995;76:1460–66.
22. Mitchell A, Morris PJ. Splenectomy for malignant lymphomas. World J Surg 1985;9(3):444–8.
23. Davidson RN, Wall RA. Prevention and management of infections in patients without a spleen. Clin Microbiol Infect 2001;7(12):657–60.
24. Benoist S. Median and long-term complications of splenectomy. Ann Chir 2000;125(4):317–24.
25. Friedman, RL, Hiatt JR, Korman JL et al. Laparoscopic or open splenectomy for hematologic disease: which approach is superior? J Am Coll Surg 1997;185:49–54.
26. Shimomatsuya T, Horiuchi T. Laparoscopic splenectomy for treatment of patients with idiopathic thrombocytopenia purpura. Comparison with open splenectomy. Surg Endosc 1999;13(6):563–6.
27. Arnoletti JP, Karam J, Brodsky J. Early postoperative complications of splenectomy for hematologic disease Am J Clin Oncol 1999;22(2):114–18.
28. Boxer MA, Braun J, Ellman L. Thromboembolic risk of postsplenectomy thrombocytosis. Arch Surg 1978; 113(7):808–9.
29. Coon WW, Penner J, Clagett P, Eos N. Deep venous thrombosis and postsplenectomy thrombocytosis. Arch Surg 1978;113(4):429–31.
30. Bisharat N, Omari H, Lavi I, Raz R. Risk of infection and death among post-splenectomy patients. J Infect 2001;43(3):182–6.
31. Cullingford GL, Watkins DN, Watts AD, Mallon DF. Severe late postsplenectomy infection. Br J Surg 1991;78(6):716–21.
32. Williams DN, Kaur B. Postsplenectomy care. Strategies to decrease the risk of infection. Postgrad Med 1996;100(1):195–8.
33. http://www.phls.org.uk/seasonal/pneumococcal/pneumol13.htm.
34. Working Party for the British Committee for Standards in Haematology Guidelines. The prevention and treatment of infection in patients with an absent or dysfunctional spleen. Br Med J 1996;312:430–4.

# 17

# Lymphomas

Mark Deakin, A. Murray Brunt, Mark Stephens and Richard C. Chasty

## Aims

To describe the types of lymphoma of the stomach, aetiology and treatment.

## Introduction

Symptoms of upper gastrointestinal (GI) lymphoma are commonly those of other upper GI malignancy, thus presenting predominantly to the gastroenterologist or surgeon for investigation.

Of the GI tract lymphomas 55–70% are gastric, 20–30% are intestinal (predominantly ileal) whilst 5–10% are colorectal. Secondary gastric involvement, however, may be seen at autopsy in up to 50–60% of advanced disseminated lymphomas.

Gastric lymphoma accounts for 2–7% of gastric malignancy. It is an extranodal lymphoma, arising in the stomach – a site which normally contains no lymphoid tissue. It is the commonest site of extranodal lymphoma and almost universally of B-cell origin. MALT or mucosa associated lymphoid tissue of the gut is involved, protecting the permeable gut mucosa that is in contact with ingested antigens. The stomach, which is normally devoid of MALT, commonly acquires it as an inflammatory response to *Helicobacter pylori* infection, i.e. *H. pylori* associated chronic gastritis.

Oesophageal lymphomas form less than 1% of oesophageal tumours although the oesophagus can be involved by gastric lymphoma at the cardia.

Primary pancreatic lymphoma is a rare form of extranodal lymphoma (less than 0.5% of pancreatic tumours) originating from the pancreatic parenchyma. A definitive diagnosis is only made at histological assessment since symptoms and radiological features are quite similar to those of other pancreatic masses.

Of primary gastric lymphoma 58% are high grade tumours (36% of these have a detectable low grade component), 38% are low grade MALT lymphomas, 1% are low grade lymphomas of non-MALT type, and 3% present as Burkitt's lymphoma. Histochemical stains may also indicate whether *H. pylori* infection is present, which has implications for the treatment options in low grade MALT type lymphomas.

Clinical features of low grade and high grade gastric lymphoma are shown in Table 17.1.

## Endoscopic Appearance of Gastric Lymphoma

- Superficial spreading
- Mass forming
- Diffuse infiltrating type
- Unclassified

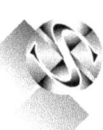

# 17 · UPPER GASTROINTESTINAL SURGERY

**Table 17.1.** Clinical characteristics of low and high grade gastric lymphoma

| Characteristics | Low grade gastric MALT (Zucca E et al Blood (2000) 96(2): 410–19) | Diffuse large B-cell gastric NHL (Cortelazzo S. et al Annals of Oncology (1999) 10: 1433–40) |
| --- | --- | --- |
| *Age (years)* | | |
| Median | 63 | 61 |
| Range | | 14–85 |
| *Sex* | | |
| Male | 50 | 52 |
| Female | 50 | 48 |
| *Main symptoms* | | |
| Pain | 53% | 76% |
| Nausea/Vomiting | 8% | 21% |
| Bleeding | 2% | 8% |
| Perforation | – | 2% |
| Weight loss | | 20% |
| Ileus | | 0.6% |
| B-symptoms | 1% | 10% |
| *Endoscopic findings* | | |
| Erythema | 30% | |
| Erosions | 23% | 10% |
| Ulceration | 47% | 67% |
| Diffuse infiltration/polypoid | | 24% |
| *Gastric localisation* | | |
| Cardia | | 5% |
| Fundus | 11% | 14% |
| Body | 12% | 49% |
| Antrum | 41% | 43% |
| Pylorus | | 4% |
| Stump | | 2% |
| Multifocal | 33% | |
| *Histology* | | |
| Low grade MALT lymphoma | 100% | |
| Diffuse Large cell | | 85% |
| Diffuse large + low grade MALT | | 15% |
| Bulky disease >10 cm | – | 19% |
| *Lugano stage* | | |
| I | 56% | 46% |
| II1 | 22% | 26% |
| II2 | 13% | 26% |
| IV | 9% | 2% |
| 5 yr Disease-free survival (DFS) | 80–95% | |
| *IPI* | | |
| 0–1 | | 65% (5-year DFS 82%) |
| 2 | | 20% (5-year DFS 48%) |
| ≥3 | | 15% (5yr DFS 35%) |

*Modified International Prognostic Index:* Age >60 years, Lugano staging ≥ II2, ECOG Performance Status ≥ 2, Increased LDH, Extranodal sites ≥ 2. (Cortelazzo S et al (1999) Annals of Oncology 10:1433–40.)

With current techniques a secure diagnosis can be made by endoscopic biopsy in at least 90% of patients.

## Basic Investigation

- Physical examination
- Full blood count and ESR
- Biochemistry profile to include creatinine, liver function tests, calcium, lactate dehydrogenase and $\beta$2-microglobulin
- Chest X-ray
- CT chest, abdomen and pelvis, to demonstrate extent, nodal and extranodal involvement
- Endoscopy with multiple biopsies and urease testing for *H. pylori*

Additional investigations which may prove useful include:

- Endoscopic ultrasound – to document extent and depth of involvement of the gastric wall and surrounding lymphadenopathy, which has implications for choice and likelihood for success of therapy.
- Additional *H. pylori* testing (antigen, breath test etc.) – to document *H. pylori* status as a basis for treatment and as a baseline to monitor effectiveness of eradication therapy.
- Upper GI series: small bowel follow-through or enema – to exclude small bowel involvement which may be difficult to detect on CT scanning.
- Bone marrow aspirate and biopsy – up to 30% of higher grade lesions can involve bone marrow.
- ($^{67}$Ga) scintigraphy – $^{67}$Ga imaging is useful in conjunction with CT and barium studies for the detection of GI NHL and for the assessment of both the extent of disease and the therapeutic effects. Lack of anatomical landmarks on scans, however, can make precise disease localisation difficult.
- (PET) scanning – availability currently limits this option in the UK.

# LYMPHOMAS

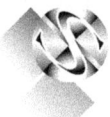

## Histopathology

The incidence of primary lymphomas of the gut is markedly different to that of the node-based tumours.

The most striking difference is that *Hodgkin's disease is exceptionally rare* in the gut (and common in the nodes). Thus for practical purposes the classification of primary gastrointestinal lymphoma is confined to non-Hodgkin's lymphoma.

Primary lymphomas occurring in the stomach are:

- MALT lymphoma
  low grade 38%
  high grade (MALT with diffuse large B-cell component) 21%
- diffuse large B-cell lymphoma 36%
- mantle cell lymphoma 1%
- Burkitt's lymphoma 3%.

Diagnosis of MALT lymphoma is made with the presence of a diffuse infiltrate of centrocyte-like cells within the lamina propria with prominent lympho-epithelial lesions or where multiple biopsies have a suspicious lymphoid infiltrate in the lamina propria with polymerase chain reaction (PCR) proving a monoclonal rearrangement of the immunoglobulin heavy chain gene.

High grade components are characterized by clusters or sheets of large atypical lymphoid cells (centroblast-like or lymphoblast-like cells). Where MALT lymphoma exists in association with a high grade component there is much debate over whether this occurs de novo or whether this represents a transition from the low grade component.

## Staging of Gastric Non-Hodgkin's Lymphoma

The applicability of the Ann Arbor staging system to gastrointestinal lymphoma has often been questioned, because of the localised site and the reduced propensity to systemic spread. The Lugano modification may have the greatest clinical utility and is now most commonly used (Table 17.2).

## Treatment

Four treatment modalities are currently available which may be applied singly or in combination: (see also Table 17.3)

- antibiotic and PPI eradication of *Helicobacter pylori*
- surgery
- radiotherapy
- chemotherapy.

**Table 17.2.** Comparison of Lugano and Ann Arbor staging for gastrointestinal lymphoma

|  | Lugano staging system for gastrointestinal lymphoma | TNM staging system adapted for gastric lymphoma | Ann Arbor stage | Tumour extension |
|---|---|---|---|---|
| Stage I | Confined to GI tract (single primary or multiple non-contiguous) | T1N0M0<br>T2N0M0<br>T3N0M0 | $I_E$<br>$I_E$<br>$I_E$ | Mucosa, submucosa<br>Muscularis propria<br>Serosa |
| Stage II | Extending into abdomen<br>$II_1$ = local nodal involvement<br>$II_2$ = distant nodal involvement | T1–3N1M0<br>T1–3N2M0 | $II_E$<br>$II_E$ | Perigastric lymph nodes<br>More distant regional nodes |
| Stage $II_E$ | Penetration of serosa to involve adjacent organs or tissues | T4N0M0 | $I_E$ | Invasion of adjacent structures |
| Stage IV | Disseminated extranodal involvement or concomitant supradiaphragmatic nodal involvement | T1–4N3M0<br>T1–4N0–3M1 | $III_E$<br>$IV_E$ | Lymph nodes on both sides of the diaphragm/distant metastases (e.g. bone marrow or additional extranodal sites) |

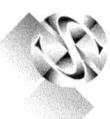

**Table 17.3.** Treatment for low grade lymphoma

| | | |
|---|---|---|
| Stage I HP+ | Eradication therapy | Restage at 3 months or earlier if recurrent or resistant symptoms |
| Stage I HP– (Stage II1 HP+/HP–) | Trial eradication therapy Or radiotherapy | Restage at 3 months or earlier if recurrent or resistant symptoms |
| Stage II2/IV | If treatment indicated No treatment indicated | Chemotherapy Observe |

Unfortunately even large national study groups have struggled to recruit more than 40–50 patients per year and hence most of the evidence base for treatment comes from historical or prospective treatment cohorts. As in other forms of lymphoma, treatment strategies will be most logically determined once consideration of histology, stage and prognostic indices are integrated.

## Low Grade Malt Lymphoma

This indolent lymphoproliferative disorder, arising in a population of lymphoid cells recruited to and maintained in the stomach as a result of inflammation, seems generally to arise in response to *Helicobacter pylori* infection. This is on the basis of a strong association with detectable *H. pylori* and almost universal evidence of current or previous *H. pylori* infection on serological testing. Lymphoma cells in tissue culture respond by proliferation when *H. Pylori* is introduced. There is no lymphoid tissue in normal gastric mucosa but individuals with *H. pylori* acquire organised lymphoid follicles. Other individuals who also develop mucosal associated lymphatic follicles are those with autoimmune diseases such as Sjögren's syndrome, patients with coeliac disease and those with infection by other *Helicobacter* species.

It is believed that there is a continual risk of clonal evolution in this acquired low grade B-cell lymphoid population which is initially dependent on T-lymphocyte help. Indeed there is evidence of a detectable clonal population of B cells developing in a small percentage of patients with gastritis alone without progression to MALT lymphoma. This may result in an autonomous low grade lympoproliferation and subsequently an autonomous high grade lymphoproliferative disorder (diffuse large B-cell lymphoma).

Cytogenetic abnormalities may develop within the lymphoid population including trisomy 3 (in up to 60% of cases) and various chromosomal translocations which may have clinical implications. t(11;18) is found in 30% of cases and t(1;14) in 5%; t (14;18) is also rarely seen. These translocations are linked to aberrant expression of Bcl10 protein. This gene belongs to a family containing caspase recruitment domains (CARD) that are involved in the apoptotic pathway. t(11;18) results in the expression of the fusion protein API2-MLT (API2-MALT1) which is associated with aberrant nuclear Bcl10 expression. Abnormal cellular localisation of Bcl10 protein which becomes nuclear rather than cytoplasmic can frequently be shown on immunohistochemistry in these tumours. Patients whose tumours are positive for t(11;18) tend to be of higher stage at diagnosis and to be less responsive to treatment by *H. pylori* eradication regimens. Cases with translocation of t(1;14) cause abnormal nuclear expression of bcl10 (an apoptotic regulatory molecule). Tumours in these cases also do not respond to antibiotic eradication therapy. Bcl10 can be identified immunohistochemically in standard tissue sections.

Whether all gastric diffuse large cell lymphomas arise from preceding low grade MALT lymphoma remains uncertain. Histology suggests this may be the case, with a detectable low grade component in up to 35% of large cell lymphomas from the stomach. However, currently some cytogenetic evidence appears to contradict this with an absence in high grade gastric lymphoma of the t(11;18) frequently seen in low grade MALT lymphoma, and the rarity of the trisomy 3 abnormality so common in low grade MALT.

Overall survival rates of 80–95% at 5 years have been reported with surgery, chemotherapy, radiotherapy or combinations. These outcome

# LYMPHOMAS

**Table 17.4.** Treatment by *H. pylori* eradication

| Pathogenesis of gastric B-NHL | | Response |
|---|---|---|
| Chronic gastric infection/inflammation | | Responds to *H.pylori* eradication |
| Development of organised gastric lymphoid tissue | Polyclonal | Yes |
| | Oligoclonal | Yes |
| Promotion/selection of B-cell monoclonality | Clonal cytogenetic abnormalities Trisomy 3, t(11,18) | Yes |
| Marginal zone lymphoma | | Yes |
| Autonomous T-cell-independent lymphoma growth | t(1,14) | Less likely |
| Large cell transformation | | Response uncertain |

figures are acceptable but optimal therapy remains to be determined.

Increasing evidence indicates that eradication therapy for *H. pylori* with antibiotics and proton pump inhibitors can be effectively employed as a sole initial therapy. Eradication of *H. pylori* is now considered to be the first choice of treatment for this type of lymphoma. Studies indicate that in up to two-thirds of cases, localised gastric MALT undergoes complete regression when the linked *H. pylori* infection is treated successfully [1]. The studies are not yet fully mature so questions remain around the allowable time to response without compromising further treatment efficacy, and the duration of even complete responses. In one study the median time to best response was 6 months with complete responses still occurring in a minority of cases up to 24 months. However, even with complete macroscopic and histological regression, PCR techniques may still show residual B-cell monoclonality in the gastric tissue biopsies. The significance of this for relapse is uncertain.

Histological assessment of response can be subject to inter-observer variation, especially where scoring systems for the presence of disease are used. There is therefore a proposal to report as either: *no change, residual disease, pathological minimal residual disease (basal lymphoid aggregates) or as complete response.*

Eradication therapy appears to be most successful in early superficial lesions (mucosal and submucosal lesions achieve 70% complete response (CR) whilst if the muscularis mucosae is penetrated a maximum 38% CR rate was achieved).

Such assessment of disease extent can be usefully performed by endoscopic ultrasound [2]. However, as the disease behaves in an indolent fashion and progression is slow, experts believe that patients' opportunity to respond to antibiotics should be maximised. Responses in the context of nodal involvement are not commonly seen.

## Endoscopic Ultrasound

The endoscopic ultrasound appearance of these tumours can classify the depth of tumour invasion in the gastric wall as *mucosal* where the lesion is localized within the first and second layers with preservation of the third layer, as *submucosal* with involvement of the third layer, or as *muscular* with involvement of the fourth layer or beyond (Figure 17.1). Peri-gastric lymphadenopathy can be shown to be present when enlarged nodes are seen with diameter greater than 1 cm.

Depth of tumour invasion as shown by endoscopic ultrasound correlates well with the effect of eradication therapy. The endoscopic appearance, however, does not necessarily correlate with the ultrasound appearance. *The presence or absence of a submucosal element correlates well with response to HP eradication* and therefore endoscopic ultrasound should be part of the staging in all cases of gastric lymphoma [7].

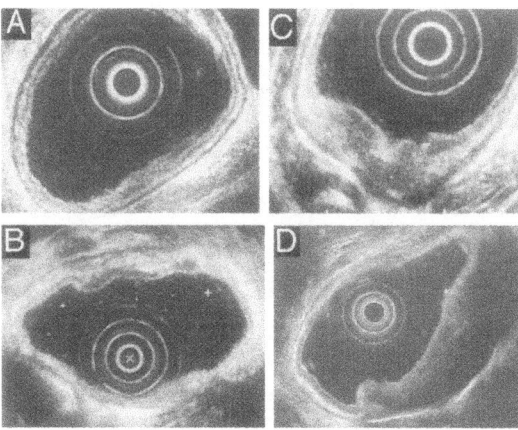

**Figure 17.1.** Pretreatment endoscopic ultrasound images of MALT showing (A) a low grade MALT lymphoma restricted to the mucosa with no significant submucosal invasion, (B) a high grade MALT lymphoma with a low grade component invading the deeper potion of the submucosa, (C) a high grade MALT lymphoma with a low grade component invading the muscularis propria and (D) a high grade MALT lymphoma with a low grade component involving the serosa. (Reproduced from Nakamura S, Matsumoto T, Suekane H, et al Predictive value of endoscopic ultrasonography for regression of grastric low grade and high grade MALT lymphomas after eradication of Helicobacter pylori M. Gut 2001;48:454–60, with permission, from the BMJ Publishing Group.)

## Features of Those Less Likely to Respond to H. pylori Eradication

- Involvement beyond the submucosa
- Evidence of nodal involvement
- Patients with chromosome 11–18 translocations

## Outcomes

Once eradication therapy has been commenced there are a series of possible outcomes on follow-up.

*Early stage disease* (stage I/II$_1$) reviewed at *3 months* after completion of eradication therapy may show:

1. *H. pylori* negative and regression of the lymphoma when observation can be repeated in 3 months.
2. *H. pylori* negative and lymphoma present. In the absence of symptoms observation for a further 3 months may allow regression but if symptomatic most would give radiotherapy or possibly single agent chemotherapy (most usually chlorambucil). Clinical judgement is required to determine how long observation can proceed to allow for lymphoma regression post *H. pylori* eradication.
3. Lymphoma regression with *H. pylori* still present when a trial of a second line eradication therapy would be indicated.
4. Lymphoma still present and *H. pylori* still detectable when if the lymphoma is stable and asymptomatic, second line eradication therapy may be reasonable. For progressive or symptomatic disease radiotherapy or single agent chemotherapy would be given.

*Early stage disease* (stage I/II$_1$) reviewed at *6 months* after completion of initial eradication therapy may show:

1. *H. pylori* negative/lymphoma negative when continued observation with repeat endoscopy 6-monthly until 2 years is appropriate (a definitive timescale for follow-up has not been the subject of randomised trials).
2. *H pylori* negative/lymphoma positive will usually indicate radiotherapy or chemotherapy, although some superficial asymptomatic lesions may still regress with further observation.
3. *H pylori* positive/lymphoma negative is a situation when further antibiotic eradication may be considered.
4. *H pylori* positive/lymphoma present will need radiotherapy and further eradication therapy.

How often to re-endoscope these patients has not been the subject of trials. However, it is suggested that possibilities 2, 3 and 4 will need repeat endoscopy again at 3 months. Histological remission precedes a normal appearance on endoscopic ultrasound. Complete responses may be followed with endoscopy every 6 months for 2 years, and possibly then yearly for life to monitor for further disease and also because these patients have an increased incidence of developing early gastric carcinoma.

As many as 50% of patients who have complete histologic remissions of MALT lymphoma after *H. pylori* eradication therapy have persisting monoclonal bands in follow-up PCR

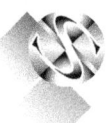

## LYMPHOMAS

monitoring. Although it is unclear as to whether monoclonality indicates the presence of minimal residual disease, patients who have persistent monoclonal bands during follow-up should be considered at risk for relapse, which may be predicted by a changing PCR pattern or clonal populations being present in basal lymphoid aggregates. Residual low grade MALT lymphoma may, however, be stable for long periods of time.

Relapses following antibiotic therapy may be treated with radiotherapy or chemotherapy. Relapses following radiotherapy may be considered for chemotherapy or surgery if still appropriately localised. Unfortunately there are no published randomised studies to help the decision. However, one non-randomised study of continuous oral chlorambucil or cyclophosphamide showed good disease control with 50% disease-free survival and 75% overall survival at 5 years [3].

Due to continuing uncertainty over optimal therapy patients should be offered entry into multicentre randomised clinical trials where available. Without clinical trials treatment should be determined by discussion at multi-disciplinary lymphoma team meetings where there is input from surgeons, gastroenterologists and oncologists/haematologists. Early intervention apart from *H. pylori* eradication might be where there is evidence of dissemination beyond the stomach and associated lymphadenpathy, where there is a significant diffuse large B-cell component, increased blasts, or associated t(11,18) with nuclear Bcl10 staining.

## Large Cell Gastric Lymphoma or Lymphoma of the Stomach with a Large Cell Component

In this aggressive lymphoma treatment modalities have again varied over time and between centres. Intuitively there can be no value for radical surgery in advanced stages II2/IV gastric non-Hodgkin's lymphoma. Diffuse large B-cell lymphoma of the stomach appears to be a highly chemosensitive disease and the previously stated advantages of preventing perforation or bleeding when chemotherapy is administered have not been confirmed when series of chemotherapy treated patients have been reviewed. The frequency of such complications appear low (0–7%) and surgery carries a significant risk of morbidity and mortality (0–9%) and can clearly delay administration of effective chemotherapy. The large study of the GELA group of large cell lymphoma showed similar outcomes for nodal and gastrointestinal large cell lymphoma, and they concluded that chemotherapy was therefore the optimal treatment [4]. Also evidence from the German Lymphoma study group has not shown different outcomes in resected and non-resected cases although follow-up remains short and the trial was not randomised [5].

It is clear, however, that 100% cure rates are not attained even in earliest stage disease and there may be a rational option in fitter early stage patients for expert surgery, followed by chemotherapy. A Canadian study of stage I/II gastric NHL treated with total macroscopic surgical resection and low dose (10–25 Gy) postoperative radiation had an 86% 10-year relapse-free survival [6]. There is currently running an IELSG (International Extra Nodal Lymphoma Study Group) trial comparing chemotherapy to complete response consolidated by two further chemotherapy courses or radiotherapy to the stomach.

Rare cases of high grade disease regression have been reported after *H. pylori* eradication therapy, so including this as a part of treatment seems rational [7]. This approach may also eliminate any persisting low grade component which could be responsible for antigen driven tumour recurrence.

## Radiotherapy

There is increasing evidence that a conservative (non-surgical) approach to gastric lymphomas can be pursued in the majority of cases. The precise role of radiotherapy as part of a conservative approach is still being defined. For high grade lymphoma the consolidative role for radiotherapy after chemotherapy is the subject of debate. A defined role for radiotherapy in the management of low grade MALT lymphoma is becoming well established. The technical aspects of radiotherapy are developing rapidly and allow a more precise treatment to be given with reduction in irradiation of other tissues.

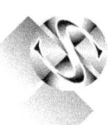

## High Grade Lymphoma

The Milan group have reported on their experience with stage I–II high grade primary gastric lymphoma in 83 patients [8]. For patients managed initially with surgery and chemotherapy, radiotherapy still added survival benefit for stage II disease ($p = 0.05$) but not for stage I disease (where survival was excellent for both approaches). The same group also reported on their experience with 21 patients managed without surgery for stage I–II and included an analysis of a further 316 cases reported in the literature [9]. Two out of 21 patients died without completing chemotherapy, the remainder achieved a complete remission. Three relapses occurred, all in patients not irradiated, but two were salvaged. None of the survivors required a gastrectomy.

The analysis of the 316 patients treated conservatively for stage I–II gastric lymphoma reports no cases of perforation and seven cases of bleeding treated without gastrectomy. Subsequent gastrectomy was performed on 3 of 120 survivors, two for local tumour progression and one for benign obstruction. Response rates recorded were between 76% and 100%, though the analysis excluded patients with low grade lymphoma or those who received radiotherapy alone. The local relapse rate was 20% (15 of 75) for chemotherapy alone and 9% (5 of 56) for chemotherapy with radiotherapy, which was statistically significant ($p = 0.03$). The 5-year actuarial survival rate ranged from 73% to 90%, but numerous non-lymphomatous deaths were recorded.

These results and those in the previous section support consideration for the use of radiotherapy in the primary management of high grade gastric lymphoma. Where possible patients should be managed in a prospective randomised controlled trial, such as the one under the auspices of the IELSG. However, many patients will have their management decided by multidisciplinary teams in non-trial settings. It would seem reasonable to include all patients in whom there was initial gastric bulk disease, stage II disease or residual disease after chemotherapy

## Low Grade Lymphoma

In a review of treatment options, supporting radiotherapy for those without evidence of H. pylori infection or persistent lymphoma after eradication therapy, the Memorial Sloan Kettering Cancer Center gave their experience [10]. Seventeen patients were irradiated and all achieved a complete response. This was maintained in all patients with a median follow-up of 27 months (range 11–68). Longer follow-up is required. Other institutions reporting even smaller numbers give the same excellent results. In the absence of an appropriate clinical trial, if there is a requirement for intervention after H. pylori eradication therapy, radiotherapy would seem to be the modality of choice.

## Radiotherapy technique

The aim of radiotherapy is to treat the whole of the stomach and appropriate nodal drainage areas. In the past this has been hampered by a variable size of target volume (stomach) and the difficulty in accurately defining the area to be treated. As a result there has been either a reluctance to irradiate or the inclusion of very large treatment fields, which for some protocols have included whole abdominal fields. The determination of the clinical target volume (CTV) has been greatly aided by the introduction of CT radiotherapy planning. This has led on to three-dimensional conformal radiotherapy (3D-CRT), which is becoming widely available, and also as it becomes available, intensity modulated radiotherapy (IMRT). 3D-CRT is the direct use of CT in radiotherapy planning combined with shaped fields to shield structures outside the CTV. 3D-CRT uses conventional radiation fields, whereas IMRT uses a beam with individually created peaks and troughs, known as a fluence profile. A dose distribution is created that irradiates the CTV and avoids normal tissue.

The above technical advances still leave the problem of a variable gastric volume. Wirth et al demonstrated both the problem and a solution [13]. The patient should be planned and treated after at least a 3-hour fast (most appropriately treated early morning) and with metoclopramide cover. This allows treatment with smaller fields and therefore reduction in morbidity, particularly to the left kidney. Dose volume histograms should record the left kidney dose, and in the majority of patients less than half of the left kidney should receive a dose above tolerance. The side effects listed in the next section are much reduced and generally acceptable in the majority of patients given the above technical advances together with modern symptomatic management.

Though dose remains a subject of debate for lymphoma generally, for high grade gastric lymphoma 40 Gy in 20–22 fractions is acceptable and supported by Ferreri et al [8,9]. Though there is slight variation between institutions, a widely accepted fractionation for low grade MALT of the stomach is 30 Gy in 20 fractions [10–13].

## Complications of Treatment

*Surgery*

- Small stomach
- Dumping
- $B_{12}$ and iron deficiency
- Adhesions

*Chemotherapy*

- Perforation
- Bleeding
- Short-term nausea/vomiting

*Radiotherapy*

- Nausea, emesis, diarrhoea
- Peptic ulceration
- Stricture
- Renal damage left kidney

## Summary

The management of gastric lymphoma has changed substantially over the last 10 years with response to *Helicobacter* eradication therapy becoming well established. As the course of this disease is often indolent, treatment in a substantial proportion of cases by *H. pylori* eradication has become first line with further research being necessary on issues such as factors predicting a poor or lack of response to indicate the need for second line therapies.

The lack of substantial trials on gastric lymphoma underlines the need for further multicentre trials including incorporation of molecular markers that may further characterize the disease. Surgery as a primary treatment has become less important but may have a role in early stage disease less likely to respond to medical management. Again the identification of potential patients that might benefit from this approach requires further research and at present gastric lymphoma cannot be considered "a surgical disease".

As with all tumours optimal treatment is best achieved and advances are more likely to occur when managed by a multidisciplinary team.

## Questions

1. What is MALT?
2. Stage lymphomas and indicate implications for treatment.
3. Do all gastric diffuse lymphomas arise from MALT lymphomas?
4. Discuss the treatment of lymphomas by eradication therapy for *H. phylori*.

## References

1. Zucca E, Roggero E, Delchier JC et al. Interim evaluation of gastric MALT lymphoma response to antibiotics in the ongoing LY03 randomised co-operative trial of observation versus chlorambucil after anti-Helicobacter therapy. Proc. Am. Soc Clin Oncol 2000;19:5a.
2. Ruskone-Fourmestraux A, Lavergne A, Aegerter PH et al. Predictive factors for regression of gastric MALT lymphoma after anti-Helicobacter pylori treatment. Gut 2001; 48:297–303.
3. Hammel P, Haioun C, Chaumette MT et al. Efficacy of single agent chemotherapy in low grade B-cell mucosa-associated lymphoid tissue B-cell lymphoma with prominent gastric expression. J Clin Oncol 1995;13: 2524–9.
4. Salles G, Herbrecht R, Tilly H et al. Aggressive primary gastrointestinal lymphomas: review of 91 cases treated with the LNH-83 regimen. A study of the GELA. Am J Med 1991;90:77–84.
5. Koch P, Del Valle F, Berdel WE et al. Primary Gastrointestinal non-Hodgkin's lymphoma: II. Combined surgical and conservative or conservative management only in localised gastric lymphoma: results of a prospective German multicenter study GIT NHL 01/92. J Clin Oncol 2001;19:3874–83.
6. Chen LT, Lin JT, Shyu RY et al. Prospective study of Helicobacter pylori eradication therapy in stage I(E) high-grade mucosa-associated lymphoid tissue lymphoma of the stomach. J Clin Oncol 2001;19:4245–51.
7. Nakamura S, Matsumoto T, Suekane H et al. Predictive value of endoscopic ultrasonography for regression of

gastric low grade and high grade MALT lymphomas after eradication of Helicobacter pylori M. Gut 2001; 48:454–60.
8. Ferreri AJM, Cordio S et al. Therapeutic management of stage I-II high-grade primary gastric lymphomas. Oncology 1999;56:274–82.
9. Ferreri AJM, Cordio S, Ponzoni M, Villa E. Non-surgical treatment with primary chemotherapy, with or without radiation therapy, of stage I-II high-grade gastric lymphoma. Leukaemia and Lymphoma 1999;33:531–41.
10. Schechter NR, Yahalom J. Low-grade MALT lymphoma of the stomach: a review of treatment options. Int J Radiation Biol Phys 2000;46:1093–103.
11. Park HC, Park W, Hahn JS et al. Low grade MALT lymphoma of the stomach: treatment outcome with radiotherapy alone. Yonsei Medical Journal 2002;43:601–6.
12. Tsang RW, Gospodarowicz MK, Pintilie M et al. Stage I and II MALT lymphoma: results of treatment with radiotherapy. Int J Radiation Biol Phys 2001;50:1258–64.
13. Wirth A, Teo A, Wittwer H et al. Gastric irradiation for MALT lymphoma: reducing the target volume, fast! Radiat Oncol 1999;43:87–90.

# 18

# Pathology of the Oesophagus and Stomach

Sukhvinder S. Ghataura and David C. Rowlands

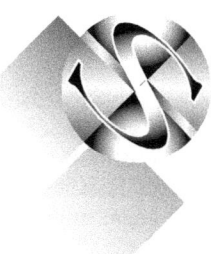

## Aims

To outline pathological lesions of the stomach.

## Structural Disorders of the Oesophagus

### Oesophageal Atresias

Abnormal foregut embryogenesis takes place between days 28 to 32 and affects 1 in 3200 pregnancies. The commoner anomalies are:

1. Oesophageal atresia with a distal tracheo-oesophageal fistula.
2. Isolated atresia.
3. Proximal tracheo-oesophageal fistula with oesophageal atresia – this variant is rare and usually associated in over 50% of fetuses with other organ abnormalities (e.g. the VACTERL syndrome). The aetiology is multifactorial and a genetic factor is implicated although no specific gene locus has been identified.

Antenatal ultrasound scanning can raise the suspicion of oesophageal atresia if the foetal stomach is consistently empty, with polyhydramnios also being seen in up to 40% of these pregnancies.

Once the diagnosis is made, the proximal pouch is kept empty with a nasogastric tube and a search for other congenital abnormalities made. Surgical repair is not an emergency unless the fetus needs to be artificially ventilated when gastric perforation can result.

### Oesophageal Diverticula

Diverticula of the oesophagus are classified into four types:

1. Congenital diverticula, a type of reduplication.
2. Pulsion diverticula, which are mucosal and caused by high intraluminal pressures associated with motor disorders of the oesophagus.
3. Traction diverticula, associated with mediastinal lymphadenopathy secondary to lymphoma or tuberculosis.
4. Pseudodiverticula.

Mid-oesophageal and epiphrenic diverticula are usually of the pulsion type and are often asymptomatic and require no treatment. They can rarely be complicated by fistula formation into the bronchial tree, into a vessel or malignant change. Larger epiphrenic ones can be a cause of dysphagia, regurgitation or nocturnal aspiration.

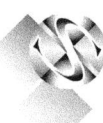

## Achalasia

This motility disorder of the oesophagus affects 1 per 90 000 of the population in the 30–60 year age group. It has been proposed that the abnormality is caused by a neurotropic virus affecting the vagal nucleus and then travelling down the vagal trunk to the oesophageal ganglia but this remains unproven [1].

In the early stages, before oesophageal dilatation has occurred, the oesophagus exhibits vigorous non-peristaltic contractions, which may cause severe chest pain and be misdiagnosed as angina pectoris. Later, as the oesophagus dilates, regurgitation of solids and liquids becomes pronounced.

Radiologically, diagnosis is made by finding a dilated oesophagus with a tapering lower segment, likened to a bird's beak, which fails to relax. Also, no gastric bubble is evident.

Manometrically, it is characterised by the absence of peristaltic waves in the oesophagus with a high resting intraluminal pressure.

Pseudoachalasia can cause diagnostic difficulties as it has similar radiological and manometric features. This can be caused by carcinoma of the lower oesophagus or cardia, or by external compression.

Overspill from the oesophagus into the bronchial tree, especially at night, can lead to bronchiectasis and lung abscess formation. Carcinoma complicates 3% of cases and is usually of squamous type, develops in the mid-oesophagus and usually carries a poor prognosis.

Treatment is designed to reduce the competence of the lower oesophageal sphincter without producing gastro-oesophageal reflux.

## Varices

Oesophageal varices are a complication of all forms of portal hypertension. Numerous collaterals are created between the portal and systemic venous systems, the most significant being between the coronary and short gastric veins towards the azygos system, with creation of oesophagogastric varices. These can be a major source of haemorrhage and mortality in patients. Approximately one-third of cirrhotic patients die from variceal haemorrhage, the risk being far greater for those with severe hepatic decompensation (Childs class C).

# Structural Disorders of the Stomach

## Hiatus Hernia

Hiatal hernias are described as two forms: sliding, in which the gastro-oesophageal junction and sphincter are above the diaphragmatic hiatus resulting in reflux symptoms, and para-oesophageal (rolling), where part of the stomach rolls up alongside the oesophagus. The majority of hernias are mixed and the symptom pattern depends on the mechanical effects of the distorted stomach, ranging from mild reflux to dysphagia and gastric outlet obstruction. Operative repair is usually effective.

## Diaphragmatic Hernia

The diaphragm forms between the fourth and eighth weeks of life. The central tendon forms from the septum transversum, the dorsal oesophageal mesentery and a circumferential margin which develops from the inner muscular chest wall. The gaps between these elements form the pleuroperitoneal canals and usually close in the eighth week. Any defects in these potential spaces can allow migration of normal or abnormally rotated bowel into the thorax and depending on the stage of development may lead to pulmonary hypoplasia if the lungs have yet to form.

## Pyloric Stenosis

The circular muscle of the pylorus becomes hypertrophic during the first 6 weeks of postnatal life and infants present at 3–4 weeks of age with projectile vomiting. The diagnosis can be made clinically or following a test feed. Treatment is surgical and a Ramstedt pyloromyotomy is usually successful.

## Heterotopic Pancreas

The most common locations for nodules of heterotopic pancreas are in the stomach and duodenum. The majority are found in the submucosa with the remainder either in the muscle wall or subserosa.

Pancreatic tissue occurs in ectopic sites either because of separation of the pancreatic anlage

# PATHOLOGY OF THE OESOPHAGUS AND STOMACH

from the primary pancreatic mass early in life or because of pancreatic differentiation of multipotent cells. Heterotopic nodules are usually incidental but can cause epigastric pain and haemorrhage.

# Oesophagitis

## Reflux Oesophagitis

The commonest cause of inflammation of the oesophageal mucosa is reflux of stomach contents. The damage is caused to the oesophageal mucosa by chemical damage from acid and/or bile. The cause of reflux is usually a functional deficit of the lower oesophageal sphincter or a hiatus hernia.

A mild or moderate degree of chemical injury to the oesophageal mucosa results in hyperplasia of the basal cells of the surface squamous epithelium and infiltration of inflammatory cells into the epithelium. This inflammatory infiltrate includes polymorphs and lymphocytes. With more severe damage ulceration of the epithelium occurs, together with a more severe inflammatory infiltrate in the adjacent epithelium and in the lamina propria beneath the ulcer.

## Columnar Lined Oesophagus

Chronic reflux damage to the lower oesophageal mucosa results in a metaplasia of the mucosa into a glandular mucosa, known as Barrett's metaplasia or columnar lined oesophagus. This mucosa typically shows a mixture of gastric and intestinal type glandular epithelia, although less commonly purely intestinal or purely gastric type glands are present. The typical mixed glandular metaplasia is morphologically identical to intestinal metaplasia in gastric mucosa as described later in this chapter. Histological proof that the biopsy came from the oesophagus rather than from a hiatus hernia or the proximal stomach depends on the pathologist demonstrating overlying squamous epithelium, underlying oesophageal submucosal glands or gland ducts. These latter features are rarely seen, and so the pathologist depends on the endoscopist's information as to where the biopsy was taken before a diagnosis of columnar lined oesophagus can be made. It is particularly important that both histological and endoscopic information is correlated in order to correctly label patients as having long segment (greater than 5 cm involvement from the gastro-oesophageal junction) on short segment (less than 5 cm of involved mucosa) columnar lined oesophagus.

Histologically in columnar lined oesophagus the mucosa contains glandular structures in which some glands are lined by gastric type epithelium and others have intestinal type epithelium. Some glands may contain both types of epithelia. Gastric epithelia has columnar cells with mucin in the cytoplasm above the nucleus. Intestinal epithelium shows a mixture of cells distended by intracytoplasmic mucin (goblet cells) and non-mucin-containing absorptive cells. This glandular epithelium often shows a degree of morphological abnormality with crowding of cells and enlargement of their nuclei. Such changes reflect increased proliferative activity, so-called regenerative changes that are a response to the continued chemical damage effected by reflux of acid and bile from the stomach. In addition, there is a variable degree of inflammatory cell infiltrate in the lamina propria. There may be mucosal ulceration also. With increasing time, there is a risk of neoplasia occurring in the metaplastic epithelium. This may manifest as dysplasia, as described later in this chapter, or as invasive adenocarcinoma.

## Other Causes of Oesophagitis

An acute inflammatory reaction is produced after ingestion of caustic substances, either accidentally or as deliberate self-harm. The cause is demonstrated by such a history. Infectious organisms causing oesophagitis include fungi and viruses. The commonest such infection is by *Candida* organisms, diagnosed by seeing a mixture of yeast and hyphal forms of the fungus. These fungal structures can be difficult to see using the standard haematoxylin and eosin stain on tissue sections, but can be demonstrated by special histochemical staining that demonstrates the walls of fungal cells. Viral infections typically occur in immunocompromised patients. In herpes simplex infection the nuclei of squamous epithelial cells show distension by pale inclusions and some infected cells become multinucleate. In cytomegalovirus infection, the nuclei of infected epithelial and endothelial cells (the cells lining small blood vessels in the mucosa) become markedly enlarged by darkly staining intranuclear inclusions. Both types of viral inclusion are best demonstrated by specific immunohistochemical stains against viral proteins.

Rarely, granulomatous inflammation can be seen in oesophageal biopsies. Causes include tuberculosis and Crohn's disease.

## Gastritis

### Helicobacter pylori *Associated* Gastritis

*H. pylori* is a Gram-negative spiral bacterium that can be seen in tissue sections on the surface epithelium and in the necks of gastric glands. The reaction to the infection starts as an inflammatory reaction with lymphocytes and plasma cells in the lamina propria and neutrophil infiltrates in the epithelium of the gland necks and mucosal surface (Figure 18.1a). The inflammation may be confined to the antrum or be distributed across the antrum and body of the stomach. Following neutrophil-induced damage to the glandular epithelium there is a reactive hyperplasia of the proliferative compartment within the gastric glands. With time there can be glandular atrophy and intestinal metaplasia. Atrophy is represented by loss of the specialised glands of the deeper layers of the mucosa. Intestinal metaplasia describes the occurrence of intestinal type goblet mucus cells and non-mucinous absorptive cells within the epithelium of necks of gastric glands and surface epithelium (Figure 18.1b). If a particular gland shows only intestinal type cells, then it is described as complete intestinal metaplasia. In incomplete intestinal metaplasia, mucin containing goblet cells are interspersed between gastric type mucin containing epithelium. Atrophy and intestinal metaplasia are often seen together. *H. pylori* can be seen on standard haematoxylin and eosin stains, but are easier to spot using a variety of special histochemical stains or by immunostaining with antibodies raised against the bacteria. It is not uncommon for antibiotics to be prescribed while the patient is waiting for an endoscopy, and so the organisms are not detected on biopsy even when the inflammation they caused remains evident.

### Autoimmune Gastritis

In autoimmune gastritis there are serum antibodies to intrinsic factor and parietal cells, and resulting in inflammation within the body mucosa. With time the body mucosa becomes atrophic with loss of specialised glands and fibrosis and chronic inflammation in the lamina propria. The epithelium typically undergoes intestinal metaplasia.

### Reactive Gastritis

Chronic chemical damage is commonly due to reflux of bile from the duodenum back into the stomach or the long-term use of non-steroidal anti-inflammatory drugs [1]. In both cases the changes seen in the gastric mucosa are similar. These consist of oedema in the lamina propria, dilatation of small vessels, a sparse inflammatory infiltrate predominantly composed of lymphocytes, tortuous elongation of the necks of the gastric glands (so called foveolar hyperplasia), and extension of smooth muscle cells from the muscularis propria up into the lamina propria. The importance of making this diagnosis is twofold. Firstly, it may help select those patients who are likely to benefit from therapy with bile-binding agents or diversionary surgery. Secondly, the finding of foveolar hyperplasia in the absence of an inflammatory component is liable to be misinterpreted as premalignant dysplasia and may have serious consequences for the patient in terms of inappropriate surgery, or at least, in unnecessary endoscopies and repeat biopsies.

### Other Causes of Gastritis

Acute gastritis can be caused by chemical injury by alcohol, drugs, or ingestion of irritant substances. It has been described also in the initial acute reaction to *H. pylori* infection. Histologically there is an inflammatory cell infiltrate with a predominance of neutrophils, degeneration of surface epithelial cells, and mucosal erosions in which there is loss of the superficial portion of the mucosa. If multiple, these erosions may cause significant blood loss.

Lymphocytic gastritis describes an infiltration of lymphocytes into the superficial epithelium of the gastric mucosa. There is an association with coeliac disease.

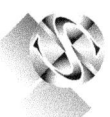

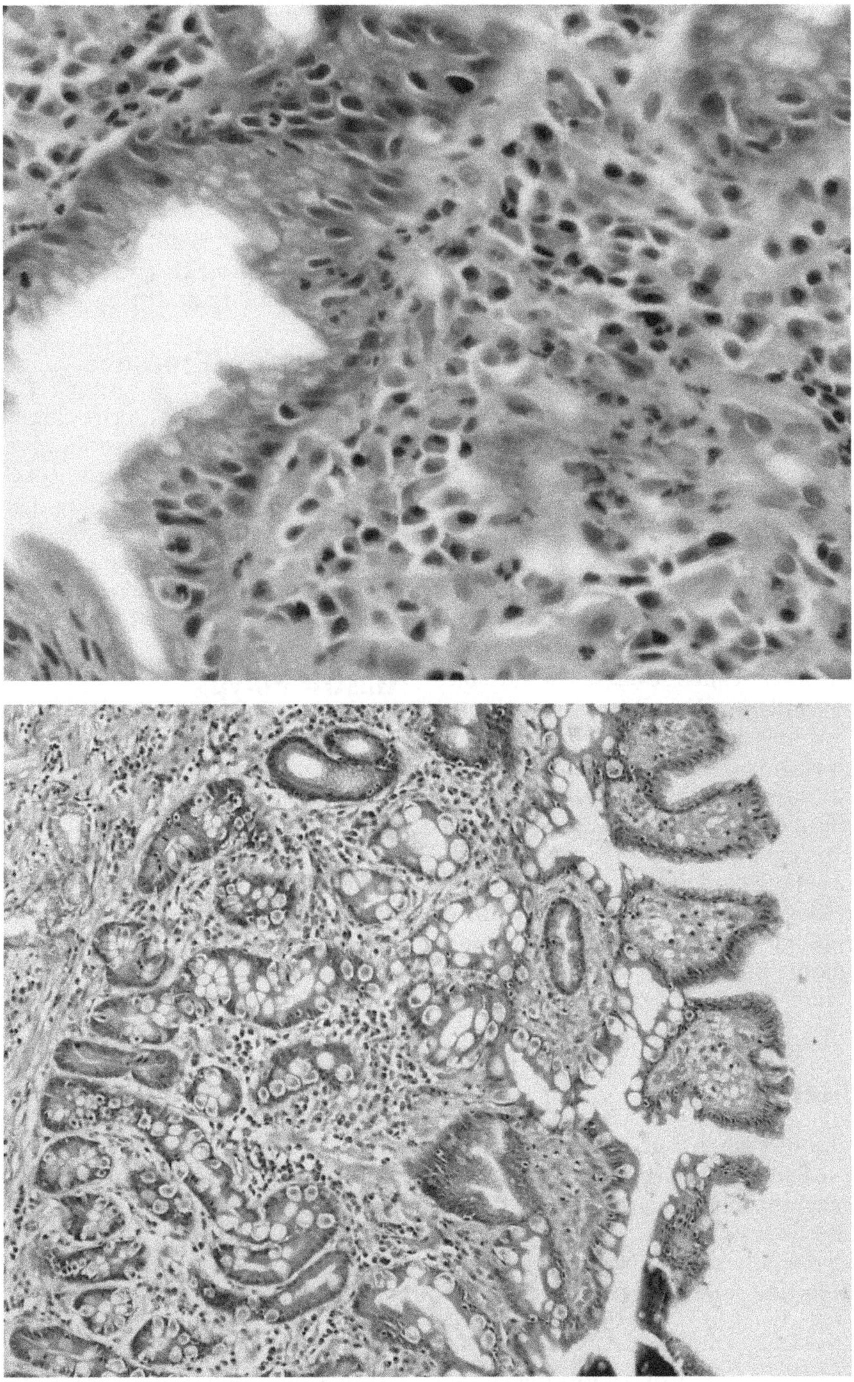

**Figure 18.1. a** Active gastritis. There is expansion of the lamina propria by a mixed inflammatory cell infiltrate that includes lymphocytes, plasma cells and macrophages. There are numerous polymorphs infiltrating the epithelium of a gland in the left half of this figure. **b** Intestinal metaplasia. A few glands lined by gastric type epithelium remain, but most glandular structures in this field show an intestinal type epithelium characterised by so-called goblet cells – cell with the cytoplasm distended by a single vacuole containing mucus.

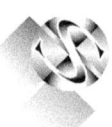

Granulomatous inflammation is seen in tuberculosis, sarcoid and Crohn's disease, although in many cases the granulomas are idiopathic.

## Sydney Classification of Gastritis

In 1990, a working party met before the World Congress of Gastroenterology in Sydney to establish guidelines for the classification and grading of gastritis. The resulting "Sydney System" had both endoscopic and histological divisions. Four years later in 1994, a group of gastrointestinal pathologists met in Houston, Texas, to reappraise the Sydney System, and overall the system was only slightly modified and the grading was aided by the provision of a visual analogue scale [2].

The system divides gastritis into three main groups – acute, chronic and specialised forms, with only the chronic type being discussed here. Various morphological variables are looked for and graded as mild, moderate or marked (previously called severe). The variables are chronic inflammation, activity, atrophy, intestinal metaplasia and *Helicobacter pylori* density and each is estimated separately. Other non-graded variables which are mentioned include surface epithelial damage, mucus depletion and erosions, presence of lymphoid follicles and foveolar hyperplasia.

The specialised category includes gastritis of various aetiologies including reactive, lymphocytic, granulomatous, eosinophilic, collagenous, radiation and various forms of infectious gastritis.

## Peptic Ulceration

Ulceration follows when there is an upset in the balance of the mucosal barrier to intraluminal acid and enzymes. Inflammation in the gastric mucosa interferes with the integrity of the mucosal barrier. Increased intraluminal acid is stimulated in the early stages of *H. pylori* induced gastritis (before intestinal metaplasia and atrophy occur). Increased acid is also seen in the Zollinger–Ellison syndrome caused by the presence of gastrin-secreting tumours, usually within the pancreas or duodenum. The ulcers may occur in both the stomach and the duodenum, where the pathological features are similar. In a typical chronic ulcer there is full-thickness replacement of the wall of the stomach with fibrous tissue with overlying inflamed granulation tissue. The ulcer can extend to erode blood vessels leading to haemorrhage, perforate through to the serosal surface producing peritonitis, or erode posteriorly into the pancreas to produce pancreatitis.

Ulcers can occur acutely, in which case a fibrotic reaction is not seen. The causes include severe acute gastritis and the stress response to severe concomitant disease.

## Ménétrier's Disease

Also known as hypertrophic gastropathy, grossly Ménétrier's disease shows a well-demarcated region of thickened mucosa in the body of the stomach. Histologically there is elongation and cystic change of the foveolae of the gastric glands, loss of specialised glands and oedema and chronic inflammation in the lamina propria.

## Gastric Polyps

Most polyps of the stomach mucosa are hyperplastic or regenerative in nature, in which there is elongation and irregular shape of the gastric gland necks and expansion of the lamina propria between glands by fibrosis and inflammatory cells. When small the predominant change in such polyps is dilatation within some of the glands, called cystic fundic gland polyps or fundic glandular cysts.

Hamartomatous polyps show a disorganised relationship of irregularly sized and shaped glandular structures admixed with an abnormal lamina propria that contains smooth muscle cells. Such hamartomas may be single or multiple, when they may represent Peutz–Jeghers syndrome. A similar appearance, but with less smooth muscle hypertrophy, is seen in so-called juvenile polyps. Multiple polyps showing cystic dilatation of foveolae on a background of similar changes and oedema in adjacent mucosa is seen in the Cronkhite–Canada syndrome.

An inflammatory fibrous polyp consists of a stromal proliferation with fibroblasts and prominent blood vessels with an accompanying inflammatory cell infiltrate. There is often ulceration of the surface.

Some true neoplasms are commonly polypoid, as discussed later in this chapter.

# Neoplasms

The histological classification of the stomach and oesohagus is shown in Table 18.1.

## Squamous Carcinoma

Squamous carcinoma is common in the oesophagus, being the predominant histological type found in tumours of the upper and middle oesophagus (Figure 18.2a). Squamous carcinomas of the stomach do occur but are rare. Aetiological associations include alcohol and cigarette smoking.

Grossly, the tumours present as a mass growing both into the lumen and out through the oesophageal wall. Central ulceration is usual. The histological features that define squamous differentiation are the production of keratin and the presence of intercellular bridges or prickles between some of the tumour cells. Squamous tumours typically grow as solid islands of cells with undifferentiated cells at the periphery of these islands and more differentiated cells towards the centre (Figure 18.3a). There may be whorls of keratin at the centre of tumour islands in better differentiated tumours. In less well differentiated carcinomas, the centre of the tumour islands undergo necrosis.

Squamous cell carcinomas are graded into three groups – well, moderate and poor – based upon the cytological features of the tumour cells, the degree of differentiation within tumour cell islands, and the degree of keratin production. There are no agreed exact criteria on where to draw the boundary between well and moderate and between moderate and poor grades. In addition, the pattern of differentiation within any one particular tumour can be very variable, and this also affects the degree of inter-observer agreement between pathologists grading these tumours.

Following radiotherapy or chemotherapy, there may be extensive death and loss of the tumour cells, being replaced by necrosis or fibrous tissue. In these circumstances tumour cells may be sparse and distributed as single cells or small groups. Sometimes a granulomatous response to keratin debris is demonstrated.

There are a number of variants of squamous cell carcinoma, and other tumour types that are related to squamous tumours.

1. Adenosquamous carcinoma. These are mixed tumours in which there is both squamous and glandular differentiation of the tumour cells. Such tumours are typically poorly differentiated, and tend to have a more aggressive clinical course with a poor prognosis. If special stains for mucin are performed upon sections of poorly differentiated squamous carcinomas, it is not uncommon to find occasional positive cells. Adenosquamous carcinoma is thus probably just one end of a spectrum of aberrant differentiation in poorly differentiated carcinomas.

2. Spindle cell carcinoma. In some tumours the cells have a spindle appearance rather than the more typical polygonal shape of squamous cells. Such tumours can wrongly be called a sarcoma rather than a carcinoma. Careful search will usually demonstrate a subpopulation of more typical squamous cells within the tumour, and these can be revealed using immunostains for cytokeratin. Such tumours are often polypoid.

3. Carcinosarcoma. This tumour is similar to spindle cell squamous carcinoma, except that there is true differentiation into mesenchymal elements such as bone or cartilage within the spindle cell component of the tumour. Carcinosarcomas

**Table 18.1.** Histological classification

| Benign | Epithelial | Squamous papilloma |
| | | Adenoma |
| | Stromal | Benign gastrointestinal stromal tumour (GIST) |
| | | Haemangioma |
| | | Granular cell tumour |
| Malignant | Epithelial | Squamous cell carcinoma |
| | | Adenocarcinoma |
| | | Small cell carcinoma |
| | | Carcinoid tumour |
| | | Undifferentiated carcinoma |
| | Stromal | Malignant gastrointestinal tumour |
| | Others | Malignant melanoma |
| | | Lymphoma |
| | Secondary tumours | |

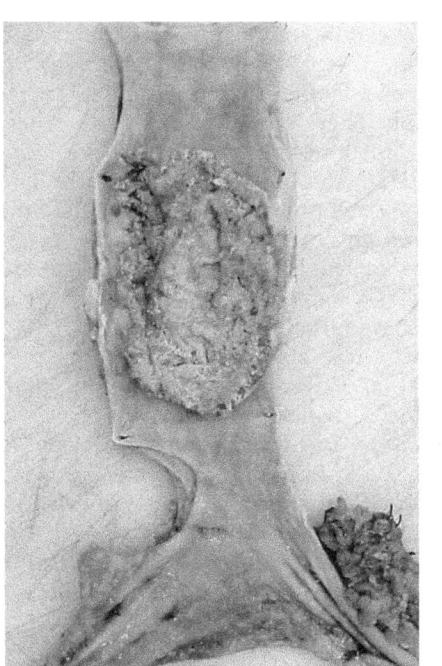
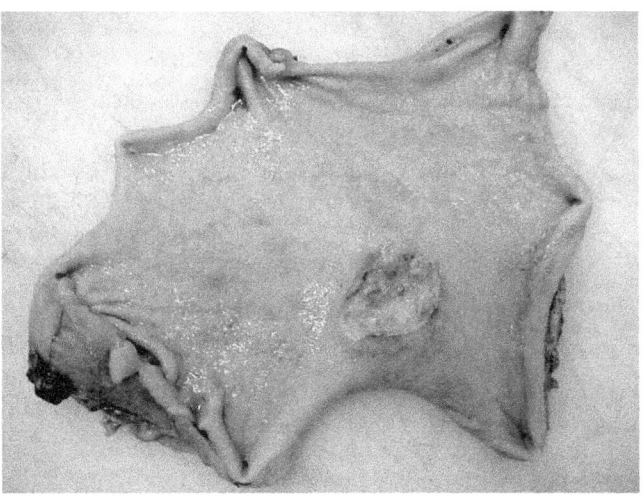
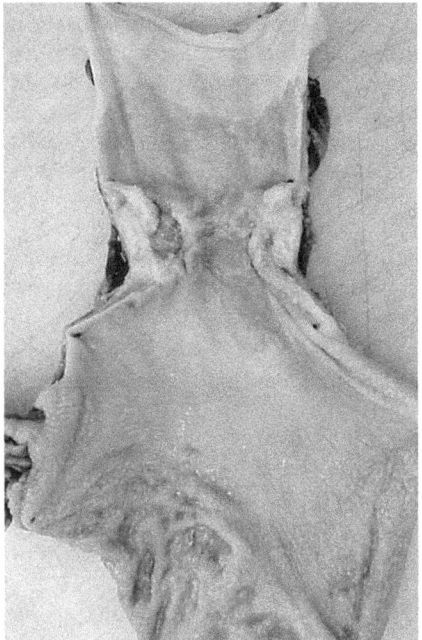
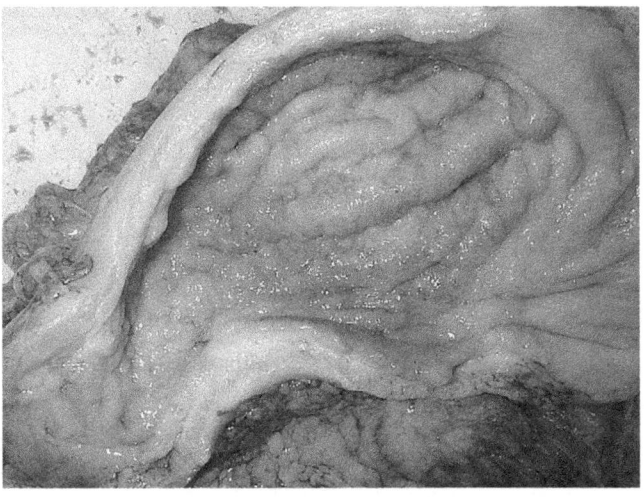

**Figure 18.2.** **a** Oesophagectomy specimen, with a narrow cuff of proximal stomach at the bottom end. In the mid-oesophagus there is a large ulcerated tumour that histologically was a squamous cell carcinoma. **b** Oesophagogastrectomy specimen that includes the lower oesophagus and proximal stomach. Just above the gastro-oesophageal junction there is an ulcerated tumour which has invaded into the thickened oesophageal wall. There is an extensive area of columnar lined oesophagus extending proximal to the tumour. The mucosa proximal to this is lined by squamous epithelium. **c** Distal gastrectomy specimen showing an ulcerated tumour with well-defined margins on the greater curve. **d** Total gastrectomy with a diffuse thickening of the gastric wall due to infiltration by a diffuse adenocarcinoma ( linitis plastica). The mucosal surface is intact but irregularly thickened.

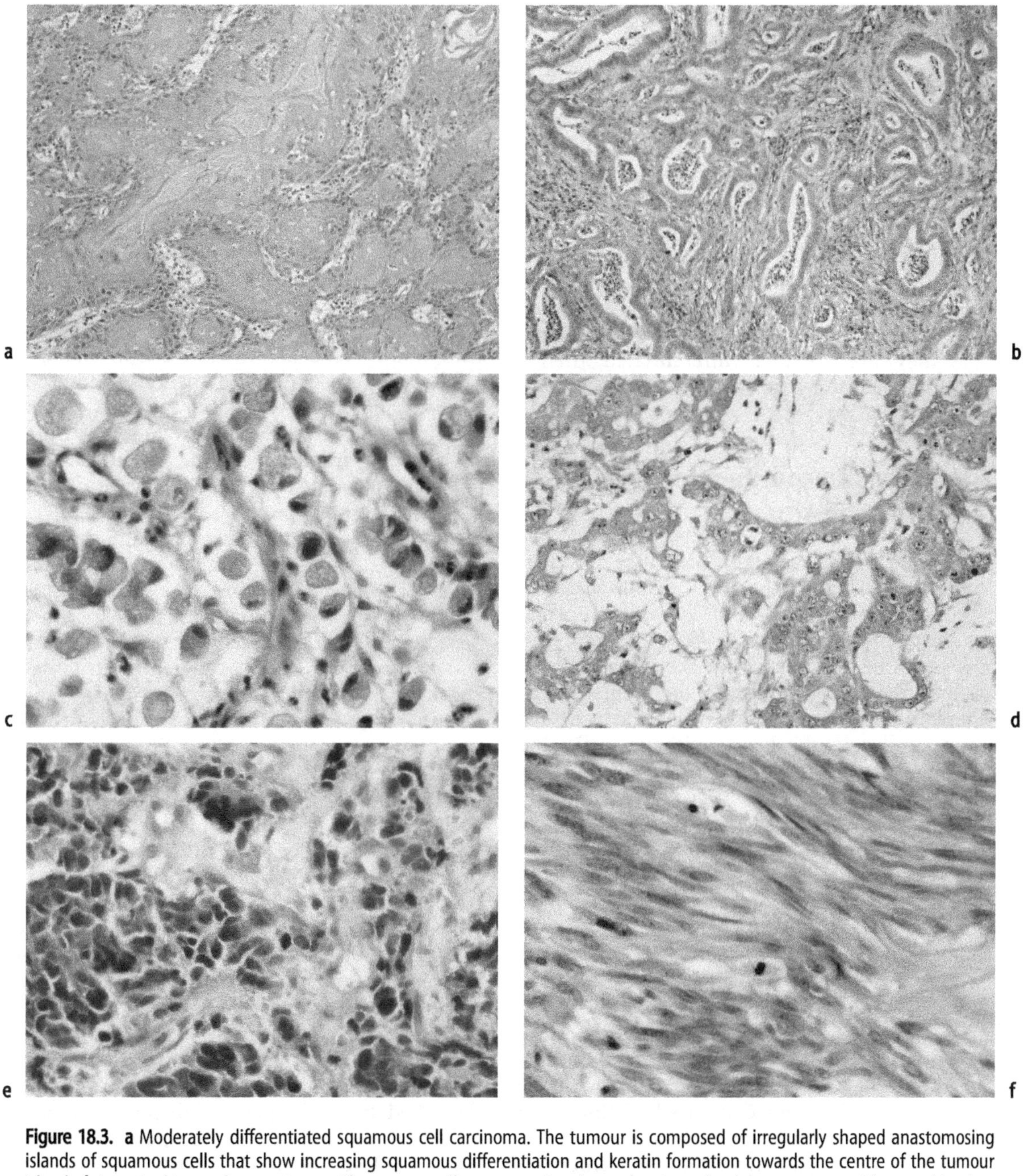

# PATHOLOGY OF THE OESOPHAGUS AND STOMACH

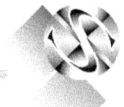

**Figure 18.3.** **a** Moderately differentiated squamous cell carcinoma. The tumour is composed of irregularly shaped anastomosing islands of squamous cells that show increasing squamous differentiation and keratin formation towards the centre of the tumour islands. **b** Intestinal type adenocarcinoma. The tumour cells are arranging themselves into glandular structures with central lumina. The glands being formed are irregular in size and shape. Between the neoplastic glands there is a cellular fibrous stroma reacting to the invasive tumour. **c** Diffuse adenocarcinoma. The tumour cells are invading through the pre-existing stromal tissues singly or in small groups. Glandular structures are not seen. In this case, many of the tumour cells have abundant cytoplasm filled with mucin. **d** Mucinous carcinoma. The tumour cells are forming glandular structures and small tumour islands. The pale material between these structures is mucin which is secreted into the surrounding stroma by the tumour cells. **e** Small cell carcinoma. The tumour cells are relatively small compared to other tumour types. They have very little cytoplasm, such that the nucleus accounts for the majority of the cell volume. **f** Malignant gastrointestinal stromal tumour. The tumour is composed of tightly packed spindle-shaped stromal cells. A cell in mitosis is present centrally.

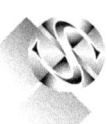

are also often polypoid, growing into the lumen of the oesophagus more than into deeper tissues of the oesophageal wall. Perhaps as a result of this architecture, spindle cell carcinomas and carcinosarcomas are associated with a better prognosis than usual squamous cell carcinoma.

4. Verrucous carcinoma. These are very well-differentiated squamous tumours that grow into the underlying tissue with an expansive margin and have thick layers of keratin on the surface. Because they are so well differentiated their malignant nature can be missed in a small biopsy.

## Squamous Dysplasia and Carcinoma in situ

A precancerous lesion that develops in squamous epithelium is recognised histologically as atypical squamous cells with loss of the normal pattern of squamous differentiation seen between the basal and surface cells. This is called squamous dysplasia of the epithelium. If there is no differentiation, when surface cells look similar to the basal epithelial cells, the change is called carcinoma in situ. Such carcinoma in situ may widely affect the epithelium of the oesophagus and upper aerodigestive tract. It is commonly seen in mucosa adjacent to a squamous carcinoma. In those affected patients who do not yet have a malignant tumour, there is a high risk of subsequent development of squamous carcinoma.

## Squamous Papilloma

Squamous papilloma is a benign lesion seen uncommonly as small polypoid masses in the oesophagus. They are composed of thickened surface epithelium forming papillary folds, often with surface keratin production. Infection with human papilloma virus can be demonstrated in many of these lesions.

## Adenocarcinoma

Adenocarcinoma is the commonest tumour type in the lower oesophagus and the stomach. They are derived from stem cells in the glandular mucosa of the stomach. In the lower oesophagus they are typically found arising within columnar lined oesophagus (Fiure 18.2b). Those oesophageal adenocarcinomas that do not have columnar change in the adjacent mucosa are thought to have overgrown and destroyed the glandular mucosa from which they arose.

Epidemiological studies demonstrate a link between *H. pylori* infection and gastric adenocarcinoma. Dietary factors may also be important in explaining the wide variation in incidence of the disease across the globe. Adenocarcinoma of the oesophagus is related to columnar metaplasia, which is due to reflux.

The gross appearance of adenocarcinomas is very variable. Early gastric carcinomas, defined as tumours confined within the mucosa and/or submucosa, may appear as slightly raised or depressed areas within the mucosa. More advanced carcinomas may be polypoid, ulcerated, or diffuse. Some ulcerated tumours have well-defined margins (Figure 18.2c), others have ill-defined margins due to irregular tumour permeation into the adjacent gastric or oesophageal wall. Diffuse tumours may extend widely through the wall of the stomach underneath the mucosa (linitis plastica) (Figure 18.2d). Large tumours may show a mixture of growth patterns.

Histologically, adenocarcinomas characteristically show formation of abnormal glandular structures and/or mucin production by the tumour cells, but neither feature is necessary for the diagnosis. A number of histological classifications of adenocarcinoma, particularly for the stomach, have been proposed. The system of the Japanese Research Society for Gastric Cancer has a large number of entities, but has been shown to have a high degree of reproducibility [3]. The WHO classification [4] has four adenocarcinoma subtypes (reduced from six in the first edition). The system proposed by Lauren described two subtypes of adenocarcinoma – intestinal and diffuse. Intestinal carcinoma, which corresponds to the tubular types of the Japanese Research Society and WHO classifications, shows the formation of glandular structures that resemble the tumours seen in the intestine (Figure 18.3b). Diffuse carcinoma typically consists of small cords and individual cells diffusely infiltrating through the pre-existing stroma of the gastric wall (Gastric 18.3c). This system has proved to relate to the epidemiology and aetiology of the disease, with intestinal type adenocarcinoma being associated with environmental factors causing the disease and accounting for the excess cancers in regions of the world where gastric cancer is more common. However, many tumours show mixed architectures, some diffuse carcinomas show formation of small irregular glands, and some adenocarcinomas are unclassifiable using Lauren's system. As a result, the degree of inter-observer agreement between pathologists is less good. A cell type seen in many diffuse tumours has abundant intracytoplasmic mucin which distends the cell and squashes the nucleus to one edge. This is called a signet ring cell. Some diffuse carcinomas consist predominantly of such cells, but others have only a few and many have none. Some diffuse carcinomas consist of small or medium-sized solid islands of cells rather than cords or single cells. Other distinct types of adenocarcinoma include papillary adenocarcinoma and mucinous carcinoma. In papillary carcinoma the tumour cells are arranged to form villi or papillae covering a thin core of stromal tissue. Mucinous carcinomas secrete large amounts of mucus into the stroma and end up as islands of cells floating in this mucus (Figure 18.3d).

Many adenocarcinomas harbour a small subpopulation of cells that immunostain positively with markers of neuroendocrine differentiation such as chromogranin. This finding is common in otherwise classical adenocarcinomas and does not indicate a diagnosis of carcinoid tumour or other endocrine carcinoma.

Adenocarcinomas may be graded into well, moderate or poorly differentiated tumours. Tubular or intestinal adenocarcinomas can be well or moderately differentiated depending on the regularity of the glandular structures they are forming. Diffuse tumours are regarded as poorly differentiated. Tumours that show two or more of the recognised adenocarcinoma subtypes are very common. In general, the histological subtype and degree of differentiation add little to the treatment decisions or prognosis of a particular tumour after staging information is taken into account. The histological parameter that has shown the best relationship with prognosis has been the shape of the invasive margin as detailed in Ming's staging system. Tumours are described as expansive or infiltrative, the former having a better prognosis.

## Glandular Dysplasia

A premalignant change in glandular epithelium, analogous to squamous dysplasia and carcinoma in situ, can be identified and is called glandular dysplasia. Low and high grade forms of dysplasia are described. Such dysplasia may arise in either the gastric mucosa or in columnar lined oesophageal mucosa.

In high grade dysplasia there is failure of normal differentiation of the glandular cells such that undifferentiated cells extend onto the surface epithelium. There is nuclear enlargement and crowding of these glandular cells, the nuclei become randomly situated at different levels from the basement membrane of the glands and the glandular structures themselves may be distorted and irregular in size and shape (Figure 18.4b). When high grade dysplasia is seen in a biopsy specimen, the risk of concurrent invasive carcinoma is very high – in some series two thirds of such patients will have an adenocarcinoma. In addition, the risk of subsequent progression to an invasive tumour is very high unless the dysplastic mucosa is resected.

Low grade dysplasia is also characterised by failure of normal differentiation in glandular epithelium, but with a lesser degree of cytological atypia and gland architecture distortion than is seen with high grade dysplasia. In addition, the nuclei of the dysplastic cells are less crowded and situated along the basal portion of the cells near to the basement membrane (Figure 18.4a). There is a lower risk of progression to invasive carcinoma. The cytomorphological and architectural changes of low grade dysplasia can be confused with regenerative and inflammatory changes in non-neoplastic glandular epithelium, particularly in intestinal metaplasia. For this reason, there can be a poor level of inter-observer agreement on the diagnosis of low grade dysplasia.

Glandular dysplasia may be seen in flat or just slightly thickened mucosa, or as a raised polyp, in which case it is called an adenoma. Adenomas may show low or high grade dysplasia and these convey a similar risk of invasive adenocarcinoma as does flat dysplasia.

In September 1998, just before the World Congress of Gastroenterology in Sydney, a workshop was held in Vienna, Austria, on early neoplasia in the gastrointestinal tract [5]. It was felt that there were large discrepancies between

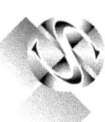

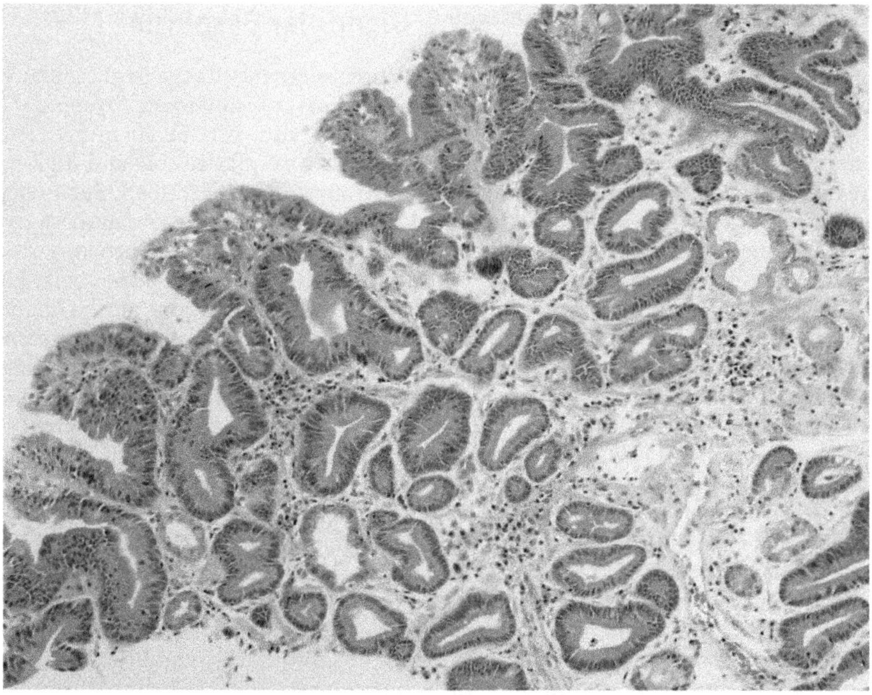

**Figure 18.4.** **a** Low grade dysplasia. The cells lining these glands show lack of normal cytoplasmic differentiation and the epithelial cell nuclei are crowded together. The nuclei are not particularly enlarged, however, and tend to be situated towards the basal portion of the cell, near the basement membrane. **b** High grade dysplasia. Compared to the picture of low grade dysplasia, the atypical glands are more irregular and many more nuclei are crowded together such that they are arranged randomly within the cells.

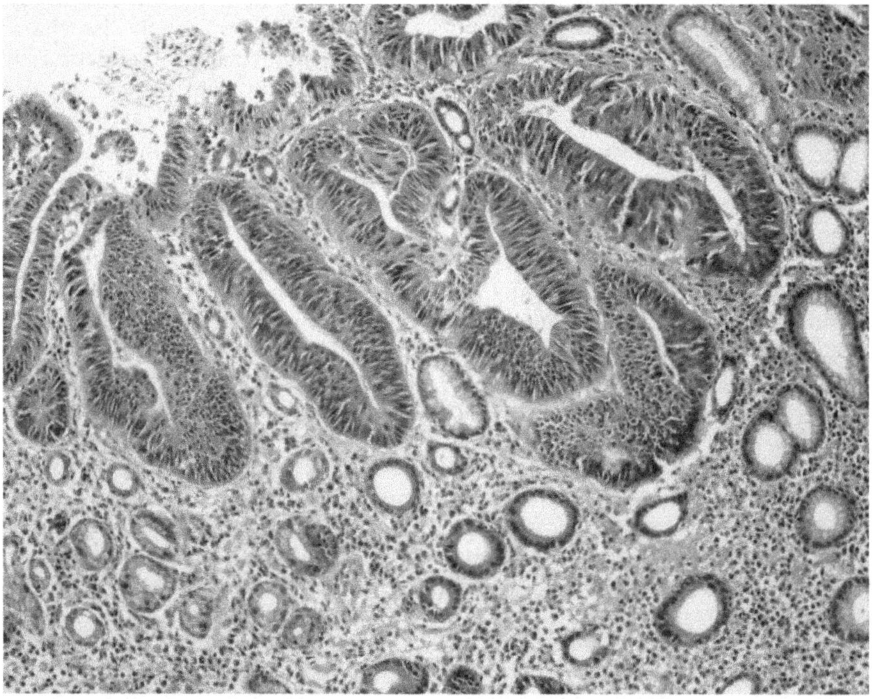

Western and Japanese pathologists in the diagnosis of adenoma/dysplasia versus carcinoma for gastric and colorectal glandular lesions and for oesophageal squamous lesions., and it was felt these called for a united effort to reach a consensus on the nomenclature used for gastrointestinal epithelial neoplastic lesions.

For biopsy diagnosis, five categories were identified:

*Category 1* – negative for neoplasia/dysplasia (including normal, reactive, regenerative, hyperplastic, atrophic and metaplastic epithelium) – further follow-up may or may not be needed, as clinically indicated.

*Category 2* – indefinite for neoplasia/dysplasia – follow-up is needed because of uncertainty about the real nature of the lesion.

*Category 3* – non-invasive low grade neoplasia (low grade adenoma/dysplasia) - neoplasia is present but the risk of developing invasive carcinoma is low. Clinicians may consider local treatment of the lesion or opt for follow-up.

*Category 4* – non-invasive high grade neoplasia – the risk of invasion and development of metastases is increased. Local treatment such as endoscopic mucosal resection or local surgical treatment would be indicated.

*Category 5* – invasive neoplasia – the risk of subsequent deeper invasion and metastases is so high that urgent treatment is indicated and should only be withheld if clinically contraindicated.

The final diagnosis rests on the examination of the resection specimen where the full extent of spread or the most severe grade of epithelial neoplasia can be documented. Thus, the pathologist's report on a biopsy diagnosis of intramucosal carcinoma is best qualified by "at least".

## Tumours Resembling Salivary Gland Carcinomas

Mucoepidermoid carcinoma and adenoid cystic carcinoma are rare tumours of the oesophagus, where they may arise from oesophageal glands. These are low grade tumours that are often small and grow and spread over a long period.

Mucoepidermoid carcinoma shows a mixture of squamous and mucin gland differentiation. A high grade version has been described, but such tumours are better regarded as adenosquamous carcinoma.

Adenoid cystic carcinoma forms small sheets of regular uniform cells which form small cystic spaces and surround globules of basement membrane like material. The tumour shows a mixture of secretory type cells and myoepithelial cells – cells that in a normal glandular duct surround the secretory cells and have contractile fibres in the cytoplasm. Adenoid cystic carcinoma commonly invades nerves and permeates along the perineural space.

## Undifferentiated Carcinoma

Some carcinomas show no recognisable pattern of differentiation at all. In the stomach these are considered to be adenocarcinomas. In the oesophagus such tumours may be either very poorly differentiated variants of squamous cell carcinoma or adenocarcinoma. If enough tissue is sampled from a resection specimen it is usually possible to find some areas with recognisable differentiation pattern allowing classification. In a small biopsy, however, the clues as to the real nature of the tumour are less likely to be evident.

## Small Cell Carcinoma

This tumour is rapidly progressive and prone to metastasis to local lymph nodes at an early stage. Morphologically and immunophenotypically it is identical to the small cell carcinomas that occur in the lung. When seen in the oesophagus it is important to consider the possibility that it represents direct spread from a primary in the lung or a metastasis in mediastinal lymph nodes. Small cell carcinoma accounts for 2% of primary oesophageal carcinomas. It is much rarer in the stomach.

Morphologically the tumour cells are small with very little cytoplasm. In biopsy specimens the tumour cells can be mistaken for lymphocytes (Figure 18.3e). The tumour cells may express a variety of neuroendocrine markers demonstrable by immunostaining, and most are immunopositive for CD56.

Rarely, tumours showing areas of small cell carcinoma admixed within areas showing adenocarcinoma are found.

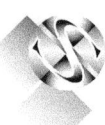

## Carcinoid Tumour

Carcinoid tumours are low grade neuroendocrine carcinomas. They are rare in the stomach and very rare in the oesophagus. They arise from the endocrine cell population scattered in the basal portion of gastric glands. Morphologically the small regular tumour cells, which have more cytoplasm than small cell carcinomas, form solid islands and trabeculae infiltrating through the stomach wall. Because these tumours are slow growing, mitotic figures are infrequent in tissue sections. The diagnosis can be confirmed by immunostaining for chromogranin, a protein component of neurosecretory granules, which is found expressed in a proportion of the tumour cells. These tumours are often small and localised at the time of diagnosis and if completely removed the prognosis is good. There may be multiple tumours in the stomach, however.

Tumours showing a mixture of carcinoid and adenocarcinoma differentiation have been described, but are very rare.

## Lymphoma

Lymphoma is very rare in the oesophagus and usually represents a deposit complicating extensive systemic disease. Lymphomas of the stomach are the commonest site for a gastrointestinal lymphoma, and most of these are specific tumours arising from mucosa associated lymphoid tissue (MALT).

Low grade MALT lymphomas are composed of cells resembling the centrocytes of germinal centres, but are in fact analogous to the marginal cells found at the periphery of germinal centres in the spleen and mesenteric lymph nodes. These cells have a B-cell phenotype. The tumour cells fill and expand the mucosa where they characteristically show destructive infiltration of glandular epithelium. Around the periphery of tumour nodules there are often many plasma cells, and deep to the tumour reactive lymphoid follicles form. With time, the abnormal neoplastic B-cell population colonise and replace the normal germinal centre cells of these lymphoid follicles. As they increase in size the lymphomatous areas in the mucosa ulcerate. These ulcers typically affect the mucosa with preservation of the underlying muscularis propria, in distinction to peptic ulcers.

Low grade MALT lymphomas have been shown to be antigenically driven by *Helicobacter pylori* infection. Eradication of *H. pylori* results in regression and long-term cure in many cases. The tumours are often multiple in the stomach, and even when the tumour is localised a population of similar atypical B cells can be demonstrated elsewhere in the gastric mucosa.

If untreated, many low grade MALT lymphomas transform into a high grade B-cell lymphoma. Such transformation can be demonstrated at the time of the initial diagnosis in some tumours, and in other patients the disease presents as a pure high grade lymphoma. These tumours do not respond to *H. pylori* eradication but do show a good response to standard chemotherapy.

Another type of lymphoma that can present in the stomach is mantle cell lymphoma. The tumour cells in this tumour can resemble low grade lymphoma arising from MALT and also have a B-cell phenotype. Mantle cell lymphoma is a more aggressive tumour, however, is more likely to be systemic and does not respond to *H. pylori* eradication. The tumour cells are immunopositive for the T-cell antigen CD5 and express high levels of cyclin-D1 in their nuclei.

Other types of lymphoma can affect the stomach as part of a systemic lymphoma of lymph nodes or other lymphoid tissues. In these cases the tumour type has usually been determined from biopsies at other sites.

## Gastrointestinal Stromal Tumour (GIST)

These tumours are composed of spindle cells arranged in interweaving bundles resembling smooth muscle. This architecture, and the observation that most of these tumours appear to arise from the muscle layers of the gut, caused them in the past to be classified as smooth muscle tumours – leiomyomas and leiomyosarcomas. In fact, most such tumours do not show a smooth muscle phenotype, and so the name of gastrointestinal stromal tumour or GIST was coined. Most GISTs are immunopositive for CD34, and more recently have been shown to be CD117 (*c-kit*) positive. The small number of morphologically similar tumours that are negative for CD117 probably represent true smooth muscle or nerve sheath tumours.

GISTs can occur anywhere along the gastrointestinal tract, and some occur elsewhere in the abdomen such as the retroperitoneum. The commonest site, however, is the stomach. Grossly, these tumours grow as solid masses that commonly expand as polypoid growths into the lumen of the stomach, covered by an attenuated mucosa which often ulcerates centrally. Microscopically the tumour cells are typically spindle in shape, although an epithelioid cell variant in which the cells have a more polygonal appearance can occur. This variant can be mistaken for a carcinoma. The degree of cellular crowding, pleomorphism, mitotic figures and tumour necrosis is very variable (Figure 18.3f).

Many GISTs behave in a benign manner, but up to a third of those in the stomach will invade adjacent structures and/or metastasise. Predicting the biological behaviour on the basis of the morphological appearance is very difficult, however. In general, cell crowding, significant pleomorphism and mitoses are more likely to be seen in malignant tumours, but some malignant tumours can appear very similar histologically to their benign counterparts. The most useful discriminators of subsequent behaviour are the tumour size and the number of mitotic figures seen on tissue sections. Different authors have used these features to derive three predictive groups – benign, borderline and malignant. The size determinants are usually based on cut-offs of 5 cm and 10 cm maximum diameter, but there is wide variation in the number of mitotic figures that are allowed before a tumour is regarded as malignant for the three different size groups. The rate of progression of the malignant tumours is often slow – recurrence or metastasis may not be evident for many years following initial diagnosis and survival with untreatable disease may be much longer than is seen with carcinomas of similar size.

## Other Stromal Tumours

Benign lipomas and haemangiomas may occur in both the oesophagus and stomach. The so-called granular cell tumour is a rare tumour most commonly seen in the upper aerodigestive tract but can also be found in the oesophagus and stomach. This tumour is composed of a diffuse infiltrate of cells extending through the tissues of the submucosa and adjacent tissue layers. The overlying mucosa is usually intact but may become secondarily ulcerated. The tumour cells have an abundant granular cytoplasm. Almost all are benign but may show local recurrence due to their diffuse nature, making local excision difficult.

Malignant sarcomas that can occur include Kaposi's sarcoma and malignant schwannoma. Other types of benign and malignant stromal tumour are described rarely.

## Malignant Melanoma

Melanocytes are seen occasionally in the normal oesophagus, and these explain the rare occurrence of malignant melanoma as a primary tumour in the oesophagus. Secondary melanoma from a previous primary in the skin or other site is more common. Some of these tumours produce melanin, and this pigment gives the diagnostic clue both on gross appearance and in histologic sections. Non-pigmented melanomas, however, can be confused with undifferentiated carcinoma. The diagnosis is best made by immunostaining with a panel of antibodies. Melanomas usually express S100 protein and stain positively with HMB45 and Melan-A, but are immunonegative for cytokeratins, which distinguishes them from carcinomas. These tumours are rapidly progressing and have a poor prognosis.

## Metastatic Tumours

Metastatic tumours in the stomach and oesophagus are rare, but should always be considered when the tumour type or morphology is unusual. A particular problem is found with metastatic lobular carcinoma of the breast which may be mistaken for a primary diffuse adenocarcinoma if the history of breast carcinoma is not made known to the pathologist.

## Staging of Oesophageal and Gastric Carcinomas

The principal staging systems for oesophageal and gastric carcinomas are based upon the TNM system [6] and the Japanese Research Society for Gastric Carcinoma [3]. There is much in common between them. The principal difference is the way that metastases to local lymph

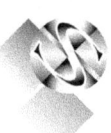

## 18 · UPPER GASTROINTESTINAL SURGERY

nodes are recorded, and in this respect there was also a change in the TMN classification between the 1992 and 1997 editions.

## The T stage

### Oesophagus

pT1: invasive tumour is in the lamina propria or submucosa.

pT2: invasion of the muscularis propria.

pT3: there is invasion beyond the muscularis propria into the adventitia around the oesophagus.

pT4: tumour invades adjacent structures such as the trachea, aorta, pleura or pericardium.

### Stomach

pT1: invasive tumour is in the lamina propria or submucosa.

pT2: invasion of the muscularis propria and/or the subserosal tissue.

pT3: tumour invades onto the peritoneal surface.

pT4: tumour invades adjacent structures such as the pancreas, liver or intestine.

The pT2 stage for the stomach differs from the oesophagus and large intestine in that invasion beyond the muscularis propria is still pT2 and invasion onto the peritoneal surface is pT3, unlike the large intestine where peritoneal invasion is called pT4. In addition, for both oesophagus and stomach there are the categories pT0 (no demonstrable tumour), pTis (carcinoma in situ), and pTX (tumour cannot be assessed).

The concept of early gastric cancer is defined as a pT1 carcinoma, irrespective of the lymph node status. The prognosis of such cancers treated by complete surgical resection is good.

## Lymph Node Staging

If the pathological status of the local lymph nodes cannot be assessed, the nodal stage is described as pNX. If all nodes are negative the stage is pN0.

For oesophageal tumours there are just two pN stages – pN0 for no node involvement and pT1 for histological demonstration of metastases in mediastinal or perigastric lymph nodes. Metastases to cervical lymph nodes or para-aortic lymph nodes (including the coeliac axis nodes) are counted as distant metastases (pM1).

The staging for stomach tumours is as follows:

pN1: 1 to 6 involved nodes.

pN2: 7 to 15 nodes involved.

pN3: 16 or more involved nodes.

Metastases to nodes in the retroperitoneum, para-aortic region and the intestinal mesentery are classified as distant metastases.

The staging system of the Japanese Research Society is based upon the distribution of involved nodes relative to the site in the stomach occupied by the tumour. Prior to the 5th edition, the nodal stage under the TNM system was also based upon the position of involved nodes being less or greater than 3 cm from the primary tumour. The simpler staging based upon number of involved nodes gives better prognostic information. However, correlation with staging based upon radiological investigations and the design of operative procedures may in future require that pathologists describe the site of the positive nodes also.

The accuracy of staging is greater the more lymph nodes are identified. The lymph nodes regional to the stomach tend to be smaller than elsewhere in the gastrointestinal tract, and involved nodes are often not enlarged, especially with diffuse adenocarcinomas. It is thus recommended that at least 15 nodes are identified in a resection specimen.

## Distant Metastasis

MX: no information on distant metastases is known.

M0: no distant metastases.

M1: distant metastases have been demonstrated.

In the oesophagus the pM stage can be split into pM1a and pM1b. pM1a represents metastases in cervical nodes for an upper oesophageal tumour, defined as above the level of the tracheal bifurcation, or in coeliac axis nodes for a lower oesophageal (the distal 8 cms) tumour. Other distant metastases are pM1b.

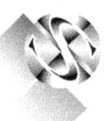

## Minimum Dataset Information

The pathology report from an oesophageal or gastric resection specimen should include the following items of data.

1. Gross description, to include the length of the individual parts of the specimen (oesophagus, lesser curve, greater curve, duodenum, omentum, spleen, pancreas and any other structures included). Fixation causes shrinkage of the specimen unless it is opened and pinned out onto a cork board, and so the state of fixation (fresh or fixed) and whether it was pinned or not should be recorded. The dimensions of the tumour, the distance to the specimen ends and the radial resection margin, any involvement of the serosal surface and the shape (polypoid, ulcerated, flat, diffuse) should be described. For gastric tumours, the site in the stomach and which wall the largest diameter of the tumour is situated on are described also.
2. Number of tumours – if more than one tumour is present, details about all the tumours should be described individually.
3. Histological type – e.g. squamous, adenocarcinoma.
4. Tumour grade – well, moderate or poor.
5. Depth of invasion – in sufficient detail to derive the pT stage. For gastric tumours, the pattern of invasion should be described as expansive or infiltrative.
6. State of the resection margins, including the specimen ends and the radial margin for oesophageal tumours. It is very unusual for the mesenteric margin to be involved in curative gastric tumour resections.
7. Vascular invasion – not seen, or present. When tumour invades vascular structures these are usually capillaries or small venules, and it is difficult to distinguish these from lymphatics. Invasion in both large and small vascular and lymphatic spaces is thus grouped under vascular invasion. Vascular invasion can be very infrequent and difficult to spot in histological sections.
8. Lymph node status – total number of lymph nodes found in the specimen and the number of nodes that are involved.
9. If biopsies of possible metastases from other sites such as the liver or peritoneum are included, the status of these should be described.
10. Background mucosal lesions – columnar lined oesophagus, gastritis, atrophy, intestinal metaplasia.

## Questions

1. Give a classification of oesophagogastric neoplasms.
2. What is dysplasia and outline its significance.
3. Describe neoplastic lesions.

## References

1. Dixon MF, O'Connor HJ, Axon AT et al. Reflux gastritis: distinct pathological entity? J Clin Pathol 1986;39:524–30.
2. Dixon MF, Genta RM, Yardley JH, Correa P. Classification and grading of gastritis, the updated Sydney System. Am J Surg Pathol 1996;20:1161–81.
3. Japanese Research Society for Gastric Cancer. Japanese classification of gastric carcinoma, 1st edn (English). Tokyo: Kanehara, 1995.
4. Watanabe H, Jass JR, Sobin LH. Histological typing of oesophageal and gastric tumours, 2nd edn. Berlin: Springer-Verlag, 1990.
5. Schlemper RJ, Riddell RH, Kato Y et al. The Vienna classification of gastrointestinal epithelial neoplasia Gut 2000;47:251–5.
6. Sobin LH, Wittekind CL. TNM classification of malignant tumours, 5th edn. New York: Wiley, 1997.

## Further Reading

Lewin, KJ, Appelman HD. Atlas of tumour pathology. Third Series Fascicle 18. Tumors of the esophagus and stomach. Washington: AFIP.

# 19

## Premalignant Lesions of the Oesophagus: Identification to Management

Andrew Latchford and Janusz A.Z. Jankowski

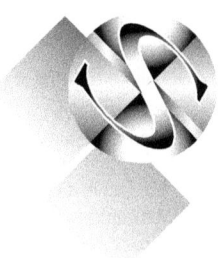

## Aims

- To identify premalignant lesions of the oesophagus.
- To discuss the pathology and malignant potential of these lesions.
- To highlight the controversies with regard to surveillance and management of these lesions.

## Introduction

Primary oesophageal tumours are classified as epithelial or non-epithelial tumours, depending on the cell of origin, and may be benign or malignant (Table 19.1). Non-epithelial tumours arise from the mesenchymal or supporting stromal tissue.

In this chapter the epidemiology, pathology and management of premalignant oesophageal lesions are discussed. Premalignant lesions have not been identified for all primary oesophageal cancers and to date only three such lesions have been identified, namely Barrett's oesophagus, squamous epithelial dysplasia and squamous papilloma of the oesophagus (Figure 19.1).

Worldwide squamous cell carcinoma remains the most common oesophageal cancer but in the Western world adenocarcinoma now predominates. The prognosis for both these oesophageal cancers is poor. This is because presentation is delayed by the fact that symptoms occur late by which time the lesion is already advanced. Early detection and treatment improves the prognosis, hence the need to identify and understand the pathology of premalignant lesions. By doing this it is hoped that those with high risk of malignant progression can be identified and intervention occur at an earlier stage.

## Barrett's Oesophagus

### Epidemiology

Barrett's oesophagus (BO) is a premalignant condition for oesophageal adenocarcinoma. The true prevalence of BO in the general population is not known but is estimated to be 1–2%. It is thought to be underdiagnosed, with only 5–30% of patients with Barrett's adenocarcinoma (BA) having BO diagnosed before the development of cancer. Post-mortem studies have reported the lifetime risk in the general adult population in the Western world as 1% [1]. The incidence of new cases in the at-risk population is 0.5–2% per year and is increasing [2]. There is a male predominance in a ratio of 4:1. The geographical distribution is still being clarified. It occurs mainly in Caucasians in the Western world and is rarely found in Afro-Americans. The incidence in the Asian subcontinent may be approaching that of Western countries.

## 19 · UPPER GASTROINTESTINAL SURGERY

**Table 19.1.** Cancers and their cell of origin

| Malignant tumour | Cell of origin |
| --- | --- |
| Squamous cell carcinoma | Squamous epithelium |
| Adenocarcinoma | Columnar epithelium |
| Adenocanthoma | Columnar epithelium with metaplasia |
| Adenoid cystic carcinoma | Oesophageal gland duct |
| Mucoepidermoid carcinoma | Oesophageal gland duct |
| Choriocarcinoma | Germ cell |
| Small cell carcinoma and carcinoid | Foregut endocrine cell |
| Malignant melanoma | Melanocytes |

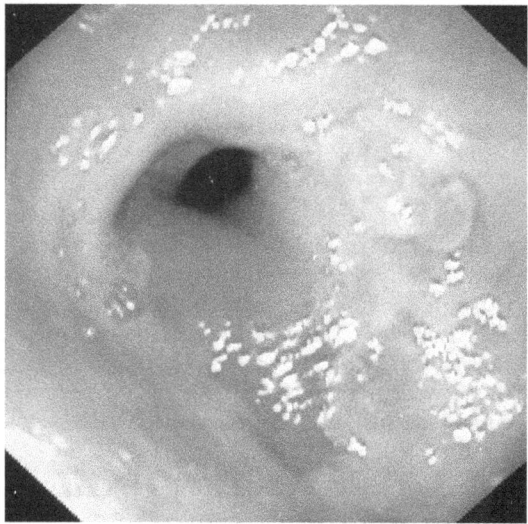

**Figure 19.1.** Barrett's oesophagus complicated by a stricture and an incidental squamous papilloma.

The definition of BO has changed from its initial definition of columnar lined esophagus. The columnar lined oesophagus can be of three types: gastric fundic gland, junctional type epithelium with cardic mucous glands and a distinct type of columnar metaplasia called specialised intestinal epithelium or intestinal metaplasia. Only intestinal metaplasia carries an increased risk of the development of carcinoma and some current definitions of BO require intestinal metaplasia to be found histologically.

Historically 3 cm of columnar epithelium was required to make the diagnosis of BO but these largely arbitary criteria have now been abandoned. BO however, is still classified into long segment (>3 cm) and short segment (<3 cm) disease.

Most if not all oesophageal adenocarcinoma arises from esophageal metaplasia, with BO carrying a 30–50-fold increased risk of adenocarcinoma over the general population. The reported incidence of oesophageal adenocarcinoma in BO ranges from 1:52 to 1:441 patient years follow-up and using pooled data the cancer risk in BO is 1% per year [3]. Debate has arisen as to whether the cancer risk in BO has been over-estimated due to publication bias. However, it is now clear that many supposed cases of BO are in reality hiatus hernia or gastric type metaplasia without the increased risk of adenocarcinoma. There is little doubt, however, that in parallel with BO there has been a large increase in the incidence of oesophageal adenocarcinoma in the last two decades in the Western population, increasing at a rate of 10% per year.

## Aetiology

Familial association and twin studies suggest that genetic factors may be important in a minority of BO [4]. However, most cases arise as a result of duodeno-gastro-oesophageal reflux disease, although any insult that causes distal oesophageal irritation (e.g. chemotherapy, radiotherapy) may predispose to metaplasia.

### Gastro-oesophageal Reflux Disease (GORD)

GORD is a common condition in the Western world: 30% of adults have symptoms of heartburn at least once a month and a third of these will have endoscopic evidence of oesophagitis; 10% of those with oesophagitis will progress to BO. There is correlation between duration of acid exposure and BO length and in addition there is both in vitro and in vivo evidence to suggest that intermittent exposure to acid causes epithelial changes which may be interpreted as selecting poorly differentiated cells with increased proliferative potential.

### Biliary Reflux

Proton pump inhibitors are highly effective at healing squamous mucosa, but do not convincingly reverse or halt progression of BO and as such interest has turned to the role of bile acids in BO. Analysis of refluxate shows that bile acid rich duodenal juice is more frequently found than previously thought. Bile acids may damage the oesophageal mucosa either alone or in conjunction with acid. Neoplastic progression of BO has been reported in patients with bile reflux but no pathological acid reflux [5], indeed worsening mucosal damage, BO appearance and extent of disease have all been correlated with bile acid exposure.

BO and dysplasia are thought to arise from stem cells of native oesophagus or adjacent oesophageal glandular tissue. Stem cells are able to self-renew as well as produce indefinite numbers of daughter cells, which have a finite capacity to divide. Stem cells are the only permanent cells of the epithelium and it is thought that chronic damage induces them to undergo altered differentiation. The location of stem cells in metaplastic Barrett's epithelium has not been identified although it is known that stem cells for squamous oesophageal mucosa are found in the basal compartment of the epithelium.

## Development of Metaplasia

Various theories exist as to the tissue of origin for BO. Squamous stem cells, oesophageal glands and transitional zone epithelium have all been proposed and for each there exists an analogy of metaplastic change in other regions. The de novo hypothesis suggests that squamous stem cells in the papillae are damaged, resulting in metaplastic change. The transitional cell metaplasia theory proposes that pluripotent transitional zone cells colonise the gastric cardia or distal oesophagus in response to noxious luminal agents, thereby creating a variable boundary between squamous and columnar epithelium. The final mechanism is supported by the ulcer-associated cell lineage, which occurs adjacent to ulceration in the gastrointestinal tract, and it hypothesises that stem cells in the glandular neck region of oesophageal ducts selectively colonise the oesophagus following squamous mucosal damage.

Differences in stem cell biology may account for regional differences in cancer risk but extrinsic factors are required to initiate and maintain clonal expansion. Reflux of gastric acid and bile acids, and cytokines produced by the inflammatory cell infiltrate found in BO are thought to be involved.

Clonal expansion is the next important step in the progression of BO once metaplasia has occurred. Normally stem cells divide to produce one stem cell and one daughter cell. However, the metaplastic stem cell may divide to produce two stem cells, which is associated with glandular bifurcation. The bifurcating glands ultimately divide again to produce a large contiguous group of epithelial cells with a common genotype. In BO this colonisation occurs rapidly with maximal proximal colonisation taking place within 3 years.

Rapid colonisation can be seen in other inflamed epithelial tissues and may occur by non-bifurcating mechanisms such as lateral migration of stem cells into neighbouring glands. This occurs in urothelial dysplasia but its role in BO is not yet clear.

## Molecular Biology

### Apoptosis

Due to their responsiveness to external stimuli and sensitivity to DNA damage metaplastic stem cells can undergo apoptosis as a result of p53-mediated mechanisms. Apoptosis may by reduced by genetic mutations such as p53 and p16 mutations, loss of heterozygosity of the adenomatous polyposis gene or aneuploidy. Mutations and deletions of the p53 gene are the most common genetic lesions in human cancers. There is overwhelming evidence that p53 gene alterations are early and frequent events in BO progression through dysplasia to adenocarcinoma, but p53 abnormality alone is not sufficient to predict progression to cancer or disease outcome. Studies have also shown p16 inactivation is present in non-dysplastic premalignant BO as well as being an important in neoplastic progression. This inactivation may occur due to loss of heterozygosity or by methylation of the p16 promoter [6,7]. It may be that inactivation of p16 has a future role as a biomarker to stratify risk of neoplastic progression. Loss of heterozygosity in the APC gene has been identified in oesophageal adenocarcinoma and high grade dysplasia but not in low grade dysplasia and non-dysplastic BO.

Other mechanisms have also been identified which may reduce apoptosis. The *bcl-2* proto-oncogene encodes a protein that blocks apoptosis and *bcl-2* expression has been shown to be increased in reflux oesophagitis, non-dysplastic BO and low grade dysplasia. It has not, however, been found in high grade dysplasia and adenocarcinoma thus indicating an early role in the dysplasia to carcinoma sequence.

Telomerase has been implicated in the immortalisation of cells in neoplastic and pre-neoplastic disorders, thus allowing accumulation of genetic mutations. Telomerase synthesises telomeric DNA located at the chromosome ends, thus preventing the loss of telomere length that occurs during normal somatic cell division. In normal squamous oesophageal mucosa little telomerase is present whereas increasing telomerase activity is seen in BO as it progresses towards carcinoma [8]. It is of interest to note that fundic and cardic-type columnar lined oesophagus are not associated with increased telomerase activity.

## DNA Content

Aneuploidy refers to numerically abnormal DNA content in a cell and it has been shown that evolution from normal oesophageal epithelium to BO is frequently associated with aneuploidy. There is some data to suggest that the presence of aneuploidy may be used to predict neoplastic progression [9] and also that Barrett's adenocarcinoma associated with aneuploidy has increased lymph node metastasis, advanced disease and poorer survival.

## Mucosal Inflammation

Another important aspect of both initiation and progression of BO is the role of an inflammatory cell infiltrate that is found in the mucosa. Initially a mixed acute inflammatory cell infiltrate is seen as a result of acid/bile acid damage but subsequently lymphocytes predominate. It is felt that this is not solely a secondary response to mucosal inflammation but is also involved in the persistence of BO, including initiation of clonal expansion. This is supported by the finding that the inflammatory infiltrate persists in BO despite acid suppression therapy and endoscopic ablative therapy.

The infiltrate may be involved by numerous mechanisms including free radical production, cytokine production and modulation of membrane receptors. High levels of free radicals have been isolated in ulcerated gastro-oesophageal mucosa and may cause DNA damage in the epithelial stem cells. In addition, free radicals can induce cytokines, which influence the extent and phenotype of the infiltrate, as well as providing growth factors for epithelial cells.

The Fas gene encodes a transmembrane protein that is involved in apoptosis. The inflammatory infiltrate may induce expression of Fas ligand on metaplastic cells, which might afford some protection from immune surveillance.

Numerous cytokines have been isolated in BO including tumour necrosis factor alpha (TNF-$\alpha$), transforming growth factor beta (TGF-$\beta$), interleukin 1beta (IL-1$\beta$) and interferon gamma (IFN-$\gamma$), which are thought to have a role in both promotion and propagation of metaplastic clones. TNF-$\alpha$ regulates proliferation in murine intestine, and mice that do not encode the TNF-$\alpha$ gene are protected from epithelial damage and cancer from environmental agents. Both TNF-$\alpha$ and IL-1$\beta$ reduce E-cadherin, which has been implicated in the neoplastic progression of BO. Tumour invasiveness and stage are both associated with reduced expression of E-cadherin [10]. In addition germline mutation of the E-cadherin gene, resulting in loss of E-cadherin expression on the cell membrane, has been found in certain cases of familial diffuse gastro-oesophageal cancer. E-cadherin associates with the cytosolic protein beta-catenin, which is involved in the transcription of various oncogenes. Transcription requires tyrosine phosphorylation of beta-catenin, which occurs by endogenously produced TGF-$\alpha$ in the neoplastic cells. This facilitates transformation and survival of abnormal cells due to the increased expression of COX-2 and cyclin D1, which are implicated in chronic inflammation, cell survival and epithelial growth. COX-2 expression is also stimulated by bile acids in vitro.

COX-2 is expressed in 70–80% of oesophageal adenocarcinomas and also in corresponding Barrett's metaplasia. Among regular aspirin users a 40% reduction in the oesophageal has been shown which is thought to represent the repression of COX-2 induction [11,12]. This requires further investigation.

## Natural History of Metaplasia and Dysplasia

It can be seen that a molecular basis is implicated in the inflammation, metaplasia, dysplasia, carcinoma pathway. It is hoped that these molecular changes may provide a basis for risk stratification to rationalise screening of individuals, but currently they are not used in routine clinical practice. Clinical risk factors for progression have been identified, but they are neither sensitive nor specific enough (Table 19.2).

Although the stepwise progression from metaplasia to dysplasia and cancer is generally accepted there are unresolved issues with regard to the natural history of this process. Ten per cent of patients with oesophagitis will develop Barrett's metaplasia of whom 24% progress to dysplasia. Neither the prevalence nor the natural history of dysplasia is clearly understood. Dysplasia is categorised into no dysplasia, indeterminate for dysplasia, low grade dysplasia (LGD), and high grade dysplasia (HGD). LGD is estimated to progress to adenocarcinoma in 18% of patients over a 1.5–4.3 year follow-up. There is also evidence that LGD may remain static for 57 months before progressing [9]. The diagnosis of HGD can only be made after minimisation of inflammation by obtaining acid suppression.

HGD requires at least two experienced pathologists to confirm the diagnosis. The rate of progression of HGD to cancer may be as fast as 5–35 months of follow-up. HGD is currently the gold standard for cancer risk and indeed in patients who undergo oesophagectomy for HGD adenocarcinoma is found in 40–75% [13]. There is some evidence to suggest that LGD and HGD may in fact regress, but many believe that this purely represents potential sampling bias or misclassification. This does, however, cast doubt on HGD being the optimal marker for cancer risk.

## Screening and Surveillance

Oesophageal adenocarcinoma has a dismal prognosis with 11% 5-year survival rates. This rises to 17% if surgically resected but falls to <1% if inoperable. As neither aggressive medical acid suppression therapy nor anti-reflux surgery induces a predictable regression nor exerts a protective effect against neoplastic progression, guidelines have been instituted for screening and surveillance in BO. It is currently recommended that patients with long-standing reflux symptoms, especially if they are over 50 years old, should undergo a screening endoscopy to look for BO. Although doubt remains as to cost-effectiveness of surveillance, it is currently recommended that all patients with BO, who are considered surgically fit, should be placed on a surveillance programme (Table 19.3). At endoscopy the location and extent of BO should be documented and four quadrant biopsies taken at intervals of 2 cm.

Methods to improve yield of detection of dysplasia at endoscopy are currently being evaluated. Methylene blue stains intestinal metaplasia and there is evidence to suggest that methylene blue directed biopsies reduce the number of biopsies, cost less and pick up significantly more dysplasia and adenocarcinoma

**Table 19.2.** Clinical risk factors for Barrett's adenocarcinoma

| |
|---|
| Male sex |
| Age (years) >45 |
| Caucasian |
| Chronicity of symptoms >10 years |
| Length of Barrett's oesophagus >8 cm |
| Ulcer/stricture in Barrett's oesophagus |
| Severe and frequent duodeno-gastro-oesophageal reflux |
| Obesity |
| Smoking |
| Drug therapy, e.g. nitrates, theophyllines, anticholinergics |
| Diet high in fatty foods |

**Table 19.3.** American Gastroenterlogical Association recommendations for surveillance of Barrett's oesophagus in relation to dysplasia

| Dysplasia | Surveillance |
|---|---|
| No dysplasia | After 2 negative endoscopies, every 2 years |
| LGD | Twice every 6 months, annually thereafter |
| HGD | Confirm by second pathologist. Either selective surgery or intensive monitoring every 3 months |

Modified from Sampliner et al (American Journal of Gastroenterology 1998;7:1028–32).

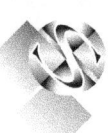

than current methods [14]. Endoscopic fluorescence techniques are also being investigated with encouraging initial results [15]. These methods use 5-ALA sensitisation, which is converted intracellularly to photoactive protoporphyrin IX and accumulates in malignant tissue preferentially due to low activity of ferrochelatase in tumour cells.

Interest in alternative biopsy analysis methods also provides hope for risk stratification of patients. Quantitative fluorescent DNA techniques, known as flow cytometry, have shown that abnormal DNA content shows a correlation with the histological diagnosis of dysplasia and carcinoma. Flow cytometry also detects a subset of patients whose biopsy samples are histologically indefinite or negative for dysplasia and carcinoma but who have DNA content abnormalities similar to those otherwise seen only in dysplasia and carcinoma. This technique has been studied prospectively and aneuploidy may be a prognostic factor for malignant transformation in BO. Seventy per cent of patients with aneuploidy in biopsy specimens at initial endoscopic evaluation developed HGD or cancer, whereas none of those without flow cytometric abnormalities showed progression to HGD or invasive carcinoma [8].

## Treatment

Treatment options in patients with BO are limited. Proton pump inhibitors are used to treat reflux symptoms and to maintain squamous mucosal healing. Long-term studies to elucidate whether this prevents progression of BO are still awaited. Patients with no, indefinite or low grade dysplasia are followed up expectantly as laid down in the surveillance programme. The management for HGD remains controversial. Current recommendations are that patients with HGD should undergo surgical resection as a high proportion will have coexistent adenocarcinoma. If HGD really does regress in a proportion of patients then a less aggressive approach may well be necessary.

Recently interest in local therapies for HGD and intramucosal carcinoma has arisen. These employ a variety of thermal or chemical ablation methods and endoscopic mucosal resection. They are based on the destruction of columnar epithelium, which in the setting of acid suppression will allow healing by squamous mucosa.

They are, however, flawed by the persistence of intestinal metaplasia under squamous islands and also by recurrent tumour after initial response. They have not been shown to reduce mortality and currently can only be recommended for those who are unfit for sugery.

## Summary

- BO is the finding of intestinal metaplasia in the oesophagus.
- BO carries a 30–50-fold increased risk of oesophageal adenocarcinoma.
- Most cases arise due to duodeno-gastro-oesophageal reflux.
- Molecular changes may help identify those at high risk of progression.
- Although contentious, firm guidelines exist with regard to screening and surveillance.
- Endoscopic fluorescence techniques and flow cytometry may improve detection of dysplasia and predict those at higher risk of progression.
- Current treatment consists of proton pump inhibitors and surgical intervention if high grade dysplasia develops.
- New, less invasive treatment modalities are being evaluated.

# Squamous Epithelial Dysplasia

## Epidemiology

Squamous epithelial dysplasia is the premalignant lesion from which squamous cell carcinoma develops. Although in the Western world squamous cell carcinoma is now less common than adenocarcinoma, worldwide there is wide geographical variation, with China, India, Iran and South Africa being areas of high incidence. In Europe and the USA the incidence is low with a male preponderance. The UK incidence is 6.5 per 100 000 for men and 3.2 per 100 000 for women. In the USA it predominantly affects Afro-Americans.

The precancerous nature of squamous epithelial dysplasia is supported by two obser-

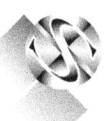

# PREMALIGNANT LESIONS OF THE OESOPHAGUS: IDENTIFICATION TO MANAGEMENT

vations. Firstly dysplasia and carcinoma often coexist in continuity. Secondly follow-up studies of dysplastic epithelium show development of carcinoma after a variable length of time. Overall 9% of patients with dysplasia will develop carcinoma over a 15-year follow-up. This risk, however, is variable according to the degree of dysplasia. The relative risk for moderate dysplasia is 15.8, 72.6 for severe dysplasia and 62.5 for carcinoma in situ during a follow-up of 3.5 years.

Squamous epithelial dysplastic cells are abnormal pleomorphic cells with disorderly arrangement. It is always present in the basal layer and involves various proportions of mucosal thickness. Large discrepancies exist in the interpretation between Western and Japanese pathologists in the diagnosis of oesophageal squamous lesions, making comparisons in incidence and prognosis difficult. Dysplasia is mild if it affects the lowest 25% of mucosa, moderate if it affects 50% and severe if up to 75% is affected. If greater than 75% is affected it is termed carcinoma in situ. Mild and moderate dyslasia are categorised as low grade dysplasia and severe dysplasia and carcinoma in situ are termed high grade dysplasia.

Dysplastic lesions may be unifocal or widespread and multifocal. In the latter multiple synchronous squamous carcinomas may be present, supporting the concept of "field carcinogenesis" in oesophageal squamous cell carcinoma.

## Aetiology

The aetiology and pathophysiology of squamous epithelial dysplasia is not fully understood and is likely to involve both environmental and genetic factors.

### N-nitrosamines

These are the only group of carcinogens recognised as effective on the oesophagus and are widely used to induce dysplasia and carcinoma in animal models. Low levels of nitrosamines and their precursors have been found in the diet of high risk areas in China and India. In addition N-nitroso compounds and aromatic hydrocarbons are found in alcohol and tobacco, which are major risk factors for the development of squamous cell carcinoma.

### Alcohol

In addition to containing carcinogens, alcohol may act in other ways to induce dysplasia. It is oxidised not only in the liver but also in the gastrointestinal tract, which has relevance in first pass metabolism and tissue-induced toxicity. Alcohol is metabolised in mucosal cells via alcohol dehydrogenase (ADH) and microsomal alcohol oxidising system. In the oesophagus there is significantly more sigma-ADH present and the local production of acetaldehyde in the oesophagus may contribute to tissue injury.

Genetic pleomorphism in the alcohol metabolising enzymes ADH3 and aldehyde dehydrogenase 2 (ALDH2) has been investigated in oesophageal multiple dysplasia in patients with head and neck cancer [16]. Mutant ALDH2 allele appears to be a risk factor for dysplasia in these patients. Accumulation of acetaldehyde due to low ALDH2 activity may play a role in cancerous changes throughout the mucosa in the upper aerodigestive tract.

### Diet

Diet is also important in squamous cell carcinogenesis. Dried foods, smoked fish and pickled foods are found in the diet in high risk areas and contain N-nitrosamines. Plants grown in soil with low levels of molybdenum contain higher levels of nitrosamines and such soil is found in areas where ther is a high incidence of squamous cell carcinoma. In addition, chronic deficiency of vitamins A, B, C, E, selenium and zinc are thought to predispose the oesophagal squamous mucosa to malignant transformation. Finally an association with a diet high in beta-carotene also exists.

## Molecular Biology

TP 53 mutations are important in the development of squamous cell carcinoma as they are in adenocarcinoma. In adenocarcinoma there is a high prevalence of G to A transitions at CpG sites, whereas in squamous cell carcinoma there is a higher prevalence of G-T transversions and mutations at A:T base pairs. TP 53 mutations have been shown to be strongly associated with tobacco smoking and alcohol consumption in squamous cell carcinogenesis. P53 protein accumulation is an early event in this carcinogenesis. In addition, P53 immunohistochemistry has been assessed in squamous dysplasia in patients with and without cancer [17]. Distinct differences were found between the groups of patients and as such may have potential to help identify possible high risk dysplasia of the oesophagus.

DNA aneuploidy is associated with dysplasia and detected in 50% of moderate to severely dysplastic cells (similar to carcinoma in situ). As with P53 immunohistochemistry, distinct differences are found in squamous cell dysplasia between patients with and without cancer when analysing DNA ploidy [17] and again this may have potential for risk stratification of squamous dysplasia for malignant progression.

Cellular adhesion relies upon cadherin–catenin complexes and in the normal squamous mucosa of the oesophagus there is membranous co-expression of E- and P-cadherin in the basal compartment, whereas suprabasal stratification is associated with preservation of E-cadherin expression but loss of P-cadherin. Squamous dysplasia and carcinoma in situ have an increase in the proportion of cells within the epithelial compartment showing co-expression of E- and P-cadherin with appropriate expression of beta and gamma catenin [18]. This increased expression of P-cadherin is found early in tumorigenesis. In addition, cadherin–catenin complexes are linked with tumour invasiveness, with loss of complexes associated with poorly differentiated, invasive cancers.

Cyclin D1 is important in controlling the progression of cells through the cell cycle. Oral-oesophageal tissue specific cyclin D1 expression with Epstein–Barr virus promoter in transgenic mice results in dysplasia. In addition, in view of the likely interplay between environmental and genetic factors in oesophageal squamous carcinogenesis, the interaction between nitrosamines and cyclin D1 expression has been assessed in the transgenic mouse [19]. It was found that cyclin D1 overexpression and nitrosamines may cooperate to increase the severity of oesophageal squamous dysplasia.

Changes in cytokeratin and lectin binding have been identified in oesophageal squamous dysplasia. These changes are found in non-atypical cells in oesophageal squamous dysplasia, which are morphologically indistinguishable from normal mucosa. This also supports the field change hypothesis in squamous cell carcinogenesis.

## Diagnosis

Squamous epithelial dysplasia may be identified by endoscopically abnormal mucosa. However, some foci can be missed using routine endoscopic examination. Various methods have been tried to improve detection of dysplastic lesions, the most widely being the dye Lugol iodine. This is a cheap, easy method with no associated severe side effects. It contains potassium iodide and iodine and has an affinity for glycogen in non-keratinised squamous epithelium, staining it dark brown. Dysplastic or malignant lesions as well as inflamed/scarred areas do not stain as they lack glycogen. Lugol iodine solution improves endoscopic detection and delineation of dysplasia and carcinoma, increasing sensitivity to 96%, albeit with some loss of specificity, for high grade dysplasia and carcinoma.

## Screening and Surveillance

In high risk areas for squamous cell carcinoma, mass screening exists. This is, however, inappropriate in the Western world. The American Society of Gastrointestinal Endoscopy has discussed surveillance guidelines for three high risk conditions. Achalasia has insufficient data to support its use but caustic ingestion and patients with tylosis should both be screened. It has also been recommended by some that surveillance should also be performed on patients with the Plummer–Vinson syndrome, previous oesophageal cancer (after curative treatment), and patients with previous oropharyngeal cancer. Unfortunately no firm guidelines are established.

## Treatment

Dysplasia and tumours confined to the mucosa have a better prognosis, as they are thought to have no risk of spread and as such less invasive procedures are being assessed for these lesions. Reports of endoscopic mucosal resection (EMR) for dysplasia and early cancer report no recurrence after 20–39 months follow-up, with few complications. Criteria have been established for those lesions in which EMR may be considered (Table 19.4).

Photodynamic therapy (PDT) has also been investigated as a treatment for early cancer or

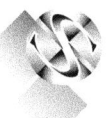

Table 19.4. Limitations and inclusion criteria for endoscopic curative treatment of oesophageal cancers defined by Lambert (Endoscopy 2000;32:322–30)

| | |
|---|---|
| Dimensions | 2 cm |
| Transverse extension | 30% |
| Histology | Squamous high grade dysplasia/cancer |
| Depth of invasion | m1, m2, m3? |
| Safety margin of resection | 2 mm |

dysplastic lesions which are non-visible and cannot be treated by EMR. Selective tumour destruction is induced after sensitising the lesion with a specialised sensitiser and then illuminating it with laser light at an appropriate wavelength. PDT for early squamous cell carcinoma has a response rate of 50–100% depending on factors such as light and drug dose. The largest series reports a 74% 5-year disease specific survival rate [20]. The sensitiser 5-ALA has been assessed in dysplasia, with a response rate of 100%. Further sensitisers, which may be more potent, are being evaluated.

Unfortunately to date there exists no randomised controlled trials comparing EMR or PDT with the gold standard treatment (surgery and radiotherapy) of dysplasia or early cancer.

## Summary

- Squamous epithelial dysplasia predisposes to squamous cell carcinoma of the oesophagus.
- There is wide geographic variation in incidence.
- Genetic, dietary and environmental factors are thought to be aetiological factors.
- Endoscopy and dye staining is very sensitive at detecting dysplasia and carcinoma.
- Mass screening programmes exist in high risk areas.
- No firm guidelines for screening exist in the Western world.
- Surgery with/without radiotherapy remains the gold standard treatment.
- Endoscopic mucosal resection and photodynamic therapy are being evaluated.

# Esophageal Squamous Papilloma

## Epidemiology

Squamous papillomas are uncommon in humans and usually discovered incidentally. They are found more frequently in animal models treated with N-nitroso compounds, where they may be precancerous or paracancerous (i.e. remain benign but coexist with separate carcinomas). They can occur at any age and have been reported in children as young as 1 month old. There is discrepancy in the reported literature as to whether or not there is a male preponderance.

Esophageal papillomas are composed of finger-like projections of hyperplastic squamous epithelium covering a connective tissue core containing small blood vessels. Most are small, measuring 2–5 mm, but lesions up to 6 cm have been described. The majority of papillomas are found in the distal oesophagus and are usually single lesions. The malignant potential of papillomas has been debated and is not fully resolved. Atypia is very rare and a papilloma has never been described as invasive. It should be noted that generally squamous cell carcinoma of the oesophagus is not associated with papillomas. Tylosis, however, is the exception to this. It is a rare autosomal dominant condition marked by hyperkeratosis of the palms of the hands and soles of the feet. It is associated with multiple oesophageal papillomas and oropharyngeal leukoplakia. Approximately 50% will develop squamous cell carcinoma by the age of 45 years and 95% by the age of 65. The gene locus for esophageal cancer in tylosis has recently been mapped to 17q25 by linkage analysis [21].

## Aetiology

The pathogenesis is not known. Chronic mucosal irritation and infection with human papilloma virus (HPV) are proposed aetiologies. Over half of papillomas can be demonstrated to contain HPV by polymerase chain reaction, most commonly types 16 and 18 [22]. In addition, most papillomas are associated with chronic and often severe forms of esophageal mucosal irritation such as oesophagitis or Barrett's oesophagus. It has also been reported that papillomas may occur as a complication of metal stent insertion, probably secondary to mucosal injury. As such the aetiology is likely to be multifactorial and it may be that mucosal irritation and HPV act synergistically in the development of papillomas.

## Treatment and Prognosis

Of the 161 reported cases of papillomas, the treatment has been described in 96. Surgery has been performed for large papillomas and a case of multiple lesions causing dysphagia. By far the majority, however, are treated endoscopically by forcep removal or diathermy snare. Follow-up observations are scant. It seems that after treatment recurrence is rare. Some patients have been left untreated and no modifications in the lesions have been found during a follow-up of between 2 months and 10 years[23].

## Summary

- Oesophageal squamous papillomas are rare.
- The malignant potential is thought to be very low.
- Human papilloma virus and chronic mucosal irritation are thought to be involved in the pathogenesis.
- Endoscopic removal is suggested and recurrence is rare.

## Questions

1. How does BO differ from columnar lined oesophagus?
2. What is the role of the mucosal inflammatory infiltrate in BO?
3. What is the role of acid suppression and antireflux surgery in the management of BO and does it prevent progression of BO?
4. Which patients with reflux symptoms should be screened for BO?
5. What is the current gold standard for cancer risk in BO and is it reliable?
6. What is the risk of progression of squamous epithelial dyslasia to cancer?
7. In what way may alcohol metabolism be involved in squamous epithelial dysplasia?
8. What changes in cadherin and catenin expression are found in squamous epithelial dysplasia?
9. In the Western world who should undergo surveillance for squamous epithelial dysplasia?
10. What aetiological links exist between squamous cell carcinoma of the oesophagus and oesophageal squamous papilloma?

## References

1. Cameron AJ, Lomboy CT Pera M et al. Adenocarcinoma of oesophagogastric junction and Barrett's oesophagus. Gastroenterology 1992;103(4):1241–45.
2. Jankowski J, Harrison R, Perry I et al. Barrett's metaplasia. Lancet 2000;356:2079–85.
3. Drewitz DJ, Sampliner RE, Garewal HS. The incidence of adenocarcinoma in Barrett's esophagus: a prospective study of 170 patients followed 4.8 years. Am J Gastroenterol 1997;92:212–15.
4. Poynton AR, Walsh TN, O'Sullivan G, Hennessy TPJ. Carcinoma arising in familial Barrett's esophagus. Am J Gastroenterol 1996;91:1855–6.
5. Jankowski J, Hopwood D, Pringle R, Wormsley K. Increased expression of EGFR in Barrett's esophagus associated with alkaline reflux: a putative model for carcinogenesis. Am J Gastroenterol 1993;56:1480–3.
6. Klump B, Hsieh CJ, Holzman K et al. Hypermethylation of the CDKNZ/p16 promoter during neoplastic progression of Barrett's esophagus. Gastroenterology 1998;115: 1381–86.
7. Wong DJ, Barrett MT, Stoger R et al. p16/NK4a promoter is hypermethylated at a higher frequency in esophageal adenocarcinoma. Cancer Res 1997;57: 2619–22.
8. Morales CP, Lee EL, Shay JW. In situ hybridisation for the detection of telomerase RNA in the progression from Barrett's esophagus to esophageal adenocarcinoma. Cancer 1998;83:652–9.
9. Reid BJ, Haggitt RC, Rubin CE et al. Flow-cytometric and histological progression to malignancy in Barrett's esophagus: prospective endoscopic surveillance of a cohort. Gastroenterology 1992;102:1212–19.
10. Richards FM, McKee SA, Rajpar MH et al. Germ-line E-cadherin gene (CDH1) mutations predispose to familial gastric and colorectal cancer. Hum Mol Genet 1999;4: 607–10.
11. Funkhouser EM, Sharp GB. Aspirin and reduced risk of esophageal carcinoma. Cancer 1995;76:1116–19.
12. Thun MJ, Namboodiuri MM, Calle EE et al. Aspirin use and risk of fatal cancer. Cancer Res 1993;53:1322–27.
13. Edwards MJ, Gable DR, Lentsch AB et al. The rationale for oesophagectomy as the optimal therapy for Barrett's

14. Canto MI, Setrakian S, Willis J et al. Methylene blue-directed biopsies improve detection of intestinal metaplasia and dysplasia in Barrett's esophagus. Gatsrointest Endosc 2000;51(5):560–8.
15. Endlicher E, Knuechel R, Hauser T et al. Endoscopic fluorescence detection of low and high grade dysplasia in Barrett's oesophagus using systemic or local 5-aminolaevulinic acid sensitisation Gut 2001;48:314–319.
16. Muto M, Hitomi Y, Ohtsu A et al. Association of aldehyde dehydrogenase 2 gene polymorphism with multiple oesophagea dysplasia in head and neck cancer patients. Gut 2000;47(2):256–61.
17. Itakura Y, Sasano F, Date F et al. DNA ploidy, p53 expression and cellular proliferation in normal epithelium and squamous dysplasia of non-cancerous and cancerous human oesophagi. Anticancer Res 1996;16(1):201–8.
18. Sanders DS, Bruton R, Darnton SJ et al. Sequential changes in cadherin–catenin expression associated with the progression and heterogeneity of primary oesophageal squamous carcinoma. Int J Cancer 1998;79(6):573–9.
19. Jenkins TD, Mueller A, Odze R et al. Cyclin D1 overexpression combined with N-nitrosomethylbenzylamine increases dysplasia and cellular proliferation in murine esophageal squamous epithelium. Oncogene 1999;18(1):59–66.
20. Sibble A, Lambert R, Souquet JC et al. Long-term survival after PDT for esophageal cancer. Gastroenterology 1995;108:337–46.
21. Risk JM, Whittaker J, Fryer A et al. Tylosis oesophageal cancer mapped. Nat Genet 1994;8:319–21.
22. Odze R, Antonioli D, Shocket D et al. Esophageal squamous papillomas. A clinicopathologic study of 38 lesions and analysis for human papilloma virus by the polymerase chain reaction. Am J Surg Pathol 1993;17(8):803–12.
23. Orlowska J, Jarosz D, Gugulski A et al. Squamous cell papillomas of the esophagus: Report of 20 cases and literature review. Am J Gastroenterol 1994;89(3):319–21.

# 20

# High Risk Lesions in the Stomach

Marc C. Winslet and S. Frances Hughes

## Aims

To identify high risk lesions and explore pathology.

## Introduction

Gastric cancer remains a common cause of death worldwide, but the incidence is declining [1]. There is evidence to support a stepwise sequence of histological changes in gastric carcinogenesis from inflammatory gastritis, gastric atrophy to intestinal metaplasia, dysplasia and finally intestinal type gastric carcinoma [2]. Dysplasia may also arise de novo in non-metaplastic glands as a precursor of diffuse type gastric carcinoma.

## Atrophic Gastritis and Gastric Atrophy

Atrophic gastritis is a common condition whose incidence increases directly with age [4]. Screening studies of a healthy Japanese population revealed atrophic gastritis in over half the study population with the vast majority related to the presence of *Helicobacter pylori* [3]. Figures of 15–30% are recorded in Western populations. One to three per cent of patients with inflamed gastric mucosa will have evidence of atrophic gastritis and cohort studies indicate this occurs almost exclusively in the presence of preceding chronic gastritis. Chronic gastritis is frequently found in association with gastric cancer, but whether it is itself precancerous is debatable. Gastric atrophy is defined as the loss of gastric acid producing glands, which develops as a progression from chronic atrophic gastritis.

Atrophic gastritis has been classified into two major groups, autoimmune type A, which is associated with pernicious anaemia, and environmental type B.

Type A chronic atrophic gastritis is an autoimmune disease associated with disorders of the thyroid and adrenal glands. The changes in type A occur predominantly in the fundus and body with antral sparing and may be found in patients with or without overt pernicious anaemia. Initially pathological changes are superficial, affecting the foveolar mucosal region, with subsequent progression to the deeper layers and destruction of parietal and chief cells. End-stage disease results in gastric atrophy, achlorhydria and hypergastrinaemia [4]. Autoantibodies to intrinsic factor result in megaloblastic anaemia due to $B_{12}$ deficiency. The incidence of gastric carcinoma in patients with pernicious anaemia is three to four times that of the general population, with 2% of patients with pernicious anaemia developing overt gastric cancer [5].

Type B atrophic gastritis is more prevalent and increases with age. It is seen with greatest

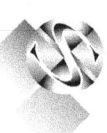

frequency in areas with the highest incidence of gastric cancer. It is multifocal in nature and usually arises from the antrum and body. In type B atrophic gastritis, gastric acid secretion may be low, normal or increased. The vast majority of patients are asymptomatic, but type B disease may be associated with non-steroidal anti-inflammatory drugs (NSAIDs), alcohol, smoking and biliary reflux. The major aetiological agent is *Helicobacter pylori* infection. The prevalence of *H. pylori* infection varies from 40 to 80% and is influenced by associated economic factors. It causes gastritis in almost all cases, irrespective of symptomatology and is strongly implicated in the pathogenesis of gastric cancer [6]. The presence of *H. pylori* results in inflammation, apoptosis and direct gland injury followed by regeneration in the majority of cases.

In others, functional glands lose the ability to regenerate, resulting in fibrosis and atrophy. Simultaneously the chief and mucus cells of the stomach are replaced by intestinal type epithelium containing goblet cells. These two markers, subsequently influenced by external factors, are the forerunner of intestinal type gastric carcinoma. The risk of developing cancer in the presence of atrophic gastritis is 10% over 10 years.

## The Influence of Bacterial, Genetic and Environmental Factors in Atrophic Gastritis and Gastric Atrophy

Cancer risk may vary with different strains of *H. pylori*, with the maximal extent of gastric atrophy associated with the cytotoxin-associated gene A (Cag A) gene product. Cag A may be associated with an exaggerated inflammatory response and increased epithelial cell proliferation, abnormal mucus secretion and mutation induction. The vacuolating cytotoxin (Vac A) gene product also has a positive influence on the development of carcinoma, with possible polymorphism influencing whether ulceration or neoplasia develops [7].

Several host factors may influence susceptibility to neoplasia. There may be a genetic susceptibility to the degree of inflammation induced by *H. pylori*. There may also be a variable response in terms of gastric acid secretion leading to severe atrophy, a reduction in parietal cell mass, increasing hypoacidity and increased (pre-) malignant potential. HLA status may influence the development of atrophic gastritis.

A variety of environmental factors have been implicated in the development of gastric atrophy. In vitro studies, have shown that sodium chloride increases mutagenicity of nitrosamine-related food as well as inflammatory changes and atrophy. It may act as a co-carcinogen with *H. pylori*. The formation of nitrosamines promotes atrophic gastritis and intestinal metaplasia. Antioxidants such as ascorbic acid and vitamin E may inhibit the conversion of nitrates to such mutagens [8].

Duodenogastric reflux promotes bacterial proliferation and mutagen production. Long-term acid suppression may increase atrophic gastritis.

## Pathology

The precise definition of atrophic gastritis, other than the absence of gastric glands, is controversial, resulting in problems in classification, diagnosis and prognosis.

Unfortunately there are few cellular markers associated with atrophic gastritis or gastric atrophy. Indirect markers of proliferation such as AgNORS (silver staining nucleolar organising regions) have been shown to be increased. There is little to confirm changes in p53 mutation in the premalignant stomach and their significance remains unclear.

Serological markers in the form of pepsinogen 1 and 2 ratio may be associated with a progression to gastric atrophy [9].

Pepsinogen 1 is normally secreted by T cells in the corpus, with low levels indicating gastric atrophy. Pepsinogen 2 normally originates in the antral glands but may also be secreted by pre-neoplastic or neoplastic cells. A low pepsinogen 1:2 ratio is a reliable marker for atrophic gastritis. This ratio is significantly lower in the presence of *H. pylori*. Serum gastrin is a marker of the degree of gastric atrophy in the presence of *H. pylori*.

## Natural History

The proportion of patients with atrophic gastritis who progress to atrophy is unknown whilst the transition from superficial gastritis to atrophic gastritis is approximately 5% per year.

The cancer risk varies and is highest in type B with extensive mulifocal involvement. The risk is proportionate to the degree of atrophy, which predisposes to intestinal metaplasia. This progression in turn is influenced by factors such as age, the presence of bile reflux and antioxidants.

## Management

There may be some benefit in recommending a reduced salt intake and increased vitamin C supplementation in high cancer risk areas but both factors may only influence the disease process at a fairly late stage.

Whilst *H. pylori* eradication may help in peptic ulcer disease, the benefits in relation to gastric cancer are controversial and unproven [10]. Eradication may cause regression of intestinal metaplasia, but similar findings for atrophic gastritis and atrophy are unconfirmed. Gastric atrophy with associated dense inflammatory infiltrate is reversible by eradication therapy unless replacement is with fibroblasts. The role for *H. pylori* eradication is convincing in association with mucosa associated lymphoid tumours (MALT) and there is a strong argument for eradication after early gastric cancer resection in order to reduce the rate of recurrence [11].

The histological interpretation of endoscopic biopsies is difficult due to surrounding inflammation. Eradication of *H. pylori* with subsequent 6-monthly biopsies is required. As the available natural history data indicates that progression from atrophic gastritis to atrophy occurs over years, as does the progression from early gastric cancer to advanced disease, the policy of serial surveillance and biopsy seems appropriate. The frequency remains controversial but 5-yearly, increasing to 3-yearly in high risk areas and individuals, may be appropriate [12].

## Intestinal Metaplasia

Intestinal metaplasia is the functional morphological transformation of gastric epithelial and glandular secretory type cells to intestinal absorptive type epithelium containing goblet cells. This is the forerunner of intestinal-type gastric carcinoma.

Intestinal metaplasia is classified according to the type of mucins produced and crypt histology. Type I or complete intestinal metaplasia resembles small bowel mucosa and produces neutral sialomucins. Type II has goblet cells containing acid mucins with columnar cells secreting sialomucins. Type III or incomplete intestinal metaplasia resembles colonic mucosa with distorted crypts and produces sulphomucins. Type III carries the highest risk of malignant transformation. Intestinal metaplasia is usually multifocal and invariably associated with *H. pylori*. Such cells are thought to arise from mutation of undifferentiated stem cells.

Intestinal metaplasia and atrophic gastritis may occur together or independently and increase with age. This may be due in part to the relationship with *H. pylori*. The relationship between intestinal metaplasia and *H. pylori* infestation is variable, with reduced positivity reported in patients with type III disease. Its overall role may be as an initiator or co-factor [13]. The relationship between intestinal metaplasia and Cag A is variable. Glycentin, an intestinal polypeptide hormone that promotes intestinal metaplasia, is increased in mucosa associated with *H. pylori*.

As with atrophic gastritis, antioxidants may play an important role in aetiology. Vitamin C inhibits the conversion of nitrates to nitrosomutagens, which encourage the progression of atrophic gastritis to intestinal metaplasia. Patients with intestinal metaplasia have reduced serum levels of Vitamin C and increased nitroso compound concentrations.

Vitamin E may also reverse intestinal metaplasia but the site of action is unknown. In Japan, a diet rich in dried fish, low in Vitamin A and with a high pickle intake also promotes intestinal metaplasia.

Bile reflux may promote intestinal metaplasia in the presence of *H. pylori* by raising the gastric pH and increasing bacterial proliferation and mutagenic expression.

## Natural History

The progression of gastric atrophy to intestinal metaplasia is dependent on alteration of the gastric milieu. The subsequent development of neoplasia in patients with intestinal metaplasia appears to be dependent on histological subtype, distribution and the expression of genotypic and phenotypic markers.

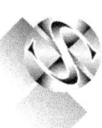

There is some evidence to suggest that the risk of cancer is increased in type III intestinal metaplasia compared to type I but this is not universally supported [14]. This uncertainty may be compounded by the progression of type I to type III intestinal metaplasia as a reflection of prolonged mucosal injury [15].

The more widespread the intestinal metaplasia, the greater the proportion of type III with possible increased malignant potential.

Various cellular markers have been advocated to identify high risk metaplasia including the presence of sulphomucins, PCNA (proliferating cell nuclear antigen) expression and mucin peptide core antigens including MUC II.

Cellular proliferation is raised in premalignant lesions, with type III intestinal metaplasia having the highest index with increased apoptosis compared to type I. Variable p53 mutations have been reported. This on the whole is a late event detectable predominantly in dysplasia and not in earlier premalignant lesions. pS2 protein expression may be an early event in the development of intestinal-type gastric cancer, with 100% positivity in type I intestinal metaplasia [16]. The transforming growth factor (TGF) beta receptor abnormalities, due to microsatellite instability, appear to be important in gastric carcinogenesis. The epidermal growth factor (EGF) R2 receptor is overexpressed in gastric cancer. TGF-$\alpha$ and EGF R1 overexpression has been observed in intestinal metaplasia with malignant change, but not in metaplasia alone.

## Management

The management strategies for intestinal metaplasia are similar to those for atrophic gastritis.

There is evidence to suggest that a diet high in the antioxidant vitamin C may be beneficial. As well as inhibiting the growth of *H. pylori*, vitamin C inhibits production of nitrosomutagens by the increased bacteria resulting from reduced gastric acidity.

Low vitamin E levels have been reported in association with gastric cancer, with evidence to suggest that regression of intestinal metaplasia may be achieved with a diet rich in vitamin E.

Regression in intestinal metaplasia has been reported after eradication of *H. pylori* but this finding was not universal. Macroscopically intestinal metaplasia appears as small grey plaques. In view of our understanding of the natural history of gastric carcinoma, there is evidence to suggest that surveillance endoscopy every 5 years may be appropriate, with increased frequency in high risk individuals and areas.

# Dysplasia

Dysplasia may be defined as an area of epithelium where atypical cellular proliferation is occurring with loss of orderly maturation of cells. The area is marked by atypical glandular formation, pleomorphic nuclei and increased mitosis dependent on degree. The grading of dysplasia into mild, moderate or severe is dependent on the severity of these changes. Several systems have been devised but considerable inter-observer variation remains [17,18].

The presence of dysplastic epithelium implies irreversible inheritable change in the genome without phenotypic expression of malignancy with regard to its ability to invade.

Dysplasia may be divided into two types. Type I or adenomatous dysplasia results from gastric atrophy via intestinal metaplasia and is a precursor for intestinal-type gastric carcinoma [17]. Type II arises in non-metaplastic glands and is associated with diffuse gastric cancer [17,18]. Non-metaplastic dysplasia may be seen in association with hyperplastic polyps, juvenile polyps and fundic gland polyps.

The presence of all grades of dysplasia increases with age. Dysplastic lesions may arise from progression of type III intestinal metaplasia or from other lesions which do not contain metaplastic cells such as polyps. Non-metaplastic dysplasia is usually identified in focal lesions of the stomach but this may represent sampling bias. Dyplasia is probably most frequently identified from macroscopically normal mucosa followed by gastric ulcers and then polypoid lesions [19].

## Aetiology

As before, disease progression is influenced by the environment, with salt, the antioxidant beta carotene and tobacco smoking being influential.

The development of gastric cancer is related to the rate of proliferation and cell maturation, and expansion of the proliferative compartment, abnormal differentiation with failure of normal cell maturation and the rate of apoptosis [20,21].

The relationship between *H. pylori* and dysplasia is unclear as previously discussed [22,23].

Previous partial gastrectomy for benign disease is associated with dysplasia in the gastric stump secondary to bile reflux, which may be premalignant. Two patterns of neoplasia have been described. Cancers in the gastric body are associated with intestinal metaplasia and dysplasia while tumours in the stump arise from non-metaplastic dysplasia.

## Markers of Dysplasia

The markers of dysplasia are those of cellular proliferation or increased apoptosis. There is evidence in well-differentiated tumours that both proliferation and apoptosis are increased whilst in poorly differentiated tumours there is an imbalance with more proliferation than apoptosis. There is evidence that apoptotic cells are more common in well rather than poorly differentiated tumours and that reduced apoptosis may contribute to tumour progression.

Abnormalities in p53 are common in dysplasia with mutation in 15–17% of cases [24]. The cell adhesion molecule E-cadherin is also lost in gastric cancer, as is catenin through which it interacts with the intracellular cytoskeleton [25].

## Natural History

Data on the natural history of dysplasia are poor but regression has been reported, ranging from 6% to 46% of cases [26,27]. This may be dependent on degree [19].

Progression of dysplasia to carcinoma is normally reported at less than 10%. This again may be influenced by degree. Progression of mild to moderate dysplasia is seen in 5% of cases whilst progression from moderate to severe dysplasia may occur in 20% [28]. The widely varying outcomes of studies of the natural history of dysplastic lesions may partly be due to sampling errors on sequential biopsies as well as different interpretation of pathological grade.

## Management

As before, chemoprevention with vitamin C may be beneficial even though nitrosomutagens are not implicated in the progression of intestinal metaplasia to dysplasia. Carotenoids may be more important in the prevalence of the development of dysplasia [29].

The management of dysplastic lesions of the stomach depends on the macroscopic appearance of the lesion and its assigned grade.

When dysplasia is identified in a macroscopically normal area, providing it is low grade, surveillance can be safely adopted in view of the rates of progression [19]. *Helicobacter pylori* should be eradicated and repeat endoscopy should be performed at 3 months surveying the whole stomach. If the stomach is macroscopically normal with no evidence of dysplasia and *Helicobacter* eradication is complete, subsequent surveillance by further endoscopy is only required for further symptoms.

The progression of moderate dysplasia to carcinoma is more common and further endoscopic surveillance should be performed at one year. The high rate of progression of severe dysplasia suggests that some form of ablation should be undertaken. If the dysplasia is localised this may allow a more limited surgical resection.

The identification of dysplasia in the presence of a discrete macroscopic lesion is managed differently. Severely dysplastic discrete gastric lesions should be removed. In the absence of invasive malignancy with lymph node involvement minimally invasive surgical or endoscopic techniques may be appropriate [30]. Eradication of *H. pylori* reduces the incidence of further dysplastic lesions after resection of early gastric carcinoma and eradication should therefore be ensured after local resection.

## Gastric Polyps

Gastric polyps have been classified into two major groups: the hyperplastic/regenerative polyps and the adenomas. The hyperplastic polyps account for 75–95% of all gastric polyps. They arise from excessive regeneration of epithelium with no distinction between the polyp and normal gastric mucosa. Malignant transformation is rare. An associated independent carcinoma, however, may be seen in between 6.5% and 25% of cases.

Adenomas account for between 8% and 25% of gastric polyps. True neoplasms have a distinct margin from surrounding mucosa with associated intestinal metaplasia and frequent mitotic figures. Malignant transformation is seen in 6–75% with a lower incidence in small flat adenomas and an increased risk in adenomas over 2 cm in diameter.

The management of gastric polyps is largely dependent on size and histological findings on biopsy. Polyps less than 2 cm in diameter have a low malignant potential and do not require removal [31]. Ginsberg et al [32], however, have suggested that in a small number of patients there was a significant incidence of dysplasia or carcinoma in situ in all polyps over 0.5 cm in size. As biopsy sampling may be non-representative, removal of all polyps greater than this size has been recommended. This area remains controversial and a pragmatic management pathway based on available criteria is required.

## Questions

1. What is the suggested pathway to development of gastric cancer?
2. What role does *H. pylori* play?
3. Describe the types of intestinal metaplasia.
4. What is recommended to treat and reverse these changes?
5. What type of gastric polyp is a high risk lesion?

## References

1. Mayers WC, Damiano RJ, Rotoro FS, Postlethwait RW. Adenocarcinoma of the stomach: changing patterns over the last 4 decades. Ann Surg 1987;205:1–8.
2. Correa P, Haenszell W, Cuello C et al. A model for gastric cancer epidemiology. Lancet 1975;ii:58–60.
3. Asaka M, Kudo M, Kato T, et al. Review article: long term *Helicobacter pylori* infection – from gastritis to gastric cancer. Aliment Pharmacol Ther 1998;12:9–15.
4. Siurala M, Lehtola J, Ihamaki T. Atrophic gastritis and its sequelae: results of 19–23 years follow up examinations. Scand J Gastroenterol 1974;9:441.
5. Hsing AW, Hansson LE, McLaughlin JK et al. Pernicious anaemia and subsequent cancer: a population based cohort study. Cancer 1993;71:745–50.
6. Parsonnet J, Friedman GD, Vandersteen DP et al. *Helicobacter pylori* infection and the risk of gastric cancer. N Engl J Med 1991;325:1127–31.
7. Atherton JC, Peek R, Tham KT et al. Clinical and pathological importance of heterogeneity in Vac A, the vacuolating cytotoxin gene of *Helicobacter pylori*. Gastroenterology 1997;112:92–9.
8. Block G. Vitamin C and cancer prevention. The epidemiological evidence. Am J Clin Nutr 1991;53:2705–825.
9. Knight T, Greaves S, Wilson A et al. Variability in serum pepsinogen levels in an asymptomatic population. Eur J Gastroenterol Hepatol 1995;7:647–54.
10. Uemura N, Mukai T, Okamoto S et al. *Helicobacter pylori* eradication inhibits the growth of intestinal type of gastric cancer in its initial stage. Gastroenterology 1996;110:A282.
11. Wotherspoon AC, Doglioni C, Diss TC. Regression of primary low grade B cell gastric lymphoma of mucosa associated lymphoid tissue after eradication of *Helicobacter pylori*. Lancet 1993;342:575–7.
12. Sjoblom SM, Sipponen P, Jarvinen H. Gastroscopic follow up of pernicious anaemia patients. Gut 1993;34:28–32.
13. Cahill, RJ, Killgallen C, Beattie S et al. Gastric epithelial cell kinetics in the progression of normal mucosa to gastric carcinoma. Gut 1996;38:177–81.
14. Huang CB, Xu J, Huang JF, Meng XY. Sulphomucin colonic type intestinal metaplasia and carcinoma of the stomach. Cancer 1986;57:1370–5.
15. Silva S, Filipe MI, Pinho A. Variants of intestinal metaplasia in the evolution of chronic atrophic gastritis and gastric ulcer. A follow up study. Gut 1990;31:1097–105.
16. Semba S, Yokozaki H, Yamamoto S et al. Microsatellite instability in precancerous lesions and adenocarcinomas of the stomach. Cancer 1996;77:1620–7.
17. Jass JR. A classification of gastric dysplasia. Histopathology 1983;7:181–93.
18. Morson BC, Sobin LH, Grundmann E et al. Precancerous conditions and epithelial dysplasia in the stomach. J Clin Pathol 1980;33:711–21.
19. Rugge M, Farinati F, Baffa R et al. Gastric epithelial dysplasia in the natural history of gastric cancer: a multicentre prospective follow-up study. Interdisciplinary group on gastric epithelial dysplasia. Gastroenterology 1994;107:1288–96.
20. Lipkin M. Biomarkers of increased susceptibility to gastrointestinal cancer: new application to studies of cancer prevention in human subjects. Cancer Res 1988;48:235–45.
21. Moss SF, Calam J, Agarwal B et al. Induction of gastric epithelial cell apoptosis by *Helicobacter pylori*. Gut 1996;38:498–501.
22. The Eurogast study group. An international association between *Helicobacter pylori* infection with gastric cancer. Lancet 1993;341:1159–62.
23. Parsonnet J, Friedman GD, Vandersteen DP et al. *Helicobacter pylori* infection and the risk of gastric cancer. N Engl J Med 1991;325:1127–31.
24. Brito MJ, Williams GT, Thompson H, Filipe MI. Expression of p53 in early (T1) gastric carcinoma and precancerous adjacent mucosa. Gut 1994;35:1697–700.
25. Shimoyama Y, Hirohashi S. Expression of E- and P-cadherin in gastric carcinomas. Cancer Res 1991;51:2185–92.
26. Coma del Corral MJ, Pardo-Mindan FJ et al. Risk of cancer in patients with gastric dysplasia. Cancer 1990;65:2078–85.
27. Di Gregorio C, Morandi P, Fante R, De Gaetani C. Gastric dysplasia. A follow up study. Am J Gastroenterol 1993;88:1714–19.

28. Kokkola A, Haapiainen R, Laxen F et al. Risk of gastric carcinoma in patients with mucosal dysplasia associated with atrophic gastritis: a follow-up study. J Clin Pathol 1996;49:979–84.
29. Haenszel W, Correa P, Lopez A et al. Serum micronutrient levels in relation to gastric pathology. Int J Cancer 1985;36:43–8.
30. Noda M, Kodama T, Atsumi M et al. Possibilities and limitations of endoscopic resection for early gastric cancer. Endoscopy 1997;29:361–5.
31. Papa A, Cammarota G, Tursi A et al. Histologic types and surveillance of gastric polyps. Hepatogastroenterology 1998;45:579–82.
32. Ginsberg GG, Al-Kawas FM, Fleischer DE et al. Gastric polyps; relationship of size and histology to cancer risk. Am J Gastroenterol 1996;91:714–17.

# 21

# Upper GI Endoscopy

Michael T. Hallissey

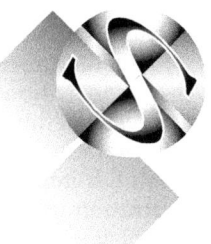

## Aims

- To identify the accuracy of endoscopy.
- To define the role of endoscopy in the assessment of upper GI disease.
- To document therapeutic opportunities in the upper GI tract.

The importance of the mucosa in the development of gastrointestinal (GI) disease has long been recognised, as has the impact of external events on mucosal behaviour. As a result, the ability to assess the mucosa of the upper GI tract has been recognised as an important part of the assessment of upper GI disease. It has been possible to visualise the upper GI tract for many years. This was initially with rigid oesophagoscopy, though semi-rigid endoscopes were developed allowing visualisation of the stomach. The latter technique was only available in selected centres with few procedures being undertaken and with limited ability to visualise the stomach.

The development of fibreoptic technology provided the opportunity to develop fibreoptic, indirect endoscopy and led eventually to the introduction of fibreoptic direct visualisation endoscopy. The recognition of the value of diagnostic endoscopy has resulted in a revolution in the ability to assess the GI tract and allow direct visualisation of and sampling of the mucosa.

From this experience, the technique of interventional endoscopy has developed with specialist therapeutic endoscopes. The introduction of modern solid-state devices has provided the next step in the development of flexible endoscopy with the introduction of video-endoscopy and most recently capsule endoscopy. This chapter outlines the value of endoscopy as a diagnostic and therapeutic tool in the upper GI tract.

## Diagnostic Upper GI Endoscopy

While rigid upper GI endoscopy still has a role in both the diagnosis and management of oesophageal pathology, fibreoptic endoscopy has become the standard method of assessing the upper GI tract.

When undertaking upper GI endoscopy, a number of systems are used to record the anatomy. In the oesophagus, position may be recorded as distance from the incisors, with the gastro-oesophageal junction normally lying at 40 cm in males and between 37 and 40 cm in females. The oesophagus can also be divided into upper, middle and lower thirds. Both of these systems are subjective and are influenced by the presence of a hiatus hernia that can vary in size between individuals and over time.

The area of the stomach can be defined either in relation to the distance from the incisors or anatomically into cardia, fundus, body and antrum. The site can also be defined by its relation to the greater and lesser curves. Despite these conventions, variations in position occur as a result of the degree of gastric distension and interpretation by individual endoscopists. As a result it is important to define the site of lesions in relation to definable landmarks such as the oesophagogastric junction and incisura.

In the duodenum, position is recorded in relation to the parts, first, second, third or fourth. While the first part is easily identified by its appearance and the papilla will mark the centre of the second part, the more distal duodenum can be difficult to define anatomically. If it is important to ensure that the distal duodenum has been fully examined, undertaking endoscopy under fluoroscopy is helpful.

These conventions help in localising lesions in the upper GI tract but there is little published evidence on interobserver variation on lesion position. Anatomical localisation is probably defined more reliably by contrast radiology.

## Diagnostic Accuracy

The available forms of imaging of the upper GI tract should be viewed as complementary. Fibreoptic endoscopy allows direct visualisation of the mucosa of the GI tract and the fibreoptic endoscopes in general use allow samples to be obtained for pathological assessment. The accuracy of fibreoptic endoscopy has been compared in a number of studies with other modalities [1,2]. There are a number of confounding factors in assessing the accuracy of the technique, particularly around defining the gold standard against which the assessment is made. An overview study of the accuracy of a contrast radiology and fibreoptic endoscopy showed that the overall accuracy of radiology was 60% while the figure for endoscopy was over 90% [1]. The final diagnosis in this study was determined following an independent review of all modalities assessed after a period of follow-up to include clinical data.

## Pathological Assessment

The accuracy of endoscopic biopsies in the diagnosis of malignancy has been evaluated. In the best series the first biopsy will provide a positive result in 93 to 95% of cases, with this figure rising to between 98 and 100% after seven biopsies. However, some series have reported an overall accuracy of 85% for initial assessment. Cytology is commonly used in conjunction with biopsy and the question of the timing of the biopsy in relation to cytology has been raised. There is no evidence to show that biopsy before or after cytology influences the diagnostic accuracy of either test and the overall accuracy for the combined test is very high and will increase overall diagnostic rates to over 95% [3-5].

## Diagnostic Adjuncts

The diagnosis of pathology at endoscopy is frequently dependent on the recognition of abnormalities in the mucosal morphology. A number of techniques have been used to improve the visualisation of mucosal abnormalities. In the oesophagus, iodine can be sprayed onto the mucosa. Normal squamous epithelial cells contain glycogen that stains a dark brown with the iodine. Areas of epithelial dysplasia and neoplasia commonly fail to stain and are easily seen as pale areas surrounded by brown-stained normal mucosa [6].

In the stomach a number of dyes have been used to improve visualisation. Indigo-carmine has been used as a contrast agent to improve recognition of the mucosal pattern and improve the recognition of abnormal mucosal patterns. In addition, methylene blue and toluidine blue have been used to stain mucosal abnormalities as well as for improving visualisation of mucosal pattern. Both have been shown to stain neoplasms while methylene blue will stain areas of intestinal metaplasia. Congo red has also been used as a marker of mucosal function as it acts as a pH indicator, and maps areas of normal parietal function. All of these have been used to map mucosal abnormalities and are reported to improve recognition of gastric cancers [7-9].

The technique of mucosal mapping involves the use of proteolytic enzymes to remove the gastric muous covering to allow the dye access to the underlying mucosa. The combination used commonly includes 50 ml of sodium bicarbonate or phosphate buffer solution, 20 000 units of protease and 20 mg of dimethylpolysiloxane. In addition, hyoscine is used to reduce gastric secretion and motility to improve visualisation. This is left in situ for 10 to 30 minutes before application of the dye. Fifteen millilitres of 0.5% methylene blue is instilled into the stomach via a nasogastric tube and the patient lies on front, back and either side for 10 minutes to obtain maximal mucosal exposure prior to endoscopy. Methylene blue has been shown to stain 92% of cancers and up to 100% of cases of intestinal metaplasia [9].

In the upper stomach, cancers can be outlined against the areas of normal acid production. Congo red is a pH indicator which can be sprayed directly onto the gastric mucosa and areas of acid production, stimulated by pentagastrin injection, are identified by conversion from red to black. This technique demonstrates both gastric atrophy and neoplasia, increasing the recognition of cancers from 40% on routine endoscopy to 86% [10]. A combination of 0.05% methylene blue together with 0.3% Congo red can be sprayed directly onto the mucosa at endoscopy to identify areas of gastric acid production in addition to improving visualisation of mucosal irregularity and staining of areas metaplasia and cancer [11].

## Complications

The complications of diagnostic endoscopy have two distinct components: those related to the sedation and/or analgesia required to undertake the procedure and those related to the procedure itself. The risks of the sedation utilised in diagnostic endoscopy has been the subject of much research. With the improvement of non-invasive monitoring, the recognition of the dangers of intravenous sedation has increased and guidelines for their safe use have been widely implemented [12]. The complications related to the procedure include perforation, bleeding and intramural haematomas. These complications are commonest in the pharynx and oesophagus, though they can be seen in any part of the upper GI tract.

Perforation of the GI tract can be either intramural or transmural. Oesophageal perforations which do not breach the mediastinal pleura can be managed conservatively and the outcome is frequently good [13]. As a result of the risk of the development of mediastinitis, oesophageal perforation carries the risk of death if not recognised immediately following the procedure and managed aggressively. Perforations of the stomach and duodenum are into the peritoneal cavity and all require aggressive management. The majority require closure of the defect to control contamination of the peritoneal cavity. The standard approach is surgery but there are reports of closure of gastric perforations with endoscopically placed clips.

Another rare complication of diagnostic endoscopy is bleeding from biopsy sites. This may be bleeding from routine biopsy of mucosal abnormalities or less frequently as a result of biopsying a vascular lesion. These range from tumours through angiomas to unrecognised varices. In addition to overt haemorrhage, intramural haematomas may develop as a result of trauma from the endoscope or biopsy forceps or as a result of an endoscopic intervention. The mortality rate for diagnostic endoscopy in an audit of a number of endoscopy units in the UK was 1 in 2000 patients [14].

## Sedation Techniques in Endoscopy

A number of techniques are available to allow endoscopy to be performed. While it is possible to undertake fibreoptic endoscopy without any medication, the commonly used medications include throat spray with lidocaine (lignocaine) and sedation with benzodiazepines either alone or in combination with opiates. Trials comparing sedation with a benzodiazepine with lidocaine throat spray in patients happy to undergo endoscopy with either technique have shown equivalent patient satisfaction and success rate.

Lidocaine throat spray provides pharyngeal anaesthesia but also reduces laryngeal sensation and as a result carries a small risk of aspiration. Patients who receive lidocaine throat spray should be kept nil by mouth for at least 1 hour following administration and patients should then be advised to try small amounts of cold fluid to ensure return of laryngeal sensation and airway protection and adequate temperature sensation.

The commonly used benzodiazepines include diazepam, either as aqueous solution or emulsion, or midazolam. It is generally accepted that the normal maximum dose of midazolam is 5 mg and in the elderly 1 or 2 mg will be adequate. It is important to ensure adequate monitoring during the procedure. This must include pulse oximetry and the ability to deliver supplemental oxygen and the nursing support must be able to recognise and act on the available monitoring. The application of this approach has reduced the number of episodes of hypoxia seen and should impact on the number of adverse events during endoscopy.

## Appropriate Criteria for Endoscopy

The value of endoscopy as the primary diagnostic method for the upper GI tract has been established. The criteria for endoscopy vary through out the world. In the UK, evidence exists for the investigation of new dyspeptic patients over the age of 40 [15] as a method of increasing the detection of operable gastro-oesophageal cancer. However, by investigating all patients with alarm symptoms (dysphagia, weight loss, anaemia and prolonged vomiting), this age could probably be safely raised to the age of 50 with little loss of sensitivity for gastro-oesophageal cancer detection. In patients under the age of 50 with dyspepsia without alarm symptoms, there are no other defined criteria to select patients for endoscopy and there is much debate about the appropriate role of endoscopy in the management of this group. The present draft guidelines from the British Society of Gastroenterology suggest a policy of test and treat and symptomatic management for this age group.

## Therapeutic Endoscopy for Benign Disease

The introduction of fibreoptic endoscopy has extended the range of interventions undertaken in all parts of the upper GI tract. An overview of these interventions will be outlined by site below.

### Oesophageal Therapy

#### Oesophageal Dilatation

Among earliest interventions undertaken in endoscopy was dilatation of oesophageal strictures. The therapeutic technique used was to pass bougies under direct vision through a rigid oesophagoscope. This was the supplemented by larger bougies without the endoscope. This technique requires a general anaesthetic for each procedure.

With the introduction of fibreoptic endoscopy, the technique of endoscopic placement of a guidewire was developed allowing the passage of dilators over the guidewire under sedation. The initial dilators included a range of sizes on the same dilator, the Tridil and Celestin dilators. With the introduction of newer polymers, the move has been to single size dilators. The results of these techniques are well reported with a documented risk of perforation. The risk of perforation is influenced by the cause of the stricture, the initial size of the lumen and the degree of dilatation [16]. The alternative method when the stricture is short and a reasonable diameter is to use Maloney bougies which use a tapered flexible tip to guide the dilator through the stricture.

The introduction of through the scope (TTS) balloons has added a new method. Initially these were single size balloons which when inflated resulted in the balloon attaining a fixed size. Newer balloons have been devised which can attain a range of sizes depending on the inflation pressure. Dilatation by balloon produces dilation by imposing a radial force and this is felt to avoid the shearing force produced by bougies [17]. However, the size of balloon must be selected at the outset whereas with bougies, a skilled operator can use the force required to dilate to determine the diameter at which to terminate the procedure.

### Variceal Management

Therapeutic interventions in portal hypertension have been developed over the past few decades. Initially sclerosants were injected into the varix as a method of controlling or preventing bleeding. A variety of sclerosants have been used which have a range of general and specific complications. Variceal ablation has also been used to prevent haemorrhage and in combination with a beta-blocker is an effective method of reducing bleeding [18]. The most recent approach has been the development of variceal banding through the flexible endoscope. This has been shown to be superior to injection sclerotherapy as a method of prevention and control of variceal bleeding [19,20].

### Endoscopic Mucosal Resection

Removal of mucosal lesions from the oesophageal mucosa is also a technique which has been undertaken with both rigid and fibreoptic endoscopes. The use of snare resection for benign polyps has a low complication rate with bleeding and perforation being the most frequent. Much work has been undertaken to develop new and safer techniques for the removal of larger sections of mucosa. Initial techniques included grasp and snare excision where an area is raised up with saline with or without adrenaline (epinephrine) and a snare applied after the lesion has been grasped to lift it. This technique requires a twin channel endoscope.

The concept of mucosal resection has been developed with the introduction of the endoscopic cap. This technique involves the area of interest being sucked up into a cap applied to the end of the endoscope. A snare is positioned on a lip inside the end of the cap and this is tightened around the base of mucosa sucked into the cap. The base of mucosa within the cap is then diathermied to divide mucosa and the specimen is removed by sucking the area into the cap. The complications include perforation and haemorrhage. Mucosal resection is performed in large numbers in areas of China where early detection programmes have been in place for some years in regions of high risk [21–23].

## Gastric Therapy

### Removal of Gastric Foreign Bodies

A variety of ingested items have been removed from the stomach. These range from button batteries to razor blade cartridges. The usual technique includes the use of an overtube, while the instruments used to retrieve the foreign body include polyp graspers and snares.

### Pyloric Dilatation

Benign gastric disease rarely requires intervention. Dilation of the pyloric channel has been used in patients with fibrous stenosis secondary to peptic ulcer disease to avoid surgery. The technique is effective in a proportion of cases but with the introduction of proton pump inhibitor therapy and *Helicobacter* eradication, this is an uncommon condition. The technique uses TTS balloons and the sizes range from 8 to 15 mm. The balloon is inserted through the pylorus which is dilated under vision. The complications include perforation, though due to the fibrous nature of the stricture this is infrequent.

### Polypectomy

True gastric adenomas are uncommon, but are suitable for endoscopic removal. Adenomas are more frequently broad based than in the colon. However, they can be resected either by simple snare resection or by using the endoscopic cap. The use of snare resection for benign polyps has a low complication rate with bleeding and perforation being the most frequent.

### Gastric Varices

Gastric varices are particularly difficult to treat endoscopically and the range of options include sclerosant injection and banding. However, the use of cynaoacrylate glue has been reported to be particularly effective in the management of gastric varies [24].

## Therapeutic Endoscopy for Malignant Disease

### Oesophageal Cancer

Therapeutic procedures in oesophageal cancer can be undertaken with either curative or palliative intent.

Intervention with curative intent is possible in cases where the incidence of nodal disease is lower than the risk of intervention. For mucosal only cancers the incidence of nodal disease is low (0–8%) while extension into the submucosa is associated with a risk of nodal disease in excess of 10%. As a result, the development of endoscopic resection has provided a mechanism for the complete removal of mucosal cancers. The techniques available to deal with different morphologies of mucosal cancers include snare resection and endoscopic caps supplemented by argon, laser and photodynamic ablation.

For patients unsuitable for curative treatment, endoscopic approaches are based on the morphology of the tumour. When the cancer is exophytic, one of the techniques of tumour ablation is useful. The techniques include snare resection, intratumoral injection of alcohol and laser and argon ablation. The reported results of

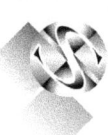

these techniques show them to be effective in the management of dysphagia though they require repeated application. Each is associated with both the general complications of endoscopy and procedure-specific complications. For techniques that use energy sources such as laser and argon plasma beam, the most significant risk is perforation due to transmural thermal injury. The techniques require multiple applications to obtain control of the tumour bulk and further applications to maintain that control.

For stenosing tumours, dilatation can palliate dysphagia. The techniques are identical to those used in benign disease, either TTS balloon or over an endoscopically placed guide-wire. The risk of perforation is higher than in benign disease and it is important to recognise that dysphagia can be the result of loss of peristalsis as well as due to the physical diameter of the stricture.

For stenosing tumours or where the frequency of therapy is too great, insertion of an oesophageal stent provides a mechanism to maintain an oesophageal lumen. These were initially rigid stents inserted using a rigid oesophagoscope. Following the introduction of the flexible endoscope, guide-wire delivered stent insertion systems were developed including the Atkinson system. The insertion of these stents is associated with specific complications in addition to the general complications of endoscopy. The specific complications include perforation during the process of insertion and stent migration that may be associated with perforation further down the GI tract. This approach dominated the 1980s until the introduction of self-expanding metal stents (SEMS) which are also delivered over a guide-wire system. The suggested benefits of the self-expanding metal stents were a reduction in the risk of perforation during insertion and the ability of the stent to transmit waves of oesophageal peristalsis. Comparison of the rates of perforation over a 5-year review of all oesophageal cancers treated in the West Midlands has shown a perforation rate of 1% in rigid stent insertion and 0% in SEMS.

The SEMS were initially uncovered but there were problems with tumour in-growth through the metal mesh and therefore plastic covering of all or part of the stent has become common. In addition, for stents that cross the gastro-oesophageal junction stents with flap valves on the distal end have been designed to prevent reflux of gastric contents through the stent. A variety of patterns of stent are currently in use with a number of deployment mechanisms.

## Gastric Cancer

Therapeutic procedures in gastric cancer can be undertaken with either curative or palliative intent.

### Endoscopic Mucosal Resection

Intervention with curative intent is possible in cases where the incidence of nodal disease is lower than the risk of intervention. For mucosal only cancers the incidence of nodal disease is low (0–5%) while extension into the submucosa is associated with a risk of nodal disease of up to 22%. As a result, the development of endoscopic resection has provided a mechanism for the complete removal of mucosal cancers. The techniques available to deal with different morphologies of mucosal cancers include snare resection and endoscopic caps supplemented by argon, laser and photodynamic ablation.

Removal of mucosal lesions from the gastric mucosa is also a technique that has been undertaken with increasing frequency for malignant conditions. The original criteria for endoscopic resection were a maximal diameter of 2 cm, mucosal only, type I, IIa or IIb, well or moderately differentiated cancer. As expertise has grown, the size of lesion that can be removed has grown and lesions of greater than 40 mm are resected in specialist centres. The techniques available for resection of mucosal cancer include lift and snare using a twin channel scope and the endoscopic cap and snare. More recently the ceramic tipped needle knife has been developed where a larger area of mucosa can be removed. In deciding when to apply endoscopic therapy, the risk of lymphatic involvement has to be lower than the risk of open surgery.

### Palliative Endoscopic Techniques

For patients unsuitable for curative treatment, endoscopic approaches include snare resection, intratumoral injection of alcohol and laser and argon ablation for exophytic lesions. The reported results of these techniques show them to effective in the management of dysphagia though they require repeated application. For stenosing tumours or where the frequency of therapy is too great, SEMS have been used to cross the gastroduodenal junction in patients with gastric outlet problems.

## Duodenal and Pancreatic Cancer

Pathology requiring therapeutic intervention in the duodenum is infrequent. Lesions requiring excision include polyps and early malignancies. Duodenal polyps can be resected by either snare or cap approach with acceptable safety. When either a duodenal or pancreatic malignancy present with gastric outlet obstruction can be treated by insertion of a SEMS inserted under combined endoscopic and fluoroscopic control.

## Enteroscopy

Evaluation of the small bowel is possible by a number of techniques. Contrast radiology is either by small bowel follow through or enema. Endoscopic assessment of the small bowel is either by fibreoptic endoscopy or by capsule endoscopy. Enteroscopy can be either push enteroscopy or balloon enteroscopy where peristalsis is used to pull the enteroscope to the distal small bowel. This technique has been shown to yield a significant number of mucosal abnormalities not evident on radiological examination of the small bowel and allows delivery of therapy for lesions such as angiodysplasia [25]. Enteroscopy allows visualisation of a limited length of the small bowel due to scope length.

Capsule endoscopy involves the ingestion of a small capsule containing a battery-powered video camera and transmitter that transmits video pictures to a receiver worn on a belt. The video is viewed subsequently to identify any mucosal pathology. This does ensure that the entire small bowel can be evaluated. While there is evidence that the technique can identify abnormalities with reliability [26], the precise role of capsule endoscopy remains to be defined and will evolve over the coming years.

## Questions

1. Comment on the overall diagnostic accuracy of upper GI endoscopy.
2. Define the requirements for safe sedation.
3. Describe the most appropriate techniques for confirmation of the nature of lesions in the upper GI tract.

## References

1. Dooley CP. Larson AW, Stale NH et al. Double contrast barium meal and upper gastrointestinal endoscopy. Ann Internal Med 1984;101(4):538–45.
2. Cotton PB. Fibreoptic endoscopy and the barium meal – results and implications. Br Med J 1973;2:161–5.
3. Singh T, Gupta NM, Bhasin DK et al. Comparison of brush before biopsy, suction cytology, brush after biopsy and endoscopic biopsy in the diagnosis of carcinoma oesophagus. J Gastroenterol Hepatol 1994;9(6): 564–6.
4. Reynolds JW, Lukeman JM, Fernandez T. Endoscopic cytology and biopsy diagnosis of esophageal carcinoma. South Med J 1982;75(10):1201–4.
5. Qizilbash AH, Castelli M, Kowalski MA, Churly A. Endoscopic brush cytology and biopsy in the diagnosis of cancer of the upper gastrointestinal tract. Acta Cytol 1980;24(4):313–18.
6. Sugimachi K, Kitamura K, Baba K et al. Endoscopic diagnosis of early carcinoma of the esophagus using Lugol's solution. Gastrointest Endosc 1992;38(6): 657–61.
7. Giler S, Kadish U, Urca I. Use of tolonium chloride in the diagnosis of malignant gastric ulcers. Arch Surg 1978;113:136–9.
8. Tatsuta M, Okuda S, Tamura H, Taniguchi H. Endoscopic diagnosis of early gastric cancer by the endoscopic Congo red-methylene blue test. Cancer 1982;50(12):2956–60.
9. Suzuki S, Suzuki H, Endo M et al. Endoscopic dyeing method for the diagnosis of early gastric cancer and intestinal metaplasia of the stomach. Endoscopy 1973;5:124–9.
10. Tatsuta M, Okuda S, Tamura A, Taniguchi H. Endoscopic determination of the extent of early ulcerated gastric cancer by the congo red test. Endoscopy 1982;14(2):41–4.
11. Tatsuta M, Okuda S, Taniguchi H, Tamura H. Gross and histological types of early gastric carcinomas in relation to the acid-secreting area. Cancer 1979;43(1):317–21.
12. British Society of Gastroenterology. Guidelines for safe sedation. 2003.
13. Haffner JF, Fausa O, Royne T. Nonoperative treatment of subcervical oesophageal perforations after forced dilatation for nonmalignant disease. Acta Chir Scand 1984;150(5):389–92.

14. Quine MA, Bell GD, McCloy RF et al. Prospective audit of upper gastrointestinal endoscopy in two regions of England: Safety, staffing and sedation methods. Gut 1995;36:462–7.
15. Hallissey M, Jewkes A, Allum W et al. Early detection of gastric cancer. Br Med J 1990;301:513–15.
16. Newcomer MK, Brazer SR. Complications of upper gastrointestinal endoscopy and their management. Gastrointest Endosc Clin North Am 1994;4(3):551–70.
17. McLean GK, LeVeen RF. Shear stress in the performance of esophageal dilation: comparison of balloon dilation and bougienage. Radiology 1989;172(3 Pt 2):983–6.
18. McCormack G, McCormick PA. A practical guide to the management of oesophageal varices. Drugs 1999;57(3):327–35.
19. Masci E, Stigliano R, Mariani A et al. Prospective multicenterr randomized trial comparing banding ligation with sclerotherapy of esophageal varices. Hepatogastroenterology 1769;46(27):1769–73.
20. Lo GH, Lai KH, Cheng JS et al. Emergency banding ligation versus sclerotherapy for the control of active bleeding from esophageal varices. Hepatology 1101; 25(5):1101–14.
21. Yoshida S. Endoscopic diagnosis and treatment of early cancer in the alimentary tract. Digestion 199859(5): 502–8.
22. Inoue H, Endo M, Takeshita K et al. Endoscopic resection of early-stage esophageal cancer. Surg Endosc 1991;5(2):59–62.
23. Makuuchi H, Machimura T, Shimada H et al. Endoscopic screening for esophageal cancer in 788 patients with head and neck cancers. Tokai J Exp Clin Med 1996;21(3):139–45.
24. Lo GH, Lai KH, Cheng JS et al. A prospective, randomized trial of butyl cyanoacrylate injection versus band ligation in the management of bleeding gastric varices. Hepatology 1060;33(5):1060–4.
25. Parry SD, Welfare MR, Cobden I, Barton JR. Push enteroscopy in UK district general hospital: experience of 51 cases over 2 years. Eur J Gastroenterol Hepatol 2002;14(3):305–9.
26. Lewis B, Swain P. Capsule endoscopy in the evaluation of patients with suspected small intestinal bleeding: results of a pilot study. Gastrointest Endosc 2002;56(3): 349–53.

# 22

## Imaging in GI Surgery

Julie F.C. Olliff and Peter J. Guest

## Aims

To explain the indications for and types of imaging available.

## Introduction

Imaging is playing an increasingly important role in the investigation and work-up of patients who present to GI surgeons. The choice of the appropriate investigation can be one of the most crucial decisions in the patient work-up. This chapter discusses the commonly used imaging methods with indications, contraindications and some discussion about technique and interpretation. Recent Ionising Radiation (Medical Exposure) Regulations (IRMER) regulations (EU) require the justification of imaging investigations that use ionising radiation. Investigations such as MRI or ultrasound that avoid the use of ionising radiation should always be considered. This becomes especially relevant in young people because of the increased risk of a lifetime cancer from ionising radiation or in patients who are going to undergo repeated imaging examination throughout the course of their illness. Examination involving ionising radiation of the lower abdomen and pelvis is not advised in patients who may be pregnant.

## Plain Radiology

### Lateral Soft Tissue Neck

Indications: Suspected radio-opaque foreign body, suspected perforation with or without retropharyngeal abscess.

### Chest

*Indications.* Suspected oesophageal perforation, suspected aspiration, suspected foreign body; perforated abdominal viscus, perforated oesophagus, achalasia.

The erect chest x-ray with the beam centred at the level of the diaphragm is the investigation of choice for detecting extraluminal intra-abdominal air (Figure 22.1). If the patient is not well enough to have an erect film, then a left lateral decubitus film of the abdomen can be performed. These films can demonstrate as little as 1–2 ml of free air (Figure 22.2).

It may take some time for small amounts of gas to collect either just below the diaphragm or lateral to the liver so ideally the film should be obtained with the patient having been in the erect position for 10 minutes or more.

Mediastinal air and/or pleural fluid should be looked for in patients suspected of oesophageal perforation following ingestion of a foreign body or instrumentation.

## 22 · UPPER GASTROINTESTINAL SURGERY

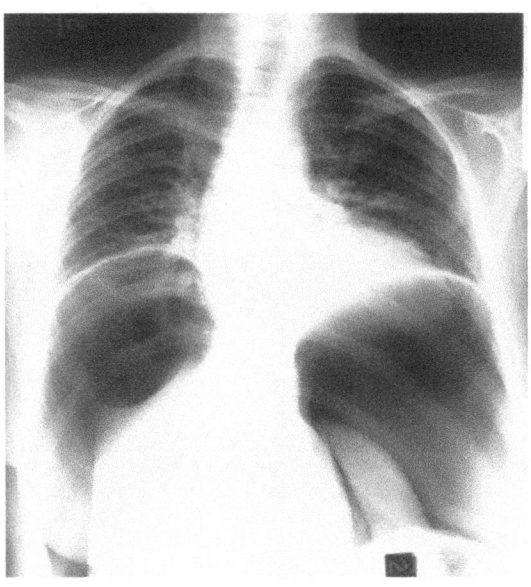

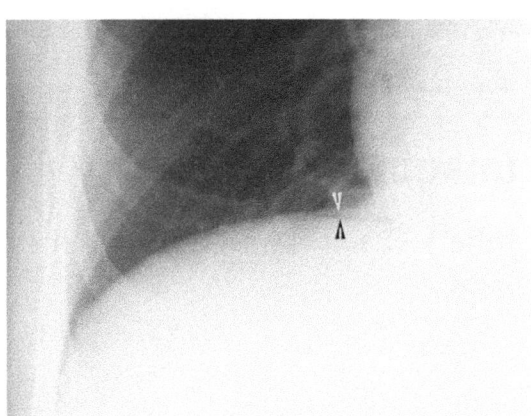

**Figure 22.2.** Erect chest X-ray demonstrates a small amount of free gas (arrowed).

**Figure 22.1.** Erect chest X-ray demonstrates a large amount of free gas below the diaphragms following caecal perforation.

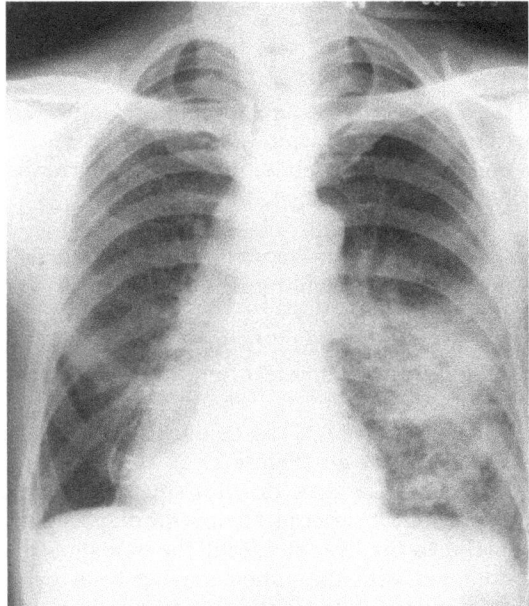

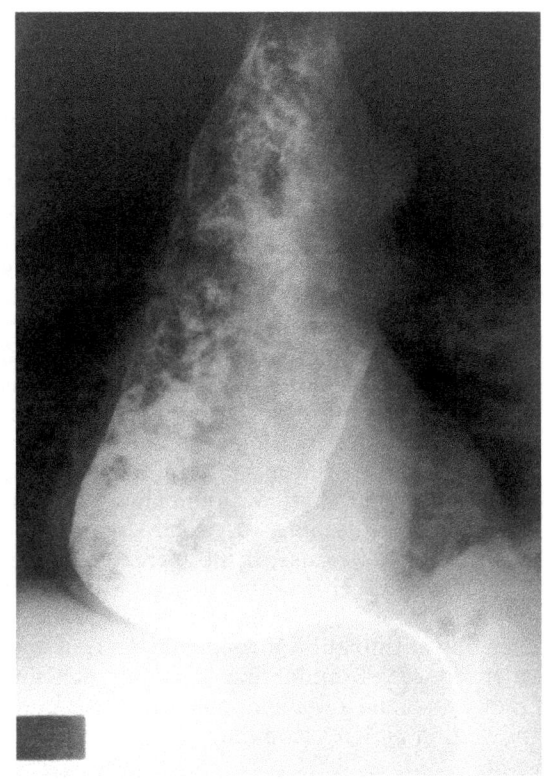

**Figure 22.3.a** Achalasia: A chest X-ray showing dilated viscus forming an extra border to the right side of the mediastinum with evidence of an aspiration pneumonia in the left lower lobe. **b** Barium swallow showing the dilated oesophagus with much food residue and the characteristic "bird beak" of the gastro-oesophageal junction.

# IMAGING IN GI SURGERY

Established achalasia may be diagnosed by the presence of a dilated oesophagus projecting beyond the normal mediastinum and containing copious fluid residue (Figures 22.3a and 3b).

## Plain Abdominal Film

*Indications.* Intestinal obstruction, detection of calcification or other radio-opaque material, suspected ischaemia, inflammatory bowel disease, intestinal transit studies.

*Contraindications.* Pregnancy.

The plain abdominal film is most helpful for detecting intestinal obstruction although the site of obstruction can be difficult to judge because of fluid-filled loops of bowel interposed between the actual obstruction and distal air-filled loops.

The normal calibre of the proximal jejunum should be less than 3.5 cm, of the mid small bowel less than 3 cm and of the ileum less than 2.5 cm (Figure 22.4a ,b and c).

Extraluminal air can also be assessed on a supine film of the abdomen. All collections of gas should be assessed for a possible extraluminal location. Triangular air collections may be extraluminal (Figure 22.5). Air may be seen in the hepatorenal space (Morrison's pouch) or outlining the fissure of the ligamentum teres (Figure 22.6). If large amounts of air are present, both sides of the bowel wall may be seen (Rigler's sign) (Figure 22.7). Retroperitoneal free gas will cause the renal outlines to appear unusually sharp (Figure 22.8).

Focal collections of air within abscesses will appear as areas of mottled gas lying outside the normal distribution of bowel or as a collection

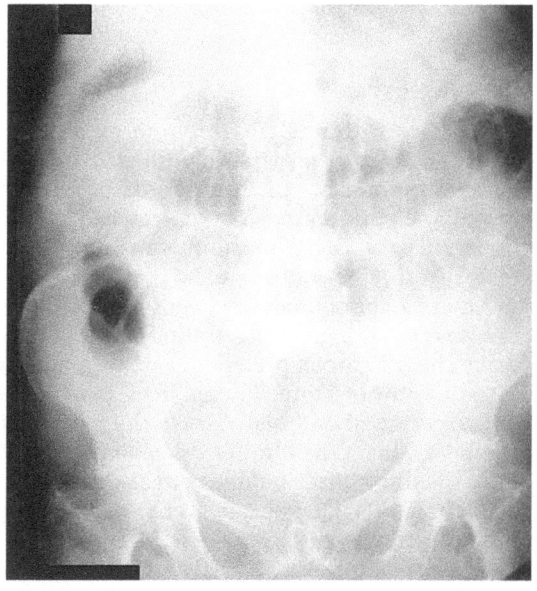

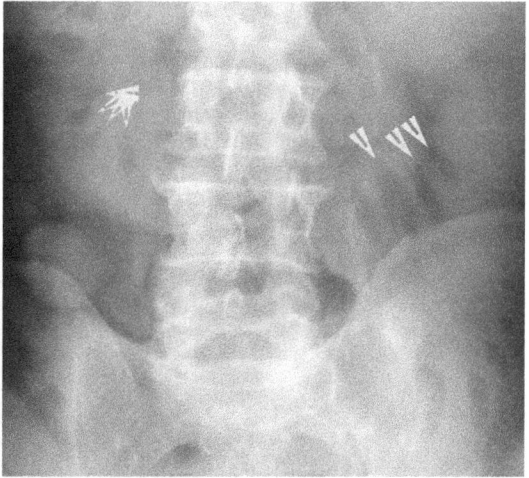

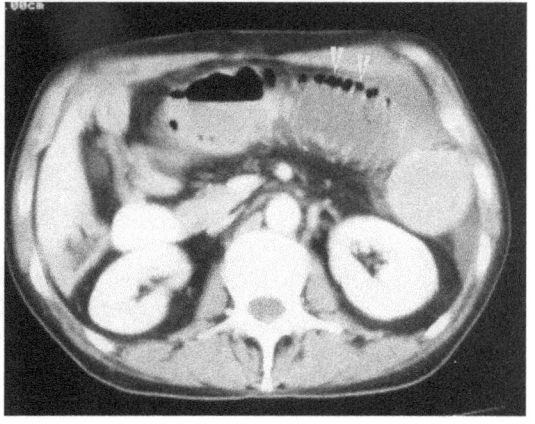

**Figure 22.4.a** Plain film of the abdomen demonstrating small bowel obstruction **b** and **c** Coned view of the abdomen (**b**) and a CT (**c**) in small bowel obstruction to illustrate the origin of the "string of beads" sign. The abdominal X-ray shows a line of gas bubbles corresponding to gas (arrowheads) trapped between the small bowel folds in dilated fluid-filled small bowel.

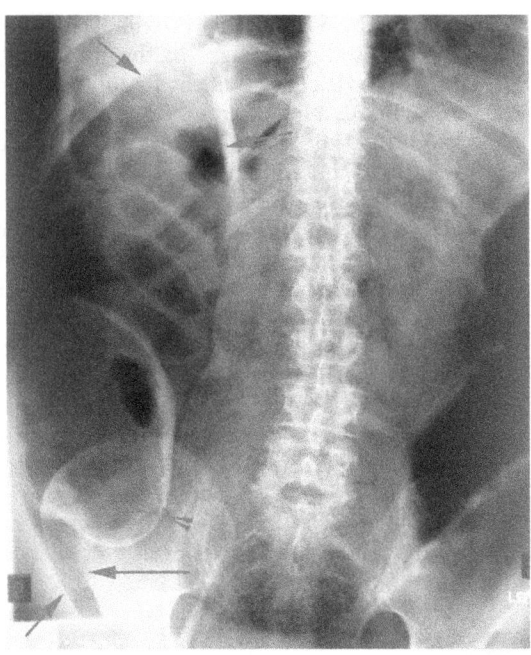

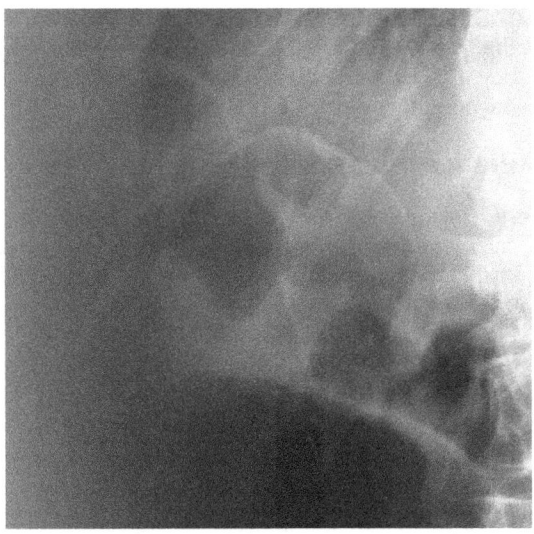

**Figure 22.7.** Close-up of an abdominal X-ray to demonstrate air on both sides of the bowel wall (Rigler's sign) as an indicator of free intra-abdominal gas.

**Figure 22.5.** Supine abdominal radiograph showing extensive free air as manifest by non-anatomical or triangular collections of air (arrows) and air on both sides of the bowel wall (Rigler's sign – arrowheads).

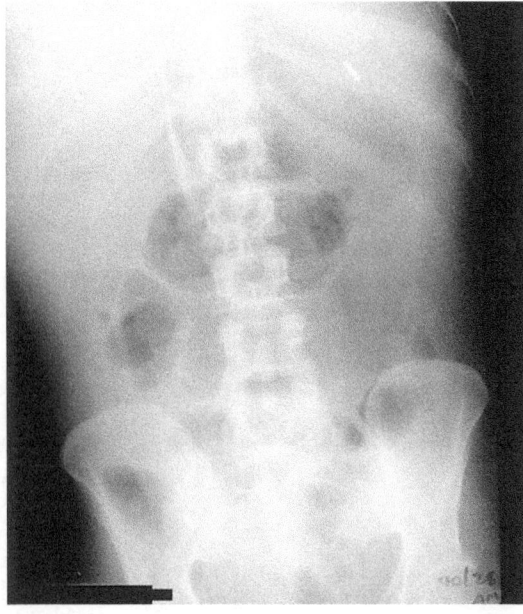

**Figure 22.6.** Plain film of the abdomen shows the falciform ligament outlined by free gas.

of gas seen within an abscess with an air fluid level. These may only be identified if they lie outside the normal distribution of bowel gas. Bowel wall thickening may be seen in conditions such as ischaemia, inflammatory bowel disease, etc.

An erect abdominal film is not needed either to assess the presence of extraluminal gas (as an erect chest X-ray is preferable) or to diagnose intestinal obstruction. Rather than fluid levels on an erect abdominal X-ray, the physician should evaluate the film for dilated bowel, or if fluid filled for linear bubbles of gas ("string-of-beads" sign) (Figures 22.4b and c) corresponding to air trapped between the small bowel folds.

Gas may be seen within the biliary tree in patients who have had sphincterotomy, have a biliary enteric anastomosis or who have recently passed a gallstone. Biliary gas appears as branching linear lucencies lying centrally. Gas in the portal veins in an adult appears as gas shadows which extend to the periphery of the liver (Figure 22.9). Gas may also be seen as splenic or mesenteric veins and within the bowel wall (Figure 22.10). This is seen in necrotising enterocololitis following umbilical vein catheterisation and in erythroblastosis fetalis. In adults it is a grave prognostic sign most

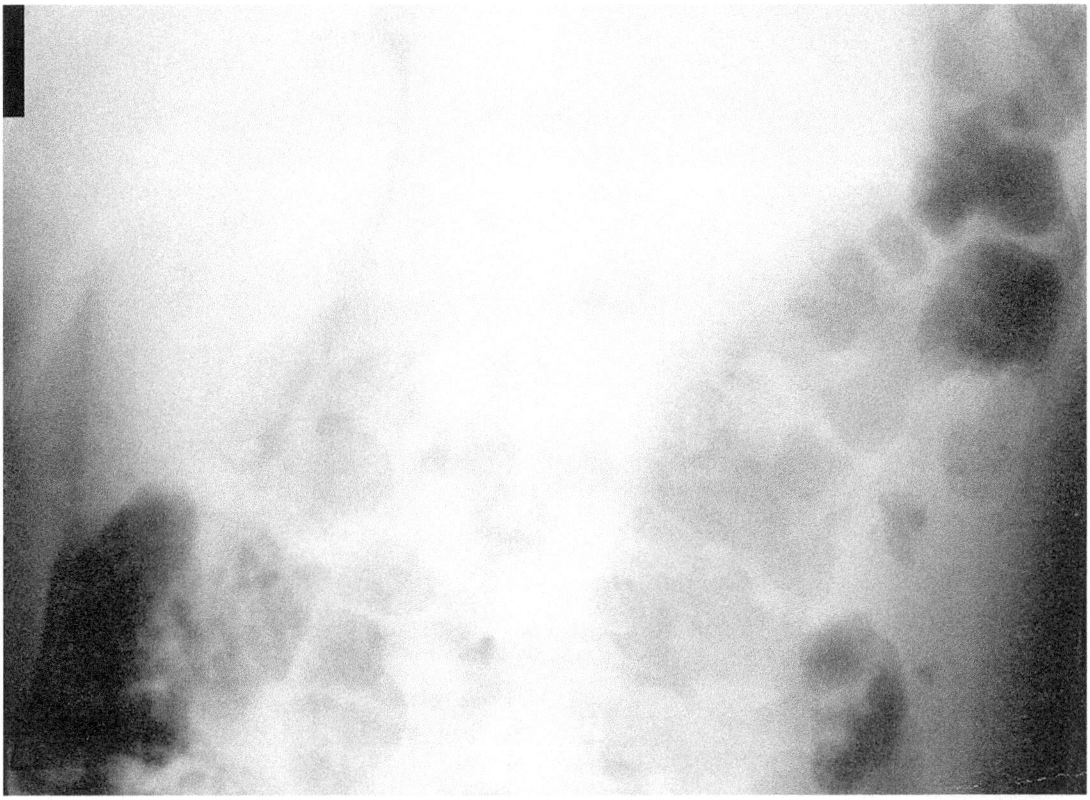

## IMAGING IN GI SURGERY

**Figure 22.8.** The right renal outline is very clearly seen due to retroperitoneal gas.

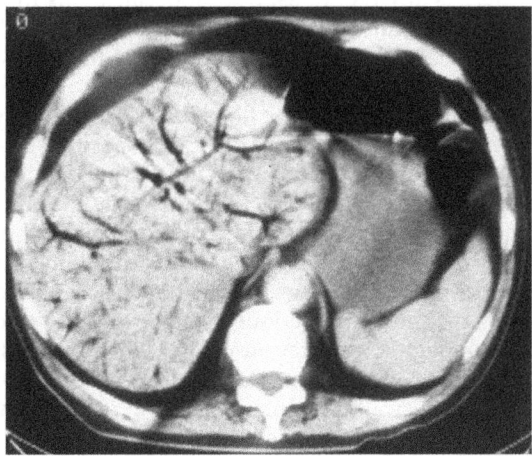

**Figure 22.9.** Portal vein gas seen on CT in a patient with ischaemic bowel.

commonly seen in critically ischaemic bowel. Rarely it may, however, be seen in patients with severely ulcerated large bowel following embolus of air during a double contrast barium enema.

Calcification should be looked for on a plain film within the gall bladder, pancreas and renal tract. Gall bladder stones are visible on a plain abdominal film in about 10% of cases, and are characteristically laminated and polygonal. Curvilinear calcification lateral to the lumbar spine raises the possibility of an aortic aneurysm which can be further assessed using ultrasound or CT.

Free intra-abdominal fluid leads to medial displacement of the colonic gas shadows from the properitoneal fat line (Figure 22.11). It also leads to a ground glass appearance.

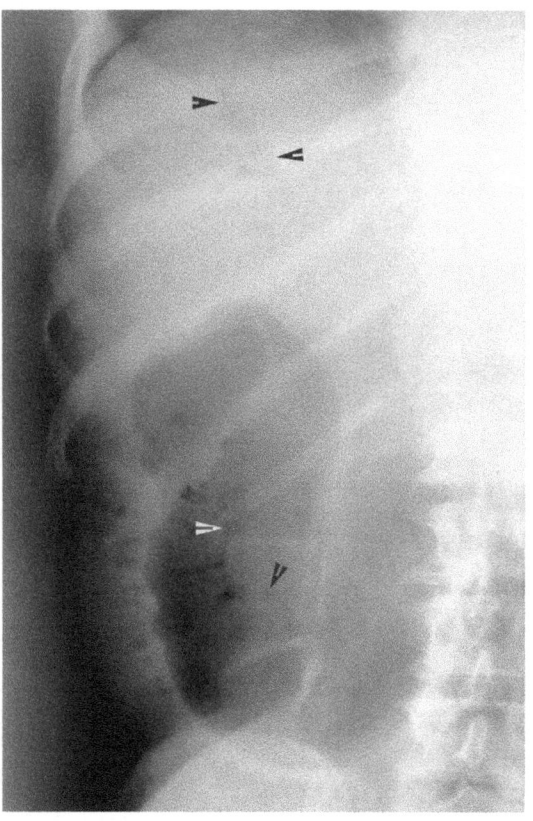

**Figure 22.10.** Coned view of a radiograph of the right flank showing gas (arrowheads) within the mesenteric arcades and the portal venous system in the liver in this patient with ischaemic gut.

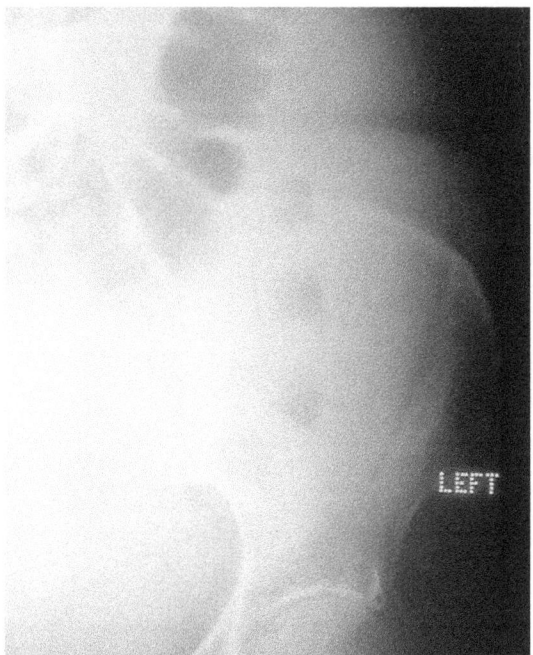

**Figure 22.11.**

## Contrast Radiography

### Oral Cholecystography

*Indications.* Suspected cholelithiasis. This method has almost completely been replaced by ultrasound. It may occasionally be needed in patients in whom ultrasound has failed usually due to obesity. It may also be used if ultra-sound is doubtful in the diagnosis of a small chronically contracted gall bladder and is useful to assess gall bladder function although this may also be done by ultrasound.

### Barium Swallow

*Indications.* Dysphagia, pain, possible motility disorder.

Barium should never be used as the oral contrast agent if there is any possibility of aspiration or leak into the peritoneum. The use of Gastrografin, which is a hyper-osmolar water-soluble contrast agent, is also contraindicated if there is any risk of aspiration because this may lead to pulmonary oedema which can be fatal. Isotonic water-soluble contrast agents should be used in these patients.

Double contrast spot films assess morphology better. The presence of gastro-oesophageal reflux may be assessed by tipping the patient head down or by asking him to cough. A double contrast barium swallow has a sensitivity of 75 to 90% in diagnosing reflux oesophagitis depending on the severity. It may also be used to diagnose infectious and drug-induced oesophagitis. Aspiration occurs when contrast medium enters the laryngeal vestibule or between swallows during normal respiration. Aspiration is associated with stasis in the pharynx. This may be due to neuromuscular disorders, tumour, pharyngeal pouch or diverticulum. Aspiration can also occur during gastro-oesophageal-reflux or may be due to an obstruction in the lower oesophagus. A prominent cricopharyngeus (Figure 22.12) is also often seen in patients with gastro-oesophageal reflux or oesophageal obstruction. It may also be due to abnormal pharyngeal peristalsis. Pharyngeal diverticulum or pouch can be demonstrated by barium swallow.

Malignant pharyngeal and oesophageal tumours may be differentiated from benign strictures by irregular narrowing of the lumen associated with mucosal destruction, ulceration and mass effect. Narrowing of the oesophagus by mediastinal tumours causes an extrinsic mass effect unless there is direct invasion. Benign strictures appear as smooth areas of oesophageal narrowing and may be due to previous radiotherapy, caustic ingestion, dermatological disorders and gastro-oesophageal reflux. High strictures or ulceration may be seen in Barrett's oesophagus.

An oesophageal web (Figure 22.12) appears as a narrow shelf-like band usually in the cervical oesophagus. Oesophageal varices may be missed if the oesophagus is distended.

Barium swallow may also be used to evaluate motility disorders of the oesophagus. These are preferably recorded as video clips or digital movie clips. Tongue movement, soft palate elevation, epiglottic tilt, laryngeal closure,

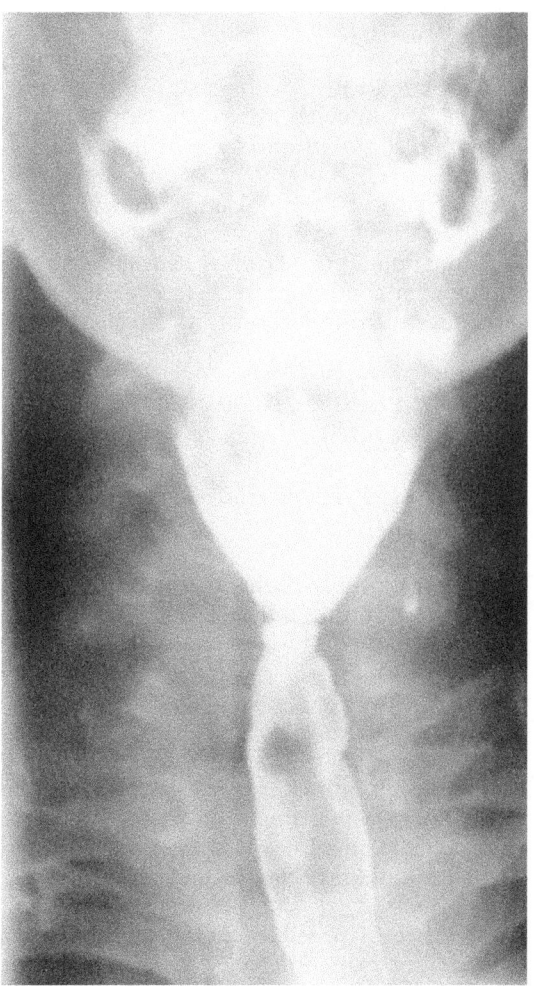
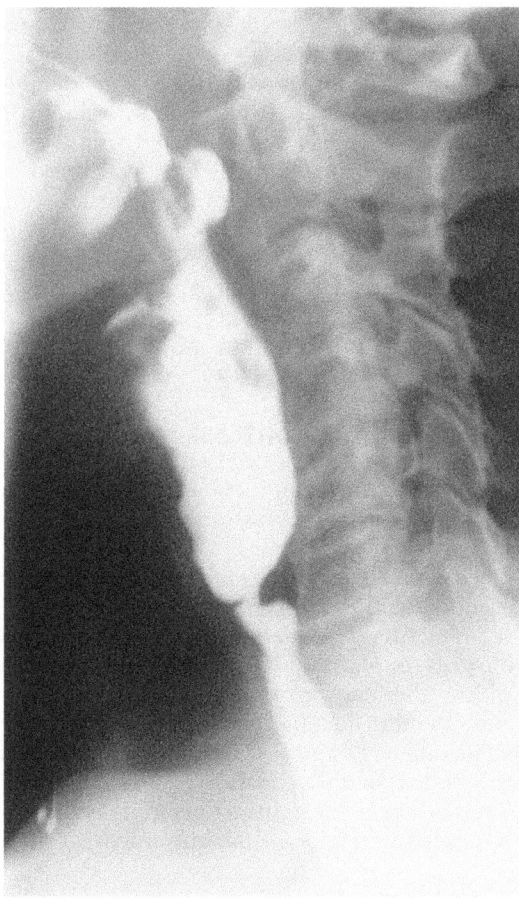

**Figures 22.12.** Anteroposterior view of a barium swallow (**a**) demonstrating a narrow linear filling defect which is shown on the lateral view (**b**) to be a well-defined shelf-like defect anteriorly consistent with a web. A prominent cricopharyngeus is noted posteriorly.

pharyngo-oesophageal segment (cricopharyngeal opening) and pharyngeal peristalsis may all be assessed.

Aspiration should be looked for early as the examination may need to be terminated.

Peristalsis should be assessed in the prone or supine position to eliminate the effects of gravity. Oesophageal peristalsis is normally rapid with a primary stripping wave propelling a liquid or solid bolus through the oesophagus. Early dysfunction is manifest as failure of this wave which may dissipate in the mid oesophagus. Secondary peristalsis may then clear the oesophagus. More advanced dysmotility is manifest as tertiary contractions which are ineffective in terms of propulsion and may be manifest as a "corksrew oesophagus". Elderly patients usually have minor dysmotility which may be asymptomatic. Patients may demonstrate a normal liquid swallow, in which case the examination should be continued with a solid bolus (bread or marshmallows if available).

Achalasia is a specific motility disorder of the gastro-oesophageal junction characterised radiologically by a dilated oesophagus, failure of relaxation of the gastro-oesophageal junction, with intermittent opening and passage of barium into the stomach (a "bird beak" appearance (Figure 22.3b)).

## Water-soluble Contrast Swallow

*Indications.* Possibility of aspiration, assessment of integrity of anastomoses.

As discussed above, water-soluble contrast agents should be used if there is any risk of aspiration. They are routinely used to assess integrity of anastomoses post surgery. Barium within the peritoneum is extremely irritant and should not be used in this instance. Unfortunately, mucosal detail is poorly seen with water-soluble contrast agents and therefore barium is the contrast agent of choice for routine examination of the gut mucosa.

## Barium Meal

*Indications.* Dyspepsia, weight loss, GI haemorrhage, high GI obstruction.

*Contraindications.* Complete large bowel obstruction, suspected site of perforation.

*Complications.* Side effects of muscle relaxants.

This investigation has been almost completely replaced by upper GI endoscopy. It is now only used on those patients who are not suitable for upper GI endoscopy or in instances where upper GI endoscopy is not available. A gas-producing agent is swallowed. The patient then drinks barium. The patient is turned to achieve adequate coating of the stomach and double contrast views are obtained. An intravenous injection of a smooth muscle relaxant (Buscopan or glucagon) is given and views of the duodenum are taken.

A barium meal may be used to diagnose gastritis and peptic ulceration. Ulcers greater than 5 mm in size are more likely to be detected on barium study than smaller ones. Imaging cannot confidently distinguish between benign and malignant ulcers but may be very suggestive (Figure 22.13). Atrophic gastritis, eosinophilic gastritis and involvement of the stomach by Crohn's disease may also be shown. Benign tumours such as hyperplastic polyps and adenomatous polyps may be demonstrated. Congenital conditions such as ectopic pancreatic rests and duplication cysts can also be seen.

## Barium Follow Through/Small Bowel Meal

*Indications.* Pain, diarrhoea, bleeding, partial obstruction.

*Contraindications.* Complete obstruction, suspected perforation unless a water-soluble contrast medium is used rather than barium sulphate.

Small bowel contrast studies are better performed as a dedicated study rather than a study following a barium meal. The relaxant given for a barium meal will hinder the passage of barium through the small bowel. An optimal study is dynamic and involves regular fluoroscopy to assess mobility of small bowel loops and take spot views of possible pathologies with compression or palpation.

Although direct enteroscopy is developing, barium radiology of the small bowel remains the main method for evaluation of this segment of bowel. It demonstrates the mucosal ulceration,

## IMAGING IN GI SURGERY

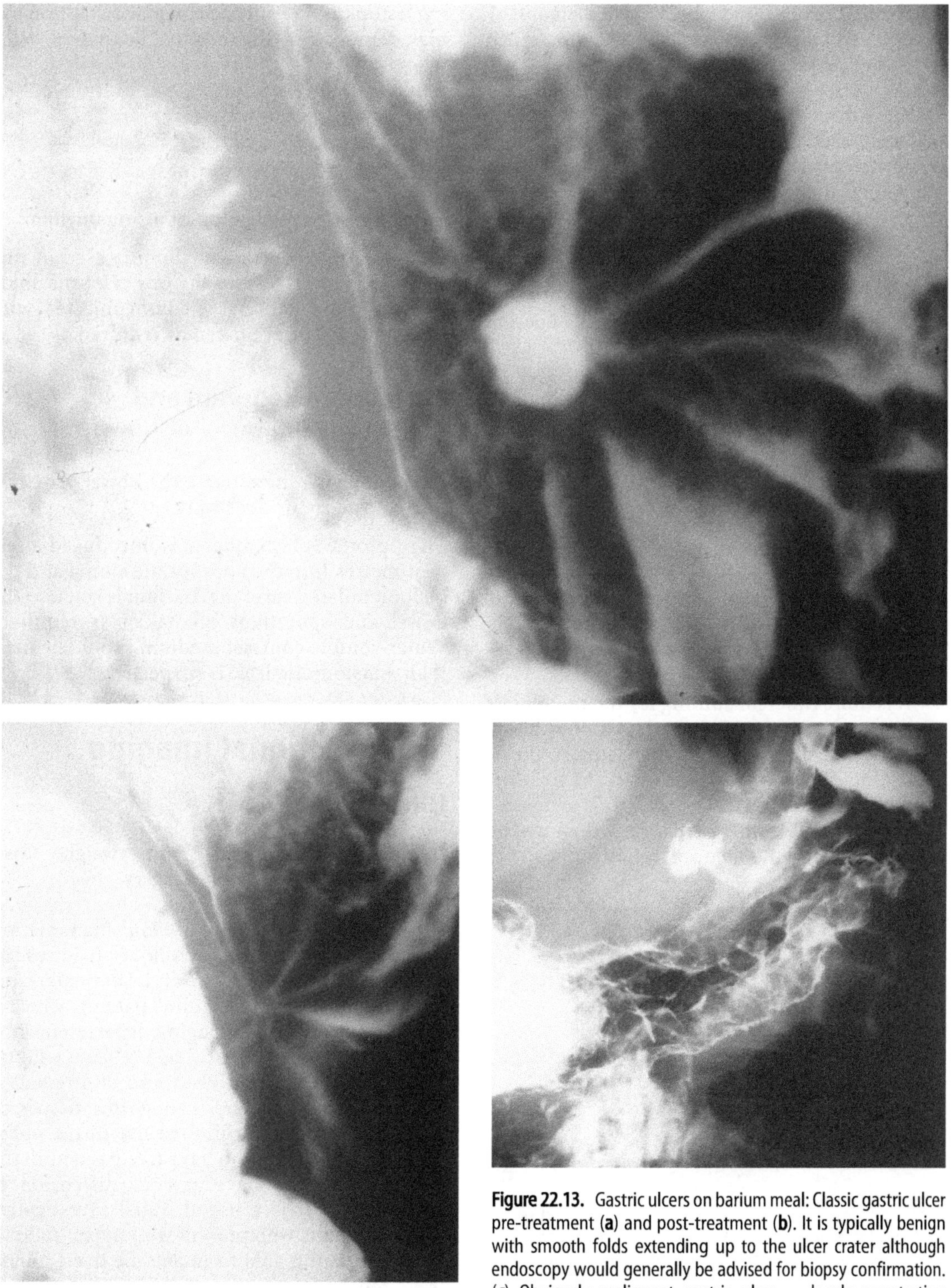

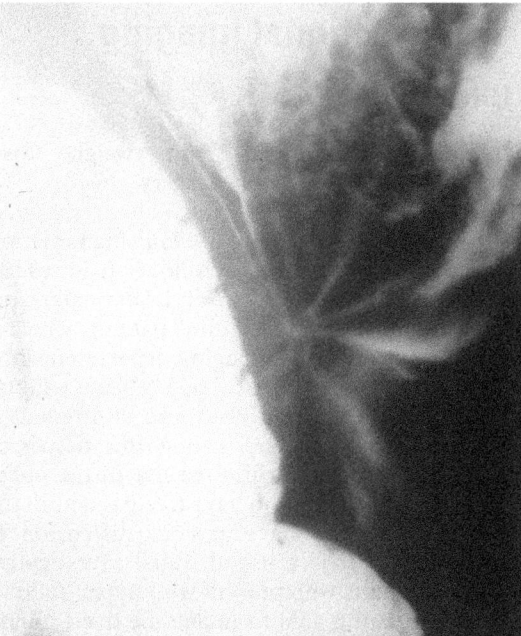

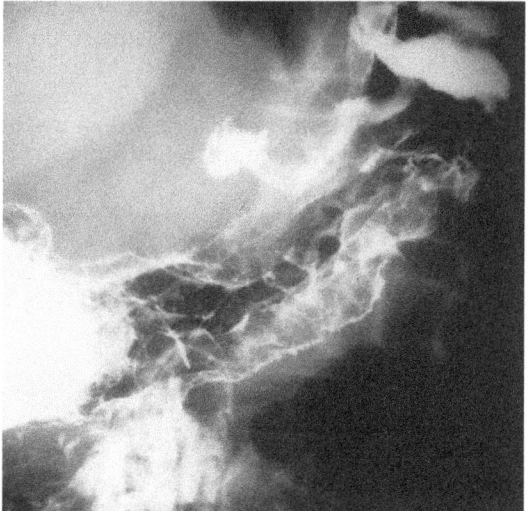

**Figure 22.13.** Gastric ulcers on barium meal: Classic gastric ulcer pre-treatment (**a**) and post-treatment (**b**). It is typically benign with smooth folds extending up to the ulcer crater although endoscopy would generally be advised for biopsy confirmation. (**c**) Obviously malignant gastric ulcer – deeply penetrating irregular lesion with associated extensive infiltration through a thickened stomach wall.

strictures, fistulas and obstructive elements of Crohn's disease (Figure 22.14) Characteristic appearances are seen in coeliac disease, systemic sclerosis, radiotherapy change etc. Malignancies such as adenocarcinoma or lymphoma are rare but usually well shown. Obstruction can be demonstrated and the cause identified although computed tomography (CT) is a competitive modality here.

## Small Bowel Enema

*Indications.* As for small bowel meal. Possible Meckel's diverticulum.

*Contraindications.* Complete obstruction, suspected perforation.

A nasojejunal tube with a guide-wire is introduced into the duodenum and advanced to beyond the duodenojejunal flexure (the level of the ligament of Treitz). Diluted barium is then run in quickly or barium followed by methylcellulose for a double contrast effect. Spot films are taken of the barium column and its leading edge at regions of interest until the colon is reached.

It is more time-consuming for the radiologist, more unpleasant for the patient but it allows better visualisation of the small bowel. Radiologists are divided, however, as to which technique is the best.

It is a more sensitive technique than a small bowel meal for the demonstration of obstructing lesions as a result of proximal distention but may demonstrate the terminal ileum less well.

*Complications.* Aspiration, perforation of the bowel by the guide-wire.

## Sinogram

*Indications.* Investigation of a sinus/fistula.

Water-soluble contrast medium is used. A fine catheter is inserted into the orifice of the sinus or fistula and contrast medium injected with screening. Films are taken as required.

## Retrograde Ileogram and Colostomy Enema

*Indications.* To investigate the bowel proximal to a colostomy or ileostomy.

The tip of a Foley catheter is introduced a few centimetres into the appropriate stoma and the balloon inflated carefully. Barium is run into the bowel and spot films are taken as required. Water-soluble contrast medium should be used if an anastomotic leak is suspected.

# Cross-sectional Imaging

## Ultrasound

*Indications.* Abdominal pain, weight loss, unexplained pyrexia post surgery.

Ultrasound (US) does not use ionising radiation and is therefore a safe technique. It is readily available in most hospitals and can be portable and therefore used to examine patients who are too ill to travel to the imaging department. It is very operator dependent. The US beam will not penetrate gas or bone well and is attenuated (weakened) as it passes through the tissues. It may therefore have a limited use in the obese patient, in patients who have free gas within the abdomen or who have gaseous distension of bowel loops. It is a useful initial investigative tool in patients who present with upper abdominal pain, being able to image the liver, biliary tree, renal tract pancreas and spleen before upper endoscopy or after a negative upper endoscopy.

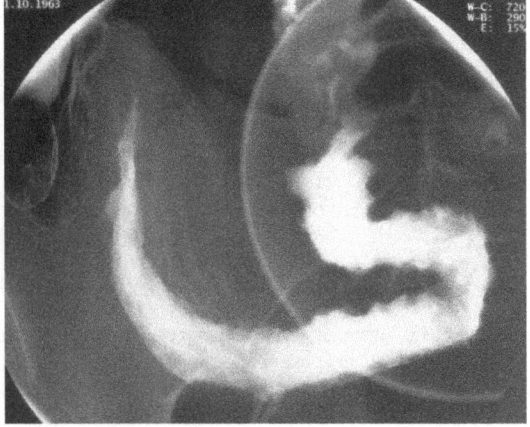

**Figure 22.14.** Terminal ileal mucosal Crohn's ulceration optimally demonstrated with a small bowel meal.

# IMAGING IN GI SURGERY

Bowel wall thickening (Figure 22.15a and b) may be detected on US in patients with inflammatory or neoplastic conditions.

It is very useful to detect fluid within the chest and abdomen. It may be used to differentiate between pleural effusions and underlying pulmonary parenchymal collapse and consolidation. It is to able to distinguish between fluid collections above and below the diaphragm and to guide diagnostic tap. If necessary US can then be used to guide pigtail catheter placement. It thus has an important role to play in the investigation of the pyrexial postoperative patient. It may not identify collections lying between gas-containing bowel loops and therefore a negative US scan in a patient suspected of having a postoperative abscess or collection needs to be interpreted with caution. In these patients it may be necessary to proceed to CT. It can be used to obtain diagnostic cytology in patients with upper GI cancers who are found to have ascites and suspected peritoneal disease.

## Endoscopic Ultrasound (EUS)

*Indications.* Local staging of oesophageal and gastric cancer, assessment of the pancreatic head and bile duct for malignancy and stone.

EUS is the most accurate method of assessing early T-stage GI tumours (Figure 22.16) and for predicting local organ invasion. Currently it is not widely available but is likely to become increasingly required to direct conservative surgery such as endoscopic submucosal resection.

## Computed Tomography

*Indications.* Staging upper GI cancer, investigation of abdominal pain, postoperative pyrexia.

Computed tomography (CT) uses ionising radiation. X-rays are attenuated by the tissues that they pass through. This attenuation is proportional to the atomic number of the tissue. Images are displayed as a grey scale with air conventionally displayed as black and bone as white. The development of spiral CT and more recently multi-slice CT enables a volume of data to be collected during a breathhold. This data may be displayed as axial slices or multiplanar reformats may be made. Upper GI CTs should use water to distend the stomach (hydro CT).

The normal oesophageal and gastric walls are thin. Abnormal thickening may be due to benign or malignant causes and therefore histology (usually from endoscopy) is needed before a diagnosis can be made. CT can, however, stage local and distant disease (Figure 22.17a, b and c), being able to image not only the extent of the local tumour but also local and distant nodal involvement, hepatic metastatic disease and peritoneal disease.

Aortic invasion by oesophageal cancer is rare (Figure 22.18) but is a contraindication to surgery. CT and MRI have similar accuracy in the assessment of aortic involvement.

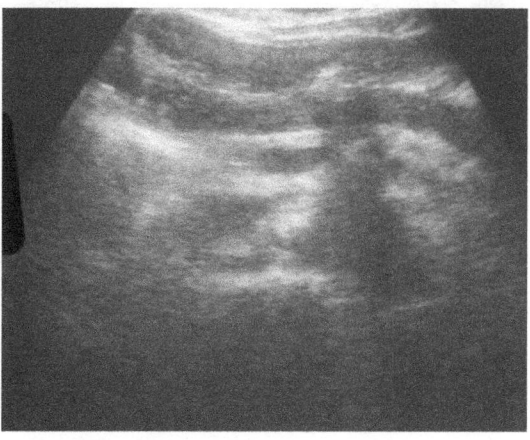
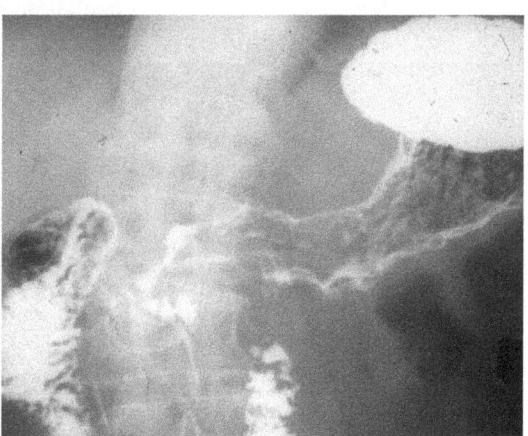

**Figures 22.15.** Gastric cancer manifest as irregular hourglass-type stricture on barium meal (**a**) and marked wall thickening on ultrasound (**b**).

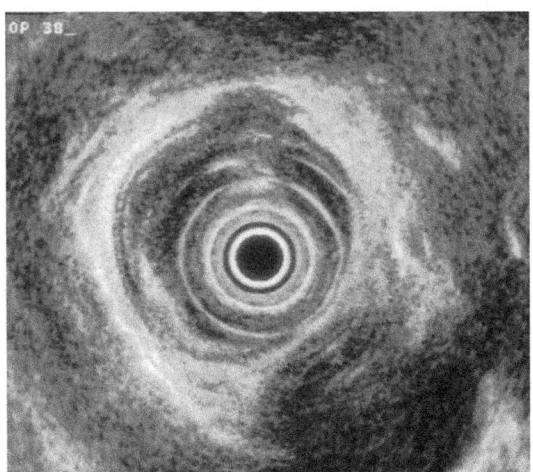
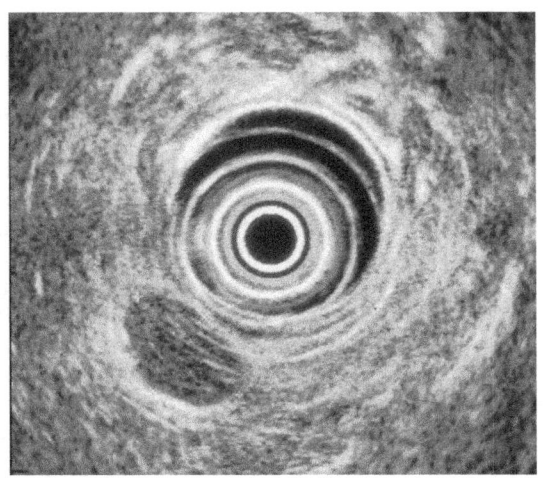

**Figure 22.16.** Endoscopic ultrasound is the most accurate method of local staging of oesophageal and gastric tumours. **a** An EUS showing a T3 tumour on the basis of the irregular external contour indicating invasion into the perioesophageal fat. **b** An enlarged local node. Involved nodes are typically round and hypoechoic. (Images courtesy of Dr Alison Maclean.)

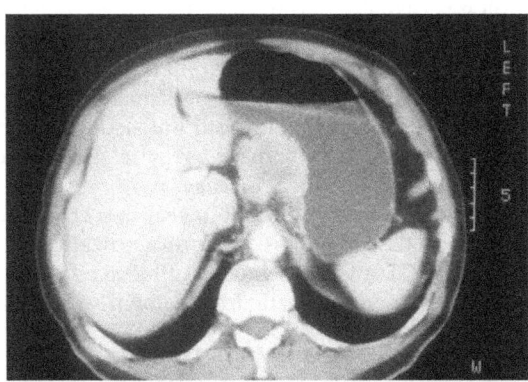
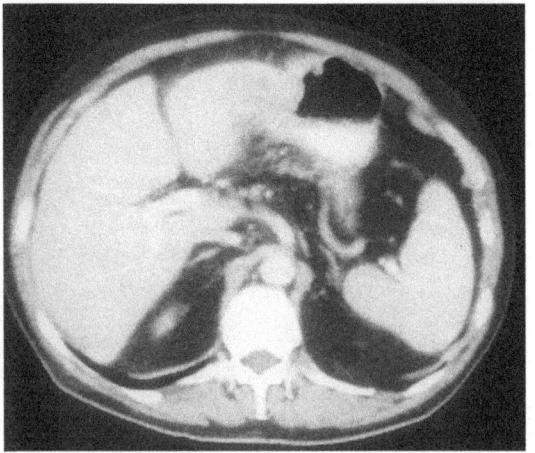
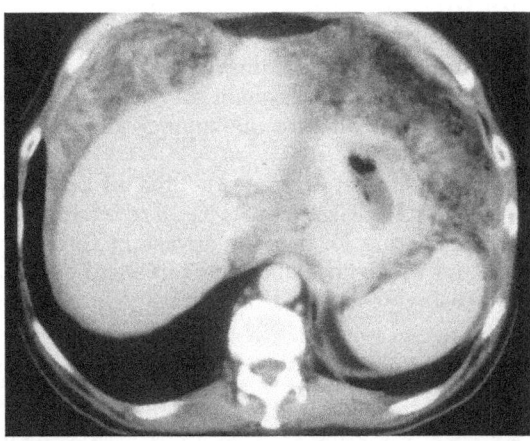

**Figure 22.17. a** CT showing a large lesser curve gastric cancer extending into the gastrohepatic ligament which is nevertheless operable. **b** Local direct liver invasion from gastric cancer on CT. **c** Advanced gastric cancer with extensive peritoneal carcinomatosis as seen on CT. Note wall thickening and a non-distensible stomach, and marked peritoneal infiltration and nodularity.

IMAGING IN GI SURGERY

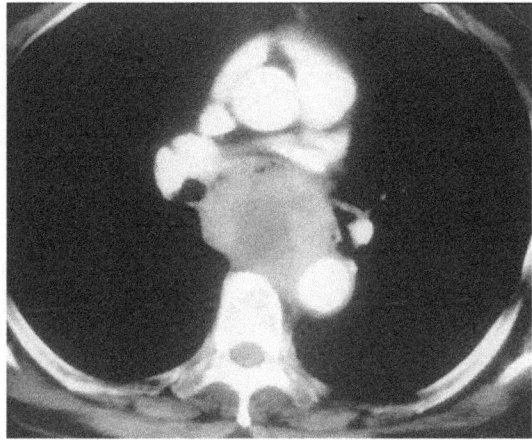

**Figure 22.18.** CT of a large oesophageal cancer subtending an angle of greater than 90 degrees on the descending aorta which is deformed. This tumour is likely to be inoperable therefore.

Nodal abnormality is assessed using size criteria with para-aortic nodes and mediastinal nodes being considered abnormal if they measure greater than 1 cm in diameter. CT can be used to diagnose and stage other small bowel tumours such as carcinoid (Figure 22.19)

CT can be used to investigate the acute abdomen in patients with suspected upper GI pathology. It can be used to determine the site and probable cause of obstruction (Figures 22.20 and 22.21). It will demonstrate not only the abnormal wall thickening seen in Crohn's disease (Figure 22.22) but will elucidate whether bowel separaration seen on barium studies is due to fibro-fatty proliferation, lymph node enlargement or to abscess/phlegmon formation. In the postoperative patient it can be used not only to identify collections but also to guide diagnostic aspiration and drainage procedures.

## Magnetic Resonance Imaging

Magnetic resonance imaging (MRI) has a relatively limited role in the upper GI tract. MRI staging of oesophageal and gastric cancer has no advantage over CT.

Magnetic resonance cholangio-pancreatography (MRCP) uses a heavily T2-weighted sequence usually with fat suppression to provide images of the water content of the biliary and pancreatic ducts. It is non-invasive, uses no contrast and is therefore no risk. It provides good images, particularly in the dilated system, and is increasingly used for diagnosis rather than endoscopic retrograde cholangiopancreatography (ERCP). However, ERCP remains essential for therapeutic manoeuvres.

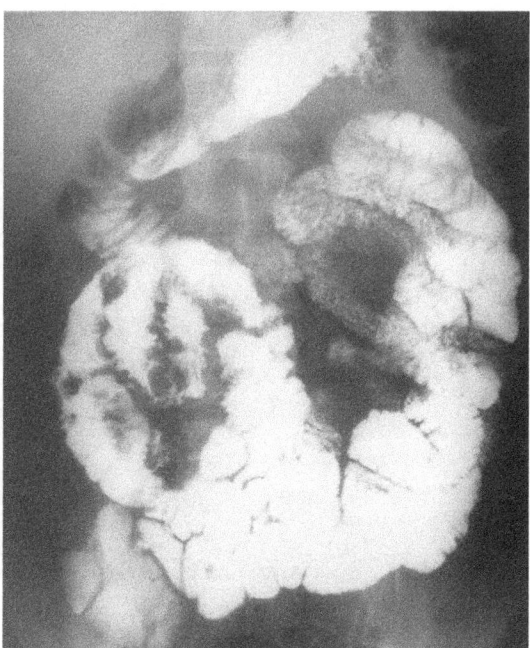

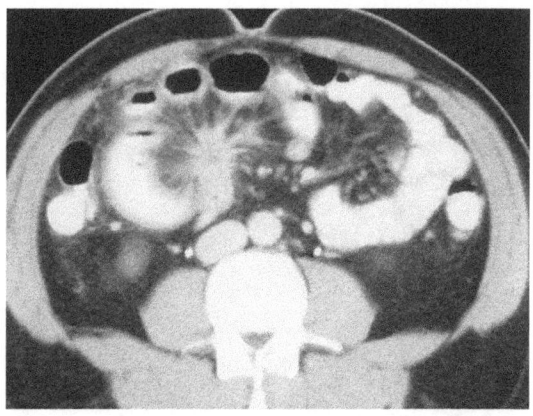

**Figure 22.19.** Carcinoid tumour as seen on a small bowel meal with barium and a CT. **a** The barium study shows irregular nodularity and fold thickening of the distal small bowel but with a normal terminal ileum. **b** The CT shows indrawing of small bowel loop by a spiculate irregular cicatrizing mesenteric nodal mass, typical of carcinoid nodal metastases.

## 22 · UPPER GASTROINTESTINAL SURGERY

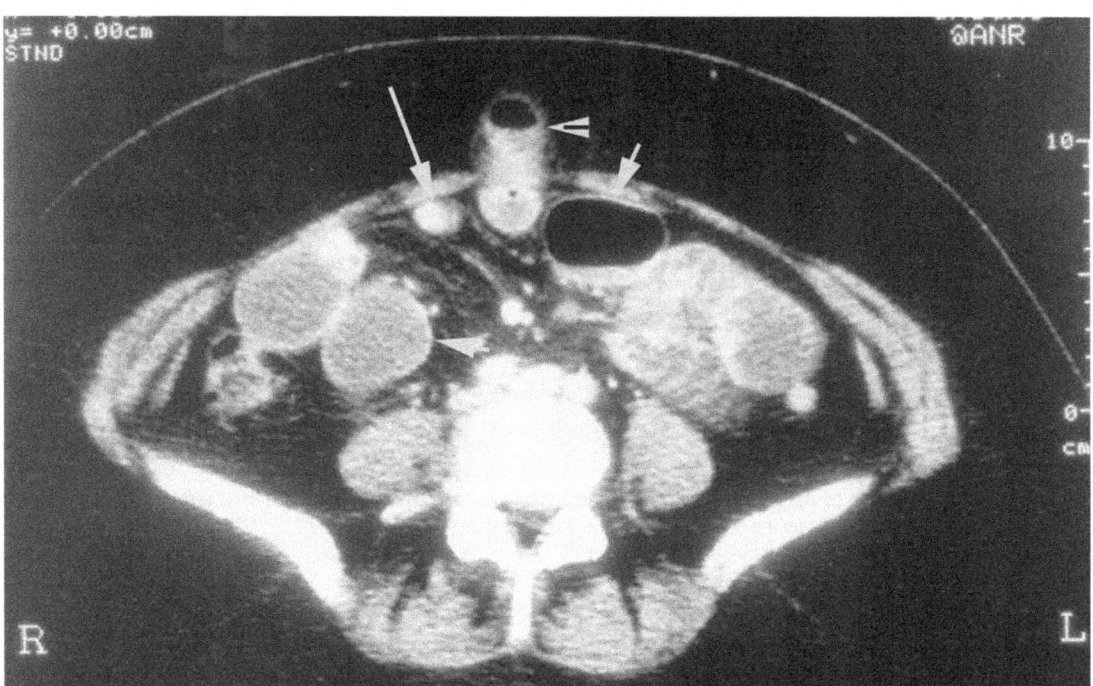

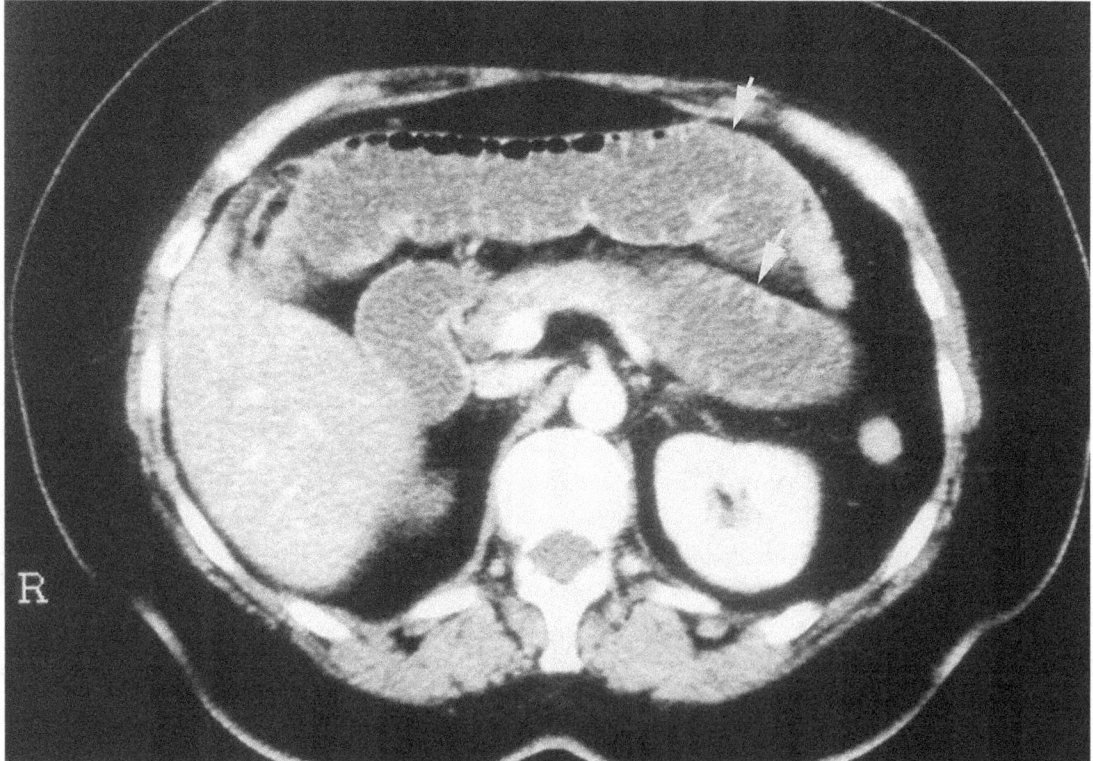

**Figure 22.20.a, b** Small bowel obstruction due to an incarcerated umbilical hernia as shown on CT: umbilical hernia (arrowhead) and dilated small bowel proximally (short arrows) and collapsed distally (long arrows).

# IMAGING IN GI SURGERY

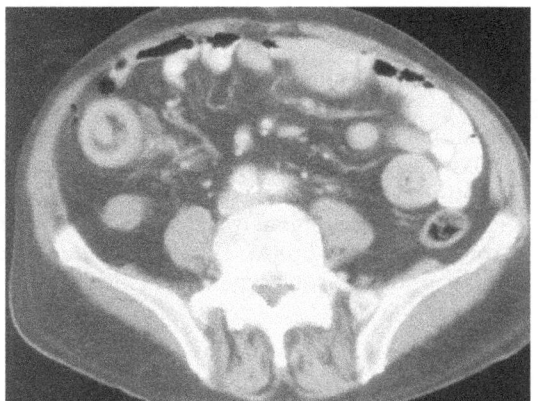
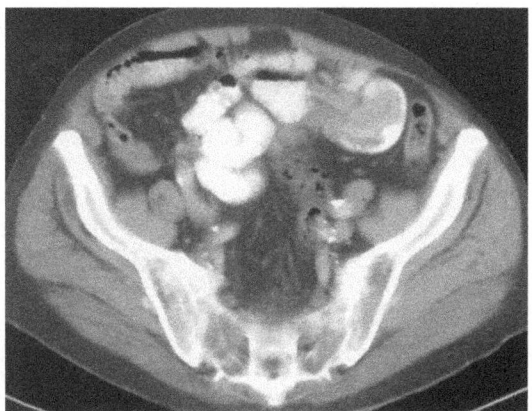
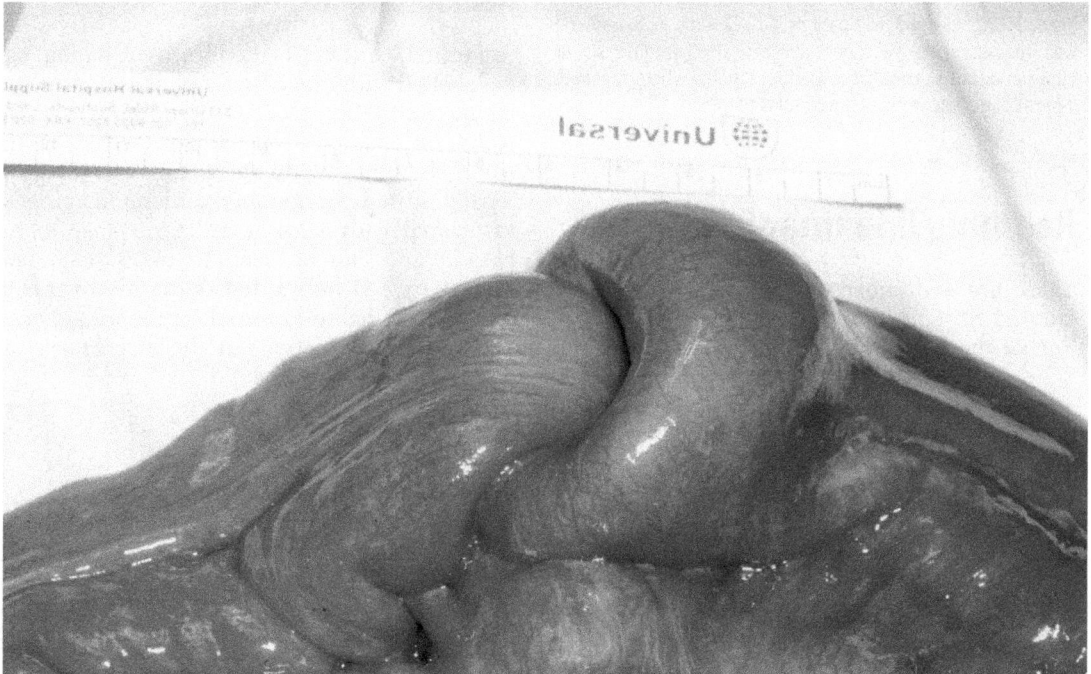

**Figure 22.21.** Intussusception due to melanoma metastatic to small bowel as shown by CT. **a** CT showing fat and mesenteric contents within the bowel lumen, and a layered appearance as a result of invagination of the bowel. **b** CT at a lower level showing the intraluminal bowel and the lead point, a picture corresponding well to the intraoperative photograph (**c**).

Magnetic resonance enteroclysis is currently undergoing evaluation for the assessment of small bowel pathology. Technique is as for a small bowel enema, i.e. a nasojejunal tube is placed and up to 2 litres of an isotonic solution infused directly into the small bowel. As for MRCP the water content of the bowel is the basis for the images. It involves no ionising radiation and because it is a cross-sectional technique has advantages over the X-ray projection images, by taking out the effect of overlying bowel loops. It demonstrates the bowel lumen but also the wall and extraluminal disease unlike barium studies. It does not, however, demonstrate mucosal detail (Figure 22.23).

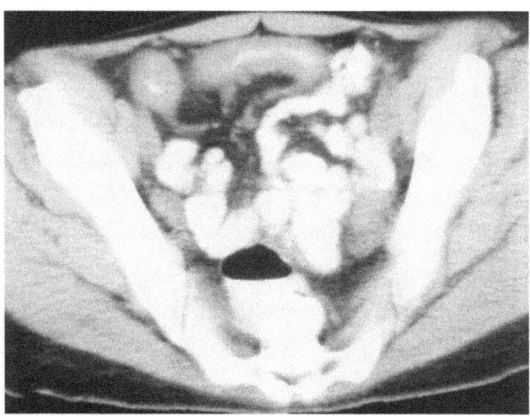

**Figure 22.22.** CT study of a patient with Crohn's. Note how the wall thickening is well seen, as with MR enteroclysis or ultrasound, but in contrast to barium studies where far more information about mucosal integrity is obtained.

imaging is best not regarded as a structural investigation as the anatomical resolution is of the order of 10 times worse than cross-sectional imaging such as US or CT. However, it provides a unique functional map of physiological processes in the body. For example, white cell scanning directly images inflammation and enables an assessment of disease activity in Crohn's disease, but does not provide good images of the morphology such as ulceration or strictures.

## White Cell Scanning Using Radiopharmaceuticals

Separated white cells taken from the patient can be labelled with one of two radionuclide agents: technetium-99m HMPAO or indium-111. The technetium agent is usually preferred as the isotope with a gamma ray energy of 140 keV is ideally suited for gamma camera imaging, is associated with a lower radiation dose to the patient and can be used to reach diagnostic images by 1–4 hours. It has the disadvantage, however, of being excreted by the biliary tract and hence bowel activity on the later images can

## Radionuclide Imaging

There are a number of radiopharmaceuticals tailored for specific purposes in the investigation of the gastrointestinal tract. Radionuclide

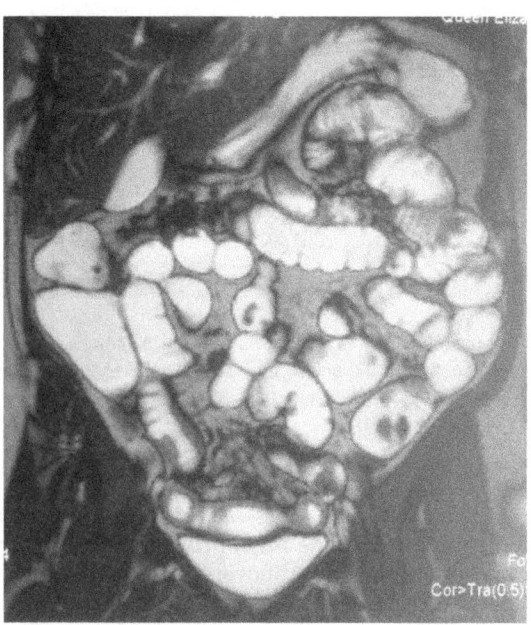
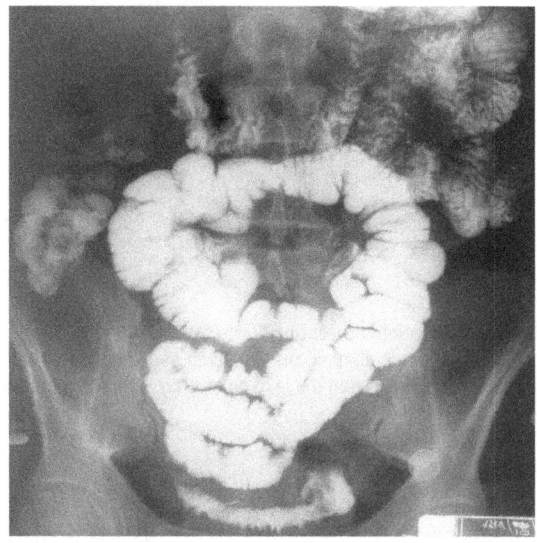

**Figure 22.23.** New techniques such as MR enteroclysis (MRE) demonstrate mural disease of the bowel to good effect as in this case of Crohn's disease (**a**) with the corresponding barium examination (**b**). Mucosal detail is not, however, seen with the MRE although the extraluminal effect, e.g. loop separation, is apparent.

# IMAGING IN GI SURGERY

cause diagnostic difficulties. Indium-111, on the other hand, may be more helpful if lower grade or chronic infection is suspected. Because of the longer half-life of the agent imaging is usually undertaken at 4–24 hours but can be extended for longer.

*Indications.* The main GI tract indication is the diagnosis and assessment of inflammatory bowel disease (Figure 22.24a and b), as the distribution of the disease and disease activity are shown.

Other indications are the investigation of unexplained pyrexia or suspected abdominal collections, but this has largely been superseded by ultrasound supplemented by CT where necessary.

## Biliary Imaging Using Radiopharmaceuticals

The usual radiopharmaceuticals are iminodiacetic acid (IDA) derivatives, e.g. HIDA or T-BIDA. These are labelled to technetium-99m and have the property of being excreted by the hepatocytes into the biliary system.

They can therefore be used for the following indications:

- bile leaks and fistulae (extraluminal collections or abnormal drainage pathways)
- bile reflux (Figure 22.25) into the stomach as a cause of biliary gastritis (gastric activity)
- afferent loop obstruction (activity retained)
- congenital anomalies, e.g. choledochal cysts, biliary atresia (delayed drainage)
- acute cholecystitis (gall bladder shows no uptake)
- suspected functional disorders of the gall bladder or sphincter of Oddi (delayed or absent gall bladder contraction or biliary drainage in response to a fatty meal or pharmacological agents such a cholecystokinin or morphine)
- characterisation of hepatic masses (e.g. follicular nodular hyperplasia characteristically shows retention of IDA derivatives).

## Meckel's Scan

A Meckel's diverticulum as a cause of unexplained gastrointestinal bleeding will always contain ectopic gastric mucosa. It will therefore show as an isolated focus of activity in the right

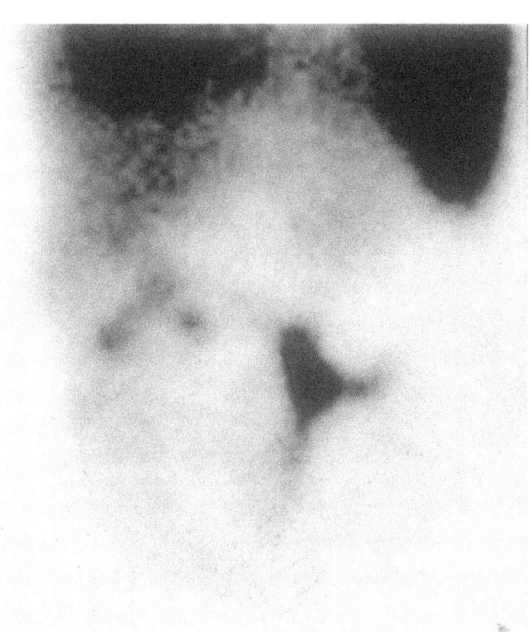

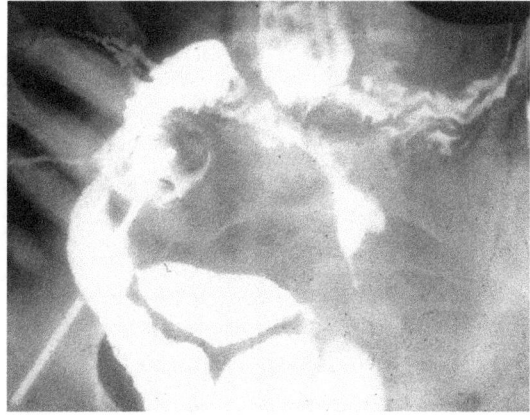

**Figure 22.24.** Technetium-99m-labelled white cell scan (**a**) showing activity in pelvic small bowel loops but with an associated non-anatomical branching pattern that can only be explained by fistula formation as shown on the corresponding small bowel meal study (**b**).

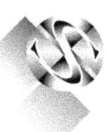

## 22 · UPPER GASTROINTESTINAL SURGERY

iliac fossa on a radionuclide scan using free technetium-99m pertechnetate.

## Octreotide Imaging

Octreotide is an analogue of somatostatin and hence when attached to an appropriate radionuclide such as indium-111 can be used to image tumours (Figure 22.26) that express somatostatin receptors – in particular neuroendocrine tumours such as carcinoids and gastrinomas.

## Transit Studies

### Oesophagus

Technetium-labelled colloid mixed with 10 ml liquid food such as tomato soup is used to obtain a dynamic assessment of oesophageal motility in patients with oesophagitis, dysphagia or atypical chest pain. The results are displayed as time activity curves for each third of the oesophagus, with combined curves for the whole oesophagus and the stomach. Transit in the upper third is about 1 second, middle third 2 seconds and the lower third 4–6 seconds. There are a number of drugs which affect motility such as metoclopramide and domperidone, and opiates, and these should generally be stopped before the test if possible.

Total and sectional transit time, ineffective peristalsis, retrograde peristalsis and gastro-oesophageal reflux can be assessed. A barium swallow dedicated to function provides similar data but is not quantitative.

### Gastric Emptying

Gastric function in response to both solid and liquid agents can be shown using technetium-99m colloid mixed with scrambled egg or orange squash respectively. This may be helpful in patients with dumping syndromes, unexplained nausea or vomiting, autonomic dysfunction or oesophagitis.

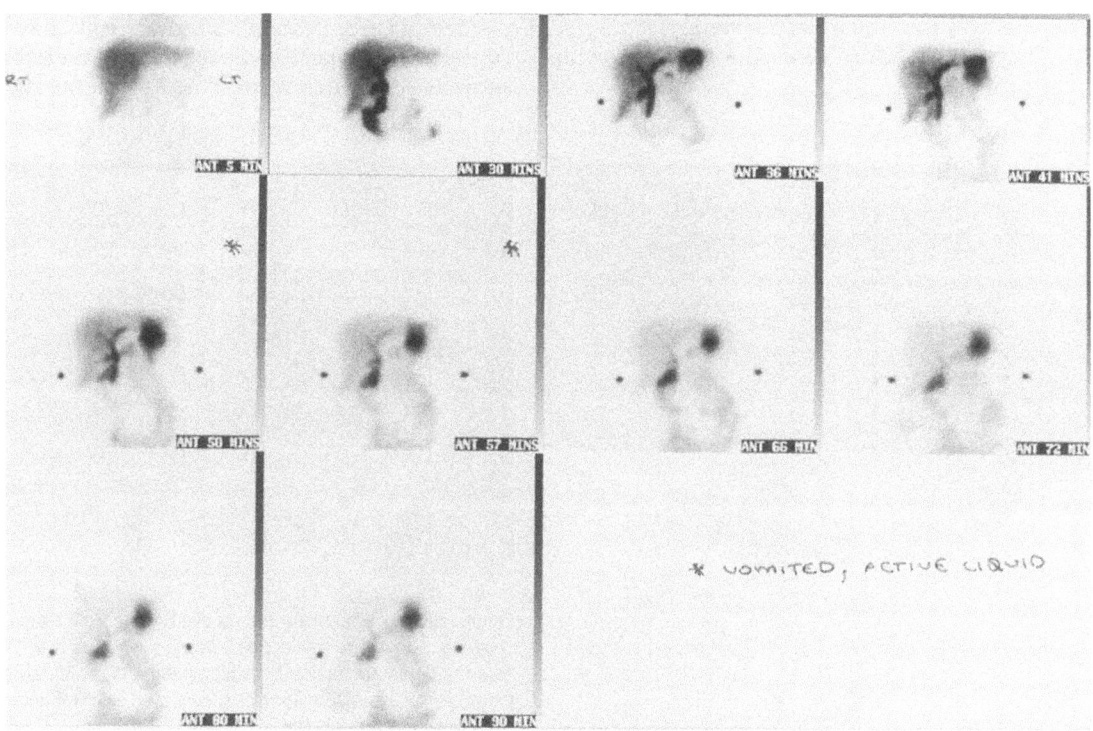

**Figure 22.25.** Radionuclide imaging: T-BIDA scan demonstrating activity excreted by the biliary tract refluxing into the stomach.

## IMAGING IN GI SURGERY

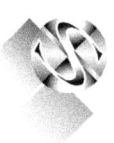

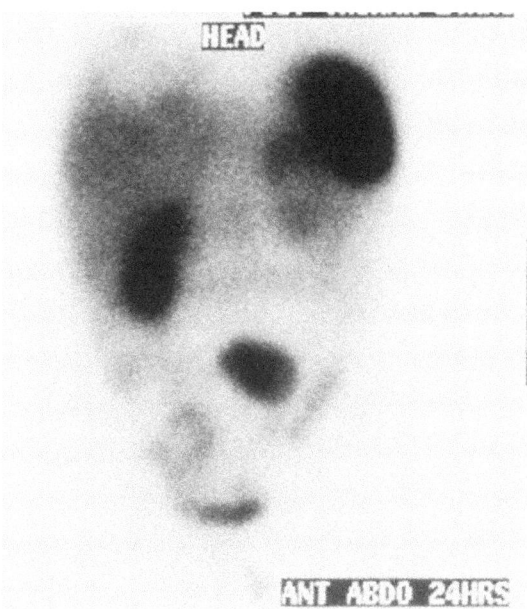

**Figure 22.26.** Radionuclide imaging: indium-111 labelled octreotide scan showing somatostatin-receptor positive tumour in the left iliac fossa, confirmed on CT (not shown). Necrotic tumour in the liver is manifest as cold lesions in the superior segments. Activity in the right flank is normal renal activity.

Dynamic images are obtained for up to 60 minutes and gastric emptying curves calculated. Normal $T_{1/2}$ for liquids is 10–20 minutes, and for solids 30–60 minutes. As for oesophageal studies, it may be necessary to withhold certain drugs.

### Small Bowel Transit

The solid gastric emptying study can be continued by taking further images at 30 minute intervals to allow calculation of the stomach to caecum transit time. There is a wide normal range and difficulties may be encountered in defining the position of the ileocaecal junction.

### Questions

1. Give indications for plain chest X-ray.
2. What contrast radiology is available?
3. What techniques should be used to stage gastro-oesophageal neoplasms?
4. Outline functional investigations.

# 23

# High Risk Lesions in the Esophagus and Nuclear Medicine

Andrew Phillip Chilton and Janusz A.Z. Jankowski

## Aims

- The scope of esophageal transit scintigraphy.
- Methodological investigational differences (advantages and disadvantages).
- The role of scintigraphy in esophageal investigations.
- Quantitative and qualitative data and its interpretation.

## Introduction

Multiple lesions within the esophagus have the potential to progress to frank neoplasia; achalasia and gastro-esophageal reflux disease (GERD) are both risk factors for the development of esophageal cancer. These pathologies are both detectable by esophageal transit scintigraphy (ETS).

ETS is a method of investigating the esophagus by measuring the passage of radiolabeled fluids or semi-solids through their esophageal transport. Kasem first described this method in 1972 [1].

Opinions on the usefulness of this method range from its proponents, who feel it offers the most precise assessment of function in the esophagus and provides a second means for diagnosis of motility disorders in patients with equivocal or near normal manometry [2], to those who feel it never fulfilled its initial promise as a simple screening test for suspected esophageal motility disorders [3].

Esophageal motility disorders frequently present with dysphagia, odynophagia and non-specific chest pain. Ambulatory manometry with 24-hour pH monitoring is recognized as the gold standard for investigation of esophageal motility disorders, but has the disadvantage of not always being readily available. It is also time-consuming and uncomfortable and requires expertise in carrying out the investigation plus the subsequent interpretation of it.

ETS allows investigation of esophageal pathology by direct monitoring of a swallowed radioactive bolus. It has excellent patient acceptance with low radiation exposure. ETS provides both quantitative data on esophageal transit, and qualitative data on esophageal function.

It must be stressed that ETS is not an investigation to be utilized in isolation in the investigation of esophageal disease, but should follow or complement endoscopic or radiologic assessment of the upper gastrointestinal tract.

## Esophageal Transit Scintigraphy

Multiple variations and test methodologies exist. However, the underlying principle remains constant. The test is affected by position (supine or upright), bolus volume [4], bolus viscosity, age [5] and method employed. Most investigators use a liquid bolus of 5–15 ml combined with 10–20 MBq of technetium-99m. Some investigators feel that a semi-solid bolus taken in the upright position is the most physiological method [6]. However, the most important tenet is that individual departments offering the investigation should establish their own "normal ranges". Jorgensen et al [7] described their method of determining normal ranges for ETS using water radiolabeled swallows in the sitting and supine positions. However, in view of the multiple different methods available it mitigates and limits comparisons between different studies.

## Method of Esophageal Transit Scintigraphy

As many investigational methodologies exist we will describe the method employed within our Nuclear Medicine department.

All pro- and anti-kinetic drugs (Table 23.1) are stopped 7 days prior to the investigation. However, if the patient is on opiates for pain relief these should be discontinued 24 hours before the examination.

Patients are fasted for at least 3 hours prior to the investigation. The patient is positioned supine or in the sitting position and administered a number of test swallows with 10 ml of unlabeled vehicle. Some investigators believe the sitting position to be more physiological. The detector is placed anteriorly (can be posterior) and the cricoid cartilage is identified and marked with a radioactive marker. Ten milliliters of a radiolabeled vehicle (in our practice tomato soup) is administered containing 20 MBq of techetium-99m. As the patient swallows the radioactive bolus, computer acquisition begins on a 64 × 64 matrix, with 0.5 seconds per frame for 30 seconds. The patient then dry swallows every 15 seconds for the remainder of the examination with one frame being taken per 15 seconds for a total of 38 frames (total test time 10 minutes). Repeated tests are better than a single investigation, as a single negative test does not exclude a functional abnormality (see ETS and Clinical Applications section below).

## Analysis of the Esophageal Transit Study

Quantitative analysis is performed over the region of interest (ROI), which extends from the cricoid to the gastro-esophageal junction. Analysis of the ROI allows for the construction of time activity curves (TAC) from which the esophageal transit time (ETT) is determined. ETTs are usually determined from the time of entry of 10% of the peak count to 90% clearance of peak count. Times are of the order of 12 to 13 seconds for the upper limit of normal. This will, however, vary depending on whether a supine or sitting position was adopted and the bolus composition (a normal range for ETT will need to be determined by the laboratory offering the investigation).

In addition, an assessment of the time taken for the esophageal contents to drop below a specified level (the activity at the start of the ROI at the initial swallow will represent 100%) can be made, or a calculation of the residual fraction can be determined at a defined time. This will provide an assessment of the amount of the original bolus retained within the esophagus. This result needs to be treated with caution in patients who reflux. A normal range for the residual fraction will need to be established for individual laboratories offering the investigation. However, upper limits of normal are between 18 and 20% (the position and method of testing will affect this, and normal ranges will need to be determined).

Qualitative assessment of the dynamic behavior of the bolus can be assessed via a cinematic or animated representation of the bolus passage through the esophagus in the sequential frames. A superior method to this is to represent the

**Table 23.1.** Drugs that may affect esophageal motility

| Pro-kinetic | Anti-kinetic |
| --- | --- |
| Dopamine antagonists (metoclopramide and domperidone) | Anticholinergic drugs |
| Cisapride | Antidepressant drugs with anticholinergic action (tricyclics) |
| | Calcium channel blockers |
| | Benzodiazepines |
| | Opiates |
| | Alpha-blockers |

# HIGH RISK LESIONS IN THE ESOPHAGUS AND NUCLEAR MEDICINE

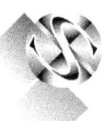

data as a single image. This is achieved by compacting the dynamic data into a condensed dynamic image (CDI), which provides spatial and temporal dimensions [8] (vertical and horizontal respectively). CDIs are not a substitute for quantitative assessment, but they facilitate the understanding of the ETT and residual fractions.

ETS provides information on:

- esophageal transit time
- residual activity
- CDI.

The ETTs derived from TACs identify abnormalities. They do not, however, characterize the nature of the abnormality. The CDI has allowed an understanding of the behavior of the bolus within its passage through the esophagus.

A variety of abnormal CDIs are recognized in different motility disorders (Table 23.2).

## Patterns of Abnormality in Condensed Dynamic Images

The CDI provides spatial temporal patterns of bolus transit and a number of morphological variations are recognized which are associated with abnormal esophageal motility.

A range of opinions exist as to ETS's ability to diagnose specific motility disorders [9]. The most common patterns seen are:

1. Uncomplicated linear descent into the stomach.
2. Division of the bolus and retrograde oscillatory motion (oscillations are usually synchronous with swallows but minimal propulsion of the test contents takes place) (see Figures 23.1 and 23.2).

Eriksen et al [10], using an esophageal egg transit study (EET), described five patterns (Table 23.2). They identified that normal patterns correlated with normal manometric findings. Patients with type II patterns (oscillatory) were significantly more likely to have serious manometric abnormalities. In a group of 21 patients with a type "" pattern, 20 had abnormal manometry and this encompassed all the patients with achalasia. In addition, patients with type III–V patterns (step delay, non-clearer, non-specific) were associated with normal manometry or non-specific manometric findings.

## Esophageal Transit Scintigraphy and Clinical Applications

ETS has an excellent sensitivity for identifying achalasia and scleroderma esophagus. Its usefulness in identifying diffuse esophageal spasm (DES) and nutcracker esophagus (NCE) is less well defined [8]. Reasons for this may be due to the episodic nature of the conditions and although high amplitude waves are experienced in NCE there is no impairment of transit to liquids through the esophagus. A further difficulty with DES is that there is a poor correlation with symptoms and manometric episodes of spasm [11]. In scintigraphic studies esophageal retention is most pronounced in achalasia and scleroderma esophagus and less so in DES and non-specific esophageal motility disorders (NSEMD).

A study by Parkman et al [12] compared ETS with the gold standard of esophageal manometry (EM). Esophageal retention, transit time and

Table 23.2. CDI patterns seen in the EET test [10]

| Type I | Normal pattern | Rapid and direct passage into the stomach |
|---|---|---|
| Type II (see Figures 23.1 and 23.2) | Oscillatory pattern | Propulsion and retropulsion of bolus, failure of bolus transit through stomach in 4 minutes |
| Type III | Non-clearance pattern | Failure to clear bolus at 4 minutes |
| Type IV (see Figure 23.3) | "Step delay" pattern | Initial normal transit followed by delay in either middle or distal third of esophagus |
| Type V | Non-specific pattern | Transit displayed an irregular pattern not classifiable into above four patterns |

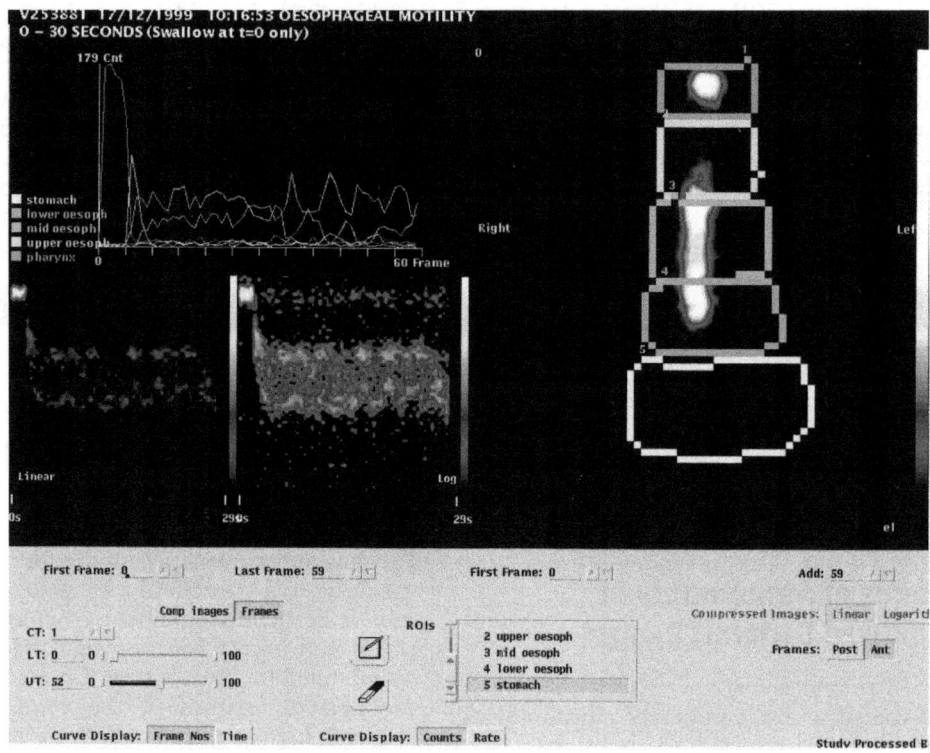

**Figure 23.1.** From a patient with achalasia. The CDI obtained from the ETS study demonstrates an oscillatory pattern (type II) and the time activity curve (TAC) show severe hold-up of the bolus in the mid and lower esophagus with failure to achieve satisfactory emptying into the stomach. This situation persists in the delayed images. See this figure in colour in the insert.

ETS diagnosis (based on retention, transit and the CDI), was compared with manometry. A significant correlation between the results of the two tests was obtained (Spearman correlation coefficient $r = 0.823, p < 0.001$). Of the 23 patient with achalasia, ETS correctly diagnosed 21 and identified all four patients with scleroderma esophagus (Table 23.3). In addition, Parkman et al proposed criteria that defined the diagnosis of abnormal motility using ETS (Table 23.4).

## ETS and Upper Esophageal Abnormalities

Partial or complete hold-up of the bolus at the level of the cricoid cartilage is usually secondary to an anatomical abnormality. In our own practice we have identified a number pharyngeal pouches responsible for this (Figure 23.4). It should, however, be stressed that ETS is an adjunct to other investigations and should not be employed as the initial primary mode of investigation.

## ETS and Esophageal Body Dysmotility

A variety of patterns are observed in body dysmotility ranging from type II to V (Table 23.2). However, the pattern should not be viewed in isolation, but in conjunction with ETT and the residual fraction. This tripartite approach will aid in making a diagnosis of the abnormality encountered (Table 23.4).

# HIGH RISK LESIONS IN THE ESOPHAGUS AND NUCLEAR MEDICINE

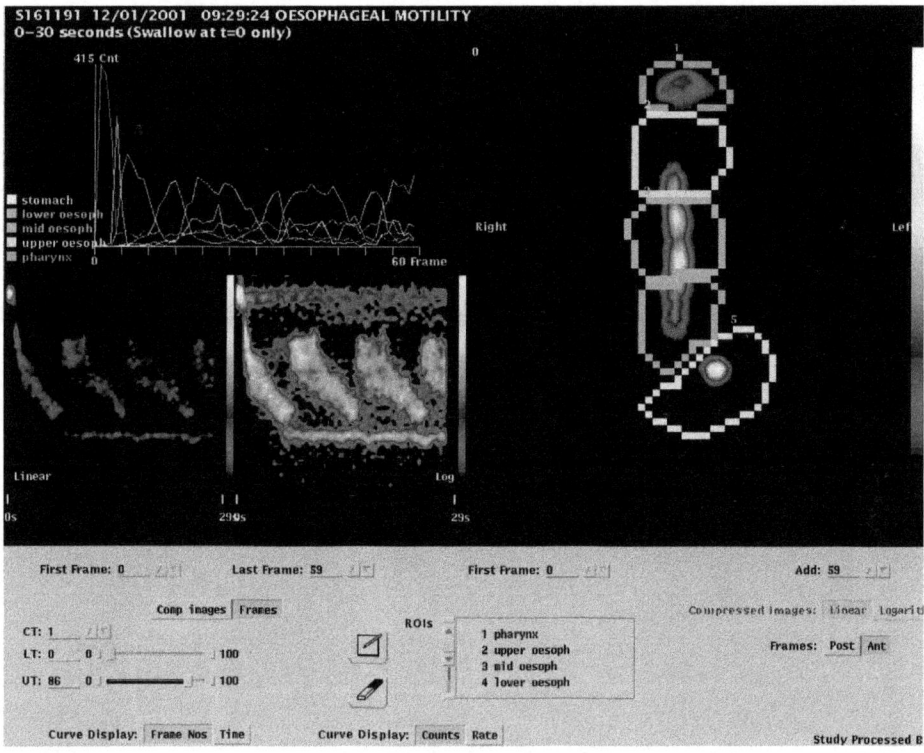

**Figure 23.2.** The time activity curve (TAC) shows relatively normal movement from the upper esophagus into the mid esophagus. Hold-up of the bolus is seen in the mid to lower esophagus with the CDI demonstrating a striking oscillatory pattern (type II). See this figure in colour in the insert.

**Table 23.3.** Comparison of ETS with esophageal manometry [12]

|  | Abnormal esophageal retention (AER) | % | Esophageal transit time (ETT) | % | ETS diagnosis (using AER, ETT and CDI) | % |
|---|---|---|---|---|---|---|
| Achalasia | 22/23 | 95 | 23/23 | 100 | 21/23 | 88 |
| Scleroderma esophagus | 4/4 | 100 | 4/4 | 100 | 3/4 | 75 |
| Non-specific esophageal motility disorder (NSEMD) | 5/21 | 25 | 13/21 | 55 | 15/21 | 76 |
| Lower esophageal sphincter dysfunction | 0/8 | 0 | 2/8 | 25 | 2/8 | 25 |
| Diffuse esophageal spasm | 3/6 | 50 | 3/6 | 50 | 2/6 | 33 |
| Normal | 1/26 | 4 | 6/26 | 22 | 17/26 | 67 |

Parkman et al [12] compared ETS with esophageal manometric diagnoses in a population of patients with esophageal motility disorders. Although numbers are small the scintigraphic diagnosis compares well with manometry in achalasia and scleroderma esophagus with prolonged transit times and abnormal retention. Transit time was calculated from the time of entry of 10% of peak radioactivity into the esophagus to 90% clearance of peak counts, esophageal retention calculated at the end of 40 swallows (10 minutes) and dubbed E-40. (Upper limit normal for transit time 13.5 seconds and upper limit of normal for E-40 was 18.3%.)

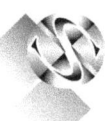

**Table 23.4.** Criteria for diagnosing esophageal motility disorders (adapted from Parkman HP et al [12])

| Motility disorder | Esophageal scintigraphy |
|---|---|
| Achalasia | Severe delay in mid/distal esophagus (ETT >30 s), severe retention >50%. No improvement in upright position |
| Diffuse esophageal spasm | Oscillatory transit throughout esophagus, mild delay in ETT, normal or mild retention (<30%) |
| Scleroderma esophagus | Severe delay in transit time (ETT >30 s), moderate to severe retention ≥ 30%, marked clearance in upright position |
| Isolated lower esophageal sphincter dysfunction | Normal transit in upper and middle esophagus with delay in distal transit, localized at gastro-esophageal junction; normal to mild retention |
| Non-specific esophageal motility disorder | Localized episode of oscillatory motion in ≥ 2 swallows, or mild delay in transit (ETT >13.5 s), or mild retention |
| Normal | Antegrade transit throughout esophagus, may have a single mild retrograde transit in one of three swallows (ETT ≥ 13.5 s) |

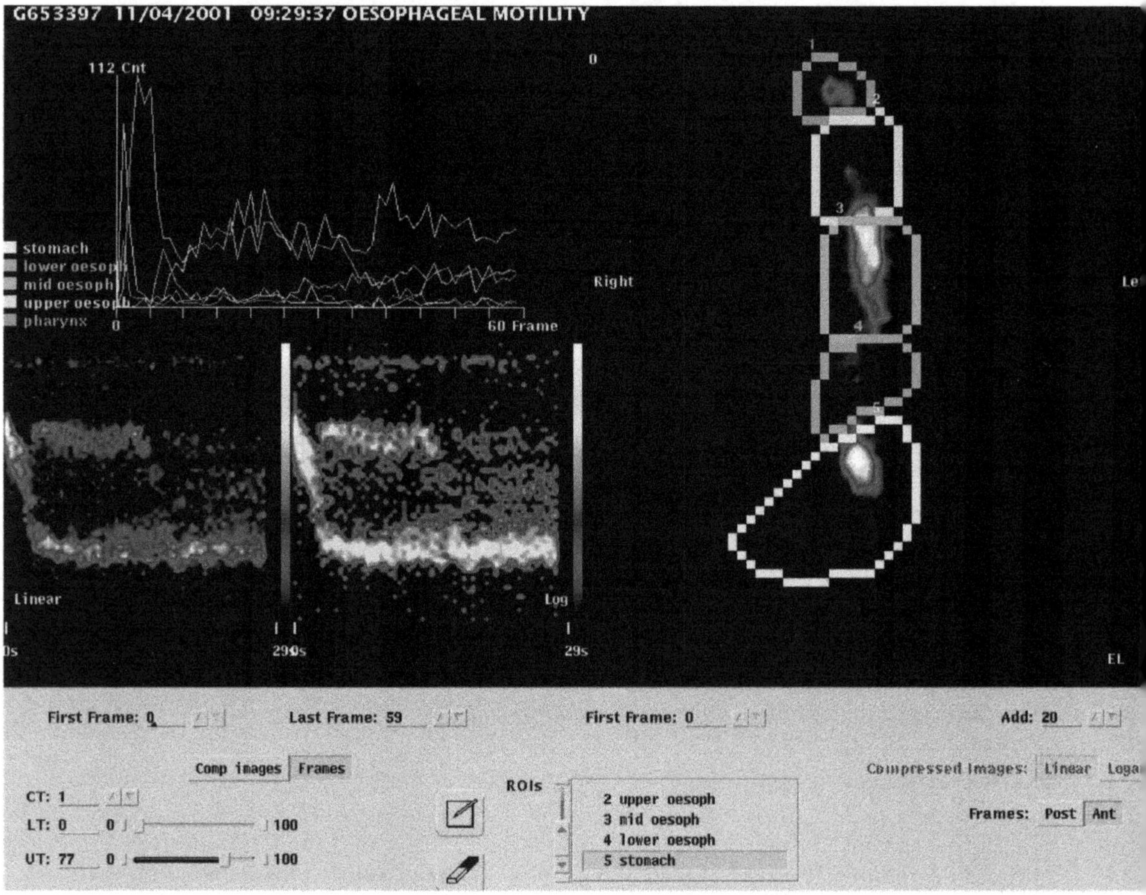

**Figure 23.3.** The CDI demonstrates a type IV step delay; the time activity curve (TAC) confirms delayed emptying in the mid esophagus. See this figure in colour in the insert.

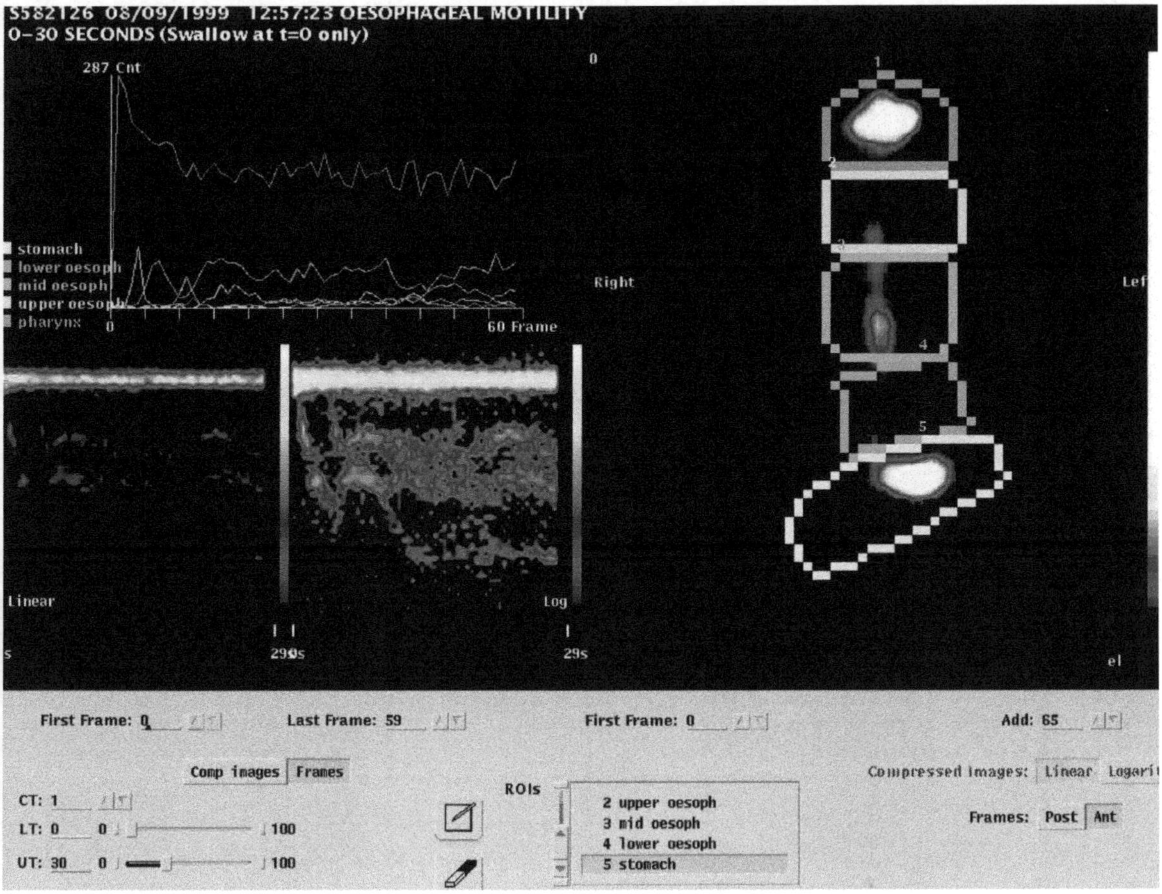

# HIGH RISK LESIONS IN THE ESOPHAGUS AND NUCLEAR MEDICINE

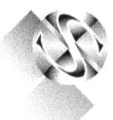

**Figure 23.4.** The CDI demonstrates a non-clearance pattern (type III). The time activity curve (TAC) shows failure of clearance of the bolus from the pharynx. Further investigation confirmed the presence of a pharyngeal pouch. See this figure in colour in the insert.

As previously detailed, ETS has an excellent sensitivity in diagnosing scleroderma esophagus, which may present as a dysmotility disorder of the esophageal body. It should, however, be stressed that the clinical manifestations of the illness should alert the individual clinician to the potential existence of the disorder (see Table 23.4 for ETS features of the disorder).

More commonly disorders of "body motility" will be secondary to NSEMD, DES and nut cracker esophagus, but with the limitations as previously described under the section ETS and Clinical Applications.

## ETS and Lower Esophageal Abnormalities

Abnormalities of the lower esophagus may be secondary to mechanical hold-up, or failure of relaxation of the lower esophageal sphincter. In the former case, mechanical obstruction should have been previously identified by either upper GI endoscopy or radiological imaging. Mechanical obstruction presents as partial or a complete hold-up of the bolus in the relevant ROI along with prolonged ETT.

In the case of failure of lower esophageal sphincter relaxation, of which achalasia is the most poignant and extreme example of a dysmotility disorder, ETS has a high sensitivity in identifying the condition. A type II pattern (Figures 23.1 and 23.2) is usually observed along with abnormal retention of the test bolus and prolonged ETT. In studies by Parkman et al and Eriksen [10,12] 21 out of 23 patients and 6 out of 6 demonstrated a type II pattern (oscillatory with pulsion and retropulsion) respectively. As for esophageal manometry is not

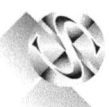

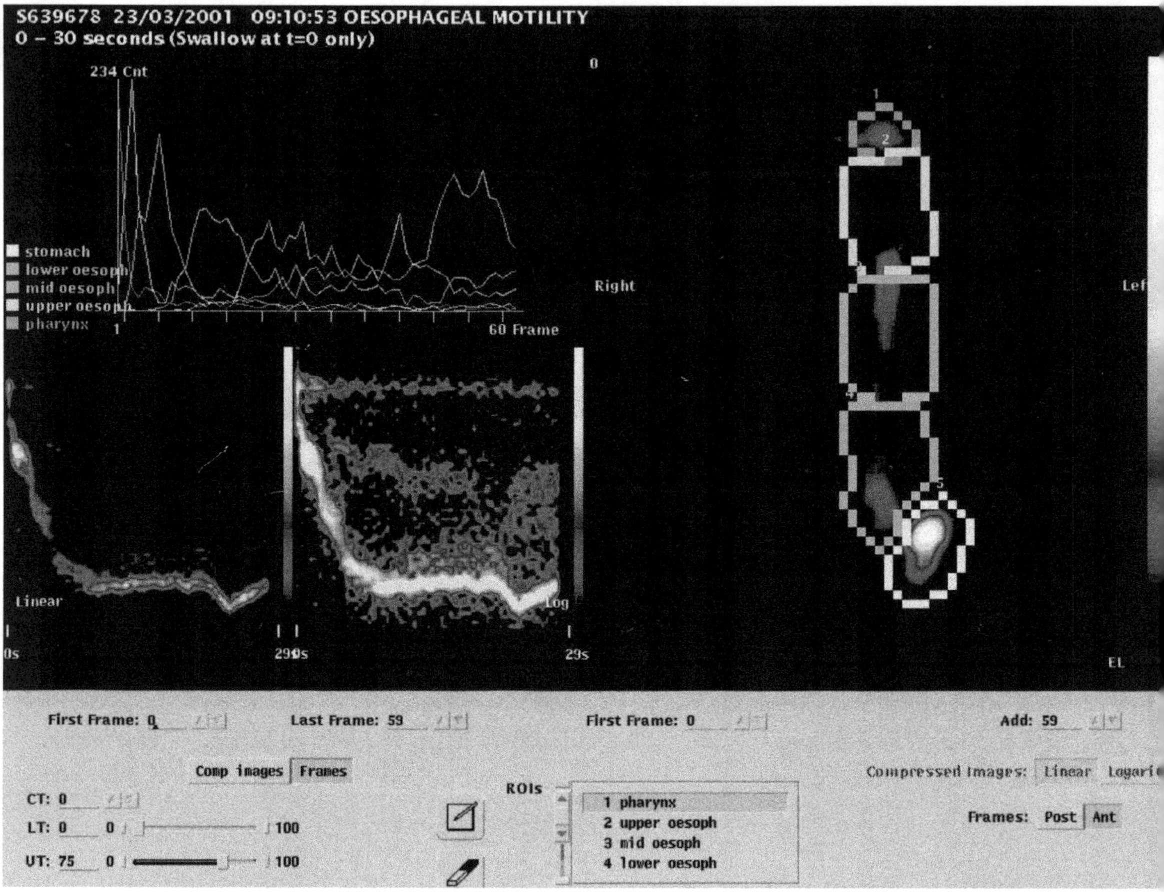

**Figure 23.5.** The CDI demonstrates a normal linear emptying pattern (type I). See this figure in colour in the insert.

always feasible some authors have suggested that initial dysmotility investigation should begin with ETS and on identification of a type II pattern these patients should be selected for manometry.

## ETS and Follow-up in Achalasia

Myotomy and pneumatic dilatation are recognized methods of managing achalasia. The impact of these treatments can be assessed with the use of ETS. Although impaired esophageal emptying will persist, quantifiable improvements are seen. This is also the case in botulinum toxin injections into the lower esophageal sphincter. However, no real effect has been observed with calcium channel blockers or other pharmacological agents.

## Esophageal Replacement

ETS has been employed in assessment of esophageal replacement in benign and malignant disease. Gastric, small bowel and colonic esophageal replacements function less well than the normal esophagus. However, gastric reconstructions function as well as normal stomachs [13,14].

## Conclusion

ETS is a well-tolerated procedure with excellent patient acceptance. It has high sensitivity in the diagnosis of achalasia and scleroderma esophagus. It is a good alternative if esophageal manometry is not available or poorly tolerated.

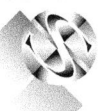

It has value as an initial screen in suspected esophageal motility disorders prior to proceeding to manometry.

## Questions

1. What is the radiation dose?
2. Should Endoscopy or contrast radiology of the upper GI tract be done before proceeding with ETS?
3. List the methods of doing examinations.
4. What conditions are best diagnosed by this method?
5. Does a single negative result exclude an abnormality?

## References

1. Kasem I. A new scintigraphic technique for the study of the esophagus. Am J Roentgenol 1972;115:681–8.
2. Bunker C. Esophageal disorders and scintigraphy: One clinician's perspective. J Nucl Med 1992;33:1301–3.
3. Baron TH, Richter JE. The use of esophageal function tests. Adv Intern Med 1993;38:361–86.
4. Ham HR, Georges B, Froideville JL et al. Oesophageal transit of liquid: Effects of single or multiple swallows. Nucl Med Commun 1985;6:263–7.
5. Van Calck H, Franken Ph, Baudoux M. Vieillissement et transit oesophagien. Etude isotopique au krypton. Rev Méd Brux 1988;9:415–17.
6. Taillefer R, Beauchamp G, Duranceau AC, Lafontaine E. Nuclear medicine and esophageal surgery. Clin Nucl Med 1986;11:445–60.
7. Jorgensen F, Hesse B, Tromholt N et al. Esophageal scintigraphy: reproducibility and normal ranges. J Nucl Med 1992;33:2106–9.
8. Klein HA, Wald A. Computer analysis of radionuclide esophageal transit studies. J Nucl Med 1984;25:957–64.
9. Blackwell JN, Hannan WJ, Adam RD, Heading RC. Radionuclide transit studies in the detection of esophageal dysmotility. Gut 1983;24:421–6.
10. Eriksen CA, Holdsworth RJ, Sutton D et al. The solid bolus egg oesophageal transit test: its manometric interpretation and usefulness as a screening test. Br J Surg 1987;74(12):1130–3.
11. Kahrilas PJ. Nutcracker esophagus: An idea whose time has gone? Am J Gastroenterol 1993;88:167–9.
12. Parkman HP, Maurer AH, Caroline DF et al. Optimal evaluation of patients with nonobstructive esophageal dysphagia: manometry, scintigraphy, or videoesophagography? Dig Dis Sci 1996;41(7):1355–68.
13. Paris F, Tomas-Ridocci M, Galan G et al. The colon as an oesophageal substitute in non-malignant disease. Eur J Cardiothorac Surg 1991;5:474–8.
14. Nishikawa M, Murakami T, Tangoku A. Functioning of the intrathoracic stomach after esophagectomy. Arch Surg 1994;129:837–41.

# 24

## Surgical Resection for Esophageal Cancer: Role of Extended Lymphadenectomy

Hubert J. Stein, Jörg Theisen and Jörg-Rüdiger Siewert

## Aims

To describe types of esophageal cancer, methods of selection for definitive treatment and the treatment itself.

## Introduction

The epidemiology of esophageal carcinoma is currently changing dramatically in the Western world. In contrast to squamous cell esophageal cancer, the incidence of esophageal adenocarcinoma has risen exponentially during the past two decades. At many institutions in Europe and the North America esophageal adenocarcinoma now outnumbers squamous cell esophageal cancer. In addition, adenocarcinoma of the distal esophagus is increasingly diagnosed at early stages because of a known precursor lesion and effective endoscopic surveillance programs. The marked differences between squamous cell carcinoma and adenocarcinoma of the esophagus in terms of pathogenesis, tumor location, tumor stage at the time of presentation, tumor biology and characteristics of the affected patients have now significantly affected surgical practice [1].

Strategies for surgical treatment of squamous cell esophageal cancer, which are mostly based on the vast experience of Japanese surgeons with extensive lymphadenectomy, cannot be applied uncritically to patients with esophageal adenocarcinoma. A more discriminate approach is required. Improvements in the treatment of esophageal cancer can thus be achieved by tailored therapeutic strategies which are based on the individual histologic tumor type, tumor location, tumor stage and consideration of established prognostic factors. A clear classification of the underlying tumor, a knowledge of the prognostic factors, and a thorough preoperative staging are essential for the selection of the optimal therapeutic modality in a given situation [1].

## Classification of Esophageal Cancer According to Topographic Tumor Location and Histologic Tumor Type

In many centers the topographic classification of esophageal cancer according to its location in the proximal, middle and distal third of the esophagus has been abandoned. A more practically oriented approach is based on a topographic anatomical assessment of the relationship between the esophageal cancer and the tracheobronchial tree, i.e. a differentiation of tumors with and without contact to the trachea or main stem bronchi. This facilitates the selection of the treatment strategy. While tumors located below the level of the tracheal bifurcation can frequently be resected with wide margins, an extensive resection of transmural tumors at or above the level of the tracheal bifurcation is usually prohibited by the proximity to the tracheo-esophageal tree. The pattern of lymphatic spread appears to have its watershed at the level of the bifurcation: the direction of lymphatic flow is primarily to the upper mediastinum and cervical region in patients with "suprabifurcal" tumors and towards the lower posterior mediastinum and celiac axis in patients with "infrabifurcal" tumors. Tumors located at the level of the tracheal bifurcation tend to metastasize in both directions (Figure 24.1).

While the vast majority of esophageal cancers located at or above the level of the tracheal bifurcation are of the squamous cell type, tumors in the distal esophagus today are usually adenocarcinomas associated with areas with specialized intestinal metaplasia (the so-called Barrett's esophagus), which is due to chronic recurrent reflux disease. Such tumors are also termed "Barrett's cancer". Since these tumors arise from within the esophagus, and thus require treatment as esophageal cancer, they need to be differentiated from other tumors arising at or below the esophagogastric junction. The topographic/anatomical classification system of adenocarcinomas of the esophagogastric junction (AEG tumors) reported by our group [2] provides a clear discrimination of the various tumors. It is now increasingly used to guide the selection of the surgical approach. Based on the anatomic location of the tumor center or, in patients with an advanced tumor, the location of the tumor mass, the following three tumor types are defined: Firstly, adenocarcinoma of the distal esophagus (AEG type I tumors), which usually arises from an area with specialized intestinal metaplasia of the esophagus, i.e. Barrett's esophagus, and may infiltrate the esophagogastric junction form above; secondly, true carcinoma of the cardia (AEG type II tumors) arising from the cardiac epithelium or very short segments with intestinal metaplasia at the esophagogastric junction; and thirdly, subcardial gastric carcinoma (AEG type III tumors), which infiltrates the esophagogastric junction and distal esophagus from below.

## Prognostic Factors

The presence of distant metastases is the single most important prognostic factor in patients with squamous cell and adenocarcinoma of the esophagus. The median survival of such patients is in the order of 6–12 months irrespective of the location of the primary tumor and can not be prolonged significantly by any of the available therapeutic modalities.

In patients without systemic metastases a complete macroscopic and microscopic tumor resection (i.e. a R0 resection according to the Union Internacional Contra la Cancrum/ American Joint Committee on Cancer (UICC/AJCC) guidelines) constitutes the most powerful independent prognostic factor. The chance of achieving a complete tumor resection is dependent on the histology and the pT category (Table 24.1).

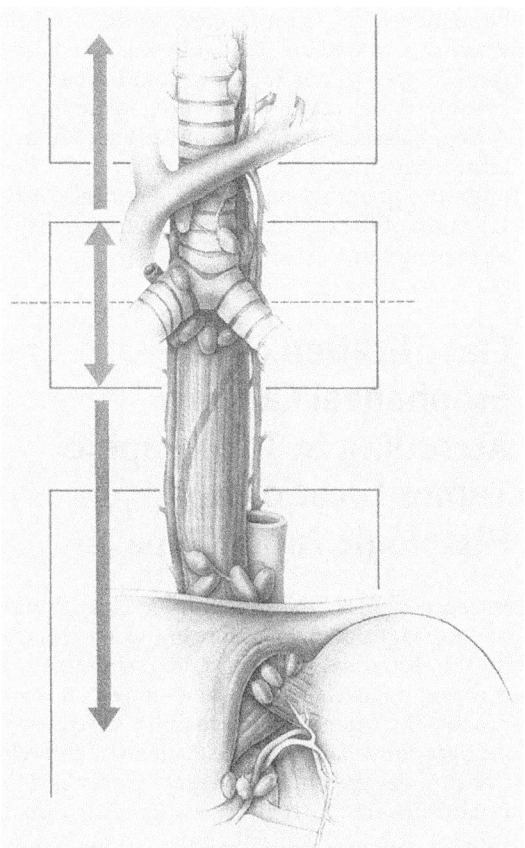

**Figure 24.1.** Direction of lymphatic flow from the esophagus.

# SURGICAL RESECTION FOR ESOPHAGEAL CANCER: ROLE OF EXTENDED LYMPHADENECTOMY

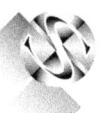

In the subgroup of patients with a complete tumor resection, the lymph node status and the number of positive lymph nodes represent the major independent prognostic factors. The prevalence of lymph node metastases is dependent on the histologic tumor type and the pT category (Table 24.2). Compared to squamous cell esophageal cancer, lymphatic spread appears to start later in patients with adenocarcinoma. In our experience with more than 250 resected early esophageal carcinomas, lymph node metastases were never found in adenocarcinoma limited to the mucosa and were significantly less common in patients with pT1b esophageal adenocarcinoma as compared with pT1b squamous cell esophageal cancer (Table 24.2). The reason for this observation is unclear, but could be related to an occlusion of submucosal lymphatic channels due to the chronic underlying reflux diseases with repeated episodes of inflammation in patients with esophageal adenocarcinoma. In recent studies, an independent prognostic effect of the so-called "micro-involvement" of lymph nodes, which were negative by routine histology, was demonstrated for patients with squamous cell carcinomas but not in patients with adenocarcinomas [3].

On multivariate analysis the histologic tumor type also constitutes an independent prognostic factor. In an analysis of more than 1000 resected esophageal cancers, adenocarcinoma was associated with a significantly better long-term prognosis than squamous cell cancer irrespective of T and N category [4].

Of the treatment-related factors the experience of the treatment center and the surgeon performing the resection have been identified as independent prognostic factors for long-term survival. The amount of perioperative blood transfusions and postoperative morbidity appear to constitute further independent prognostic factors. The concentration of esophageal cancer surgery in centers with large experience and a documented history of excellence is therefore recommended [3,5].

No overall survival benefit has been demonstrated for extended lymphadenectomy in squamous cell and adenocarcinoma of the esophagus. Nevertheless, several studies indicate that

**Table 24.1.** Rate of complete macroscopic and microscopic tumor resections (R0 resections according to the UICC/AJCC definition) in squamous cell and adenocarcinoma of the esophagus in relation to the UICC/AJCC pT category (data from the Chirurgische Klinik und Poliklinik, Klinikum rechts der Isar, Technische Universität München)

|  | Squamous cell carcinoma of the esophagus (%) | Adenocarcinoma of the distal esophagus (%) |
|---|---|---|
| pT1 |  |  |
|   mucosa | 100 | 100 |
|   submucosa | 91 | 100 |
| pT2 | 84 | 84 |
| pT3 | 70 | 68 |
| pT4 | 48 | 59 |

**Table 24.2.** Prevalence of lymph node metastases (including micrometastases documented by immunohistochemical techniques) in squamous cell and adenocarcinoma of the esophagus in relation to the UICC/AJCC pT category (data from the Chirurgische Klinik und Poliklinik, Klinikum rechts der Isar, Technische Universität München)

|  | Squamous cell carcinoma of the esophagus (%) | Adenocarcinoma of the distal esophagus (%) |
|---|---|---|
| pT1 |  |  |
|   mucosa | 11 | 0 |
|   submucosa | 40 | 22 |
| pT2 | 79 | 67 |
| pT3 | 84 | 85 |
| pT4 | 93 | 89 |

extended lymphadenectomy may improve survival in a subgroup of patients with a limited number of positive lymph nodes or early stages of lymphatic spread, i.e. lymph node microinvolvement. The lymph node ratio, i.e. the ratio between positive and removed nodes, constitutes a parameter to estimate the extent of lymph node dissection in relation to lymphatic spread. A lymph node ratio <0.2 constitutes an independent prognostic factor for patients with squamous cell and adenocarcinoma [6,7]. The potential benefit of extended lymphadenectomy may, however, be nullified if there is an associated increase in postoperative morbidity.

## Staging as a Prerequisite for Tailored Surgical Therapy

A tailored therapeutic approach requires precise staging for selection of the appropriate treatment modality [8]. After histologic confirmation and classification of the tumor type, determination of the presence or absence of distant metastases (M category), depth of tumor infiltration into the organ wall (T category) and the lymph node status (N category) thus becomes essential.

In the past percutaneous ultrasonography, plain chest X-rays and CT scanning have been routinely employed to assess for distant metastases. These are today increasingly being replaced by positron emission tomography and, in patients with locally advanced adenocarcinoma of the distal esophagus, diagnostic laparoscopy.

The pT category of an esophageal carcinoma can today be predicted by endoscopic ultrasound (EUS) with a diagnostic accuracy of about 85% in experienced hands. However, problems still arise in the differentiation of T2 from T3 category and T1a from T1b category. The presence and extent of tumor infiltration into neighboring organs is best be assessed by high resolution modern generation multi-slice spiral CT scanning. If the primary tumor has contact to the tracheobronchial tree bronchoscopy is mandatory to exclude or diagnose infiltration.

None of the available imaging non-invasive techniques (CT, MRI, endoscopic ultrasound) can today reliably predict the presence of lymph node metastases. The problem with these techniques is that lymphatic spread can only be inferred by the documentation of enlarged nodes. Recent studies indicate that lymph node metastases distant from the primary tumor may reliably be detected by positron emission tomography. Whether the use of diagnostic thoracoscopy, laparoscopy or the technologies of sentinel node detection for preoperative determination of the lymph node status will have an impact on the management of patients with esophageal cancer, will have to be shown in ongoing studies.

Since esophagectomy and reconstruction of the alimentary tract continuity constitutes a major surgical insult, a thorough evaluation of the physiologic reserve and the general status of the patients is essential to make sure that they can withstand a potentially prolonged and complicated postoperative course. In our experience a detailed risk analysis employing a dedicated organ function scoring system has proved helpful in selecting such patients [9].

## Aims of Surgical Resection

Most surgeons agree that complete resection of the tumor and its entire lymphatic drainage has the best potential for long-term survival [10]. In patients with incomplete tumor resection the procedure must be considered palliative. These patients have no survival benefit form surgical resection. Palliation of dysphagia in patients with irresectable esophageal cancer is better achieved by endoscopic intervention or radiochemotherapy. A complete macroscopic and microscopic tumor resection must consequently be the aim of any surgical approach to squamous cell and adenocarcinoma of the esophagus. Intended palliative resections or bypass procedures have been abandoned at most institutions.

With standardized resection and reconstruction techniques, advances in postoperative management and careful patient selection a transthoracic or transmediastinal esophagectomy with en-bloc two-field lymphadenectomy can today be performed with a postoperative mortality below 5%. In our experience postoperative mortality could be decreased to below 2% by consequent application of a procedure-

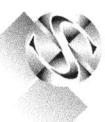

specific risk scoring system and exclusion of high risk patients from surgery (Figure 24.2). Such results can, however, only be achieved in experienced centers with a high patient load ("high volume centers").

## Lymphadenectomy for Esophageal Cancer

Although the principle of lymphadenectomy for tumors of the gastrointestinal tract was introduced more than 100 years ago, the value of lymph node dissection in patients with esophageal cancer still remains controversial. While extensive lymphadenectomy is advocated by some in order to reduce the rate of local recurrences and prolong survival, others argue that the claimed benefits of extensive lymph node dissection in patients with esophageal cancer have not been proven and that lymphadenectomy may in fact increase the morbidity and mortality of esophageal resection [7].

## Pattern of Lymphatic Spread of Esophageal Cancer

An intimate knowledge of the lymphatic drainage system is the prerequisite for any approach to lymph node dissection. Key to the understanding of the lymphatic drainage of an organ is the comprehension of its embryogenesis. The esophagus originates from two different tissue sources, i.e. the branchial arches and pharyngeal pouches orally and the splanchnic mesoderm aborally. Both join during the embryonic and fetal development but keep a delimitation at the level of the tracheal bifurcation even during adult life. This results not only in a bilateral oral and aboral vascular supply but also in a corresponding bilateral lymphatic drainage (Figure 24.1).

In patients with early stage esophageal cancer the pattern of lymph node spread follows these anatomical pathways. The location of the primary tumor thus determines the direction of lymphatic drainage and, consequently, the location of lymph node metastases. Tumors located above the level of the tracheal bifurcation

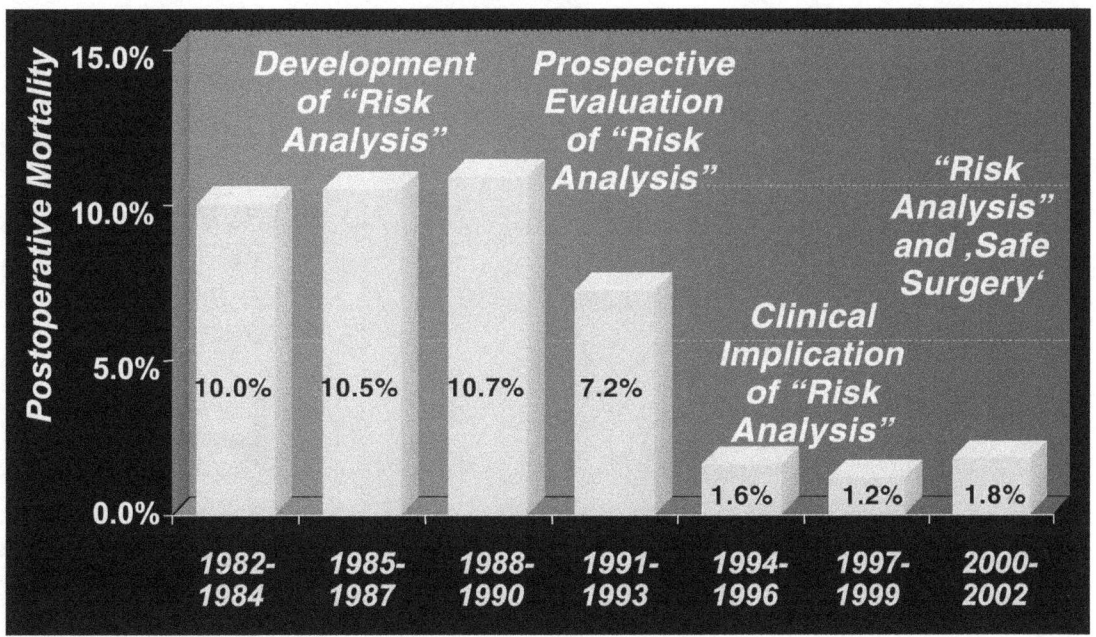

**Figure 24.2.** Decreasing postoperative mortality after esophagectomy for esophageal cancer at the Chirurgische Klinik und Poliklinik, Klinikum rechts der Isar, Technische Universität München.

preferentially metastasize orally to the upper mediastinal and neck lymph nodes, while tumors located below the level of the tracheal bifurcation follow the aboral lymphatic drainage of the splanchnic mesoderm towards the celiac axis. Tumors located at the level of the tracheal bifurcation can metastasize in both directions. In early tumors skipping of lymph node stations is rare. The location of the primary tumor is therefore of the utmost importance for surgical lymph node dissection.

Of particular importance is the extensive longitudinal submucosal lymphatic network. This allows communication between the two separate lymphatic drainage systems of the proximal and distal esophagus. A redirection of lymphatic drainage is possible when the primary lymphatic pathway is blocked, i.e. in patients with advanced tumors and extensive lymphatic metastases. In this situation an extra-anatomic pattern of lymph node metastases can be observed.

This pattern of lymphatic spread is reflected in our prospective analysis of the location of lymph node metastases in patients with resected squamous cell and adenocarcinoma of the esophagus. In patients with squamous cell cancer, lymph node metastases were most commonly found in the area of the tracheal bifurcation, the upper mediastinum, the lower mediastinum, and the left and right paracardial region, followed by lymph nodes along the left gastric artery, the cervical region and at the celiac axis (Figure 24.3). The pattern was different for adenocarcinoma of the distal esophagus. In these patients lymph node metastases

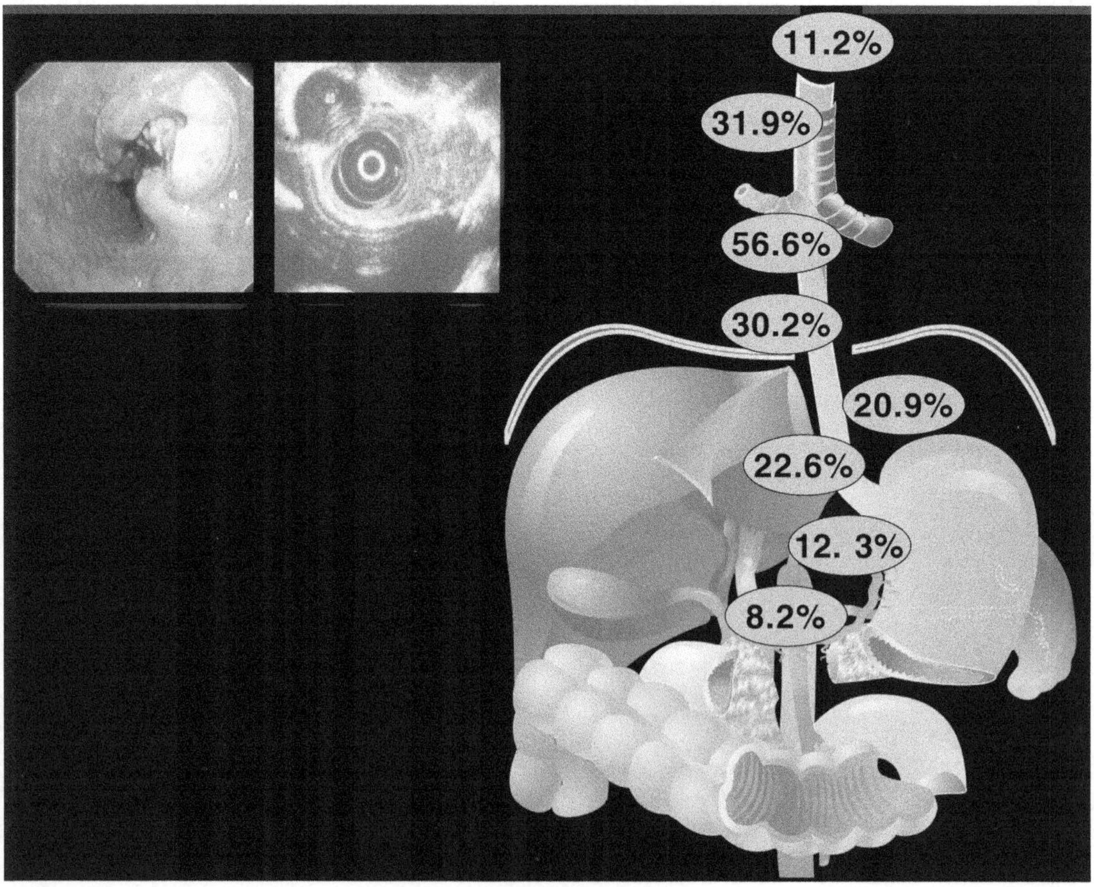

**Figure 24.3.** Distribution of lymph node metastases in squamous cell esophageal cancer (data of 100 consecutive patients resected at the Chirurgische Klinik und Poliklinik, Klinikum rechts der Isar, Technische Universität München).

# SURGICAL RESECTION FOR ESOPHAGEAL CANCER: ROLE OF EXTENDED LYMPHADENECTOMY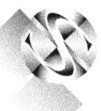

occurred in decreasing order in the paracardial region, the posterior lower mediastinum, the lesser curvature side of the stomach, and along the left gastric artery towards the celiac axis. Lymph node metastases in the region of the tracheal bifurcation, the upper mediastinum or cervical region occurred only in patients with locally advanced adenocarcinoma who also had numerous positive loco-regional nodes (Figure 24.4).

## Definition of the Extent of Lymphadenectomy for Esophageal Cancer

The understanding of lymphadenectomy for esophageal cancer has also long been compromised by confusion in terminology and nomenclature used when describing the extent of lymph node dissection. According to a consensus conference of the International Society for Diseases of the Esophagus (ISDE) the term *two-field lymphadenectomy* should be used for removal of abdominal and mediastinal lymph nodes, while the term *three-field lymphadenectomy* describes an abdominal, mediastinal and cervical lymph node dissection [11].

Today there is a wide consensus on the extent of abdominal lymphadenectomy for esophageal cancer. Most experts agree that removal of the compartment II lymph nodes of the gastric cancer classification is essential. In addition, the lymph nodes along the lesser curvature should be removed down to the so-called "crawfoot", due to the high number of lymph node

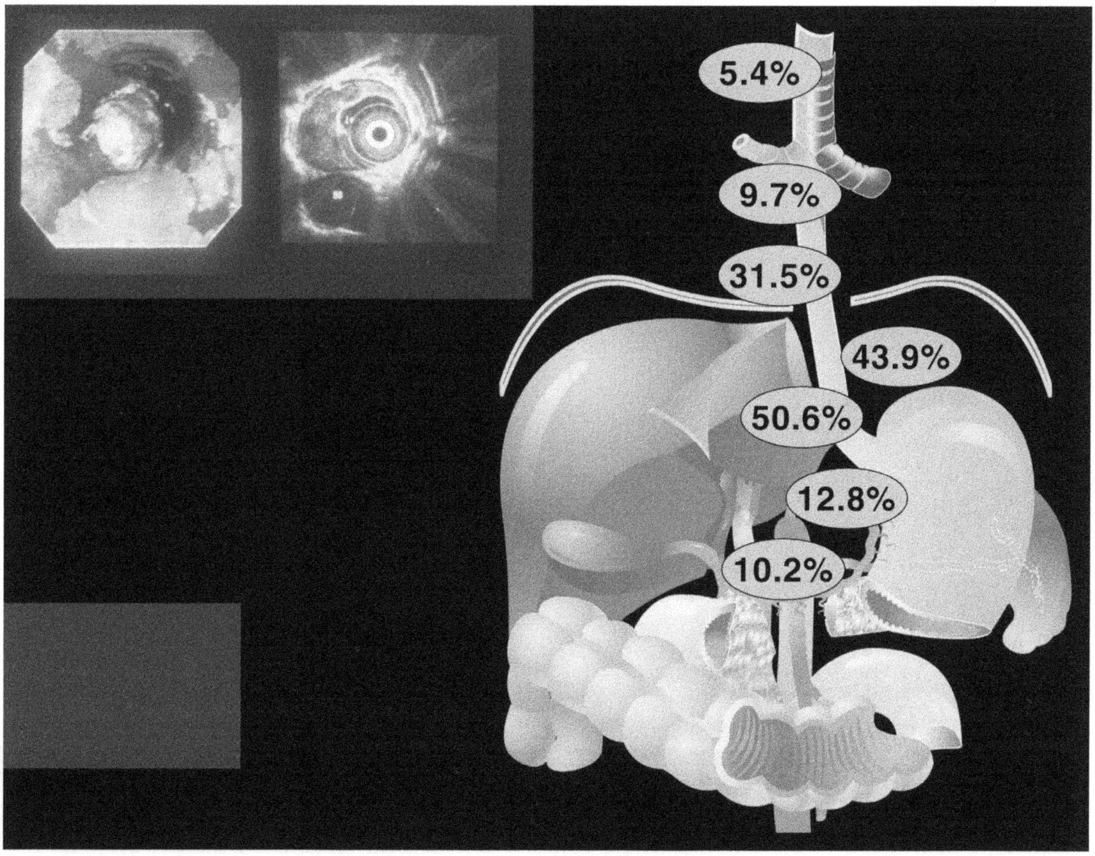

**Figure 24.4.** Distribution of lymph node metastases in adenocarcinoma of the distal esophagus (data of 100 consecutive patients resected at the Chirurgische Klinik und Poliklinik, Klinikum rechts der Isar, Technische Universität München)

metastases in this area. Abdominal lymphadenectomy is usually performed together with the proximal gastric resection and preparation of the stomach for interposition.

Most experts also agree that, as a minimum, a complete lymphadenectomy of the lower posterior mediastinum should be performed. This is termed a "standard mediastinal lymphadenectomy". An extension of the lymphadenectomy along the right side of the trachea is termed "extended mediastinal lymphadenectomy". Lymphadenectomy of the left paratracheal, left recurrent laryngeal nerve and subaortic nodes in addition to the extended mediastinal lymphadenectomy is termed a "total mediastinal lymphadenectomy" (Figure 24.5) [11]. The term "cervical lymphadenectomy" includes removal of the central cervical lymph nodes and bilaterally the lymphatic drainage along the large vessels.

Further advances in the understanding of lymphatic spread and standardization of lymphadenectomy for esophageal cancer may in the future be achieved by combination of several closely related lymph node groups into so-called compartments, similar to the classification of lymphatic metastases of gastric carcinoma. Based on the work of Fujita et al [12] the Japanese Research Society for Esophageal Cancer is currently evaluating a classification of lymph node groups into three compartments defined according to the sequence of lymph node metastases for tumors at various locations. This predicts the prevalence of lymph node

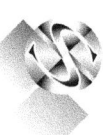

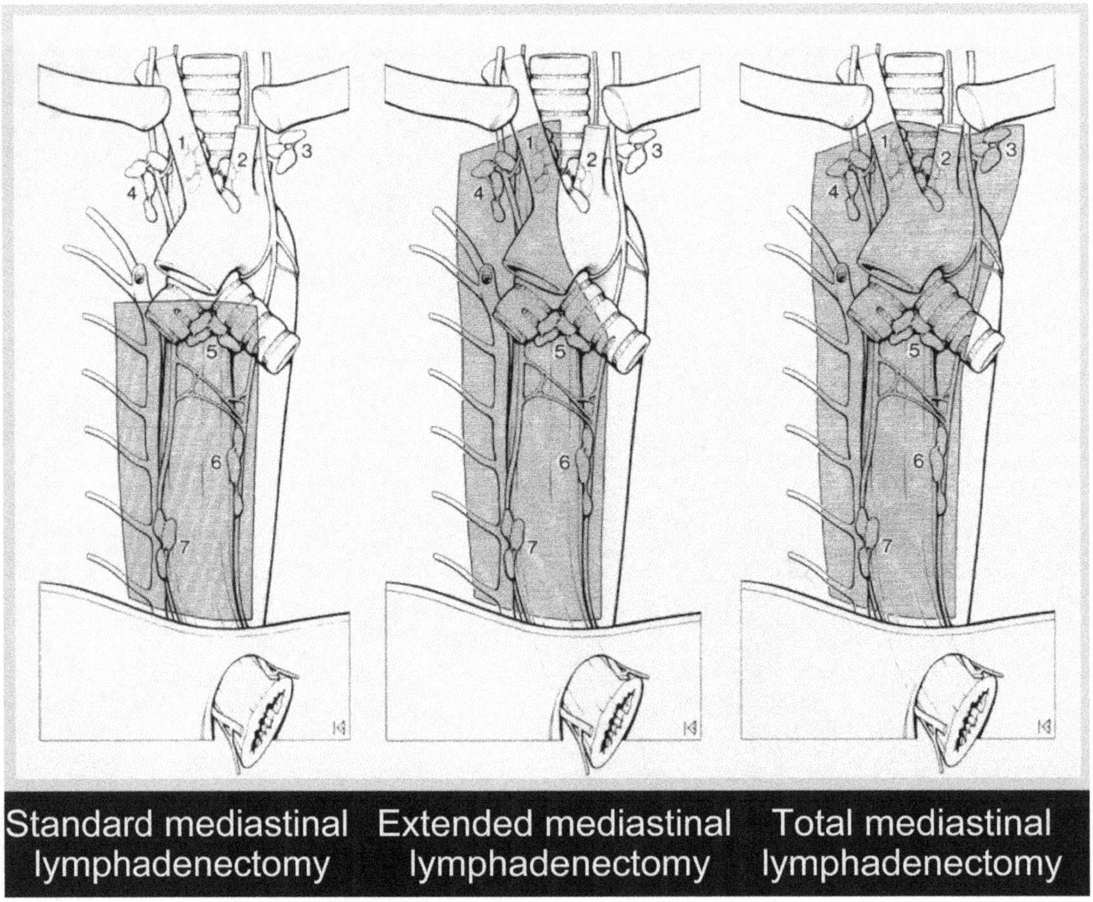

**Figure 24.5.** Nomenclature of the extent of mediastinal lymphadenectomy according to a consensus conference of the International Society for Diseases of the Esophgus (ISDE)[11].

metastases in the various compartments based on the tumor location and can be used to tailor the extent of lymph node dissection. The individual lymph node compartments for tumors located below and above the level of the tracheal bifurcation are depicted in Figure 24.6. When the widely accepted experience with lymphadenectomy for gastric carcinoma is transferred to the esophagus, a resection of lymph node compartments I and II, the so-called "D2-resection", must then, at least theoretically, be recommended as the standard therapy for esophageal cancer. This would comprise dissection of lesser curvature, celiac axis, para-esophageal, lower mediastinal and bifurcation lymph nodes for tumors located below the level of tracheal bifurcation and resection of the para-esophageal, bifurcation, left and right paratracheal, and cervical lymph nodes in patients with tumors located above the level of the tracheal bifurcation.

## Basic Considerations of Lymph Node Dissection in Esophageal Cancer

The value of lymph node dissection in gastrointestinal cancers can be considered under two premises [13]:

- The first is based on the assumption that the primary tumor metastasizes in a stepwise fashion. Due to the dense lymphatic drainage of the esophageal submucosa, lymphatic spread to peritumoral lymph nodes occurs relatively early and can be documented already in up to 40% of patients with pT1b squamous cell cancer and about 20% of patients with pT1b adenocarcinoma (Table 24.2). The tumor then metastasizes along the lymph node groups according to the anatomical position. Hematogenous metastases occur late in the course of lymphatic spread except in the rare situation of venous tumor invasion.
- In the second hypothesis lymphatic metastases are considered a marker for systemic spread of the tumor. With this concept, lymph node dissection is only of diagnostic value and any surgical resection in patients with lymph node metastases is only palliative.

An aggressive surgical approach with extended lymphadenectomy in esophageal carcinoma only makes sense if the first hypothesis is followed. Under this premise, systematic lymph node dissection can stop tumor spread on its way to systemic disease provided the correct lymph nodes, i.e. the nodal groups that anatomically comprise the lymphatic drainage of the tumor-bearing organ, are removed completely.

Quality control of the therapeutic procedure thus becomes essential to assess the efficacy of lymph node dissection. There are two ways to assure the quality of the lymph node dissection provided the lymph node dissection is correctly performed anatomically. One method, which is popular in Japan, requires that the surgeon dissects the individual lymph node stations separately and documents removal of the lymphatic groups according to anatomical regions. In this situation the pathologist only evaluates individual lymph nodes for the presence of metastatic tumor. For legal reasons the surgeon may not perform the work-up of the removed specimen in many Western centers. Here the pathologist has to assure the quality of the lymph node dissection. The prerequisite for this second method of quality control is an en-bloc preparation of the esophagus and its lymphatic drainage, correct identification of the borderline lymph nodes, and delivery of a complete specimen to the pathologist. The extent of lymphadenectomy can then be assessed by an accurate count of the removed lymph nodes. The updated version of the UICC/AJCC staging system has taken this into account by requiring a minimum of six regional nodes for staging [14]. An even higher number of removed node, i.e. at least 15 nodes, was thought to be required by the participants of an ISDE consensus meeting [10]. Adequate lymphadenectomy and lymph node staging thus comprises both quality and quantity aspects, i.e. removal of a sufficient number of lymph nodes at the anatomically correct position.

With this approach it is, important to realize that lymphatic spread is often more advanced than can be detected with routine histology techniques. Immunohistochemical staining with monoclonal cytokeratin antibodies can show lymph node microinvolvement in a substantial portion of patients staged as pN0 with

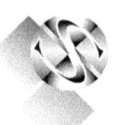

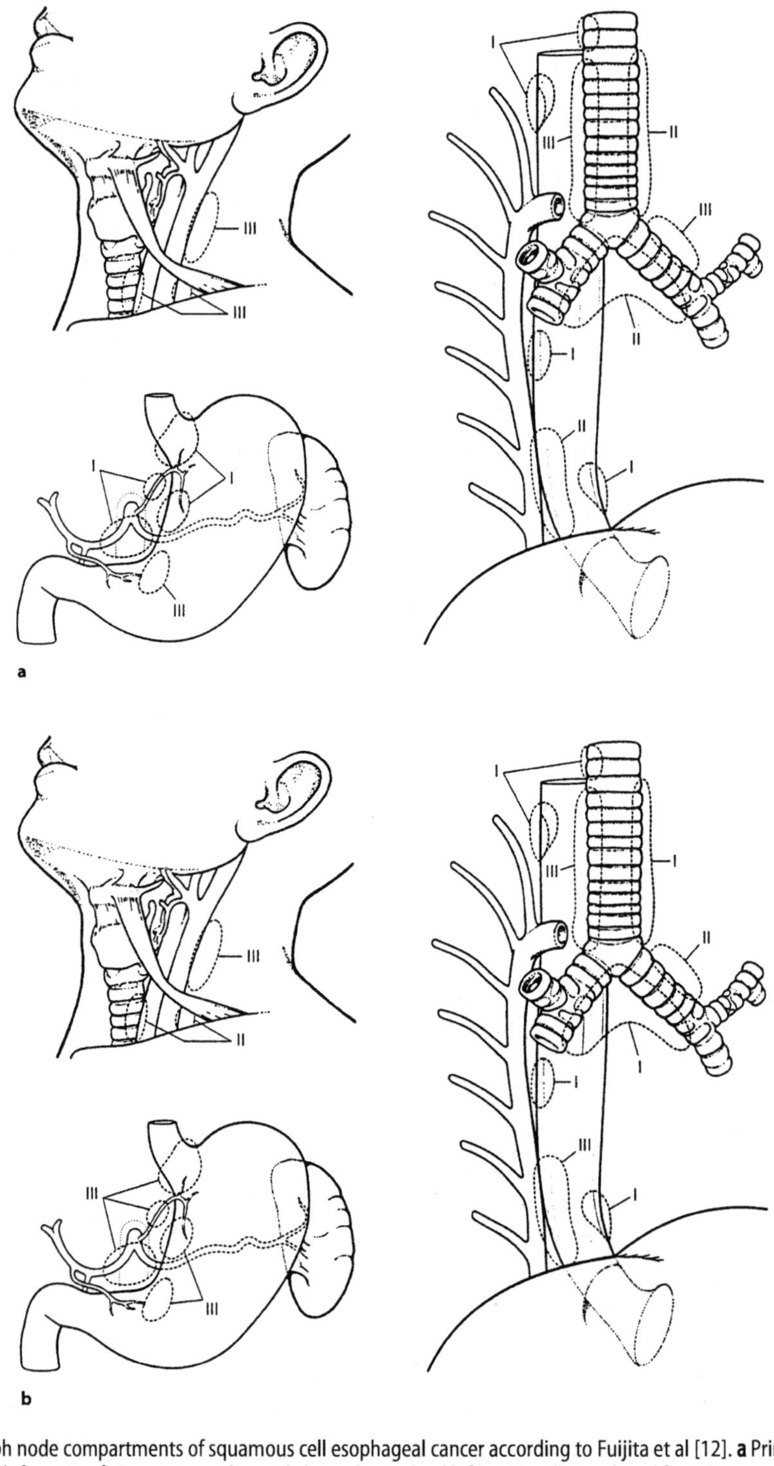

24 · UPPER GASTROINTESTINAL SURGERY

**Figure 24.6.** Lymph node compartments of squamous cell esophageal cancer according to Fuijita et al [12]. **a** Primary tumor located below the tracheal bifurcation. **b** Tumor tumor located above the tracheal bifurcation. (Reproduced from Siewert JR, Stein HJ, Sendler A, Fink U. Ösophaguskarzinom. In: Siewert JR (ed) Praxis der Viszeralchirurgie: Onkologische Chirurgie. Springer Verlag, Berlin, 2001, pp 407–38, Abbildung 26.10,a,b.)

standard histology techniques. Similar to the primary tumor, a safety margin is therefore also essential in the area of the lymphatic drainage to assure a complete tumor resection. The required safety margin of lymphadenectomy can be estimated by the so-called lymph node ratio, i.e. the ratio between positive and removed nodes. Cure is still possible in a patient with esophageal cancer when the lymph node ratio is below 0.2, i.e. less than 20% of the removed nodes are positive [6]. For clinical practice this means that the number of removed nodes must exceed the number of positive nodes by a factor of 5. In patients with a limited number of positive regional nodes this can only be achieved by a formal lymphadenectomy of the upper abdominal and mediastinal compartments.

Based on these concepts a further extension of the lymph node dissection (three-field lymphadenectomy) appears theoretically reasonable because this further increases the safety margin in the area of the lymphatic drainage and improves the lymph node ratio. Radicality of lymph node dissection for esophageal cancer is limited by anatomical borders, vital structures and a marked increase in morbidity and mortality with more extensive procedures. Furthermore distant lymph node metastases may reflect systemic tumor dissemination rather than loco-regional disease. Thus only a subgroup of patients with incipient lymph node metastases or a limited number of positive regional lymph nodes will benefit from an extensive lymphadenectomy. Lymphadenectomy must thus not be considered an independent therapeutic principle. Rather it constitutes an important component of the surgical procedure with the aim to achieve a complete local tumor removal, the primary goal of any surgical approach to malignant disease.

"Stage migration" (also termed the "Will Rogers phenomenon") [15] is a problem that has not been addressed in the analysis of lymphadenectomy studies in patients with esophageal cancer. Removal of a higher number and more distant lymph nodes improves the accuracy of lymph node staging. This results in an up-staging of the lymph node category in a number of patients. The extent of lymph node dissection therefore determines tumor staging. Based on these observations the survival benefit observed in patients with a higher number of removed lymph nodes may not be real but rather reflect under-staging in patients with less extensive lymph node dissection. When comparing survival data between procedures one must be sure that the accuracy of tumor staging is similar for both groups.

## Results of Lymphadenectomy for Squamous Cell Esophageal Cancer

In the Western world the benefits of lymphadenectomy for squamous cell esophageal cancer have not been proven in a large and well-designed prospective randomized trial. A comparison of the results from various centers employing different strategies for lymphadenectomy indicates that formal two-field lymphadenectomy can improve the prognosis in patients with an early stage of lymphatic metastases [7]. In our own experience a transthoracic en-bloc esophagectomy with two-field lymphadenectomy (abdominal lymph node dissection and extended mediastinal lymphadenectomy) results in an overall 10-year survival rate of about 20% (Figure 24.7). The lymph node ratio, i.e. the ratio between positive and removed nodes, constituted one of the major independent predictors of survival in this analysis [6]. The prognosis is dismal if more than 20% of the removed lymph nodes contain metastatic tumor on routine histologic assessment. If less than 20% of the removed lymph nodes are involved by tumor, long-term survival

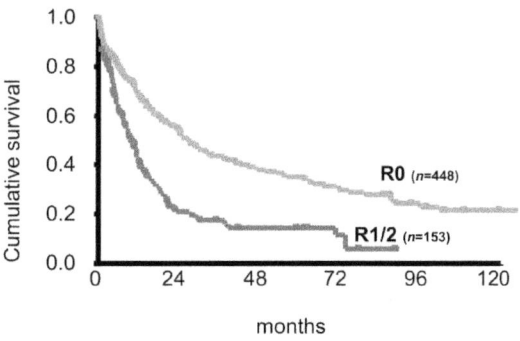

Figure 24.7. Overall 10-year survival rates for squamous cell esophageal cancer with two-field lymphadenectomy according to the R category (data of the Chirurgische Klinik und Poliklinik, Klinikum rechts der Isar, Technische Universität München).

is possible after two-field lymphadenectomy. The prognostic gain that can be achieved with lymph node dissection is highest in patients with early stages of lymphatic spread, i.e. only a limited number of positive lymph nodes.

Considerable experience with a more extended lymphadenectomy has been reported from various Japanese centers. Although a number of retrospective series gave evidence for an improvement of survival and a reduction of local recurrence rates after extended three-field lymphadenectomy, recent prospective studies indicate that this may only be the case for patients with tumors located in the proximal esophagus and patients with fewer than five positive lymph nodes [7,16]. In a randomized Japanese trial comparing two- and three-field lymphadenectomy, extended lymph node dissection prolonged survival time, but the difference to two-field lymph node dissection, did, however, not reach statistical significance [17]. Importantly, in most of the recent series that extended three-field lymph node dissection was associated with a marked increase in pulmonary complications and recurrent laryngeal nerve injuries requiring tracheotomy (Table 24.3). This limits the potential benefits of three-field lymphadenectomy.

In the Western world patients with squamous cell esophageal cancer located at or above the level of tracheal bifurcation, who may theoretically benefit from three-field lymph node dissection, are usually submitted to multimodal therapies with neoadjuvant or primary combined radiochemotherapy [18]. Since extended lymph nodes dissection will further increase the morbidity of esophagectomy after preoperative combined radiochemotherapy, it is unlikely that three-field lymphadenectomy will gain wide popularity in the West.

## Results of Lymphadenectomy for Adenocarcinoma of the Distal Esophagus

Three-field lymphadenectomy for patients with adenocarcinoma of the distal esophagus has so far been reported in only a few case series [19]. As with squamous cell esophageal cancer, the morbidity of this ultra-radical approach was high. In addition, lymphatic spread to the cervical lymph nodes in patients with adenocarcinoma of the distal esophagus appears to be a late event indicating systemic spread. Therefore three-field lymphadenectomy currently has no firm place in the surgical treatment of adenocarcinoma of the distal esophagus in the Western world.

The current discussions on lymphadenectomy in patients with distal esophageal adenocarcinoma center around the extent of

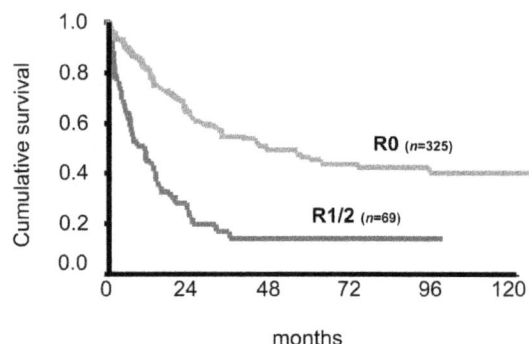

**Figure 24.8.** Overall 10-year survival rates for adenocarcinoma of the distal esophagus according to the R category (Data of the Chirurgische Klinik und Poliklinik, Klinikum rechts der Isar, Technische Universität München).

**Table 24.3.** Complications after three-field lymphadenectomy and two-field lymphadenectomy for squamous cell esophageal cancer [17]

|  | Three-field lymphadenectomy | Two-field lymphadenectomy |
| --- | --- | --- |
| Pulmonary complications | 6/32 (19%) | 5/30 (17%) |
| Recurrent nerve palsy | 18/32 (56%) | 9/30 (30%) |
| Phrenic nerve palsy | 4/32 (13%)* | 0/30 (0%) |
| Incidence of tracheostomy | 17/32 (53%)* | 3/30 (10%) |
| Leakage | 2/32 (6%) | 6/30 (20%) |

* $p < 0.001$

# SURGICAL RESECTION FOR ESOPHAGEAL CANCER: ROLE OF EXTENDED LYMPHADENECTOMY

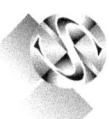

mediastinal dissection, i.e. the need for a thoracotomy to achieve complete mediastinal lymph node clearance. While resection of the primary tumor in the distal esophagus and a lymphadenectomy in the lower posterior mediastinum can be achieved by an abdominal approach after splitting the diaphragmatic hiatus (i.e. radical transmediastinal esophagectomy), the removal of bifurcation and paratracheal nodes can only be performed through a thoracotomy. A recent Dutch prospective randomized trial compared transmediastinal and right transthoracic esophagectomy for distal esophageal adenocarcinoma [20]. In this study, as in the authors' experience, morbidity was substantially higher with the transthoracic approach. Although on long-term follow-up patients with transthoracic resection appeared to have a better prognosis, the survival advantage was not significant as compared to patients who had a transmediastinal resection. This matches the experience at the authors' institution (Figure 24.9).

The value of extended mediastinal lymphadenectomy for adenocarcinoma of the distal esophagus is currently supported only by theoretical arguments and the experience of individual centers. Detailed subgroup analyses identifying patients who most benefit from an extension of the lymph node dissection are still lacking.

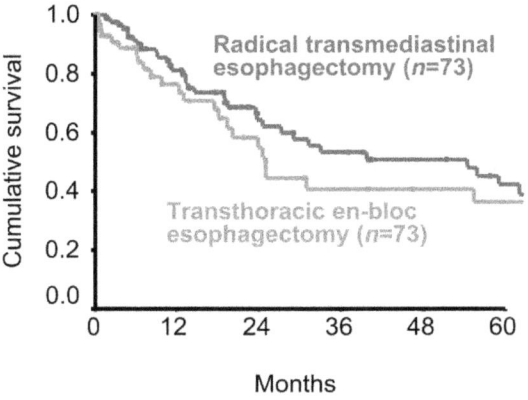

**Figure 24.9.** Overall survival rates with radical transmediastinal and transthoracic esophagectomy in patients with adenocarcinoma of the distal esophagus (case-control data of the Chirurgische Klinik und Poliklinik, Klinikum rechts der Isar, Technische Universität München).

## Surgical Approach to Esophageal Cancer

Based on these concepts a surgical resection should be considered in all patients with potentially R0-resectable esophageal cancers (based on preoperative staging) who are in good general condition (based on detailed preoperative risk analysis). This includes T1 and T2 tumors located at or above the level of the tracheal bifurcation and T1, T2 and T3 tumors located in the distal esophagus. If based on preoperative staging a complete (R0) resection appears unlikely but the patient is in good general condition, multimodal preoperative radiochemotherapy or chemotherapy protocols are applied. These patients proceed to surgery only if the response evaluation (done by positron emission tomography) shows good remission of the tumor [21]. All other patients with esophageal cancer are included in nonsurgical protocols.

The surgical approach and extent of the lymphadenectomy are tailored based on the histological tumor type, location of the primary tumor, and the expected prevalence and location of the lymph node metastases. Irrespective of these factors the spleen is preserved whenever possible.

## Surgical Approach to Squamous Cell Esophageal Cancer

Based on concepts an abdomino-right transthoracic esophagectomy with two-field lymphadenectomy is the procedure of choice for patients with resectable squamous cell esophageal cancer at the authors' institution [1]. Subtotal esophagectomy is always performed because of a high likelihood of a longitudinal, submucosal tumor spread and multicentric disease. The lymphadenectomy includes the following:

- the periesophageal lymph nodes above the diaphragm and along the vena cava superior
- the lymph nodes at the tracheal bifurcation
- the paratracheal lymph nodes together with the nodes along the left recurrent nerve and

- the abdominal suprapancreatic lymphatic compartment along the celiac axis.

This corresponds to a D2 lymphadenectomy according to the Japanese classification.

Because of early lymphatic spread in squamous cell esophageal cancer, lymphadenectomy is performed in patients with T1 tumors. In the authors' opinion there is no place for a limited resection in patients with squamous cell cancer. Limited surgical or endoscopic procedures, as proposed by some Japanese centers, are only indicated in patients with high grade squamous cell dysplasia. This situation is as rarely seen in Western countries.

Reconstruction after transthoracic esophagectomy is usually done by gastric pull-up with a cervical esophagogastrostomy. An important decision relates to the positioning of the interponate. Two routes are possible, either in the natural esophageal bed in the posterior mediastinum or substernally. After a safe R0 resection in patients with early tumor stages (T1/2), reconstruction in the posterior mediastinum is recommended. A reconstruction within the posterior mediastinum leads to better postoperative swallow function. In patients with advanced tumor stages (T3/4) or patients included in multimodal therapy protocols, where postoperative radiation therapy is likely, the reconstruction should be done in the anterior mediastinum – retrosternal route. In the case of a necessary operative revision the retrosternal route has the advantage of better access to the cervical anastomosis.

Because the sequelae of an anastomotic leak are much more severe if the anastomosis is placed in the chest rather than the neck, only the following special situations justify a high intrathoracic anastomosis in patients with squamous cell carcinoma of the esophagus:

- a history of previous neck radiation (e.g. carcinoma of the hypopharynx or thyroid cancer)
- the absolute necessity of the preservation of the recurrent nerve function (singer, speaker etc).

An intrathoracic anastomosis can only be done in the posterior mediastinum, i.e. in the area of the original tumor location. Therefore this alternative should not be chosen in patients with advanced tumor stages.

After neoadjuvant chemotherapy or radiochemotherapy it maybe difficult to differentiate scars from residual tumor during the surgical procedure. The extent of resection after neoadjuvant chemotherapy or combined radiochemotherapy therefore matches that of the primary surgical resection. The postoperative course after combined radiochemotherapy appears to be more severe than after neoadjuvant chemotherapy without radiation or after a primary resection. A radiation-induced compromise in immune function appears to account for this observation [22]. This has prompted the authors to perform the reconstruction after esophagectomy in patients who had neoadjuvant radiochemotherapy after a delay of 1–2 weeks in order to increase the safety of the procedure. In our experience this "safety concept" has resulted in a marked decrease in postoperative mortality after neoadjuvant combined radiochemotherapy [23].

## Surgical Approach to Adenocarcinoma of the Distal Esophagus

Submucosal spread to the proximal esophagus and multicentric disease outside the area with intestinal metaplasia are relatively rare in patients with adenocarcinoma of the distal esophagus. Subtotal esophagectomy therefore is not a "must" in patients with distal esophageal adenocarcinoma. Multicentric disease within the area of intestinal metaplasia is, however, common. Consequently the entire segment of intestinal metaplasia has to be removed with any surgical approach to Barrett's cancer. In order to achieve a complete resection a careful preoperative endoscopic assessment of the length of the Barrett's esophagus is necessary since during the operation it might be difficult to diagnose the length of the Barrett's esophagus.

Based on the currently available data it remains unclear whether an extended mediastinal lymphadenectomy prolongs survival in patients with adenocarcinoma of the distal esophagus. The alternatives for patients with Barrett's cancer therefore include a radical transmediastinal esophagectomy with fundectomy, an abdomino-right transthoracic approach or an abdomino-left transthoracic approach [1]. The latter has the disadvantage of a limited exposure proximally (i.e. the upper mediastinum) and distally (i.e. lymphadenectomy at the lymph nodes 12 and 13). Consequently we prefer the radical transmediastinal esophagectomy with fundectomy or the abdomino-right thoracic approach. The transmediastinal approach is chosen in elderly patients (reduction of the operative risk by sparing the thoracotomy) and patients after neoadjuvant chemotherapy with partial response (usually patients with locally advanced disease). The abdomino-right thoracic approach is the procedure of choice in patients with potential lymph node metastasis at the tracheal bifurcation or above (diagnosed by CT or PET scan) who are young and healthy.

Radical transmediastinal esophagectomy is performed via a generous upper abdominal incision and wide anterior splitting of the diaphragmatic hiatus. The use of special retractors then provides an adequate overview of the posterior mediastinum (Figure 24.10).

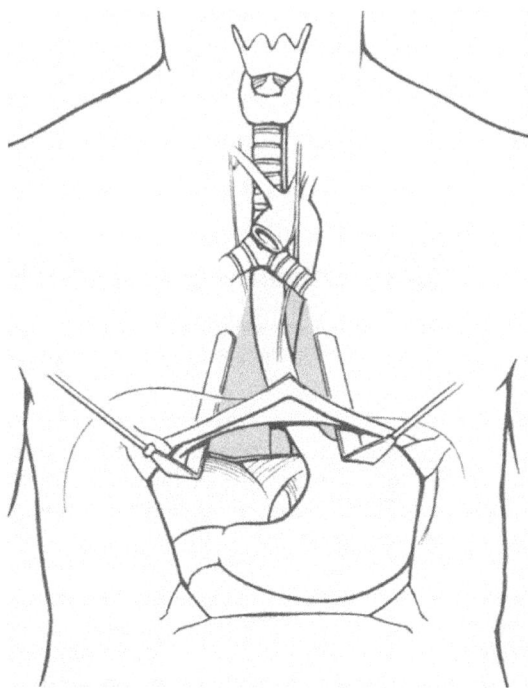

**Figure 24.10.** Exposure of the hiatus and extent of lower mediastinal lymphadenectomy with radical transmediastinal esophagectomy.

The extent of resection includes:

- resection of parts of the diaphragm in the area of the tumor
- mediastinectomy along the pericardium with resection of the mediastinal pleura on both sides
- dissection of the tissue on the anterior wall of the aorta and lymphadenectomy up to the pulmonary vein

This provides an "en-bloc" specimen of the esophagus and its surrounding tissue in the lower posterior mediastinum. The cervical esophagus is dissected through an incision along the anterior part of the left sternocleidomastoid muscle. Mobilization of the esophagus between the tracheal bifurcation and the upper thoracic aperture is done by blunt dissection from the abdomen and through the cervical incision. The lymphadenectomy in the abdomen includes the suprapancreatic and celiac nodes as described above.

If an abdomino-right transthoracic esophagectomy for distal esophageal adenocarcinoma is chosen, a high intrathoracic anastomosis is suitable because there is no need to perform a (sub-)total esophagectomy.

## Limited Surgical Approach to Early Adenocarcinoma of the Distal Esophagus

The substantial morbidity and poor postoperative quality of life associated with extended esophagectomy has stimulated efforts to assess more limited forms of resection for early adenocarcinoma of the distal esophagus. Because of the virtual absence of lymph node metastases in patients with early distal esophageal adenocarcinoma more limited forms of surgical and endoscopic resection have recently been evaluated [24,25]. We have assessed a limited transabdominal resection of the distal esophagus, gastroesophageal junction and proximal stomach with a regional lymphadenectomy. To avoid postoperative reflux, reconstruction is performed by interposition of a pedicled jejunal segment (Figure 24.11) [24]. In our experience with more than 50 such procedures for tumors staged as uT1 on endoscopic ultrasound, a complete resection (R0) resection could be achieved in all cases. There was no evidence of lymph

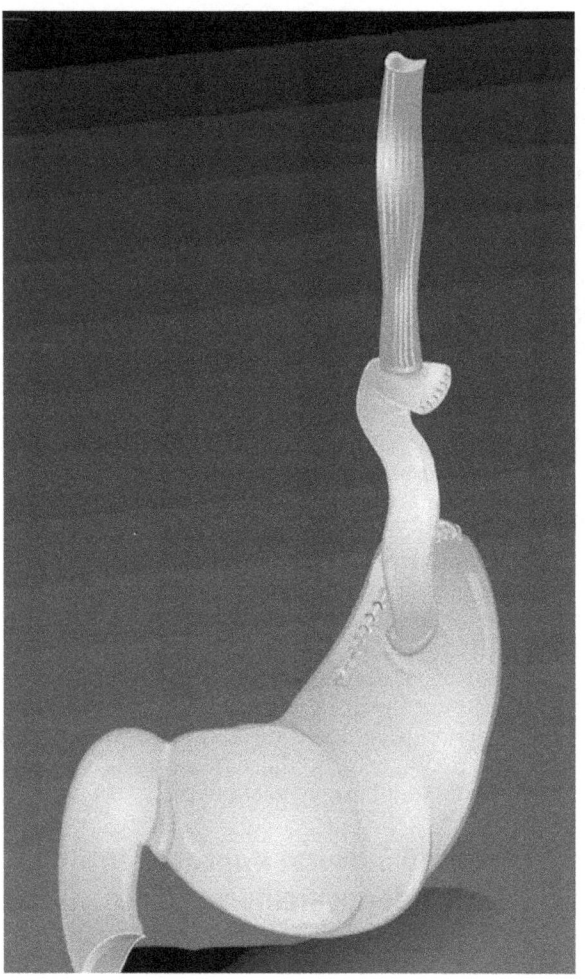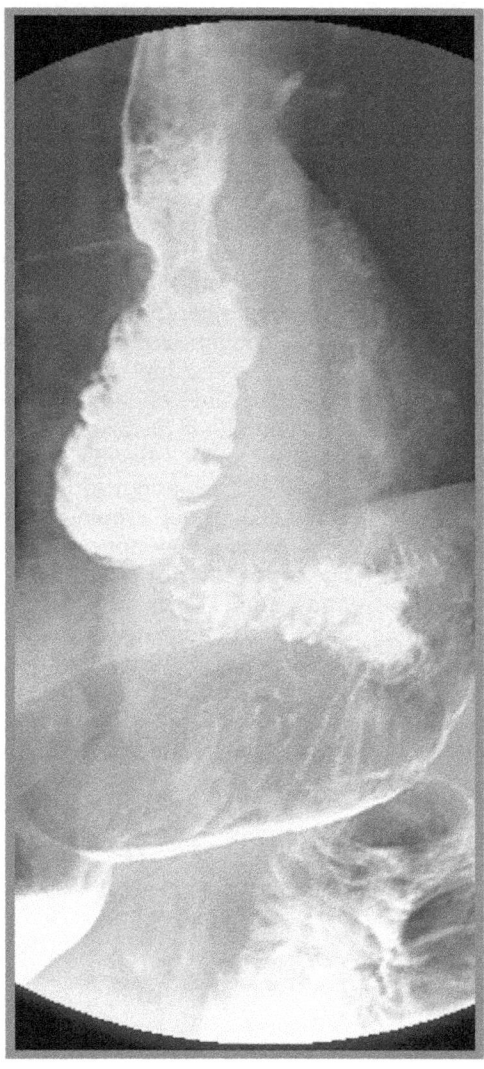

**Figure 24.11.** Limited resection of the distal esophagus with jejunal interposition. **a** Resection specimen with Barrett's esophagus and multiple areas with early cancer. **b** Schematic depiction of the reconstruction with jejunal interposition. **c** Postoperative contrast radiography.

node metastases or micrometastases in a mean of 19 removed nodes per patient. During a short follow-up there have been no recurrences or deaths. Quality of life assessment showed no evidence of gastroesophageal reflux and good to excellent swallowing function in more than 90% of the patients. Similar encouraging data with limited resection in patients with early tumors at the esophagogastric junction are also reported from several other centers, particularly when the vagus nerve can be preserved during the resection [26].

Endoscopic mucosa resection offers an even more limited approach to early tumors of the distal esophagus [25]. Since a lymphadenectomy is not possible with this technique, endoscopic mucosa resection can only be recommended in patients with high grade dysplasia or pT1a tumors. The frequent multicentric tumor growth, the inaccuracy of current preoperative staging modalities to differentiate mucosal from submucosal tumors, and the persistence of precancerous lesions (i.e. Barrett's esophagus) with a high rate of tumor recurrences, currently limits the broad clinical application of this limited procedure.

## Sentinel Lymphadenectomy for Early Barrett's Cancer

In recent years the concept of sentinel lymphadenectomy has been successfully used for breast cancer and malignant melanoma and is increasingly being evaluated for tumors of the gastrointestinal tract. The principle is based on the assumption that regional lymph nodes are affected in a stepwise fashion and that the first lymph node station in the area of the lymphatic drainage from the primary tumor (the so-called "sentinel node") gives reliable information on the presence or absence of lymph node metastases. Because of the complex lymphatic drainage from the thoracic esophagus, some early Japanese reports on frequent "skip metastases" and erratic lymphatic spread in squamous cell cancer the validity of this approach in esophageal cancer has been questioned. As discussed above, the biology and pattern of lymphatic spread from early adenocarcinoma located in the distal esophagus, however, markedly differs from that of squamous cell cancer located in the thoracic esophagus. In contrast to squamous cell cancer, lymphatic spread in patients with Barrett's cancer appears to follow certain rules. Lymphatic spread is closely correlated to the pT category of the primary tumor, starts only after infiltration of the submucosa and is initially limited to the regional lymph nodes. Distant lymph node metastases are almost exclusively found in patients with multiple positive regional nodes; skipping of regional lymph nodes is rare.

These observations set the stage for tailored lymphadenectomy strategies in patients with early esophageal adenocarcinoma based on the "sentinel lymphadenectomy" concept [27,28]. A number of studies assessing sentinel lymphadenectomy for Barrett's cancer are currently on the way. Provided sentinel node identification is possible and reliable in such patients much of the morbidity associated with lymphadenectomy for esophageal cancer could be avoided. This would then open the door for truly individualized concepts of lymphadenectomy.

## Questions

1. Type tumors at the gastro-esophageal junction.
2. Define the staging procedures.
3. What are the important prognostic factors?
4. Outline the types of lymphadenectomy.
5. Outline methods to assess quality of excision.
6. Discuss the results of trials of different centers.
7. Describe surgical lymphadenectomies for squamous cell cancer.

## References

1. Siewert JR, Stein HJ, Sendler A et al. Esophageal cancer: Clinical management. In: Kelsen DA et al (eds) Gastrointestinal oncology: principles and practice. Philadelphia: Lippincott Williams & Wilkins, 2002; 261–88.
2. Siewert JR, Feith M, Werner M, Stein HJ. Adenocarcinoma of the esophagogastric junction: results of surgical therapy based on anatomical/topographic classification in 1002 consecutive patients. Ann Surg 2000;232: 353–61.
3. Stein HJ, Feith M. Cancer of the esophagus. In: Gospodarowicz M et al (ed) Prognostic factors in cancer. New York: Wiley-Liss Inc, 2001; 237–49.
4. Siewert JR, Stein HJ, Feith M, et al. Tumor cell type is an independent prognostic parameter in esophageal cancer: Lessons learned from more than 1000 consecutive resections at a single institution in the Western world. Ann Surg 2001;234:360–9.
5. Birkmeyer JD, Siewers AE, Finlayson EV et al. Hospital volume and surgical mortality in the United States. N Engl J Med 2002;346:1128–37.
6. Roder JD, Busch R, Stein HJ et al. Ratio of invaded to removed lymph nodes as a predictor of survival in squamous cell carcinoma of the oesophagus. Br J Surg 1994;81:410–13.
7. Siewert JR, Stein HJ. Lymphadenectomy for esophageal cancer. Langenbecks Arch Surg 1999;384:141–8.
8. Stein HJ, Brucher BL, Sendler A, Siewert JR. Esophageal cancer: patient evaluation and pre-treatment staging. Surg Oncol 2001;10:103–11.
9. Bartels H, Stein HJ, Siewert JR. Preoperative risk analysis and postoperative mortality of esophagectomy for resectable esophageal cancer. Br J Surg 1998;85:840–4.
10. Fumagalli U and Panel of Experts. Resective surgery for cancer of the thoracic esophagus. Results of a consensus conference. Dis Esoph 1996;9:3–19.
11. Bumm R, Wong J. Extent of lymphadenectomy in esophagectomy for squamous cell esophageal cancer: How much is necessary? Dis Esoph 1994;7:151–5.

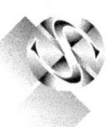

12. Fujita H, Kakegawa T, Yamana H, Shima I. Lymph node compartments as guidelines for esophageal carcinoma. Dis Esoph 1994;7:169–77.
13. Sigurdson ER. Lymph node dissection: Is it diagnostic or therapeutic? J Clin Oncol 2003;21:965–7.
14. Sobin LH, Wittekind C. TNM classification of malignant tumors, 6th edn. New York: Wiley-Liss, 2002.
15. Feinstein AR, Sosin DM, Wells CK. The Will Rogers phenomenon. Stage migration and new diagnostic techniques as a source of misleading statistics for survival in cancer. N Engl J Med 1985;312:1604–8.
16. Fujita HH, Sueyoshi SS, Tanaka TT, Shirouzu KK. Three-field dissection for squamous cell carcinoma in the thoracic esophagus. Ann Thorac Cardiovasc Surg 2002;8:328–35.
17. Nishihira T, Hirayama K, Mori S. A prospective randomised trial of extended cervical and superior mediastinal lymphadenectomy for carcinoma of the thoracic esophagus. Am J Surg 1998;175:47–51.
18. Stein HJ, Sendler A, Fink U, Siewert JR. Multidisciplinary approach to esophageal and gastric cancer. Surg Clin North Am 2000;80:659–82.
19. Altorki N, Kent M, Ferrara C, Port J. Three-field lymph node dissection for squamous cell and adenocarcinoma of the esophagus. Ann Surg 2002;236:177–83.
20. Hulscher JB, van Sandick JW, de Boer AG et al. Extended transthoracic resection compared with limited transhiatal resection for adenocarcinoma of the esophagus. N Engl J Med 2002;347:1662–9.
21. Brücher BLDM, Weber W, Bauer M et al. Neoadjuvant therapy of esophageal squamous cell carcinoma: Response evaluation by positron emission tomography. Ann Surg 2001;233:300–9.
22. Heidecke CD, Weighardt H, Feith M et al. Neoadjuvant treatment of esophageal cancer: Immunosuppression following combined radiochemotherapy. Surgery 2002; 132:495–501.
23. Stein HJ, Bartels H, Siewert JR. [Esophageal carcinoma: 2-stage operation for preventing mediastinitis in high risk patients] Chirurg 2001;72:881–6.
24. Stein HJ, Feith M, Mueller J et al. Limited resection for early Barrett's cancer. Ann Surg 2000; 232:733–42.
25. Ell C, May A, Gossner L. Endoscopic mucosal resection of early cancer and high-grade dysplasia in Barrett's esophagus. Gastroenterology 2000;118:670–7.
26. Banki F, Mason RJ, DeMeester SR et al. Vagal-sparing esophagectomy: a more physiologic alternative. Ann Surg 2002;236:324–35.
27. Kitajima M, Kitagawa Y. Surgical treatment of esophageal cancer – the advent of the era of individualization. N Engl J Med 2002;347:1705–9.
28. Kitagawa Y, Fujii H, Mukai M et al. Intraoperative lymphatic mapping and sentinel lymph node sampling in esophageal and gastric cancer. Surg Oncol Clin N Am 2002;11:293–304.

# 25

# Surgical Resection of the Stomach with Lymph Node Dissection

Mitsuru Sasako, Takeo Fukagawa, Hitoshi Katai and Kateshi Sano

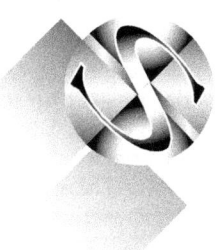

## Aims

- To describe the techniques of radical lymph node clearance in gastric cancer surgery.
- To identifiy the aspects of surgery associated with significant morbidity.
- To define the use of pancreatic and splenic resection in gastric cancer surgery.

## Type of Gastric Resection

### Commonly Used Types of Resection

As gastrectomy is now rarely indicated for benign disease of the stomach, this chapter focusses on gastrectomy for gastric malignancies. For gastric cancers, several types of resection are commonly used. For proximal advanced tumours or large tumours, a total gastrectomy (TG) is usually used. For a distally located tumour which does not involve the proximal third of the stomach, a distal (DG) or distal subtotal gastrectomy (DSG) is the preferred type of gastric resection. In the 1980s, proximal gastrectomy (PG) was for a while abandoned because of the high incidence of reflux oesophagitis and in pursuit of radical surgery. However, with the identification of an increasing number of small T1/2 tumours located near the cardia, interest in the role of proximal gastrectomy has been renewed. For similar tumours in the middle of the stomach, pylorus preserving distal gastrectomy (PPG) is being undertaken in an attempt to improve quality of life after surgery [1].

### Total Versus Subtotal Gastrectomy

The concept of total gastrectomy as the appropriate radical surgical management of gastric cancer was promoted by some enthusiasts in the West during the 1970s. This concept has been described as "gastrectomie totale en principe". In Japan, however, TG was carried out only when it was required to allow an R0 resection to be achieved while DG was carried out for many antral tumours, with satisfactory results. To establish the role of the extent of gastric resection, several trials have been carried out to evaluate TG in principle.

There have been two randomised controlled trials comparing TG with DG for antral tumours. In France between 1980 and 1985, 201 patients were randomized between TG and DSG to test if TG could increase 5-year survival rate from 30% after DSG to 50%. After excluding 32 ineligible cases, 84% of randomised patients were included in the analysis; no differences in postoperative morbidity and mortality or in 5-year survival rates were demonstrated [2]. A similar trial was carried out in Italy enrolling 648 patients between 1982 and 1993 [3]. This trial was set up to test the equivalence of DSG and TG, i.e. DSG should show 5-year survival rates no worse than −10% of the results of TG (50%). There was no significant difference in postoperative death (1.2% after DSG and 2.3% after TG) and 5-year survival rate after DSG was better than after TG (65% versus 62%), confirming the equivalence of the two methods for antral tumours. A further trial has compared DSG with D1 nodal dissection versus TG with D3 dissection [4]. The sample size was small (55 patients) and hypothesis tested included both the extent of gastric resection and extent of lymphadenectomy; as a result the trial is difficult to evaluate. The results demonstrated no significant differences in outcome though the survival curve after DSG was better than after TG.

Theoretically, the oncological gain provided by TG over DSG lies in the reduction in the risk of positive resection margins, the removal of missed second primaries and increasing the extent of lymphatic clearance. The extent of nodal dissection increases the dissection of the left cardiac nodes, short gastric artery nodes, splenic hilum nodes and distal splenic artery nodes. The pattern of lymphatic spread in antral cancers would indicate that removal of these node groups is unlikely to improve outcome. The problem of positive margins is mainly due to inaccurate diagnosis of proximal extension of tumours. For cancers in the mid body on the greater curve, the risk of lymphatic involvement of the splenic hilar and distal splenic artery nodes might support a need for total gastrectomy. For such cases, negative sampling of the nodes at the root of the left gastroepiploic artery or the sentinel nodes may safely allow surgeons to avoid TG.

## Indications for Proximal Gastrectomy (PG)

In 1970s, PG was abandoned for two reasons: a high incidence of local failure in the remnant stomach and frequent and severe reflux oesophagitis due to bile reflux when reconstruction was by oesophagogastrostomy. A dramatic increase in junctional tumours small cancers at the cardia, has been observed in the West. For small tumours located at the cardia as well as T1 tumours in the proximal third of the stomach, PG has been revived in both hemispheres during the 1990s. For T1 tumours of the proximal stomach, PG with extended D1 (D1 plus proximal splenic, coeliac and common hepatic artery nodes) is carried out, followed by a reconstruction with short segment jejunal interposition (modified Merendino's operation: Figure 25.1). For large tumours involving the cardia, because of intramural distal extension to the antrum and the significant incidence of nodal metastasis to the lower lesser curvature and infrapyloric nodes, a TG should be carried out. Harrison et al [5] claimed that TG is not necessary for proximal gastric cancer but the average size of the tumours treated by PG in their series was just 4 cm, much smaller than those treated by TG. Their method of reconstruction was traditional oesophagogastrostomy. As they did not evaluate the quality of life (QOL) of patients, especially in terms of reflux oesophagitis, their technique cannot be justified.

## Pylorus Preserving Gastrectomy (PPG)

Due to the increasing recognition of early gastric cancer in Japan, several surgical techniques have been recently tested to reduce

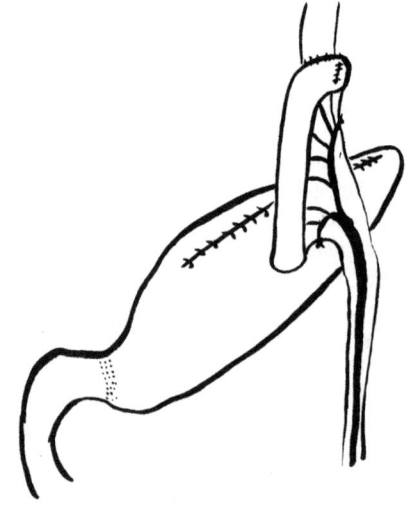

**Figure 25.1.** Modified Merendino's operation of proximal partial gastrectomy with jejunal interposition.

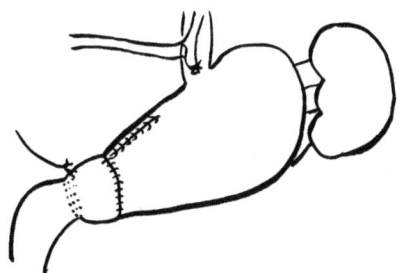

**Figure 25.2.** Pylorus preserving distal partial gastrectomy.

the incidence of postgastrectomy symptoms. Pylorus preserving gastrectomy is one of these options. This procedure was originally described by Maki as a surgical treatment for benign gastric ulcer [6]. By preserving the pylorus with a small part of the gastric antrum, rapid emptying of the stomach, causing the dumping syndrome, should be reduced. In the 1990s, this technique was introduced in patients with early gastric cancer of the middle part of the stomach [1]. There is now experience with hundreds of patients who have undergone this operation with satisfactory results, in terms of QOL and survival. The original method preserved 1.5 cm of the distal antrum but the preference now is to preserve at least 3 cm of the antrum for better gastric emptying (Figure 25.2).

# Concept, Classification and Efficacy of Lymph Node Dissection for Gastric Carcinoma

## Concept

The initial description of lymph node dissection for cancer treatment was in breast cancer by Halsted and the work was developed by Haagensen. The primary aim of this procedure is to avoid local failure in axillary lymph nodes. Originally all systemic metastasis was thought to occur via lymphatic spread. In this theory, called the Halstedian cancer model, cancer cells spread initially to the nearest nodes and then to farther nodes step by step, and eventually to various distant sites. Therefore the wider the nodal dissection, the better the survival that should be achieved. Local recurrence should be rare after adequate nodal dissection. However, cancer metastases occur not only via lymph stream but also primarily via the bloodstream and sometimes directly through the pleural or peritoneal cavity. In breast cancer, 20–30% of node-negative patients develop systemic recurrence [7]. Local recurrence sometimes occurs as a part of systemic recurrence in high grade tumours. Prognosis of patients with multiple nodal metastases worsens steeply as the number of metastatic nodes increases [8]. All these facts demonstrate that regional lymph nodes do not form an effective barrier to cancer dissemination. Several clinical trials have shown nodal dissection does not contribute to better survival for breast cancer and nodal metastasis is an indicator of poor prognosis. Nodal disease is indicative of a high risk of the presence of systemic disease (systemic disease model).

Unlike breast cancer, gastric cancer more closely follows the requisites for the original Halstedian model. Those having no or limited spread of nodal metastasis have a good prognosis if peritoneal seeding does not occur. Five-year survival rates of those having 4, 6, 8, 10 nodal metastases are 52.3%, 43.5%, 37.7%, 29.9%, respectively (unpublished data from National Cancer Center Hospital Tokyo). Systemic/distant metastases are quite rare in T1 and T2 tumours, whereas lymph node metastases are already frequent in these stages (Table 25.1) [9]. Thus in gastric cancer, nodal metastasis is the primary site of metastatic spread in most cases and systemic recurrence after curative operation in node-negative patients is rare. The commonest type of recurrence of advanced tumours is peritoneal seeding after formal nodal dissection [10]. However, recurrence after limited surgery occurs most frequently in the gastric bed and, with regional peritoneal seeding, accounts for over 90% of recurrences [11]. These differences between breast and gastric cancers might be explained by the following. First, the stomach is located in the portal venous system, with bloodborne metastases occurring most frequently via the portal vein to the liver rather than through the lympho-venous connection in the neck. Second, the high intraluminal bacteria count is associated with an abundant lymphatic system including mucosa associated lymphoid tissue.

Most of the reported adjuvant chemotherapy trials have failed to prove any efficacy over surgery alone [12]. Recently a clinical trial comparing surgery plus radiochemotherapy versus surgery alone showed significantly better survival for the radiochemotherapy group [13]. In this study, 90% of the patients underwent either D0 or D1 lymph node dissection. This could be interpreted as showing that adjuvant chemotherapy may be effective when the local regional lymph node metastases are well controlled by radiotherapy. However, the survival results of the radiochemotherapy group in this study could not reach the level of the results achieved by D2 dissection alone. Therefore it is still uncertain whether D0/1 surgery plus radiochemotherapy can replace D2 dissection or not. In fact, retrospective analysis of the patients in this trial suggests that surgical undertreatment undermined survival [14].

## Classification

Of the two commonly used classifications for gastric cancer, the Japanese classification [15] and the Union Internacional Contra la Cancrum (UICC) TNM classification, only the former includes a method for classification of the extent of lymph node dissection. The regional lymph nodes are topographically classified from the first to third tier nodes, according to the tumour location in the stomach. In general terms, perigastric nodes are usually classified as the first tier and lymph nodes in the suprapancreatic area with splenic hilum nodes comprise the second tier; nodes in the hepatoduodenal ligament, retropancreatic and para-aortic nodes are the third tier. Nodal dissection is defined as D1, D2 and D3. D0 is defined as excision which fails to remove all of the first tier nodes. D1 includes all first tier stations but not all of the second tier stations. D2 dissection includes all first and second tier stations but not all the third tier nodes. D3 means dissection including all first, second and third tier stations.

## Efficacy

Many retrospective comparisons of lymph node dissection, D1 versus D2, have shown better survival for D2 (Table 25.2). The results of D1 have never reached the level of D2 dissection in terms of long-term survival according to stage. When the results of surgery are compared according to TNM stage, stage migration confounds comparisons. The wider the dissection, the more accurate the stage diagnosis, thus resulting in an increase in the number of cases at advanced stages and improvement of the results by stage in each category, stage migration. Therefore, for gastric cancer, the results of two groups who underwent different nodal dissection should be compared by T stage, which is not influenced by type of nodal dissection. Even in such comparisons, D2 always shows better results than D1. However, randomised controlled trials (RCTs) have never proven the superiority of D2 dissection over D1. Table 25.2 shows the results of these RCTs. Furthermore the two large-scale RCTs, the MRC trial [16] and the Dutch trial [17], showed significantly higher postoperative hospital mortality after D2 than D1. Initially these results we interpreted as pointing to an

**Table 25.1.** Metastases at the time of operation, 5-year survival, and haematogenous recurrence after resection in 4683 patients at National Cancer Center Hospital Tokyo, 1972–1991

| Tumour depth | n | LN | Liver | Peritoneum | 5Y SR (%) | Haematogenous rec. |
| --- | --- | --- | --- | --- | --- | --- |
| pT1(m) | 1063 | 3.3 | 0 | 0 | 93.3 | 2 (0.2%) |
| pT1(sm) | 881 | 17.4 | 0.1 | 0 | 88.9 | 9 (1.0%) |
| pT2(mp) | 436 | 46.7 | 1.1 | 0.5 | 81.3 | 26 (5.9%) |
| pT2(ss) | 325 | 63.6 | 3.4 | 2.2 | 65.8 | 31 (9.5%) |
| pT3 | 1232 | 79.9 | 6.3 | 17.8 | 35.5 | 149 (12.1%) |
| pT4 | 724 | 89.7 | 15.5 | 41.6 | 10.1 | 106 (14.6%) |
| All | 4683 | 47.8 | 4.5 | 11.5 | 60.3 | 318 (6.8%) |

n. number: LN. lymph node: 5Y SR. 5-year survival rate, Rec, recurrence
Reproduced with permission from Mitsuru Sasako, What is reasonable treatment for gastric adenocarcinoma? J Gastroenteroc 2000; 35 [suppl XII]: 117.

inherently greater risk in D2 dissection. However, precise analyses of these trials and other reports elucidated surgical inexperience in those undertaking D2 dissection in these trials. Moreover, the only single arm study to assess the safety and effectiveness of D2 dissection, which was started after the publication of the results of MRC and Dutch trials, has demonstrated the safety of D2 dissection if done in high volume hospitals in the West. These trials provide important lessons around the importance of quality assurance in phase trials in surgery. The issue of timing of trial initiation has been raised, with suggestions that this should be determined on the basis of demonstration that individuals are near to the plateau of their learning curve of a difficult technique. Inexperience can produce large biases when comparing technically demanding surgical procedures.

Survival results of these trials in comparison to other studies are shown in Table 25.3. This table compares exclusively the results of D2 surgery, to avoid the stage migration effect. Sometimes, the results of the Dutch trial and MRC trials are interpreted as real evidence of non-superiority of the D2 dissection for gastric cancer. However, these are not trials set up to show the equality of D1 and D2 and with the factors pointed out above, the question is still unsolved. However, from the experience in these trials, it is obvious that D2 dissection should not be carried out by surgeons with insufficient experience of this technique and inexperienced surgeons should carry out this procedure strictly under the supervision of experienced surgeons.

## Indications for Extended lymph Node Dissection (D2 Dissection)

### Tumour Factors

This procedure should not be undertaken in incurable patients because of the increased morbidity associated with the technique. For T1

**Table 25.2.** D1 versus D2 5-year survival rates

| Author | 5-year survival rate D1 | 5-year survival rate D2 | Reference |
|---|---|---|---|
| Pacelli F, et al | 50.1 | 65.4 | Br J Surg 1993;80:1153–6 |
| Onate-Ocana LF, et al | 35.1 | 64.0 | Ann Surg Oncol 2000;7:210–17 |
| De Manzoni G, et al | 28 | 63 | Br J Surg 1996;83:1604–7 |
| Lee WJ, et al | 34.8 | 41.5 | World J Surg 1995;19:707–13 |
| Sue-Ling H | 18 | 45 | Eur J Surg Oncol 1994;20:179–82 |
| Gall FP, et al | 43.6 | 51.8 | Eur J Surg Oncol 1985;11:219–25 |

**Table 25.3.** D2 Surgery: trial results

| | | | | 5-Year survival rates (%) | | | | | | |
|---|---|---|---|---|---|---|---|---|---|---|
| Author | No. of patients | # patients/y/h | PO mortality | Overall | IA | IB | II | IIIA | IIIB | IV |
| Siewert | 803 | 14 | 5.0 | NM | 84 | 68 | 57 | 32 | 14 | 13 |
| Pacelli | 157 | 16 | 3.8 | 65 | 86 | → | 66 | 49 | → | none |
| Sue-Ling | 207 | 10 | 6 | 54 | 87 | → | 65 | 24 | → | NM |
| Cuschieri | 200 | 1 | 13.0 | 33 | 58 | → | 31 | 11 | → | none |
| Bonenkamp | 331 | 1 | 9.7 | 47 | 81 | 61 | 42 | 28 | 13 | 28 |
| Sasako | 2541 | 254 | 0.3 | 66 | 92 | 90 | 76 | 59 | 37 | 8 |
| Jatzko | 345 | 33 | 4.9 | 58 | 98 | 84 | 56 | 49 | 8 | 11 |
| Hundahl * | 32 532 | NM | NM | 28 | 78 | 58 | 34 | 20 | 8 | 7 |

* Results of National Data Base, most cases are treated by D0/1, NM, not mentioned; none, no patient included; →, stage IB is included in stage IA and stage IIIB is included in stage IIIA; # patients/y/h, number of patients treated per year per hospital; PO mortality, postoperative mortality.

tumours, the risk of second tier node involvement is 5% and therefore in Western practice where the postoperative mortality is of the order of 5% in experienced centres, a D1 resection would be appropriate. This is dependent on the assumption that preoperative assessment of the depth of invasion is accurate.

For T4 tumours, a D2 dissection should be applied only when the entire tumour can be resected by the resection of neighbouring organs involved by the primary tumour. It remains unclear whether D2 dissection is of value in linitis plastica because of the frequency of recurrence in the peritoneal cavity despite an even higher incidence of nodal metastases in the second tiers than in other types. Indeed some authors claim that surgery is not indicated for this type of tumour. However, about 20% of cases of linitis plastica can be cured by D2 dissection combined with adjuvant chemotherapy when an R0 resection can be achieved. Although the recurrence rate in the peritoneum is high, cure without resection is not realistic and therefore D2 dissection remains an option in curable linitis plastica. As most tumours involve the greater curvature of the body and often the gastrosplenic ligament, splenectomy is usually required in addition.

## Patient Factors

Postoperative hospital mortality after D2 dissection is over three times greater in aged patients and mortality after total gastrectomy is over five times greater in patients over 80 years old compared with those under 70. The results of the Dutch trial showed much higher mortality after D2 in aged patients. D2 total gastrectomy for aged patients should be carried out only in high volume hospitals by experienced surgeons.

As D2 dissection includes the meticulous dissection of lymph nodes in the suprapancreatic area, in obese patients the risks are increased as the pancreas is embedded in thick adipose tissue, hindering recognition of the border of the organ and increasing the risk of injury to either the parenchyma or the vessels to the pancreas.

Patients with impaired liver function are regarded as high risk for D2 dissection, especially cirrhotic patients. The development of massive and often uncontrollable ascites after D2 dissection occurs frequently and is often fatal. These patients have increased lymphatic flow surrounding the liver and D2 dissection disturbs the lymph circulation of these patients enormously.

After D2 dissection, fluid retention in both the abdominal and the retroperitoneal space is very great and maintenance of fluid balance following surgery can be difficult. Thus pneumonia or cardiac failure during the resorptive phase can occur and this phase requires intensive management. D2 should be undertaken with caution in those with impaired respiratory and cardiac function.

## Combined Organ Resection for Lymphadenectomy

In the history of radical resection of cancers, combined resection of organs surrounding the primary tumour is based on the idea of en-bloc resection, which means complete resection of all the tissues through which draining lymph vessels pass. In gastric cancer surgery, complete bursectomy and omentectomy, pancreaticosplenectomy were based on the same idea. In en-bloc resection of the gastric bed with vascular pedicle, Appleby's operation, three-quarters of the pancreas distal to the portal vein, spleen, coeliac artery with its branches are resected en bloc [18]. Until 1980, pancreaticosplenectomy was a standard part of the D2 radical total gastrectomy. However, comparison of the survival benefit against the increased morbidity and mortality and the high incidence of diabetes mellitus led many surgeons to abandon pancreas resection. As a result, pancreas-preserving total gastrectomy became the standard in Japan during the 1990s [19]. It is now recognised that good survival rates can be achieved in node-positive patients without en-bloc resection of these neighbouring organs.

Two large clinical trials comparing D1 versus D2 showed that combined resection of spleen and pancreas largely accounted for the increased morbidity and mortality in a D2 dissection [16,17]. The remaining question is whether splenectomy alone increases the risk of operative mortality and whether it contributes to improved survival. Although in these trials splenectomy was associated with a worse prognosis, the close correlation with tumour site and histology (more proximal tumour and more

# SURGICAL RESECTION OF THE STOMACH WITH LYMPH NODE DISSECTION

diffuse type) confounds unbiased comparison. Therefore, this can be answered only by an RCT comparing D2 TG with or without splenectomy. The Japanese Clinical Oncology Group started such a trial in 2002 aiming to accrue 500 patients to demonstrate non-inferiority of splenic preservation.

Combined resection of the entire or a part of organs invaded by the primary tumour is accepted as the only way to achieve R0 resection for some cases. For these T4 tumours, radiotherapy has not yet been proven to be as effective as surgical resection.

## Techniques of D2 Dissection

### Standard D2 TG: Pancreas Preserving TG

First an extensive mobilisation of the duodenum and the head of the pancreas is carried out to observe and palpate the para-aortic area. If there are nodes which are suspicious, sampling for frozen section should be carried out. If they are negative for cancer, radical D2 dissection is started. Complete omentectomy with resection of the anterior sheet of mesocolon is carried out (Figure 25.3). Many T3 tumours have lymphatic spread in the omentum, complete omentectomy remains a part of the standard D2 dissection. Similarly, T3 tumours adhering to the anterior sheet of the mesocolon and/or the pancreatic capsule may necessitate the resection of these structures and frequently turn out to be invading them. Complete bursectomy avoids tumour exposure in such cases. By carrying out this procedure, the accessory right colic vein is identified and followed proximally. It joins with the right gastroepiploic vein, forming Henle's surgical trunk which flows into the superior mesenteric vein (Figure 25.4). The right gastroepiploic vein is ligated and divided at its origin. For antral tumours, nodes on the superior mesenteric vein are also dissected. As the layer exposed by the bursectomy continues to the posterior aspect of the pancreas, the layer of the dissection should be changed to the anterior surface of the pancreas. Several vessels coming from behind the pancreas towards the anterior

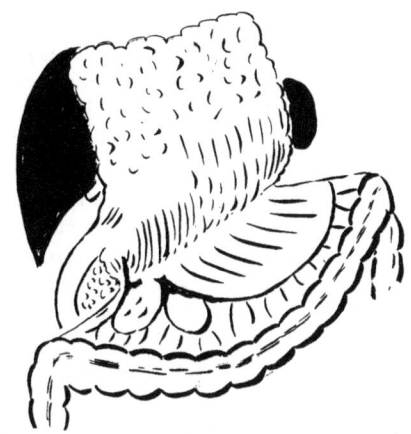

**Figure 25.3.** Elevation of greater omentum with anterior leaf of transverse mesocolon.

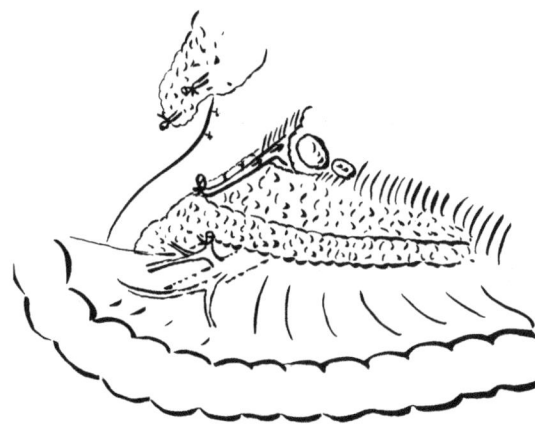

**Figure 25.4.** Division of right gastro-epiploic vein at Henley's trunk.

sheet of the mesocolon should be ligated at the inferior border of the pancreas.

The capsule of the pancreas is now dissected from the parenchyma in the middle part of the organ first, then toward the tail and the head, until the gastroduodenal artery is recognised. Following this artery, the root of the right gastroepiploic artery is found. After ligation and division of this artery at its origin, the stomach is lifted up to divide the back surface of the proximal duodenum from the pancreas and the gastroduodenal artery is followed cranially until the bifurcation of the common hepatic artery is recognized (Figure 25.4). The stomach is laid back to the natural position and the lesser omentum is divided near the lateral segment of the liver from the left edge of the hepatoduodenal ligament to the oesophageal hiatus (Figure 25.5). This line is extended on the hepatoduodenal ligament to the left side of the common bile duct, where this incision is turned caudally towards the duodenum. Then the supraduodenal vessels, usually three or four in total, are ligated and divided close to the duodenal wall (Figure 25.6). This procedure makes a window above the duodenum, through which the gastroduodenal artery can be clearly seen. The connective tissue containing the lymph nodes in the hepatoduodenal ligament left of the common bile duct is dissected from right to left, from the duodenum towards the hepatic hilum along the gastroduodenal and then the hepatic artery.

By doing so, the origin of the right gastric artery is easily identified, ligated and divided (Figure 25.6). Now the duodenum is divided a couple of centimetres from the pylorus by a linear type stapler. Pulling up the stomach from right to left and/or cranially, the suprapancreatic lymph nodes, common hepatic, coeliac, left gastric and splenic artery nodes are dissected, starting from the lymph nodes on the left side of the portal vein towards the nodes along the splenic artery. Downward traction of the pancreas by an assistant is extremely useful (Figure 25.7). During this procedure, the left gastric vein is encoun-

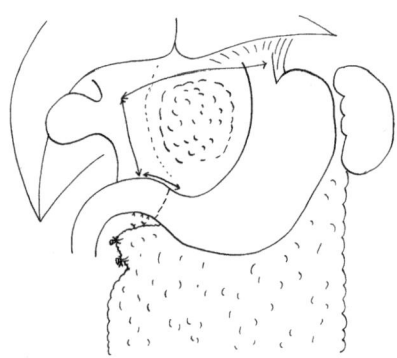

**Figure 25.5.** Line of division of the lesser omentum and duodenal clearance.

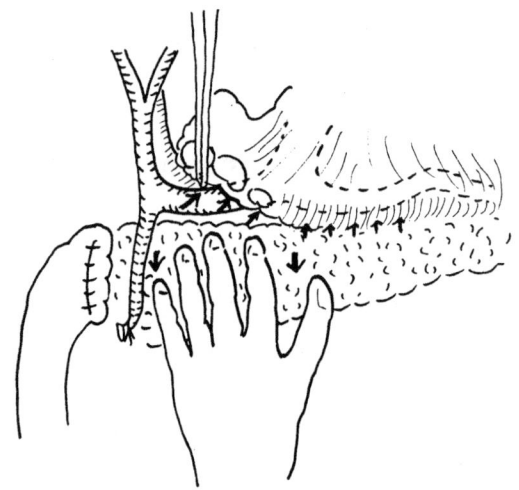

**Figure 25.7.** Clearance of suprapancreatic nodes along hepatic artery, celiac axis and splenic artery and peritoneum over pancreas. Note downward tension provided by assistant.

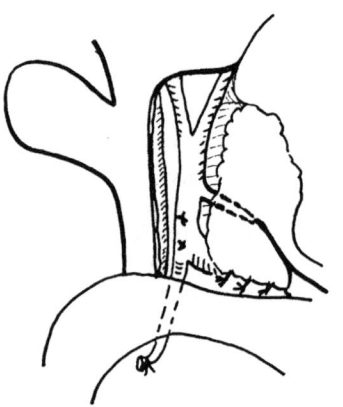 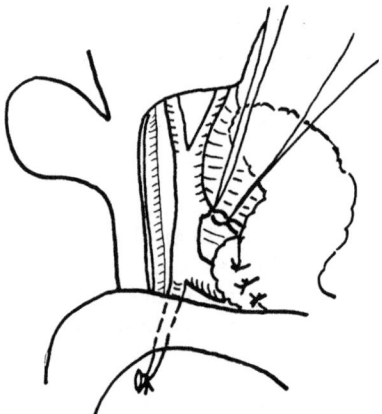

**Figure 25.6.** Identification and ligation of right gastric artery.

tered, most commonly behind the common hepatic artery (Figure 25.8). As a second frequent variation, this vein crosses over the common hepatic or splenic artery, flowing into the splenic vein. This vein is carefully found and then ligated and divided near its origin. The adipose tissue and thick nerve structures on the crus surrounding the oesophageal hiatus are divided from the crus, thus skeletonising the right side of coeliac artery and the origin of the left gastric artery. When the left hepatic artery is a branch of the left gastric artery, it should be preserved up to the origin of the hepatic artery in poor risk patients, to avoid necrosis of the lateral segment. Otherwise it should be ligated and divided at its origin.

The splenic artery nodes are dissected from the splenic artery around the origin of the posterior gastric artery (Figure 25.9). Near the origin of the posterior gastric artery, the great pancreatic artery branches off and comes into the pancreatic parenchyma. The splenic artery is now ligated and divided distal to the origin of the great pancreatic artery. In most cases, one of the large branches of the splenic vein appears on the anterior surface of the pancreatic tail. Then the pancreatic tail is mobilised completely from the retroperitoneum along Toldt's retropancreatic fascia. Traditionally the mobilisation started lateral to the spleen and the spleen is mobilised medially, pulling the spleen up with the operator's left hand. In this technique, the dissection on the left adrenal gland is carried out blindly, sometimes injuring the gland. To avoid this and the loss of the plane of dissection, it is better to mobilise the pancreatic body along Toldt's fascia at the upper border of the organ and continue towards the spleen. The lateral retroperitoneum is incised last (Fig 25.10). When the pancreas left of the coeliac artery is completely mobilised, the lymph nodes on the posterior surface of the pancreatic tail are dissected carefully, preserving the branches of splenic vein to the pancreas (Figure 25.11). All the branches from splenic vein to the stomach are carefully ligated and divided. After the pancreatic tail vein is preserved, the trunk of the splenic vein is ligated and divided. The vein commonly divides before the tip of the pancreatic tail and the branches are ligated separately. Now the pancreatic tail is naked and separated completely from the stomach and the spleen (Figure 25.12). The last step of the procedure is to dissect the left side of the oesophageal hiatus

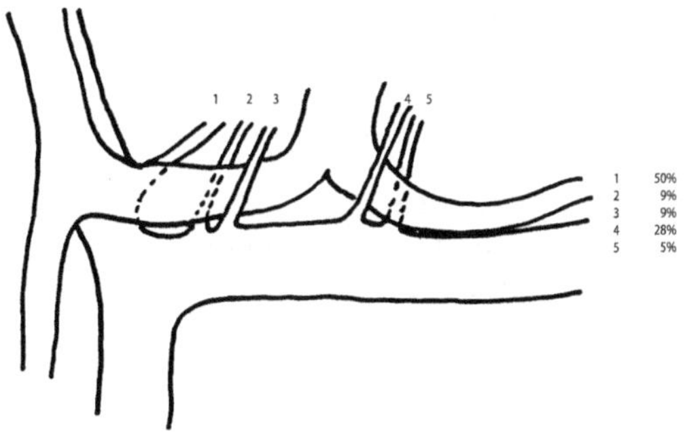

**Figure 25.8.** Variations in anatomy of left gastric vein.

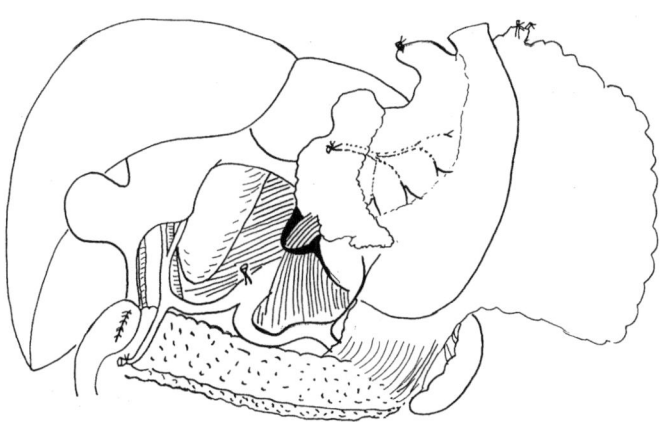

**Figure 25.9.** Origin of posterior gastric artery, defining point of division of splenic artery.

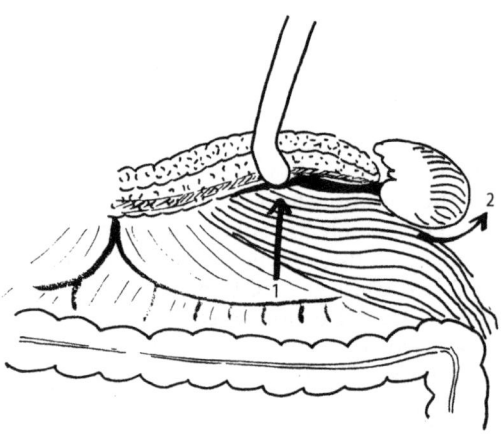

**Figure 25.10.** Mobilisation of the pancreatic tail along Todt's fascia.

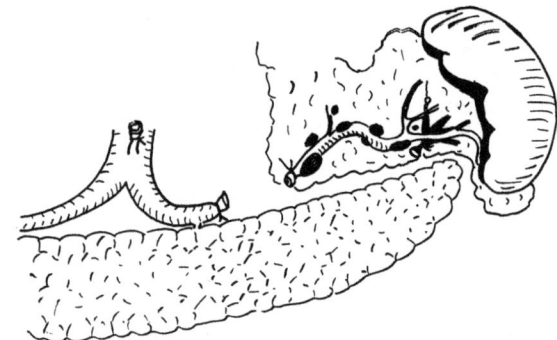

**Figure 25.12.** Separation of distal splenic artery and spleen following division of branches from splenic vein to spleen and stomach.

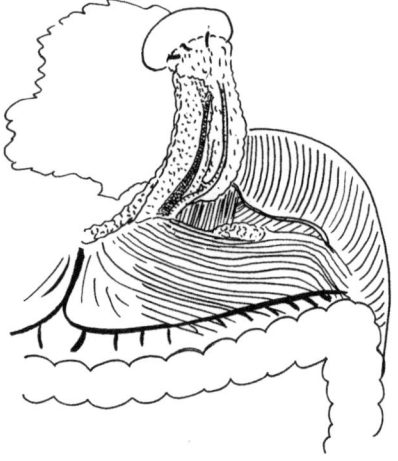

**Figure 25.11.** Dissection of pancreas to region of celiac axis preserving venous drainage to pancreas.

by ligating the oesophagocardiac branch of the inferior phrenic vessels. Both vagal nerves are divided 2–3 cm proximal to the cardia and the abdominal oesophagus is transected. An alternative technique is to divide the oesophagus as the primary step and the splenic artery nodes are dissected by pulling the entire specimen downward.

There are several methods of reconstruction of the digestive tract after total gastrectomy. The commonest and simplest method is Roux-en-Y reconstruction. Another commonly used method is jejunal interposition. Reconstruction using a pouch in conjunction with either method has been trialled but the advantage of these techniques over simple reconstruction is not clear. The oeophagojejunal anastomosis should be end to side and can be carried out using a circular stapler, with a leakage rate of 1–2% [20]. In cases where the anastomosis lies in the mediastinum, it may be necessary to divide one or two jejunal arteries from their trunk, keeping the peripheral arcade intact, to allow the jejunum to reach the anastomotic site without tension.

## TG with PS

In a conventional D2 total gastrectomy with pancreaticosplenectomy, the pancreas is transected near the coeliac artery. The indications for a combined resection are a T4 tumour invading the pancreas, bulky nodal metastases in the suprapancreatic area or metastatic nodes invading the pancreas. In these cases, the pancreas is transected adjacent to the portal vein. When the pancreas is resected, the splenic artery is ligated and divided at its origin, preserving the common hepatic artery, and then the splenic vein is divided at the resection line of the pancreatic parenchyma or its origin from the portal vein. The remainder of the procedure is the same as pancreas preserving total gastrectomy.

## Standard Distal Gastrectomy

Most of the procedure is as described for total gastrectomy. A crucial issue in the procedure of

## SURGICAL RESECTION OF THE STOMACH WITH LYMPH NODE DISSECTION

distal subtotal gastrectomy is splenectomy. In the MRC and the Dutch trials, some surgeons carried out splenectomy in distal gastrectomy. In D2 dissection, where the left gastric artery is ligated and divided at its origin, the blood supply to the remnant stomach is provided by the short gastric vessels, posterior gastric vessels and cardio-oesophageal branch from the inferior phrenic vessels. As the latter two are sometimes absent, the short gastric vessels are crucial to the viability of the remnant. Splenectomy should be avoided in distal gastrectomy, despite many textbooks of surgical technique showing all short gastric vessels ligated in distal subtotal gastrectomy. Mortality after D2 distal gastrectomy with splenectomy was 50% in the Dutch trial.

Another technical point is the dissection of right cardiac nodes in distal gastrectomy. These nodes are embedded in adipose tissue loosely attached to the gastric wall and easily divided from the wall without breaking the membrane enveloping the adipose tissue. All small branches to the gastric wall are divided, anterior and posterior branches separately (Figure 25.13) together with numerous small vagal fibres. The last technical point is how to dissect the greater curvature nodes along the left gastroepiploic vessels. These vessels are most commonly the last branch of the splenic vessels.

At the tip of the pancreas, near the splenic hilum, they arise from the inferior border of the organ running toward the stomach in the splenogastric ligament (Fig 25.14). Unlike the right gastroepiploic artery and vein, these vessels do not have a main trunk but three or four long branches in a palm-like shape. Sometimes, the inferior polar branch of the splenic artery comes from the gastroepiploic artery. In such cases, ligation of the left gastroepiploic artery renders a small part of the spleen ischemic but rarely causes any serious problems.

## PPG

PPG was originally advocated by Maki [6] as surgical treatment for benign gastric ulcer, to avoid dumping syndrome, the most important long-term sequela of distal gastrectomy. As a result of the remarkable increase in early gastric cancer in Japan, this technique was introduced in the 1990s for early gastric cancers located near the incisura. A 3 cm antral remnant is preserved and anastomosed to the proximal gastric remnant close to the greater curvature. By preserving the hepatic branch of the anterior vagal trunk and subsequently the pyloric branch, gastric emptying function is well preserved. As a result, the suprapyloric nodes are not systematically dissected in this operation as early gastric cancers in the middle part of the stomach have a less than 1% risk of these nodes being involved. Other nodal stations in D2 distal gastrectomy can be dissected as usual. Precise evaluation of this technique in terms of both

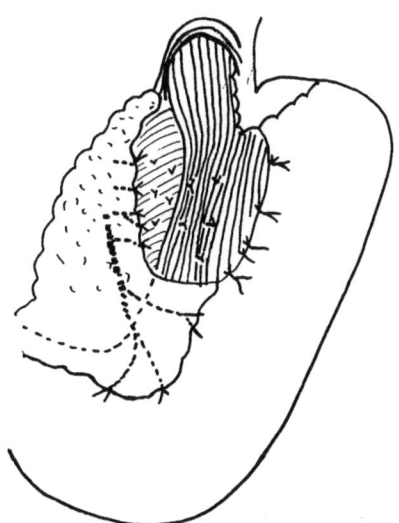

**Figure 25.13.** Clearance of right cardia nodes in distal gastric resection.

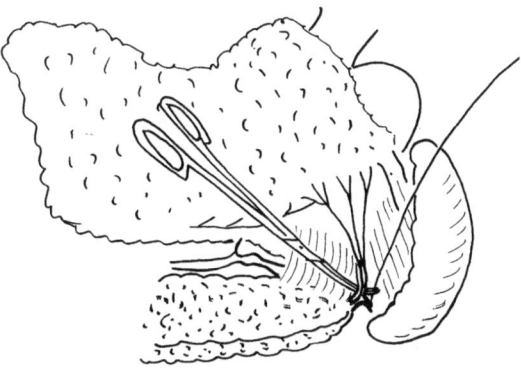

**Figure 25.14.** Identification of left gastro-epiploic vessels, usually last branch of splenic vessels.

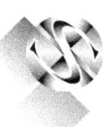

survival and quality of life after gastrectomy should be available in the near future.

## Para-aortic Nodal Dissection

In patients with advanced gastric cancer, the incidence of metastases in the para-aortic lymph nodes is reported in as many as 30% of cases. While there are reports of long-term survivors in this group the value of routine dissection remains unproven. Therefore, a randomized controlled trial was carried out by the Japanese Clinical Oncology Group (JCOG), recruiting 523 patients with curable advanced gastric cancer. Four out of 523 patients died in hospital postoperatively; thus the overall postoperative mortality rate was 0.8%, in contrast with the MRC and Dutch trials. Long-term survival evaluation will be carried out in 2006.

## Postoperative Care after D2 Dissection

Morbidity after D2 dissection in the Dutch trial and after D2 or D4 in JCOG trial is shown in Table 25.4. The most important complications after D2 or more extended gastrectomy are those related to pancreatic resection or nodal dissection around the pancreas, including splenectomy. Therefore, prophylactic use of drainage tubes and careful drain handling is recommended. The management of pancreatic leakage is complex with outcome dependent on skilled management. This includes high volume continuous irrigation or continuous suctioning together with somatostatin analogues [21]. In low volume hospitals learning how to treat pancreatic complications after D2 dissection is difficult and, in the Dutch D2 study, many patients who developed such complications died. Anastomotic leakage used to be the most important and frequent complication after a total gastrectomy but the availability of staple guns has been instrumental in reducing this to very low levels [20]. One remarkable difference between the results of the Dutch and JCOG trials is the low mortality after major complications. All participating hospitals in the JCOG trial are high volume hospitals, whereas many of those in the Dutch trial were not. In the publication of the results, it was concluded that D2 dissection should not be carried out as the standard treatment in low volume hospitals and that gastric cancer patients should be treated in specialist centres in low incidence countries.

## Questions

1. What are the indications for choosing the extent of gastric resection?
2. What are the consequences of splenic resection in partial gastrectomy?
3. What are the patient factors which determine whether extended nodal dissection is feasible?

## References

1. Sawai K, Takahashi T, Fujioka T et al. Pylorus-preserving gastrectomy with radical lymph node dissection based on anatomical variations of the infrapyloric artery. Am J Surg 1995;170:285–8.
2. Gouzi JL, Huguier M, Fagnier PL et al. Total versus subtotal gasterctomy for adenocarcinoma of the gastric antrum. A French prospective controlled study. Ann Surg 1988;209:162–6.
3. Bozzetti F, Marubini E, Bonfanti G et al and the Italian Gastrointestinal Tumor Study Group. Ann Surg 1999;230:170–8.
4. Robertson CS, Chung SCS, Woods SDS et al. A prospective randomized trial comparing R1 subtotal gastrectomy with R3 total gastrectomy for antral cancer. Ann Surg 1994;220:176–82.
5. Harrison LE, Karpeh MS, Brennan MF. Total gastrectomy is not necessary for proximal gastric cancer. Surgery 1998;123:127–30.

**Table 25.4.** Postoperative complications

| Type of complication | Incidence (%) | |
| --- | --- | --- |
| | Dutch (D2) | JCOG (D2/4) |
| Surgical | | |
| Haemorrhage | 5 | 0.6 |
| Wound infection | 9 | 1 |
| Anastomotic leak | 9 | 2 |
| Intra-abdominal infection | 17 | 5 |
| Pancreatic leak | 3 | 4 |
| Non-surgical | | |
| Cardiac | 5 | 0.1 |
| Pulmonary | 15 | 4 |
| Urinary tract | 2 | 0.4 |
| Thromboembolic | 2 | 0.4 |

6. Maki T, Shiratori T, Hatafuki T, Suganuma K. Pylorus-preserving gastrectomy as an improved operation for gastric ulcer. Surgery 1967;61:838–45.
7. Johnson H, Masood S, Belluco C et al. Prognostic factors in node-negative breast cancer. Arch Surg 1992;127:1386–91.
8. Yeh IT, Fowble B, Viglione MJ et al. Pathologic assessment and pathologic factors in operable breast cancer. In: Breast cancer treatment.
9. Sasako M. What is reasonable treatment for gastric adenocarcinoma? J Gastroenterol 2000;35(suppl XII):116–20.
10. Katai H, Maruyama K, Sasako M et al. Mode of recurrence after gastric cancer surgery. Dig Surg 1994;11:99–103.
11. Gunderson LL, Sosin H. Adenocarcinoma of the stomach: Areas of failure in a re-operation series (second or symptomatic look) clinicopathological correlation and implications for adjuvant therapy. Int J Radiat Oncol Biol Phys 1982;8:1–11.
12. Hermans J, Bonenkamp JJ, Boon MC et al. Adjuvant therapy after curative resection for gastric cancer: meta-analysis of randomized trials. J Clin Oncol 1993;11:1441–7.
13. Macdonald JS, Smalley SR, Benedetti J et al. Chemoradiotherapy after surgery compared with surgery alone for adenocarcinoma of the stomach or gastroesophageal junction. N Engl J Med 2001;345:725–30.
14. Hundahl SA, Macdonald JS, Benedetti J, Fitzsimmons T, for the Southwest Oncology Group and the Gastric Intergroup. Surgical treatment variation in a prospective, randomized trial of chemoradotherapy in gastric cancer: The effect of undertreatment. Ann Surg Oncol 2002;9:278–86.
15. Japanese Gastric Cancer Association. Japanese classification of gastric carcinoma, first English edn. Tokyo: Kanehara, 1995.
16. Cuschieri A, Fayers P, Fielding J et al for the Surgical Cooperative Group. Postoperative morbidity and mortality after D1 and D2 resections for gastric cancer: preliminary results of the MRC randomized controlled surgical trial. Lancet 1996;347:995–9.
17. Bonenkamp JJ, Hermans J, Sasako M, van De Velde CJH, for the Dutch Gastric Cancer Group. Extended lymph-node dissection for gastric cancer. N Engl J Med 1999;340:908–14.
18. Appleby LH. The celiac axis in the expansion of the operation for gastric carcinoma. Cancer 1953;6:704–7.
19. Maruyama K, Sasako M, Kinoshita T et al. World J Surg 1995;19:532–6.
20. Nomura S, Sasako M, Katai H et al. Decreasing complication rates with stapled esophagojejunostomy following a learning curve. Gastric Cancer 2000;3:97–101.
21. Sasako M, Katai H, Sano T, Maruyama K. Management of complications after gastrectomy with extended lymphadenectomy. Surg Oncol 2000;9:31–4.

# 26

# Chemotherapy of Upper GI Neoplasms: Proven/Unproven

Niall C. Tebbutt and David Cunningham

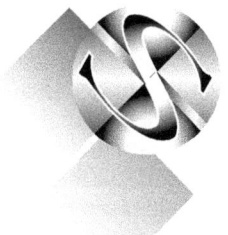

## Aims

To establish the role of chemotherapy for gastro-oesophageal tumours using currently available evidence.

## Introduction

In solid tumours, chemotherapy is frequently used both for palliation of advanced disease and also as an adjuvant therapy in order to improve the results of surgery in those patients with operable early stage disease. This chapter discusses the role of chemotherapy in upper gastrointestinal tract neoplasms, which comprise gastric and oesophageal cancers.

## Advanced Disease

In the Western world, the majority of cases of oesophagogastric cancer present with advanced stage disease. Whilst loco-regional therapies such as surgery are the only treatments capable of achieving cure in early stage disease, they have an extremely limited role in advanced stage disease. Chemotherapy is used to control symptoms, maintain quality of life and prolong survival. Since advanced oesophagogastric cancer is incurable, it was important to ascertain the benefit attributable to the use of chemotherapy in this setting. Table 26.1 summarises the results of trials comparing combination chemotherapy regimens with best supportive care. Although these trials incorporate small numbers of patients, they have shown that chemotherapy achieves a statistically significant prolongation in median survival. It has also been demonstrated that the quality of life is also significantly improved in patients receiving chemotherapy, and financial analyses have shown that attainment of these benefits is cost effective [1]. It is now, therefore, accepted that patients with advanced oesophagogastric cancer who are sufficiently fit to receive chemotherapy should be considered for this treatment.

## Single Agent Chemotherapy

A variety of chemotherapy agents have been evaluated using phase II studies in advanced

Table 26.1. Randomised trials comparing combination chemotherapy with best supportive case (BSC) in patients with advanced gastric cancer

| Regimen | Number of patients | Median survival (months) | p |
|---|---|---|---|
| ELF | 10 | 10 | <0.02 |
| BSC | 8 | 4 | |
| FAMTX | 30 | 10 | <0.001 |
| BSC | 10 | 3 | |
| FEMTX | 17 | 12 | <0.001 |
| BSC | 19 | 3 | |

ELF, epirubicin, leucovorin, 5FU; FAMTX, 5FU, adriamycin, methotrexate; FEMTX, 5FU, epirubicin, methotrexate.

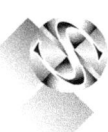

oesophagogastric cancer [2]. Results achieved in these studies are shown in Table 26.2. Most studies include relatively small numbers of selected patients. Whilst it is difficult to compare the results between studies, it does provide an indication of which agents may have the greatest activity. The results demonstrate that relatively few agents can achieve response rates of greater than 25% in previously untreated patients.

## Combination Chemotherapy Regimens

In an attempt to improve the results of chemotherapy, combination regimens consisting of those agents with the highest activity have been devised. Fluorouracil (5FU) has been a key component of many of these regimens because of its activity and its modest toxicity profile particularly when administered by infusion schedules. An early combination regimen (FAM) consisted of 5FU, adriamycin and mitomycin-C (MMC). This combination regimen was established based on impressive response rates in phase II studies. The activity of this combination regimen was confirmed in a randomised phase III study comparing treatment using FAM with adriamycin and MMC and 5FU, adriamycin and methyl-CCNU in patients with advanced gastric cancer [3]. The FAM combination regimen achieved the highest response rates (39%) and was also associated with the longest median survival (7.5 months).

Further chemotherapy regimens were devised in an attempt to improve on the FAM regimen. The FAMTX regimen incorporated high dose methotrexate instead of MMC. A randomised study showed that FAMTX achieved superior response rates (41% versus 9%; $p = 0.0001$) and more prolonged median survival times (9.7 months versus 6.7 months; $p = 0.004$) than FAM [4]. More recently, two other combination regimens have been found to be equivalent to FAMTX in advanced gastric cancer. The response rates achieved using etoposide, leucovorin and bolus 5FU (ELF), infused 5FU and cisplatin (FP) and FAMTX were 9%, 20% and 12% respectively and were not significantly different. The median survival times were 7.2 months with ELF, 7.2 months with FP and 6.7 months with FAMTX [5]. The authors concluded that all of these regimens had modest activity and that new strategies for advanced disease should be considered.

The combination of epirubicin 50 mg/m$^2$, cisplatin 60 mg/m$^2$ and protracted venous infusion 5FU 300 mg/m$^2$/day was developed at the Royal Marsden Hospital, United Kingdom. This regimen also achieved an impressive response rate of 71% in a phase II study involving 128 patients [6]. This led to comparison of ECF with FAMTX in a randomised phase III study involving 274 patients with advanced oesophagogastric cancer. The response rate in this study with ECF was superior to FAMTX (45% versus 21%; $p = 0.0002$) and overall survival was also superior (8.9 months versus 5.7 months; $p = 0.0009$). This study also included patients with locally advanced inoperable disease as well as patients with metastatic disease. The response rate in patients with locally advanced disease was 58% and a proportion of responding patients were able to proceed to surgery and subsequently underwent macroscopic and microscopic complete resection of the tumour (R0 resection).

A second randomised study has confirmed the activity of ECF. In this study ECF was compared with MCF, where MMC was combined with cisplatin and a larger dose of infused 5FU than is administered in ECF. In this study the response rates (42% versus 44%) and median survival time (9.4 months versus 8.7 months) for patients receiving both ECF and MCF were equivalent [7]. Whilst these measures of efficacy appeared equivalent, global quality of life was superior for patients receiving ECF. This is an

**Table 26.2.** Response rates achieved in phase II studies of various chemotherapy agents in advanced oesophagogastric cancer

| Chemotherapy agent | Number of patients | Response rate (%) |
| --- | --- | --- |
| 5FU (infusion) | 13 | 31 |
| 5FU (bolus) | 392 | 21 |
| Mitomycin-C | 211 | 30 |
| Epirubicin | 61 | 26 |
| Doxorubicin | 68 | 25 |
| Docetaxel | 37 | 24 |
| Paclitaxel | 33 | 17 |
| Irinotecan | 60 | 23 |
| Cisplatin | 129 | 19 |
| Carboplatin | 57 | 5 |
| Methotrexate | 28 | 11 |

important measure for a treatment that is given with palliative intent and this has led to the conclusion that ECF is the superior regimen.

## ECF is the Most Active Combination Chemotherapy Regimen in Oesophagogastric Cancer

The evidence therefore indicates that the ECF regimen is the most active combination chemotherapy regimen for patients with advanced oesophagogastric cancer. Although this regimen is widely accepted as standard treatment, its acceptance has not been universal. The reluctance to accept ECF has arisen for a number of reasons and various criticisms of the ECF versus FAMTX study have been raised to account for this reluctance. Firstly, there was a perception that the patients receiving FAMTX in the trial comparing FAMTX with ECF had fared badly. Further randomised studies using FAMTX now suggest that the median survival achieved using FAMTX of approximately 6 months is comparable to other studies. Secondly, more patients receiving ECF proceeded to a potentially curative surgical resection, which may have biased the results of this study. Whilst many would regard this result likely to be due to the superior activity of ECF, the role of neoadjuvant ECF in patients with locally advanced disease has never been formally assessed in a randomised study. Thirdly, the administration of ECF requires the insertion of long-term indwelling venous catheters and results in a relatively modest prolongation of median survival in comparison with regimens such as FAMTX.

ECF achieves a modest median survival duration in patients with advanced oesophagogastric cancer, with a median survival time of approximately 9 months. The relatively short survival times highlight the need for ongoing improvement in the treatment of patients with advanced oesophagogastric cancer. This is particularly the case for elderly and less fit patients for whom the side effects of intensive combination chemotherapy may be significant.

## Future Studies

In order to attempt to improve the results achieved using chemotherapy, several randomised studies incorporating novel agents are currently in progress. A multicentre study coordinated by the Royal Marsden Hospital is using ECF as the standard arm and is comparing this with substitution of cisplatin by the third generation platinum agent oxaliplatin and substitution of 5FU with the oral fluoropyrimidine capecitabine. The use of capecitabine in this fashion avoids the requirement for indwelling venous catheters.

Novel agents with activity in oesophagogastric cancer include the taxanes and the topoisomerase I inhibitor irinotecan (CPT11). Phase II studies have suggested that CPT11 plus 5FU is an active regimen (response rate 42%) [8]. Similarly, the combination of docetaxel, cisplatin and 5FU appears active (response rate 44%) [9]. These regimens are now being compared to standard treatment in randomised phase III clinical trials.

## Biological Therapies

Further strategies currently being evaluated in an effort to improve the results in patients with advanced oesophagogastric cancer include the use of biological therapies directed at pathways perceived to be important in the pathogenesis of gastric cancer. One of these approaches involves the use of marimastat, a matrix metalloproteinase (MMP) inhibitor. The MMP enzymes constitute a family of proteolytic enzymes. Elevated levels of MMP enzymes have been associated with a poor prognosis in gastric cancer. A randomised study comparing marimastat with placebo in patients with gastric cancer demonstrated prolongation of failure-free survival and after protracted follow-up an overall survival advantage, especially for those patients who had received prior chemotherapy. However, the prolongation in survival was modest at approximately 1 month and overall quality of life was not improved [10]. Therefore further evaluation of the role of marimastat is likely to be required in order to define a role for this drug in patients with advanced gastric cancer.

Other possible approaches include agents targeted to the epidermal growth factor receptor (EGFR). Antibodies to EGFR and drugs inhibiting the EGFR kinase domain are currently being evaluated in oesophagogastric cancer as well as other tumour types.

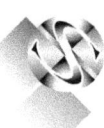

## Adjuvant Therapy

Although a proportion of patients may be cured by surgical resection of primary oesophageal or gastric tumours, 70% or more of patients will subsequently develop recurrent disease. This is due to the presence of unresected micrometastasis. Adjuvant treatment aims to eliminate residual tumour cells and increase the proportion of patients achieving long-term disease-free intervals and overall survival benefit. Instituting treatment soon after surgery may have a number of advantages. The tumour burden is low and the likelihood of development of chemotherapy-resistant cell clones smaller. The knowledge of the range of agents with activity in advanced disease raises the possibility of utilisation of these agents in the adjuvant setting.

### Gastric Cancer

The majority of studies of adjuvant therapy after resection of gastric cancers have failed to demonstrate any benefit for this treatment. A number of meta-analyses have also failed to indicate any benefit for adjuvant therapy, although a more recent analysis has suggested that there may be a small benefit [11]. An important caveat in interpretation of the data is that many of the studies used suboptimal adjuvant chemotherapy regimens, with many involving treatment using single chemotherapy agent regimens. In addition, many of the studies included relatively small numbers of patients and therefore there would need to be substantial differences in outcome for these to be statistically significant. Adjuvant chemotherapy is therefore regarded as an unproven treatment after surgical resection of gastric cancer and eligible patients should be considered for adjuvant chemotherapy trials.

### Oesophageal Cancer

Adjuvant chemotherapy after surgical resection of squamous cell carcinoma of the oesophagus has been evaluated in two randomised studies using the combinations of cisplatin with vindesine and cisplatin with 5FU given for two cycles [12-14]. In each study, there was no impact on overall survival for the group receiving chemotherapy. Like the results of the gastric cancer trials, relatively small numbers of patients have been studied and the chemotherapy regimens are not necessarily optimal. For example, it is unlikely that two cycles of chemotherapy would have a dramatic impact on micrometastatic disease. However, at this stage it must be concluded that postoperative adjuvant chemotherapy remains an unproven treatment for oesophageal carcinoma.

## Adjuvant Chemoradiotherapy

### Gastric Cancer

Since both local as well as systemic recurrence represents a common problem after gastric cancer resection, a North American Intergroup trial evaluated a combined modality adjuvant regimen compared with observation. This incorporated postoperative chemotherapy involving one cycle of 5FU and leucovorin (LV) followed by two cycles of 5FU/LV administered concurrently with radiotherapy followed by two further cycles of 5FU/LV. The schema of treatment is outlined in Figure 26.1 [15]. The results of this adjuvant treatment showed that this therapy led to a 10% survival advantage after 3 years (52% versus 41%; $p = 0.03$). Failure-free survival was 49% for the treatment arm compared with 32% for no adjuvant therapy ($p = 0.001$). Whilst this treatment is now regarded as standard therapy in North America, it has not yet been widely accepted in Europe because of concerns about toxicity with abdominal chemoradiation and the adequacy of surgery. In the trial 41% and 32% of patients suffered grade 3 and 4 toxicities respectively and 54% of patients received less than a D1 resection.

## Neoadjuvant Treatment

Neoadjuvant therapy involves the administration of systemic treatment before loco-regional therapy such as surgery. This approach to the treatment of oesophagogastric cancer offers a number of potential advantages. It allows systemic treatment to be delivered as early as possible, which may have advantages from the

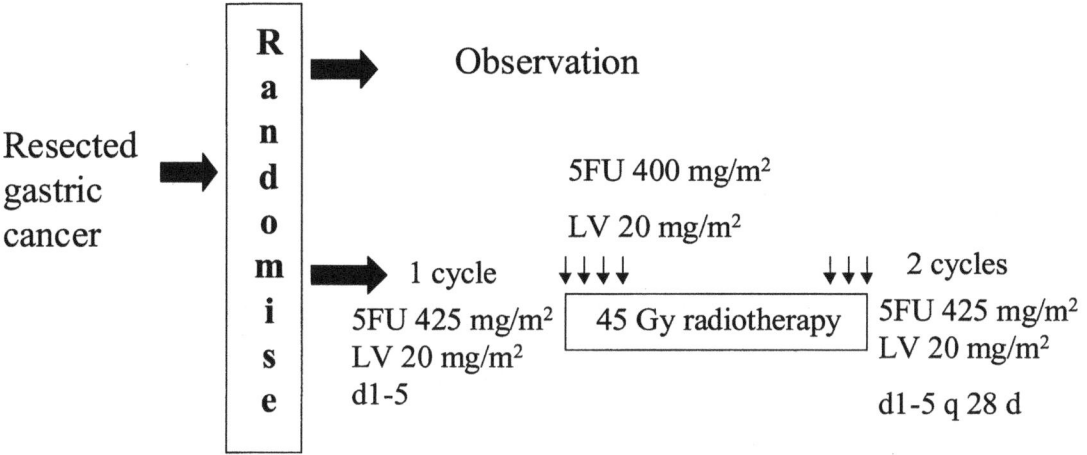

Figure 26.1. Outline of trial comparing postoperative chemoradiotherapy with observation after resection of gastric cancer.

perspective of treatment of micrometastatic disease. In addition, it allows the possibility that inoperable locally advanced tumours may be downstaged, thereby rendering these tumours amenable to potentially curative surgical resection. It also provides prognostic information, with tumour response to neoadjuvant chemotherapy representing the most important prognostic factor for prolonged survival in gastric cancer [16]. The principal disadvantage of neoadjuvant chemotherapy is the possibility that tumour progression may occur during the course of treatment, thereby rendering the tumour inoperable and allowing the risk of dissemination of disease.

## Gastric Cancer

Phase II studies have demonstrated that neoadjuvant chemotherapy is an effective strategy in selected patients with gastric cancer. A current Medical Research Council (MRC) study is comparing the results after three cycles of ECF neoadjuvant chemotherapy followed by surgical resection followed by a further three cycles of ECF adjuvant chemotherapy with surgical resection alone for patients with cancers of the stomach or oesophagogastric junction. The design of this trial is illustrated in Figure 26.2. This study is close to completing accrual and should provide valuable information about the role of neoadjuvant chemotherapy in gastric cancer.

## Oesophageal Cancer

In the case of oesophageal cancer, preoperative approaches have included neoadjuvant chemotherapy or neoadjuvant chemoradiation. The neoadjuvant chemotherapy studies have often included relatively small numbers of patients receiving a variety of chemotherapy regimens. However, two large studies have recently been reported, one of which has shown a significant benefit for this approach. The results of all these studies are summarised in Table 26.3. A recent MRC study involving 800 randomised patients compared preoperative chemotherapy using two cycles of cisplatin 80 mg/m$^2$ and 5FU 1000 mg/m$^2$ d1-4 with no preoperative treatment [17]. The trial design is illustrated in Figure 26.3. Preoperative chemotherapy was feasible and resulted in a higher rate of macroscopic complete resection (84% versus 71%). The R0 resection rate was 60% in the chemotherapy arm compared with 55% in the surgery arm. This constitutes an important outcome, as only patients who achieve an R0 resection would be anticipated to be able to achieve long-term survival. Importantly, there was no increase in perioperative complications or deaths after preoperative chemotherapy. There was a statistically significant improvement in both progression-free and overall survival, with 2-year survival being 45% in the combined modality arm compared with 35% in the surgery alone arm.

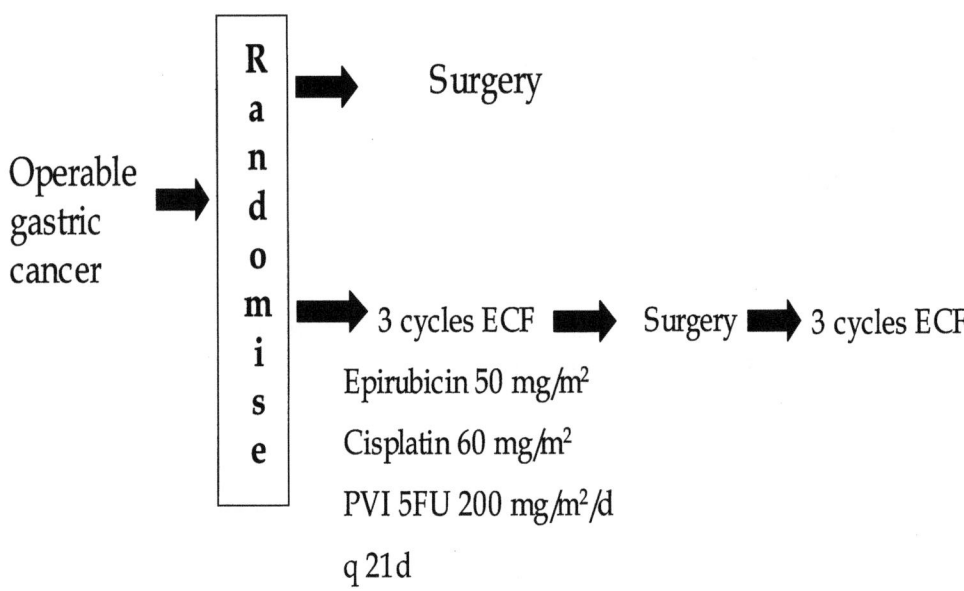

**Figure 26.2.** Outline of MRC study evaluating neoadjuvant chemotherapy in operable gastric cancer.

**Table 26.3.** Results of randomised studies of neoadjuvant chemotherapy in oesophageal carcinoma

| Trial | Number of patients | Histology | Chemotherapy | Median overall survival (months) Chemotherapy | Surgery |
|---|---|---|---|---|---|
| Roth et al | 39 | Squamous | Cisplatin, vindesine, bleomycin | 8 | 9 |
| Nygaard et al | 91 | Squamous | Cisplatin, bleomycin | 8 | 8 |
| Schlag et al | 77 | Squamous | Cisplatin, 5FU 3 cycles | 10 | 10 |
| Kok et al | 160 | Squamous | Cisplatin, etoposide 2–4 cycles | 18.5* | 11 |
| Kelsen et al | 440 | Squamous/ adenocarcionma | Cisplatin, 5FU 3 cycles | 14.9 | 16.1 |
| MRC OEO2 | 802 | Squamous/ adenocarcinoma | Cisplatin, 5FU | 17.6* | 13.6 |

\* $p < 0.01$.

A similar schedule of preoperative treatment has also been evaluated in a large American study [18]. This trial compared the results of surgery after preoperative chemotherapy using three cycles of cisplatin and fluorouracil with surgery alone. Preoperative chemotherapy achieved a small although not statistically significant improvement in the R0 resection rate. However, this did not result in any impact on overall survival.

It is difficult to explain the different results from these two studies. Nevertheless, the large number of patients enrolled in the MRC study makes the results of this trial quite compelling. It is likely that there are subgroups of patients who derive most benefit from such a neoadjuvant treatment approach. These may be identified based on more accurate staging techniques such as endoscopic ultrasound or based on the molecular genotype of the tumour. However,

## CHEMOTHERAPY OF UPPER GI NEOPLASMS: PROVEN/UNPROVEN

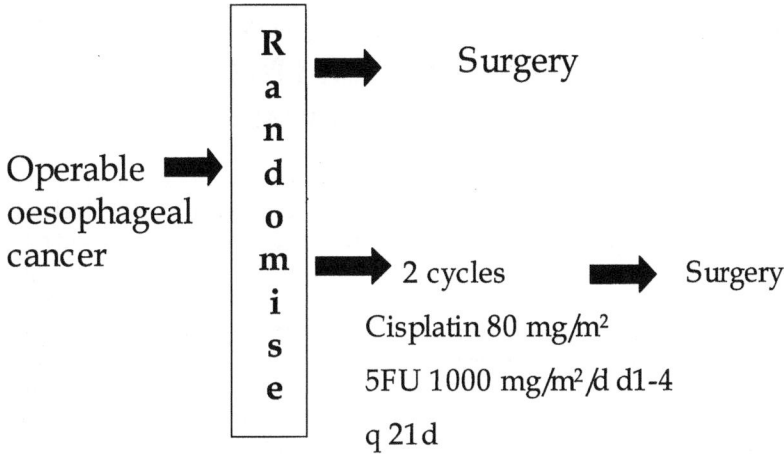

**Figure 26.3.** Outline of MRC study evaluating neoadjuvant chemotherapy in operable oesophageal cancer.

until these groups are identified it would be reasonable to consider neoadjuvant chemotherapy in patients who were being considered for radical resection of oesophageal carcinoma.

## Neoadjuvant Chemoradiotherapy

### Oesophageal Cancer

A randomised study has compared chemoradiotherapy with radical radiotherapy as definitive treatment for oesophageal carcinoma. This study compared two cycles of cisplatin 75 mg/m$^2$ and 5FU 1000 mg/m$^2$ d1-4 given concurrently in weeks 1 and 5 with 50 Gy radiotherapy followed by two further cycles of the same chemotherapy with 64 Gy radiotherapy alone (Figure 26.4) [19]. The majority of cases were squamous cell carcinomas, but adenocarcinomas were included. Median survival was 14 months in the combined modality arm compared with 9 months in the radiotherapy arm. The 5-year survival rate was 27% for the combined modality therapy versus 0% for radiotherapy.

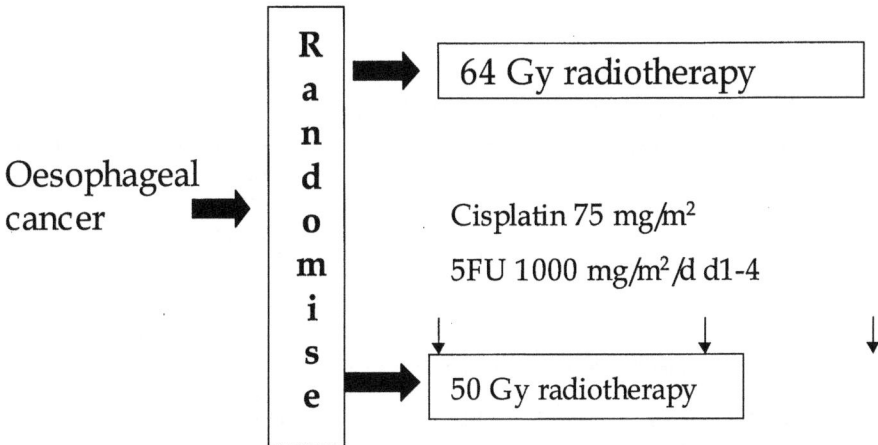

**Figure 26.4.** Outline of trial comparing radical radiotherapy with chemoradiotherapy as definitive treatment for oesophageal cancer.

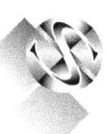

The positive results of this study have led to acceptance of chemoradiotherapy as a possible treatment option for those patients who are not surgical candidates. This may apply for those patients who are not candidates for surgical resection on the grounds of concurrent medical disorders or because the anatomical location of the primary tumour renders surgery technically difficult, such as tumours arising in the cervical oesophagus. Nevertheless, the local failure rate with such an approach is significant (47%). This has stimulated trials which incorporate chemoradiotherapy in addition to surgery.

Whilst a variety of regimens have been studied, most randomised studies evaluating these regimens have been negative. These results are summarised in Table 26.4. Whilst the study by Walsh et al has reported improved survival with neoadjuvant chemoradiotherapy prior to surgery compared with surgery alone, this study has been criticised because of the relatively poor outcomes achieved in the surgery alone control arm [20]. A limitation of chemoradiotherapy is toxicity, which is increased with such therapy. For instance, in the trial reported by Urba et al, neutropenic sepsis occurred in 39% of patients and 63% of patients required feeding tubes in order to maintain nutrition because of radiation oesophagitis [21]. Therefore, in the absence of any significant benefit attributable to this approach, neoadjuvant chemoradiation prior to surgery for oesophageal carcinoma is currently regarded as an unproven treatment.

# Improvements in Adjuvant and Neoadjuvant Therapies

As new agents are evaluated further in the advanced setting, it is likely that those agents with the highest activity will be used in the adjuvant and neoadjuvant setting. However, even the use of these agents is unlikely to benefit all patients. It is likely that only selected patients will derive benefit from adjuvant or neoadjuvant therapy. These are patients who only have micrometastatic disease and whose tumours are responsive to chemotherapy.

## Exclusion of Patients with Metastatic Disease

Conventional staging procedures do not exclude a number of patients with metastatic disease. However, the use of positron emission tomography (PET) scans has been shown to provide a useful adjunct to conventional staging using CT scans and endoscopic ultrasound examination [22]. The inclusion of PET scans could allow radical surgery and chemotherapy to be targeted at those patients who are most likely to benefit.

**Table 26.4.** Results of randomised studies of neoadjuvant chemoradiotherapy in oesophageal carcinoma

| Trial | Number of patients | Histology | Chemotherapy | Radiotherapy dose | Chemotherapy | Surgery |
|---|---|---|---|---|---|---|
| Le Prise et al | 86 | Squamous | Cisplatin, 5FU | 20 Gy, 10 fractions | 10 | 10.5 |
| Nygaard et al | 88 | Squamous | Cisplatin, bleomycin | 35 Gy in 20 fractions | 9 | 8 |
| Bosset et al | 282 | Squamous | Cisplatin, 2 cycles | 37 Gy in 10 fractions | 18.6 | |
| Walsh et al | 113 | Adenocarcinoma | Cisplatin, 5FU 2 cycles | 40 Gy in 15 fractions | 16* | |
| Urba et al | 100 | Squamous/ adenocarcinoma | Cisplatin, vinblastine, 5FU 2 cycles | 45 Gy in 30 fractions | 16.9 | |

\* $p < 0.01$.

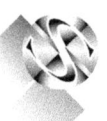

## Prediction of Tumour Response Using Molecular Markers

There has been considerable interest in the use of molecular markers to identify tumours which are most likely to respond to chemotherapy. This has not been extensively evaluated in oesophagogastric cancers. However, studies involving small numbers of patients with gastric cancer showed that patients whose tumours had elevated levels of the enzyme thymidylate synthase (TS) were resistant to 5FU. Similarly, tumours with elevated levels of mRNA encoding the DNA repair gene ERCC1 were more likely to be resistant to cisplatin [23]. Further evaluation of the role of molecular markers may allow the identification of patients who are most likely to benefit from chemotherapy, and who could potentially be targeted to receive adjuvant or neoadjuvant chemotherapy. This type of strategy is advantageous as it ensures that only those patients who are likely to derive benefit from chemotherapy actually receive that treatment, thereby sparing toxicity in those who do not derive benefit.

## Conclusions

Combination chemotherapy is proven to benefit patients with advanced oesophagogastric cancer. It is hoped that improvements in the treatment of advanced stage disease together with careful case selection will allow more patients with early stage disease to benefit from adjuvant or neoadjuvant chemotherapy or chemoradiotherapy.

## Questions

1. What are the goals of palliative chemotherapy in advanced oesophagogastric cancer?
2. Which combination chemotherapy regimen is considered most active in advanced oesophagogastric cancer?
3. Which adjuvant therapy has shown a survival advantage after resection of gastric cancer?
4. What are the potential advantages and disadvantages of neoadjuvant chemotherapy in oesophageal cancer?
5. Which neoadjuvant chemotherapy regimen has achieved a survival advantage in operable oesophageal cancer?

## References

1. Glimelius B, Hoffman K, Graf W et al. Cost-effectiveness of palliative chemotherapy in advanced gastrointestinal cancer. Ann Oncol 1995;6(3):267-74.
2. Hill ME, Cunningham D. Medical management of advanced gastric cancer. Cancer Treat Rev 1998;24(2):113-18.
3. Douglass HO, Jr, Lavin PT, Goudsmit A et al. An Eastern Cooperative Oncology Group evaluation of combinations of methyl-CCNU, mitomycin C, Adriamycin, and 5-fluorouracil in advanced measurable gastric cancer (EST 2277). J Clin Oncol 1984; 2(12):1372-81.
4. Wils JA, Klein HO, Wagener DJ et al. Sequential high-dose methotrexate and fluorouracil combined with doxorubicin – a step ahead in the treatment of advanced gastric cancer: a trial of the European Organization for Research and Treatment of Cancer Gastrointestinal Tract Cooperative Group. J Clin Oncol 1991; 9(5):827-31.
5. Vanhoefer U, Rougier P, Wilke H et al. Final results of a randomized phase III trial of sequential high-dose methotrexate, fluorouracil, and doxorubicin versus etoposide, leucovorin, and fluorouracil versus infusional fluorouracil and cisplatin in advanced gastric cancer: A trial of the European Organization for Research and Treatment of Cancer Gastrointestinal Tract Cancer Cooperative Group. J Clin Oncol 2000;18(14):2648-57.
6. Findlay M, Cunningham D, Norman A et al. A phase II study in advanced gastro-esophageal cancer using epirubicin and cisplatin in combination with continuous infusion 5-fluorouracil (ECF). Ann Oncol 1994; 5(7):609-16.
7. Ross P, Nicolson M, Cunningham D et al. A prospective randomised trial comparing MCF with ECF in advanced oesophago-gastric cancer. Submitted 2001.
8. Pozzo C, Bugat R, Peschel C et al. Irinotecan in combination with CDDP or 5FU and folinic acid is active in patients with advanced gastric or gastro-oesophageal junction adenocarcinoma: Final results of a randomised phase II study. Proc Am Soc Clin Oncol 2001; 20(abstr).
9. Van Cutsem E, Ayani J, Tjulandin S et al. Docetaxel in combination with cisplatinum with or without 5-fluorouracil in patients with advanced gastric or GE junction adenocarcinoma: Preliminary results. Ann Oncol 2001;11(S4)(abstr).
10. Fielding J, Scholefield J, Stuart R et al. A randomized double-blind placebo-controlled study of marimastat in patients with inoperable gastric adenocarcinoma. Proc Am Soc Clin Oncol 2000;19(abstr).

11. Mari E, Floriani I, Tinazzi A et al. Efficacy of adjuvant chemotherapy after curative resection for gastric cancer: a meta-analysis of published randomised trials. A study of the GISCAD (Gruppo Italiano per lo Studio dei Carcinomi dell'Apparato Digerente). Ann Oncol 2000;11(7):837–43.
12. Webb A, Cunningham D, Scarffe JH et al. Randomized trial comparing epirubicin, cisplatin, and fluorouracil versus fluorouracil, doxorubicin, and methotrexate in advanced esophagogastric cancer. J Clin Oncol 1997;15(1):261–7.
13. Ando N, Iizuka T, Kakegawa T et al. A randomized trial of surgery with and without chemotherapy for localized squamous carcinoma of the thoracic esophagus: the Japan Clinical Oncology Group Study. J Thorac Cardiovasc Surg 1997;114(2):205–9.
14. Ando N, Iizuka T, Kakegawa T et al. A randomized trial comparing surgery to surgery plus postoperative chemotherapy for localised squamous cell carcinoma of the thoracic esophagus. Proc Am Soc Clin Oncol 1998;17. (abstr).
15. Macdonald JS, Smalley S, Benedetti J et al. Postoperative combined radiation and chemotherapy improves disease-free survival (DFS) and overall survival (OS) in resected adenocarcinoma of the stomach and GE junction. Results of Intergroup Study INT-0116 (SWOG 9008). Proc Am Soc Clin Oncol 2000; 19 (abstr).
16. Lowy AM, Mansfield PF, Leach SD et al. Response to neoadjuvant chemotherapy best predicts survival after curative resection of gastric cancer. Ann Surg 1999;229(3):303–8.
17. Clark P. Surgical resection with or without pre-operative chemotherapy in oesophageal cancer: an updated analysis of a randomised controlled trial conducted by the UK Medical Research Council Upper GI tract cancer group. Proc Am Soc Clin Oncol 2001;20(abstr).
18. Kelsen DP, Ginsberg R, Pajak TF et al. Chemotherapy followed by surgery compared with surgery alone for localized esophageal cancer. N Engl J Med 1998;339(27): 1979–84.
19. Herskovic A, Martz K, al Sarraf M et al. Combined chemotherapy and radiotherapy compared with radiotherapy alone in patients with cancer of the esophagus. N Engl J Med 1992;326(24):1593–8.
20. Walsh TN, Noonan N, Hollywood D et al. A comparison of multimodal therapy and surgery for esophageal adenocarcinoma. N Engl J Med 1996;335(7):462–7.
21. Urba SG, Orringer MB, Turrisi A et al. Randomized trial of preoperative chemoradiation versus surgery alone in patients with locoregional esophageal carcinoma. J Clin Oncol 2001;19(2):305–13.
22. Flamen P, Lerut A, Van Cutsem E et al. Utility of positron emission tomography for the staging of patients with potentially operable esophageal carcinoma. J Clin Oncol 2000;18(18):3202–10.
23. Metzger R, Leichman CG, Danenberg KD et al. ERCC1 mRNA levels complement thymidylate synthase mRNA levels in predicting response and survival for gastric cancer patients receiving combination cisplatin and fluorouracil chemotherapy. J Clin Oncol 1998;16(1): 309–16.

# 27

## Radiotherapy in Upper GI Tract Neoplasms

MS Anwar, Ju Ian Geh and David Spooner

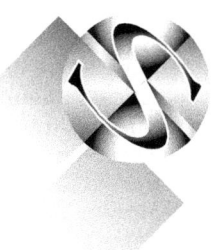

## Aims

This chapter aims to provide an evidence-based review of the role of radiotherapy in upper gastrointestinal malignancy. Multidisciplinary team working is the key to optimal management of these patients. This involves close collaboration amongst surgeons, oncologists, gastroenterologists, radiologists, pathologists, palliative care physicians, specialist nurses and dieticians. Each discipline should have an understanding of the clinical evidence that supports the use of the various treatment options available. Potential future developments in translational research and ongoing clinical trials are also discussed briefly.

## Oesophagus

Oesophageal cancer is the third commonest gastrointestinal malignancy and the tenth commonest cancer in the world. Its incidence is 7.5 per 100 000 in the UK. In the Western world, there has been a significant increase in adenocarcinoma of the lower oesophagus and gastro-oesophageal junction over the last 15 years. This is now more common than squamous carcinoma. At the time of diagnosis, the presence of locally advanced disease or distant metastases render approximately 60% of the patients surgically incurable. In a literature review of 122 papers of oesophageal cancer surgery, published between 1953 and 1978, the pooled 5-year survival of all 83 783 patients treated was 4% (range 1% to 13%) [1]. Despite improvements in surgical technique and postoperative intensive care, the survival from oesophageal cancer remains poor. A further literature review of 46 692 patients treated between 1980 and 1988 showed a 5-year survival of 10% [2].

## Radiotherapy

### Preoperative (Neoadjuvant) Radiotherapy

Preoperative radiotherapy has been used in an attempt to improve resection rates and to decrease the risk of local recurrence. Five randomised trials have failed to demonstrate increased resectability or improved overall survival. A subsequent meta-analysis of these trials using updated individual patient data also failed to show a statistically significant survival benefit from preoperative radiotherapy [3].

### Radical Radiotherapy

Radical radiotherapy can result in long-term survival of patients who are not suitable for resection. In a literature review of 49 papers published between 1954 and 1979, the pooled 5-year survival of 8489 patients receiving radiotherapy was 6% (range 0% to 21%) [4]. Two small randomised trials of resectable

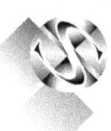

oesophageal cancer have compared radical radiotherapy with surgery and have showed a statistically significant survival advantage in favour of surgery [5,6]. A third trial by the Medical Research Council (MRC) failed to accrue.

## Postoperative (Adjuvant) Radiotherapy

Radiotherapy has been used postoperatively to reduce the risk of local recurrence. In a University of Hong Kong trial, 130 patients were randomised to radiotherapy (49 Gy if curative resection or 52.5 Gy if palliative resection) or to no further treatment following oesophagectomy [7]. Although there was a lower risk of local recurrence in the palliative resection group receiving radiotherapy (20% vs 46%), patients receiving radiotherapy had a worse overall survival (median 8.7 months vs 15.2 months; $p = 0.02$). This was due to treatment-related deaths from gastric ulceration and haemorrhage, and was probably related to the large radiation doses given per fraction (3.5 Gy/fraction).

The second trial was carried out by the French University Association for Surgical Research [8]. A total of 221 patients with squamous carcinoma were randomised to receive postoperative radiotherapy (45 to 55 Gy) or no further treatment following resection. Overall survival in both arms was identical (median 18 months).

## Chemoradiotherapy (CRT)

The use of synchronous chemotherapy with radiotherapy, known as chemoradiotherapy (CRT), has been established in a number of gastrointestinal tract cancers including oesophagus [9], pancreas [10], stomach [11], rectum and anus. In addition, there is convincing evidence that CRT improves survival in squamous carcinomas of the uterine cervix and head and neck when compared with radiotherapy alone.

### Preoperative (Neoadjuvant) Chemoradiotherapy

The intentions of delivering CRT prior to attempted surgical resection would include: improving loco-regional disease control by increasing curative resection rates and reducing the risk of loco-regional recurrence

- reducing the risk of distant metastases
- improving the nutritional status of the patient by rapid relief of dysphagia which may optimise physical condition for surgery
- making the effectiveness of CRT assessable by histological examination of the resected oesophagus.

In a review of preoperative CRT in oesophageal cancer [12], pooled data from 46 non-randomised studies totalling 2704 patients showed that the resection rate following CRT was 74%. Overall survival of the patients treated ranged from 8% to 55% at 3 years with a median range of 8 to 37 months. Of the patients undergoing resection, 32% achieved pathological complete response (pCR), as defined by the reporting pathologist being unable to identify viable tumour cells within the specimen. Pathological CR was associated with improved survival (29–92% at 3 years) and a low risk of loco-regional recurrence (3%).

There have been seven completed randomised trials comparing preoperative CRT followed by surgery with surgery alone [13–19] (Table 27.1). Only one trial has demonstrated a statistically significant survival improvement from trimodality treatment [16]. In this trial, only patients with adenocarcinoma were included and the survival of the surgery-only arm was considered to be poor (6% at 3 years). Although the EORTC trial [17] failed to show an improvement in overall survival, patients receiving preoperative CRT had superior disease-free survival. The higher postoperative mortality from trimodality treatment (12% vs 4%) had negated any survival benefit achieved. The latest and second largest (256 patients) trial to report was conducted in Australasia (AGITG/TROG) [19]. Of the 105 patients who had resection following preoperative CRT, 15% achieved pCR. This was more likely to occur in patients with squamous carcinoma (26%) than adenocarcinoma (9%). However, there was no difference in overall survival between the two groups (median of 21.7 months for preoperative CRT vs 18.5 months for surgery alone; $p = 0.38$). The US Intergroup (NCCTG-C9781) trial closed due to a failure to accrue.

Any potential benefit from trimodality treatment has to be weighed against the risk of increased treatment-related morbidity and mortality. The pooled postoperative mortality of patients treated with preoperative CRT followed by surgery was 9%, but this ranged from 0% to 29% [12]. Although the risk of postoperative death was significantly higher for patients receiving CRT in the EORTC trial [17], the other randomised trials showed no increase in risk [14–19]. Adult respiratory distress syndrome, anastomotic leak and breakdown, pneumonia and sepsis were the commonest causes of postoperative death.

## Definitive Chemoradiotherapy

A pilot study by the Toronto group of 35 patients with unresectable squamous carcinoma treated by CRT (45–50 Gy with mitomycin-C and fluorouracil (5FU) reported a 2-year survival of 28% [20]. This appeared superior to a 2-year survival of 15% achieved in a similar cohort of patients who received radiotherapy alone.

In a review of the role of definitive CRT in oesophageal cancer (radiation doses from 40 to 70 Gy and synchronous 5FU and either mitomycin-C or cisplatin) [21], the 2-year survival ranged from 28% to 72% in squamous carcinoma and 14% to 29% in adenocarcinoma. Many of these patients had unresectable disease. Several investigators have compared their results of definitive CRT with surgical controls (with or without CRT) and found no differences in survival.

The Radiation Therapy Oncology Group trial (RTOG 85–01) randomised 123 patients (88% with squamous carcinoma) to CRT (50 Gy with two cycles of synchronous cisplatin and 5FU followed by two further cycles of adjuvant chemotherapy) or radiotherapy alone (64 Gy) [9]. At interim analysis, the median survival of patients receiving CRT was superior (14.1 months vs 9.3 months; $p < 0.001$). This led to early termination of the trial. Updated data of this trial as well as the results of a further cohort of 69 patients treated with the same CRT regimen were subsequently published [22]. The 3-year survival was 30% and 26% for patients receiving CRT in the randomised and non-randomised trial respectively versus 0% for radiotherapy alone.

The Eastern Cooperative Oncology Group (ECOG) randomised (EST-1282 trial) 119 patients with squamous carcinoma to receive either CRT (radiotherapy with mitomycin-C and 5FU) or radiotherapy alone [23]. At 40 Gy, all patients were assessed for surgery or for definitive CRT (non-randomised). Forty-six patients (23 in CRT arm and 23 in radiotherapy arm) underwent resection. The median survival in the CRT arm was superior (14.8 months vs 9.2 months; $p = 0.04$). Despite the selection bias in favour of patients undergoing surgery, there was no difference in survival between resected and non-resected patients (Table 27.2).

Although the results of CRT appear to be superior to radiotherapy alone, the reported loco-regional failure rate as defined by persistent disease or subsequent recurrence following definitive CRT is 40% or more. In an attempt to improve loco-regional control, the next US Intergroup randomised trial (INT 0123) of CRT compared a higher radiation dose of 64.8 Gy with the standard dose of 50.4 Gy [26]. A total of 236 patients were entered (86% with squamous carcinoma). There was no difference in median (13.0 months vs 18.1 months) or 2-year (31% vs 40%) survival between high-dose and standard-dose treatment. However, there was an inexplicable excess of deaths during treatment in the high-dose arm (10% vs 2%), the majority of events occurring before the dose escalation was delivered.

Given the fact that survival following definitive CRT appeared equivalent to surgery alone, several investigators have questioned the routine role of surgery in resectable oesophageal cancer. To date, no randomised trial has compared CRT with surgery alone. Murakami [27] reported a study of 40 patients with resectable squamous carcinoma who received induction CRT (44 Gy with cisplatin and 5FU). The patients ($n = 30$) who achieved a good initial response were selected to complete treatment with further CRT and the remaining proceeded to surgery. The overall 3-year survival was 56% with no difference between the two groups. Comparable results were reported in another similar study of 32 patients (median disease-free survival of 16.1 months) [28]. A recently closed EORTC trial (FFCD 9102) randomised 259 patients (89% with squamous carcinoma) who had achieved a clinical response to induction CRT, to surgery or to further CRT [29]. The early results showed no difference in median survival (17.7 vs 19.3 months respectively) or 2-year survival (34% vs

**Table 27.1.** Randomised trials of preoperative chemoradiotherapy and surgery vs surgery alone in resectable oesophageal carcinoma

| Trial | Randomisation | No. | Histology SCC | Adeno | Radio-therapy | Chemo-therapy | Resection Rate (%) | Postoperative Mortality | PCR (%) | Median Survival (months) | 2-year Survival (%) | 3-year Survival (%) |
|---|---|---|---|---|---|---|---|---|---|---|---|---|
| Nygaard et al [13] | CRT + S | 47 | 47 | 0 | 35 Gy | Cis, Bleo | 66 | 24 | NS | 7 | 23 | 17 |
|  | Chemo + S | 50 | 50 | 0 | Nil | Cis, Bleo | 58 | 15 | NS | 6 | 6 | 3 |
|  | RT + S | 48 | 48 | 0 | 35 Gy | Nil | 54 | 11 | NS | 10 | 25 | 21 |
|  | S only | 41 | 41 | 0 | Nil | Nil | 68 | 13 | – | 6 | 13 | 9 |
|  |  |  |  |  |  |  |  |  |  | $p = 0.3$ |  |  |
| Le Prise et al [14] | CRT + S | 41 | 41 | 0 | 20 Gy | Cis, 5FU | 85 | 8 | 10 | 10 | 27 | 19 |
|  | S only | 45 | 45 | 0 | Nil | Nil | 84 | 7 | – | 11 | 33 | 14 |
|  |  |  |  |  |  |  |  |  |  | $p = 0.6$ |  |  |
| Apinop et al [15] | CRT + S | 35 | 35 | 0 | 40 Gy | Cis, 5FU | 74 | 12 | 20 | 9.7 | 30 | 26 |
|  | S only | 34 | 34 | 0 | Nil | Nil | 100 | 15 | – | 7.4 | 23 | 20 |
|  |  |  |  |  |  |  |  |  |  | $p = 0.4$ |  |  |
| Walsh et al [16] | CRT + S | 58 | 0 | 58 | 40 Gy | Cis, 5FU | 90 | 10 | 22 | 16 | 37 | 32 |
|  | S only | 55 | 0 | 55 | Nil | Nil | 100 | 4 | – | 11 | 26 | 6 |
|  |  |  |  |  |  |  |  |  |  | $p = 0.01$ |  |  |
| Bosset et al [17] | CRT + S | 143 | 143 | 0 | 37 Gy | Cis | 78 | 12 | 20 | 18.6 | 48 | 36 |
|  | S only | 139 | 139 | 0 | Nil | Nil | 68 | 4 | – | 18.6 | 42 | 34 |
|  |  |  |  |  |  |  |  |  |  | $p = 0.8$ |  |  |
| Urba et al [18] | CRT + S | 50 | 13 | 37 | 45 Gy | Cis, 5FU, Vinblast | 90 | 2 | 28 | 16.9 | 40 | 30 |
|  | S only | 50 | 12 | 38 | Nil | Nil | 90 | 0 | – | 17.6 | 34 | 16 |
|  |  |  |  |  |  |  |  |  |  | $p\ 0.15$ |  |  |
| Burmeister et al [19] | CRT + S | 128 | 92* | 157 | 35 Gy | Cis, 5FU | NS | 3.1 | 15.2 | 21.7 | NS | NS |
|  | S only | 128 |  |  | Nil | Nil | NS | 4.6 | – | 18.5 | NS | NS |

SCC, squamous cell carcinoma; Adeno, adenocarcinoma; PCR, pathological complete response; CRT, chemoradiotherapy; S, surgery; Chemo, chemotherapy; RT, radiotherapy; Cis, Cisplatin; Bleb, bleomycin; NS, not stated; 5FU, fluorouracil; Vinblast, vinblastin; * mixed/undifferentiated.

Table 27.2. Recent randomised trials of definitive chemoradiotherapy versus radiotherapy in unresectable oesophageal carcinoma

| Trial | Randomisation | No. of patients total | SCC | Adeno | Radiotherapy | Chemotherapy | Median survival (months) | 2-year survival (%) | 3-year survival (%) | 5-year survival (%) |
|---|---|---|---|---|---|---|---|---|---|---|
| Araujo et al [24] | CRT | 28 | 28 | 0 | 50 Gy | Bleo, Mito, Cis | 15 | 38 | 22 | 16 |
|  | RT | 31 | 31 | 0 | same | Nil | 15 | 22 | 12 | 6 |
|  |  |  |  |  |  |  | $p = 0.16$ |  |  |  |
| Roussel et al [25] | CRT | 110 | 110 | 0 | 40 Gy | Cis | 7.8 | 20 | NS | 8 (4-year) |
|  | RT | 111 | 111 | 0 | same | Nil | 10.5 | 16 | NS | 10 (4-year) |
|  |  |  |  |  |  |  | $p = 0.17$ |  |  |  |
| Smith et al [23] | CRT | 59 | 59 | 0 | 40–60 Gy | Mito, 5FU | 14.8 | NS | 27 | 9 |
|  | RT | 60 | 60 | 0 | same | Nil | 9.2 | NS | 12 | 7 |
|  |  |  |  |  |  |  | $p = 0.04$ |  |  |  |
| Herskovic [9], | CRT | 61 | 52 | 9 | 50 Gy | 5FU, Cis | 14.1 | 36 | 30 | 26 |
| Al-Sarraf [22] | RT | 62 | 56 | 6 | 64 Gy | Nil | 9.3 | 10 | 0 | 0 |
| Cooper et al | CRT (Non-R) | 69 | 55 | 14 | 50 Gy | 5FU, Cis | 17.2 | 35 | 26 | 14 |
|  |  |  |  |  |  |  | $p = 0.0001$ |  |  |  |

SCC, squamous cell carcinoma; Adeno, Adenocarcinoma; CRT, chemoradiotherapy; RT, radiotherapy; Bleo, bleomycin; Mito, mitomycin; Cis, cisplatin; NS, Not stated; 5FU, 5fluorouracil; Non-R; non-randomised.

40%). However, there were more deaths within 3 months of commencing CRT in the surgery arm (9% vs 1%; $p = 0.002$). Therefore, there is good evidence to support the use of definitive CRT in resectable squamous carcinoma of the oesophagus as an alternative to surgery [23, 27–29].

The majority of available data on CRT in oesophageal cancer used synchronous 5FU with either cisplatin or mitomycin-C. Since then, many more chemotherapy drugs have been incorporated into routine use for cancer therapy. The assessment of these as potentially useful radiosensitisers has produced interesting results. Paclitaxel appears safe in oesophageal cancer and high pCR rates can be achieved with CRT given preoperatively. Other promising agents include irinotecan and oxaliplatin.

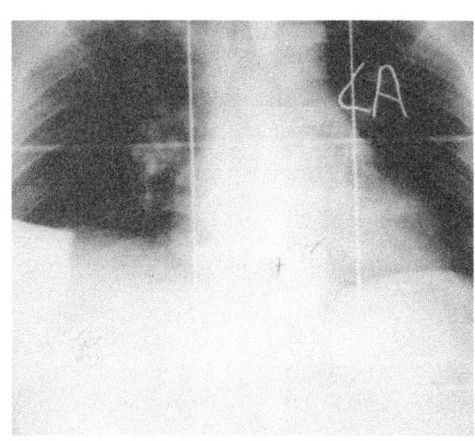

**Figure 27.1.** A simulator film during barium swallow to delineate the target volume for radiotherapy in cancer of the oesophagus.

## Radiotherapy Technique

Precise identification of the site and local extent of the primary tumour and the involved lymph nodes is essential. The gross tumour volume (GTV) can be defined by a combination of cross-sectional imaging (CT and/or MRI), endoscopic ultrasound and barium swallow. Radiotherapy planning is usually performed by CT localisation of the tumour and oesophagus. The clinical target volume (CTV) is the volume defined to encompass the GTV, the likely microscopic extension beyond the GTV and the immediate draining lymph nodes. The planning target volume (PTV) includes a final margin which is added to compensate for daily variations in patient positioning and organ movement with respiration (Figures 27.1 and 27.2). The treatment is planned to encompass the entire PTV. At the same time, the dose received by the surrounding organs such as the spinal cord, lungs and heart will need to be limited to within their normal tissue tolerance. The use of conformal and intensity modulated radiotherapy (IMRT) should enable improved sparing of normal organs, by better conformation of the high dose volume around the tumour. These techniques require three-dimensional computer planning and linear accelerators fitted with multileaf collimators (MLC). These may allow radiation dose escalation to the tumour without unacceptable toxicity to the surrounding organs. There may also be a future role for non-conventional radiotherapy scheduling such as

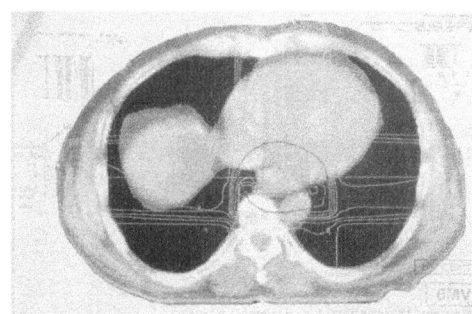

**Figure 27.2.** CT planning for cancer of the oesophagus. Computer-generated isodose distribution of the radiation beams is also shown on this CT slice.

acceleration (over a shorter treatment duration) or hyperfractionation (treatment more than once a day).

## Toxicity of Radiotherapy and Chemoradiotherapy

Acute side effects of radiotherapy include radiation-induced mucositis of the oesophagus. This can become secondarily infected by candida and will require antifungal therapy. Symptoms of odynophagia, altered taste and anorexia are common and usually commence 10 to 14 days after starting radiotherapy. Maintenance of nutritional status is essential to support patients through their treatment.

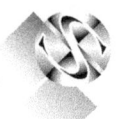

# RADIOTHERAPY IN UPPER GI TRACT NEOPLASMS

Nasogastric or parenteral feeding may need to be commenced if significant weight loss continues after commencement of radiotherapy. Patients are encouraged to cease smoking and alcohol during radiotherapy as these may exacerbate acute and long-term toxicity. Radiation-induced tracheitis can cause a persistent cough associated with thick mucus production. Acute pneumonitis can occur within the first 3 months and may cause a dry cough, dyspnoea and low grade pyrexia. Acute radiation mediastinitis is a rare complication causing chest pain, pyrexia and dyspnoea. In severe cases, hospital admission is necessary to exclude an oesophageal perforation.

The commonest long-term toxicity of radiotherapy is oesophageal stricture formation. The most likely contributing cause is the extensive tumour destruction and subsequent treatment-related fibrosis. A tracheo-oesophageal fistula can occasionally develop but again, this is more commonly due to direct tumour invasion. Radiotherapy is as safe and effective in sufficiently fit elderly patients as it is in a younger population.

## Palliative Treatment

For patients deemed incurable, short courses of palliative radiotherapy may be effective in improving symptoms of dysphagia and/or pain. Radiation doses of 20 Gy in 5 fractions or 30 Gy in 10 fractions are usually tolerated well and are associated with a low risk of serious toxicity. This can be given in combination with other interventions including oesophageal dilation, laser ablation and stenting. In addition, chemotherapy may be useful in delaying further disease progression and in prolonging survival. This is discussed in Chapter 26.

The insertion of radioactive sources (usually iridium-192) into the oesophagus, known as brachytherapy, can be an effective means of delivering high doses of radiation to the intraluminal component of the tumour with relatively low doses to surrounding structures. Using a high dose rate (HDR) selectron machine, 16 Gy in two fractions or 18 Gy in three fractions given weekly have been shown to offer excellent palliation. Brachytherapy in combination with laser ablation may reduce the frequency of required endoscopic dilatations in selected patients.

The selection of the treatment modality used to palliate a particular patient should take into account the site of disease, related symptoms, general physical condition and social circumstances. An additional factor is the level of expertise and technology available locally for each of these interventions.

## Other Histological Types

*Small cell carcinoma* is occasionally seen in the oesophagus. Its clinical behaviour of early systemic spread is similar to small cell carcinoma of the lung. Multidrug combination chemotherapy with or without radiotherapy is probably the optimum treatment. Surgery may be considered for selected patients. The role of CRT is yet to be defined.

*Carcinoma of the oesophagus with adenoid cystic differentiation* has been reported to be clinically and morphologically distinct from adenoid cystic carcinoma arising from salivary glands. Surgical resection is the mainstay of treatment.

*Primary oesophageal T-cell non-Hodgkin's lymphoma* is rare. Most cases present with evidence of widespread disease and chemotherapy would be the appropriate treatment. When truly localised, radiotherapy alone can be successful.

## Summary and Future

Although surgery remains the standard against which new treatments must be compared, there is emerging evidence that stage for stage, the survival from CRT alone is equivalent to surgery alone [30]. Salvage oesophagectomy following CRT failure is feasible in some cases and the results are encouraging [27]. Although commonly given, the role of preoperative CRT remains unproven and therefore can only be recommended in the context of a clinical trial. There is no proven role for postoperative radiotherapy.

It is clear that different treatment modalities are appropriate for different patients, but the means of selecting the appropriate treatment for the individual patient is lacking. The standard of care for surgery has also progressed. Two cycles of preoperative cisplatin and 5FU chemotherapy (without radiation) have been shown to increase curative resection rates (60% vs 54%) and overall survival at 2 years (43% vs

34%) in an MRC randomised trial of 802 patients [31]. In the future, the management of adenocarcinoma and squamous carcinoma is likely to diverge. Patients who achieve pCR following CRT for squamous carcinoma are unlikely to benefit from resection, but at the present time there is no reliable test to predict for this. Further research is needed to develop these tests. However, a non-surgical approach will enable organ preservation [30] and may lead to lower treatment-related mortality [28] and improved quality of life [32]. This can only be justified if there is no survival penalty.

Improving pretreatment loco-regional staging by the routine use of endoscopic ultrasound and multislice CT scanning in regional gastro-oesophageal cancer units should be the standard. The use of 18-fluorodeoyxglucose (FDG) positron emission tomography (PET) to detect distant metastases not identified by CT scan will help spare approximately 20% of patients from a non-curative resection or an "open and shut" procedure. Serial FDG-PET scanning may also be useful in detecting early response to radiotherapy.

In order to improve loco-regional control of this cancer, the optimum combination of chemotherapy and radiotherapy needs to be defined by refining existing regimens, assessing new agents and improving radiation dose delivery. Prevention of systemic recurrence remains an elusive target but new chemotherapy drugs and combinations are being explored for the future. In the next decade, there will be an expansion of research into the molecular biology of malignant tumours and their response to chemotherapy and radiotherapy. The development of in vitro predictive testing may help to tailor treatment strategies to achieve the best responses. Cyclin D1 immunoreactivity and metallothionein expression both appear to correlate with sensitivity to CRT in oesophageal cancer.

## Stomach

Although there has been a decrease in the incidence of gastric adenocarcinoma involving the body and pylorus in the Western world, that of cardia and gastro-oesophageal junction tumours has increased markedly. The overall 5-year survival of all patients with gastric carcinoma remains poor (between 5% and 15%). Although the mainstay of treatment remains surgical resection, the ultimate risk of recurrence is high. Adjuvant treatments are an attempt to improve outcome.

## Radiotherapy

Radiotherapy to the stomach is limited by the mobility and variation in size of this organ. In addition, the radiation dose that can be safely delivered is also limited by the presence of surrounding radiosensitive organs including the small bowel, liver, kidneys and spinal cord (Figure 27.3).

In a Chinese trial, 370 patients with adenocarcinoma of the gastric cardia were randomised to receive radiotherapy (40 Gy) prior to surgery or surgery alone [33]. Patients in the radiotherapy arm had higher resection rates (89% vs 79%; $p < 0.01$) and an improved 5-year survival (30.1% vs 19.7%; $p = 0.009$).

The British Stomach Cancer Group Trial randomised 436 patients who had undergone resection for adenocarcinoma of the stomach to receive postoperative radiotherapy (45–50 Gy), chemotherapy (mitomycin-C, doxorubicin and 5FU) or no further treatment [34]. There was no difference in survival between the three arms (median 12.9 months vs 17.3 months vs 14.7 months; 5 years 12% vs 19% vs 20%; $p = 0.14$).

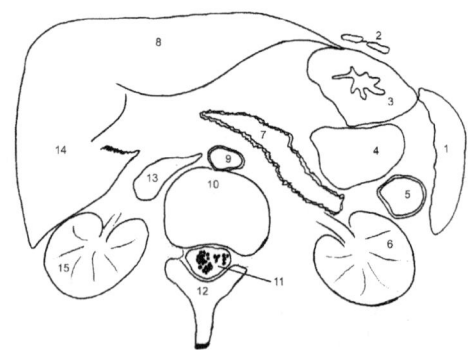

**Figure 27.3.** A schematic diagram of the cross-section of the abdomen at the level of the L1 vertebral body showing stomach and other anatomic organs in its vicinity that may be at risk of radiation damage during radiotherapy to the stomach. 1, spleen; 2, small bowel; 3, stomach; 4, transverse colon; 5, descending colon; 6, left kidney; 7, pancreas; 8, left lobe of liver; 9, abdominal aorta; 10, L1 vertebral body; 11, spinal cord/cauda equina; 12, spinal process of L1; 13, inferior vena cava; 14, right lobe of liver; 15, right kidney.

## Chemoradiotherapy

The role of postoperative combined chemotherapy and radiotherapy has been assessed by the US Intergroup in a randomised trial (INT 0116) which compared CRT with no further treatment in 556 patients who had undergone curative resection for locally advanced adenocarcinoma of the stomach and gastro-oesophageal junction [11]. In the treatment arm, the patients received one cycle of 5FU and folinic acid, followed by CRT (45 Gy with synchronous 5FU and folinic acid), followed by a further cycle of 5FU and folinic acid. Most patients had tumours involving the distal stomach and 85% had lymph node involvement on histological examination of the resection specimen. Of note, 54% of the patients had undergone a D0 dissection, meaning a less than complete dissection of the N1 lymph nodes. The median survival was 36 months for the CRT arm compared with 27 months for the surgery alone arm ($p = 0.005$), with a 3-year survival of 50% versus 41% respectively.

The Gastric Surgical Adjuvant Radiotherapy Consensus Report [35] has outlined the factors to be considered for planning postoperative CRT. These include anatomy, pathways of tumour spread, patterns of failure and surgical techniques. Nevertheless, the implementation of such complex and resource consuming individual planning can be justified by improved results in selected patients who are motivated and are of sufficiently good physical condition.

## Mucosa Associated Lymphoid Tissue (MALT) Lymphoma

The stomach is the commonest site of gastrointestinal non-Hodgkin's lymphoma. The commonest subtype is the MALT lymphoma. This is commonly associated with *Helicobacter pylori* infection. Antibiotic therapy has resulted in complete remissions in many patients with early disease [36]. A combination of chemotherapy and involved field radiotherapy in the management of Ann Arbor stage I and II MALT lymphomas is associated with good response rates and survival.

## Small Bowel

Although a wide variety of benign and malignant neoplasms can arise from the small intestine, the numbers are exceedingly small and the role of radiotherapy negligible. Primary malignant tumours range from adenocarcinoma through varieties of sarcomas and lymphomas to carcinoid tumour. Radiotherapy is unlikely to be useful not only because small bowel is difficult to target due to its mobile nature but also because of its radiosensitivity. Palliative radiotherapy may be considered to control acute or chronic haemorrhage.

## Questions

1. Outline the arguments for either surgery or radiotherapy for squamous carcinoma of the oesophagus.
2. Criticise the trial suggesting possible benefit of chemoradiotherapy for cancer of the stomach.

## References

1. Earlam R, Cunha-Melo JR. Oesophageal squamous cell carcinoma: I. A critical review of surgery. Br J Surg 1980;67:381–90.
2. Muller HM, Erasmi H, Stelzner M et al. Surgical therapy of oesophageal carcinoma. Br J Surg 1990;77:845–57.
3. Arnott SJ, Duncan W, Gignoux M et al. Preoperative radiotherapy in esophageal carcinoma: a meta-analysis using individual patient data (oesophageal cancer collaborative group). Int J Radiat Oncol Biol Phys 1998;41:579–83.
4. Earlam R, Cunha-Melo JR. Oesophageal squamous cell carcinoma: I. A critical review of radiotherapy. Br J Surg 1980;67:457–61.
5. Fok M, McShane J, Law SYK, Wong J. Prospective randomized study on radiotherapy and surgery in the treatment of oesophageal carcinoma. Asian J Surg 1994;17:223–9.
6. Badwe RA, Sharma V, Bhansali MS et al. The quality of swallowing for patients with operable esophageal carcinoma; a randomized trial comparing surgery with radiotherapy. Cancer 1999;85:763–8.
7. Fok M, Sharm JST, Choy D, Cheng SWK, Wong JW. Postoperative radiotherapy for carcinoma of the oesophagus: a prospective randomized controlled trial. Surgery 1993;113:138–47.
8. Teniere P. Hay JM, Fingerhurt A, Fagniez P-L. Postoperative radiation therapy does not increase survival after curative resection of squamous cell carcinoma of the middle and lower oesophagus as shown by a multi-centre controlled trial. Surg Gynecol Obstet 1991;173:123.
9. Herskovic A. Martz K, al-Sarraf M et al. Combined chemotherapy and radiotherapy compared with radio-

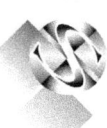

therapy alone in patients with cancer of the esophagus. N Eng J Med 1992;326:1593-8.
10. Moertel CG, Frytak S, Hahn RG et al. Therapy of locally unresectable pancreatic carcinoma: a randomized comparison of high dose radiation (6000 rads) alone.
11. Macdonald JS, Smalley SR, Benedetti J et al. Chemoradiotherapy after surgery compared with surgery alone for adenocarcinoma of the stomach or gastroesophgeal junction. N Engl J Med 2001;345:725-30.
12. Geh JI, Crellin AM, Glynne-Jones R. Preoperative (neoadjuvant) chemoradiotherapy in oesophageal cancer. Br J Surg 2001;88:338-56.
13. Nygaard K, Hagen S, Hansen HS et al. Preoperative radiotherapy prolongs survival in operable oesophageal carcinoma: a randomized, multicentre study of preoperative radiotherapy and chemotherapy. The second Scandinavian Trial in esophageal cancer. World J Surg 1992;16:1104-10.
14. Le Prise E, Etienne PL, Meunier B et al. A randomized study of chemotherapy, radiation therapy and surgery versus surgery for localized squamous cell carcinoma of the esophagus. Cancer 1994;73:1779-84.
15. Apinop C, Puttisak P, Preecha N. A prospective study of combined therapy in esophageal cancer. Hepatogastroenterology 1994;41:391-3.
16. Walsh TN, Noonan N, Hollywood D et al. A comparison of multimodal therapy and surgery of esophageal adenocarcinoma. N Engl J Med 1996;335:462-7.
17. Bosset JF. Gignoux E, Triboulet JP et al. Chemoradiotherapy followed by surgery compared with surgery alone in squamous cell cancer of the esophagus. N Engl J Med 1997;337:161-7.
18. Urba SG, Orringer MB, Turrisi A et al. Randomized trial of preoperative chemoradiation versus surgery alone in patients with locoregional esophageal carcinoma. J Clin Oncol 2001;19(2):305-13.
19. Burmeister BH, Smithers BM, Fitzgerald L et al. A randomized phase III trial of preoperative chemoradiation followed by surgery (CR-S) versus surgery alone (S) for localized resectable cancer of the esophagus. Proceedings of 38th Annual Meeting of American Society of Clinical Oncology 2002;21:A518.
20. Keane TJ, Harwood AE, Elhakim T et al. Radical radiation therapy with 5-flourouracil infusion and mitomycin C for oesophageal squamous carcinoma. Radiother Oncol 1985;4:205-10.
21. Geh JI. The use of chemoradiotherapy in oesophageal cancer. Eur J Cancer 2001;38:300-13.
22. Al-Sarraf M, Martz K, Herskovic MA, et al. Progress report of combined chemoradiotherapy versus radiotherapy alone in patients with esophageal cancer: An intergroup study. J Clin Oncol 1997;15:277-84.
23. Smith TJ, Ryan LM, Douglass HO et al. Combined chemoradiotherapy vs radiotherapy alone for early stage squamous cel carcinoma of the esophagus: a study of the Eastern Cooperative Oncology Group. Int J Radiat Oncol Biol Phys 1998;42:269-76.
24. Araujo CMM, Souhami L, Gil RA et al. A randomized trial comparing radiation therapy versus concomitant radiation therapy and chemotherapy in carcinoma of the thorac esophagus. Cancer 1991;67:2258-61.
25. Roussel A, Haegele P, Paillot B et al. Results of the EORTC-GTCCG phase III trial of irradiation versus irradiation and CDDP in inoperable esophageal cancer. Proc Am Soc Clin Oncol 1994;13:583 (abst).
26. Minsky BD, Pajak TF, Ginsberg RJ et al. INT 0123 (Radiation Therapy Oncology Group 94-05) phase III trial of combined modality therapy for esophageal cancerr: high-dose versus standard-dose radiation therapy. J Clin Oncol 2002;20(5):1167-74.
27. Murakami M, Kuroda Y, Okamoto Y et al. Neoadjuvant concurrent chemoradiotherapy followed by definitive high-dose radiotherapy or surgery for operable thoracic esophageal carcinoma. Int J Radiat Oncol Biol Phys 1998;40:1049-59.
28. Wilson KS, Lim JT. Primary chemo-radiotherapy and selective oesophagectomy for oesophageal cancer: goal of cure with organ preservation. Radiother Oncol 2000;54:129-34.
29. Bedenne L, Michel P, Bouche O et al. Randomized phase III trial in locally advanced esophageal cancer: radiochemotherapy followed by surgery versus radiochemotherapy alone (FFCD 9102). Proceedings of 38th Annual Meeting of American Society of Clinical Oncology 2002;21:A519.
30. Murakami M, Kuroda Y, Nakajima T et al. Comparison between chemoradiation protocol intended for organ preservation and conventional surgery for clinical T1-T2 esophageal carcinoma. Int J Radiat Oncol Biol Phys 1999;45(2):277-84.
31. Medical Research Council Oesophageal Cancer Working Party. Surgical resection with or without preoperative chemotherapy in oesophageal cancer: a randomised controlled trial. Lancet 2002;359:1727-33.
32. Blazeby JM, Farndon JR, Donovan J, Alderson D. A prospective longitudinal study examining the quality of life of patients with esophageal carcinoma. Cancer 2000;88:1781-7.
33. Zhang Z-X. Gu X-Z, Yin W-B et al. Randomised clinical trial on the combination of preoperative irradiation and surgery in the treatment of adenocarcinoma of gastric cardia (AGC). Report on 370 patients. Int J Radiat Oncol Biol Phys 1998;42(5):929-34.
34. Hallissey MT, Dunn JA, Ward LC, Allum WH. The second British Stomach Cancer Group trial of adjuvant radiotherapy or chemotherapy in resectable gastric cancer: five year follow-up. Lancet 1994;343:1309-12.
35. Smalley SR, Gunderson L, Tepper J et al. Gastric surgical adjuvant radiotherapy consensus report: rationale and treatment implementation. Int J Radiat Oncol Biol Phys 2002;52:283-93.
36. Wotherspoon AC, Doglioni C, Diss TC et al. Regression of primary low-grade gastric lymphoma of mucosa-associated lymphoid tissue type after eradication of *Helicobacter pylori*. Lancet 1993;342:575-7.

# Index

## A

Abdomen, effect of diaphragmatic contraction of 51–52
Abdominal muscles, contraction of, relationship with trunk stability and respiration 56
Abdominal oesophagus, anatomy of 4–5
Abdominal plexus, of the diaphragm 49
Abnormalities
  lower oesophageal, evaluating with oesophageal transit scintigraphy 313–314
  oesophageal, association with defects in other organ systems 2
  of the small intestine 43–44
  upper oesophageal, evaluating with oesophageal transit scintigraphy 310
  *See also* Congenital abnormalities
Abscess, splenic 137–138
Absorption, from the stomach 33
Accessory spleens 132–134
Accuracy, of upper gastrointestinal endoscopy 280
Acetylcholine, binding to G cells, effect on gastric secretion 33–34
Achalasia 242
  of the cardia, failure of the oesophageal sphincter to relax in 8
  diagnosis of, with contrast radiography 294
    with plain radiology 289
  as a failure of oesophageal motility 79–83
  oesophageal transit scintigraphy for identifying 307, 309
Achlorhydria, effect of, on fasting levels of gastrin 32
Acid reflux, measurement of 13–14
Acid sphingomyelinase (ASM), deficiency of, in Niemann-Pick disease 145
Acquired immunodeficiency syndrome (AIDS), risk of small bowel malignancy associated with 196
Adaptation, of the small bowel, after surgery 113
Adenocarcinoma
  of the distal oesophagus, limited surgical approach to 331–332
  of the oesophagogastric junction (AEG tumours) 318
  of the oesophagus 156, 250–251
    association with gastro-oesophageal reflux disease 73
    Barrett's oesophagus as a premalignant condition for 259–264
    glandular dysplasia as an indicator of 251
    increasing incidence of, in men and women 188–192
    outcomes of lymphadenectomy for 328–329
    surgical approach to 330–331
    surgical management of 164
  of the small bowel, comparison with adenocarcinoma of the duodenum 193
    management of 201–202
  of the stomach 250–251
  risk factors for 190–191
Adenoid cystic carcinoma 253
Adenomas
  of Brunner's gland 201
  endoscopic removal of 283
  of the oesophagus 251
Adenomatous polyps (adenomas), of the small bowel, management of 201
Adenosquamous carcinoma, of the oesophagus 247
Adjuvant therapy
  for gastric cancer, chemoradiotherapy 352
  for oesophageal cancer, postoperative radiotherapy 360
  for oesophagogastric cancer 352
Adriamycin, as part of a combination regimen for treating gastric cancer 350
Aetiology
  of asplenism 135
  of Barrett's oesophagus 260–261
  of Crohn's disease 101–102
  of epithelial dysplasia, squamous 265
  of gastric cancer 169–170
  of gastro-oesophageal reflux disease 70
  of intestinal metaplasia 274–275
  of oesophageal cancer 156
  of oesophageal squamous papilloma 267–268
  of peptic ulcer disease 91
  of small bowel neoplasms 194–195

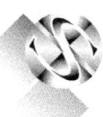

Aetiology (*cont.*)
   of splenic artery aneurysms 146
   of splenic rupture 147–148
Age/aging
   changes within muscle fibres with 54
   and incidence of achalasia 79–83
   and incidence of atrophic gastritis 271
   and mortality rate after total gastrectomy and D2 dissection 340
Alcohol
   association of atrophic gastritis type B with 272
   effect of, on gastric cancer development 170
   as a risk factor in squamous cell carcinoma of the oesophagus 182, 247
   role in squamous epithelial dysplasia and carcinoma development 265
Alkalosis, hypokalaemic metabolic, in pyloric stenosis 95
Alveolar hypoplasia, effect of, on foramen ovale closure in neonates 121
American Association for the Surgery of Trauma, Organ Injury Scaling of 65
American Joint Committee on Cancer (AJCC), TNM staging system of, for determining prognosis in small bowel adenocarcinoma 202
American National Cancer Database, data on small bowel cancer 194
American Society of Gastrointestinal Endoscopy, surveillance guidelines for squamous cell carcinoma 266
Amine precursor uptake and decarboxylation (APUD) cells, of the stomach 27
   cardiac zone 29
Aminosalicylates, for treating Crohn's disease 105–106
Ampicillin, for treating typhoid enteritis 110
Amyloidosis
   involving the spleen 145
   splenomegaly due to 61
Anaemia
   autoimmune haemolytic, diagnosis and treatment of 63–64
   iron-deficiency, web associated with 84
   pernicious, association with autoimmune atrophic gastritis 271
      risk of gastric cancer in 98
   *See also* Haemolytic anaemia
Anatomy
   of the diaphragm 45–46
   macroscopic, of the stomach 20–21
   oesophageal, in adults 2–8
   of the small intestine 39–40
   of the spleen 59–60, 127–128
   of the stomach 17–30
Aneuploidy
   in Barrett's oesophagus 262
   in squamous epithelial dysplasia development 266

Aneurysm, splenic artery 146
Angiomas
   littoral cell 222–223
   small bowel 205
Angiosarcoma, splenic 222
Ann Arbor staging system, application to gastrointestinal lymphoma 233
Anterior vagus nerve
   of the stomach 25–26
Anterosuperior surface, of the stomach 20
Antibiotics, in Crohn's disease 106
Antibodies
   IgA, proliferative disorder of, in the small intestine 203
   IgG, directed towards platelet-associated antigen 61–62
   IgM, synthesis in the spleen 60, 131–132
   production by the spleen 134–135
Antidiarrhoeal agents, for medical treatment of Crohn's disease 105
Antioxidants, role in the aetiology of intestinal metaplasia 273–274
Antiplatelet factor, immune thrombocytopenic purpura caused by 61–62
Antireflux mechanism, physiology of 13–14
Antireflux surgery, for gastro-oesophageal reflux disease 73–76
Antral cancer, association of, with *Helicobacter pylori* infection 92
Aortic opening, in the diaphragm 48, 118
APC gene, loss of heterozygosity in oesophageal adenocarcinoma 262
Aphthoid ulceration, in Crohn's disease 102–103
Apoptosis
   of metaplastic stem cells in Barrett's oesophagus 261–262
   mutation of genes involved in, Bcl10 234
Appleby's operation, defined 340
Arcuate ligaments, and structure of the diaphragm 45–46
Argentaffin cells
   of the pyloric zone of the stomach 30
Argyrophilic cells, of the pyloric zone of the stomach 30
Armed Forces Institute of Pathology, data on metastatic neoplasms of the small bowel 205
Arteries
   carrying blood supply to the diaphragm 49
   carrying blood supply to the stomach 21–23
   of the foregut 2
   gastroepiploic 22, 60
   mesenteric, blood supply to the midgut through 43–44
   musculophrenic 48
   nutrient, of the oesophagus 7
   pancreatic 23, 128
      dorsal 128
   of the small intestine 40

# INDEX

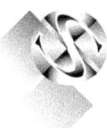

of the spleen 59–60
splenic 128
  aneurysm of 146
  superior mesenteric, blood supply to the midgut through 43–44
Asian oesophageal cancer belt 181–182
Aspirin
  damage to the stomach by 30
  reduction of oesophageal COX-2 by 262–263
Asplenia 134–135
Atelectasis, pulmonary, after splenectomy 227
ATPase, $H^+$-$K^+$, for transport of protons onto the luminal surface of the stomach 31
Atresia
  developmental, in the small intestine 44
  oesophageal 2, 85–86
    arising during embryogenesis 241
Atrophic gastritis 271–273
Atrophy, glandular, in *Helicobacter pylori* infection of the stomach 244
Attachments
  diaphragmatic 45–46
  of the oesophagus 5
Auerbach's plexus 8
  oesophageal motility disorder in 82–83
Autoimmune disorders, gastritis 244
  atrophic 271
Autoimmune haemolytic anaemia (AIHA), diagnosis and treatment of 63–64
Autosplenectomy, in sickle cell disease 140
Autotransfusion, due to contraction of the spleen 131
Autotransplantation, splenic 147–148
  to manage post-splenectomy infections 66
Azygos vein, anatomy of 4
  passage through the diaphragm 48

## B

Babesiosis, as a complication of splenectomy, 66
Bacteria, 66
  polysaccharide-encapsulated, elimination by the spleen 131–132
  in the small intestine and large intestine 41
  *See also Helicobacter pylori*
Balloon dilatation, oesophageal 282
Balloon testing, of oesophageal reaction 71
Barium enema, double contrast, for evaluating large bowel Crohn's disease 105
Barium radiology
  for diagnosing small bowel tumours 200
  meal for contrast radiography evaluation 294
  of the small bowel 295–296
Barium swallow
  for diagnosing oesophageal cancer 157
  for gastrointestinal evaluation 292–294
Barrett's cancer, early, sentinel lymphadenectomy for 333

Barrett's metaplasia, defined 243
Barrett's oesophagus 156
  adenocarcinomas associated with 318
  columnar metaplasia of the lower oesophagus in 6
  gastro-oesophageal reflux disease associated with 72–73
  identifying on endoscopy 70
  incidence of, and scleroderma 83
  location of the squamocolumnar junction in 5
  premalignant potential of 187–188, 259
B-cell lymphoma, transformation of mucosa associated lymphoid tissue 254
Benign tumours, oesophageal 86–87
Benzodiazepines, for sedation in endoscopy 281–282
Bezoars, gastric, managing 98
Bicarbonate-chloride exchange, in the interstitium of the stomach 31
Bile reflux
  aetiology of Barrett's oesophagus in 261
  as an atrophic gastritis risk factor 272
  after Billroth II reconstruction 177
  intestinal metaplasia promotion by 273
  reactive gastritis due to 244
Bile salt, malabsorption of, after resection of the small bowel 113
Biliary ducts, embryonic development of 19
Biliary imaging, with radiopharmaceuticals 303
Biliary tree, gas seen within, plain abdominal film 290–291
Billroth II gastrectomy
  for bleeding gastric ulcers 94
  for gastric cancer 177
Biological therapies, for oesophagogastric cancer 351
Biopsy
  bleeding from the site of, in diagnostic endoscopy 281
  value of, in gastric cancer diagnosis 172
Bleeding
  from gastrointestinal stromal tumours 211–212
  from peptic ulcers 93–94
  from schwannomas 209
  from small bowel tumours 198
  *See also* Haemorrhage
Blind loop syndrome 112
Blood flow
  altered splenic, splenomegaly due to 61
  diaphragmatic, during inspiration 56
Blood supply
  of the diaphragm 49
  of the oesophagus 7–8
  of the small intestine 39–40
  of the spleen 128
  of the stomach 21–24

Blood tests
    for evaluating Crohn's disease 104
    for evaluating oesophageal cancer 158
B lymphocytes
    IgA-producing 203
    increase in Crohn's disease 102
    of the white pulp of the spleen 60
Bochdalek hernia 119
Bochdalek's foramen, defined 117
Body, oesophageal 5–6
Body dysmotility, oesophageal transit scintigraphy for evaluating 310–313
Body mass index
    gastro-esophageal junction cancer associated with 188
    oesophageal adenocarcinoma risk and 182
    See also Obesity
Boerhaave's syndrome, site of 5
Bombesin (gastrin-releasing peptide), effect of, on gastrin release from G cells 34
Bowel preparation, before surgery for Crohn's disease 107
Brachytherapy, for delivering high doses of radiation 365
Branches, of the anterior vagus nerves of the stomach 26
Breast cancer, metastasis to the small bowel 205
Breathing, quiet, contraction of the diaphragm during 50–51
Bristol Royal Infirmary, study of the resistance of the small bowel to carcinogens 194
British Stomach Cancer Group
    comparison of radiotherapy, chemotherapy, and no further treatment, in stomach cancer 366
    evaluation of chemoradiation after gastric cancer surgery 179–180
Bronchoscopy, for diagnosing oesophageal cancer 158
*Brucella melitenesis*, infection by, of the liver and bone marrow 144
Brucellosis, splenic involvement in 143–144
Brunner's gland
    adenoma of 201
    mucus production by 41
Buffering, of gastric secretions, in the duodenum 40
Burkitt's lymphoma, primary gastric 231
Bursectomy, to avoid tumour exposure 341

C

Cadherin-catenin complexes, changes in, with squamous epithelial dysplasia 266
Cajal cells, gastrointestinal stromal tumour origin in 208
Calcification, viewing, on plain film for gastrointestinal evaluation 291
Calcitonin, release from C cells of the thyroid gland, effect on gastric activity 35

Calcium, reabsorption of, in the stomach 97
Calcium channel blockers, for treating diffuse oesophageal spasm 81
Calcium ion ($Ca^{2+}$) pumping, by the sarcoplasmic reticulum, in relaxation of the diaphragm muscle 53–54
Cancer
    at the gastro-esophageal junction 181–192
    oesophageal 155–156
    See also Carcinoma; Gastric cancer
*Candida* infection, oesophagitis due to 77, 243
Capecitabine, in a multiple drug regimen for treating oesophagogastric cancer 351
Capsule endoscopy 285
Carbonic anhydrase, of the mucosa of the stomach 31
Carcinoid syndrome 204
Carcinoid tumours
    defined 254
    of the small intestine, association with coeliac disease 196, 203–204
Carcinoma
    bronchiogenic, metastasis to the small bowel 205
    of the cardia 318
    oesophageal, metastasis of 7
        small cell 253
        squamous, in achalasia 242
    risk of, in high grade dysplasia 251–252
    salivary gland, tumours resembling 253
    undifferentiated 253
    See also Cancer; Neoplasms
Carcinoma in situ, of the oesophagus and upper aerodigestive tract 250
Carcinosarcoma, of the oesophagus 247–250
Cardiac orifice, communication of the oesophagus with the stomach via 20
Cardiac zone, of the gastric mucosa 29
Cardiovascular defects, association with oesophageal malformations 2
ß-Carotene, diet level of, and incidence of squamous epithelial dysplasia and carcinoma 265
Carotenoids, role in development of intestinal metaplasia of the stomach 275
Catenin
    ß, over-expression of, and outcome in gastric cancer 169
    role in diffuse gastric cancer 275
Caustic injury, oesophagitis due to 76–77
Caval foramen, of the diaphragm 118
Central tendon, of the diaphragm 46
Cephalic phase, of gastric acid secretion 33–34
C-erbB2 over-expression, association with intestinal cancer 169
Chagas' disease, achalasia caused by 79
Chemoradiotherapy (CRT) 360–366
    for adenocarcinoma of the duodenum 193–194
    definitive, for oesophageal cancer 361–364
    for oesophageal cancer 163–164

# INDEX

preoperative, for adenocarcinoma of the duodenum and pancreas 202
for stomach cancer 367
Chemotherapy
adjuvant, in adenocarcinoma of the small bowel 193–194
after antibiotic therapy for mucosal associated lymphoid tissue lymphoma 237
combination regimens, for oesophagogastric cancer 350–351
for gastric cancer 179
for immunoproliferative small intestinal disease 203
palliative, for gastric cancer 180
for oesophageal cancer 162
after surgery for adenocarcinoma of the stomach, randomised trial 366
for upper gastrointestinal neoplasms 349–358
Chest, imaging with plain radiology 287–289
Chimeric monoclonal antibody, mouse-human, for treating Crohn's disease 106
China, incidence of oesophageal cancer in 182
Chloramphenicol, for treating typhoid enteritis 110
Chloroquine, perioperative administration of, in the tropics 143
Cholecystography, oral 292
Cholecystokinin (CCK)
effects of, on pancreatic enzymes and bile production 42
production of, in crypts of the intestine 40
release in the intestine, suppression by somatostatin 32
release in the small intestine, effect on gastric activity 35
Cholesterol, accumulation of, in Niemann-Pick disease 145
Cholestyramine, for bile salt diarrhoea in Crohn's disease 105
Cholinergic excitation, in peristalsis 11
Chromosomes
3, trisomy in mucosal associated lymphatic disorders 234
5q, gene for adenomatous polyposis coli on 197
6, IBD3 locus of, association with Crohn's disease 102
9p13.3, association with Peutz-Jeghers syndrome 197
12, IBD2 locus of, association with Crohn's disease 102
13, association of trisomy with congenital diaphragmatic hernias 119
14, IBD4 locus of, association with Crohn's disease 102
15, association of trisomy with congenital diaphragmatic hernias 119
16, IBD1 locus of, association with Crohn's disease 101
17q25, gene for oesophageal cancer in tylosis at 267
18, trisomy association with congenital diaphragmatic hernias 119
translocations in mucosal associated lymphoid tissue lymphoma 234
*See also* Genes; Genetic disorders
Chronic lymphocytic leukaemia (CLL) 63
splenomegaly in 223–224
Chronic myeloid leukaemia (CML), splenomegaly in 223
Chronic obstructive airway disease, pneumatosis cystoides intestinalis associated with 111
Chylothorax, from damage during mobilisation of the oesophagus 4
Cimetidine, effects of, on acid secretion 34
Cisplatin
in a definitive chemoradiotherpy trial 361
for management of gastric cancer, in a combination regimen 350
for palliation in oesophageal cancer 162
c-KIT positive gastrointestinal neoplasms
origins of 212–214
as stromal tumours 208
treating with imatinib mesylate 215
C-*kit* positive tumours, gastrointestinal stromal tissue 254
Classification
for gastric cancer 338
Lauren, for gastric tumours 167–169, 250
Revised European-America Lymphoma (REAL), 203
TNM 157–158
for oesophageal lymph nodes 8
Clinical presentation
of Brunner's gland adenoma 201
of Crohn's disease 103–104
of eosinophilic oesophagitis 77
of gastric lymphoma 232
of gastrointestinal stromal tumour 210–212
of lymphomas 224
of oesophageal cancer 157
of oesophageal perforation 87
of oesophageal tumours 86–87
of small bowel tumours 198
Coeliac artery, supply of blood to the stomach by 21
Coeliac axis, embryology of 2
Coeliac disease (non-tropical sprue)
lymphocytic gastritis associated with 244
as a predisposing factor for gastrointestinal malignancies 196, 203–204
Coeliac plexus, nerves supply of the stomach derived from 26–27
Colon cancer, resection of the spleen in 225
Colonisation, in progression of Barrett's oesophagus, after metaplasia occurs 261

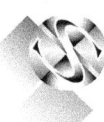

Colostomy enema 296
Complement activation, in the spleen 60
Complications
  after achalasia surgery 81
  acute gastric dilatation, after upper abdominal surgery 98
  of antireflux surgery 76
  of diagnostic endoscopy 281
  of gastrectomy 176–177
  of gastric lymphoma treatment 238
  of gastric surgery 96
  of gastro-oesophageal reflux disease 72–73
  of intestinal fistulas 112
  after oesophageal stent insertion 284
  of oesophagectomy 164
  of peptic ulcers 91, 93–95
  of radiotherapy for managing oesophageal cancer 364–365
  of reflux, and desirability of surgery 74
  of splenectomy 66–67, 150–151, 227
    in the tropics 143
  of stricturoplasty 108
Computed tomography
  for confirming traumatic diaphragmatic rupture 125
  for diagnosis, of oesophageal cancer 159
    of small bowel tumours 199–200
    of splenic artery aneurysm 146
    of splenic neoplasms 225
    of splenic cysts 137
  for staging, in gastric cancer 173
    in upper gastrointestinal cancer 297–299
Condensed dynamic image (CDI), from oesophageal transit study data 309
Congenital abnormalities
  affecting the diaphragm, table 120
  diaphragmatic hernia 118–122
  familial adenomatous polyposis 196–197
  Gaucher's disease 145
  haemolytic anaemias 63
  hereditary non-polyposis colorectal cancer 197
  involving the stomach 19, 91
  Meckel's diverticulum 111
  Niemann-Pick disease 145
  oesophageal 85–86
  Peutz-Jeghers syndrome 197
  sickle cell disease 139–140
  spherocytosis, hereditary, 141
  of the spleen 132–138
  tylosis, association with oesophageal squamous papilloma 267
  von Recklinghausen's disease, adenocarcinoma of the small bowel and 197–198
  *See also* Chromosomes; Genetic disorders
Congenital diaphragmatic hernia (CDH) 118–122
Congo red, as a marker of mucosal function 280

Contractions
  of the diaphragm 50–53
  tertiary, in swallowing 10
Contraindications
  to antireflux surgery 74–75
  to infliximab therapy 106
  to laparoscopic splenectomy 64, 227
Contrast radiography, gastrointestinal 292–296
Costal elements, of the diaphragm 117
Costodiaphragmatic recesses, formation of 47–48
COX-2 expression, in Barrett's metaplasia and oesophageal adenocarcinomas 262–263
Cricopharyngeus (upper oesophageal sphincter) 5
Criteria, for endoscopy 282
Crohn's disease (regional ileitis) 101–109
  as a predisposing factor for small bowel neoplasms 195
Cross-sectional imaging, gastrointestinal 296–302
Crural diaphragm
  attachment of 45–46
  development from muscle fibres 47
  repair of 75
  in the sphincter mechanism at the oesophagogastric junction 13
Culling, of red cells from the blood 128, 135
Curvatura ventriculi, major and minor, anatomy of 20
Curvatures, of the stomach 20
Cyclin D1, interaction with nitrosamines, in squamous epithelial dysplasia 266
Cysts, of the spleen 136–137
Cytogenetic abnormalities, in the lymphoid population 234
Cytokeratin, changes in binding of in squamous epithelial dysplasia 266
Cytokeratin antibodies, monoclonal, for immunohistochemical staining of lymph nodes 325–327
Cytokines
  in Barrett's oesophagus 262
  release of, in *Helicobacter pylori* infection 92
Cytology, for staging in gastric cancer 173
Cytomegalovirus (CMV) infection
  oesophagitis associated with infection by 77
  oesophagitis caused by 243–244
Cytotoxin-associated gene A (Cag A), gastric atrophy related to 272

## D

D cells, of the islands of Langerhans, gastrin production in 32
Definition, of the extent of lymphadenectomy for oesophageal cancer 323–325
Demographics
  of gastro-esophageal junction cancer 181
  of oesophageal cancer 156
Deprivation, economic, variation in stomach and oesophageal cancer incidence with 183–186

# INDEX

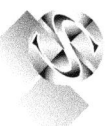

Desmoid tumours, association with adenomatous polyposis coli 197
Developmental anomalies, affecting the diaphragm, table 120
Diagnosis
   of achalasia 242
   of diaphragmatic rupture 124–125
   of eventration of the diaphragm 123
   of gastric cancer 171–172
   of gastrointestinal stromal tumours 212–214
   of mucosal associated lymphoid tissue lymphoma 233
   of neoplasms involving the spleen 225–226
   of oesophageal cancer, tests for 157
   of peptic ulcers 92
   of perforation in gastric ulcer 95
   of phrenic palsy 123
   of small bowel tumours 198–201
   of squamous epithelial dysplasia 266
   with upper gastrointestinal endoscopy 279–282
Diaphragm
   anatomy of, surgical 117–126
   anatomy and physiology of 45–58
Diaphragmatic apertures 48
Diaphragmatic attachments 45–46
Diaphragmatic hernia 242
Diarrhoea
   in Crohn's disease 103–104
   after gastric surgery 96
Diet
   and risk of chronic gastritis 170
   role in squamous epithelial dysplasia and carcinoma development 265
   *See also* Nutrition
Dieulafoy syndrome, gastrointestinal bleeding in 94
Differential diagnosis
   of spleen lesions 222
   of tropical splenomegaly syndrome 142
Differentiation, of gastric cancers 167–169
Diffuse oesophageal spasm (DES), oesophageal transit scintigraphy for identifying 309
Dilatation
   for achalasia 80–81
   oesophageal 282
   palliative, in oesophageal cancer 162
   pyloric 283
Disc batteries, burns from the alkaline anode of 76–77
Dissection
   D1 versus D2, in gastric cancer 175
   D2, techniques of 341–346
   lymph node, in oesophageal cancer, prospective evaluation of 325–327
     in stomach cancer 335
Diverticula
   in the jejunum and ileum 111
   in the oesophagus 83–84, 241
Diverticular disease, small bowel 111

DNA repair gene, ERCC1, resistance to cisplatin by tumours with high levels of 357
Docetaxel, in a multiple drug regimen for treating oesophagogastric cancer 351
Dor fundoplication, for treating achalasia 81
Dorsal mesogastrium, embryonic development of 18–19
Dorsal yolk sac, development of the oesophagus from 1–2
Drainage. *See* Lymphatic drainage
Drugs
   capecitabine, for oesophagogastric cancer 351
   chloramphenicol, for treating typhoid enteritis 110
   chloroquine, perioperative administration of, in the tropics 143
   cholestyramine, for bile salt diarrhoea in Crohn's disease 105
   cimetidine, effects on acid secretion 34
   cisplatin, in a definitive chemoradiotherpy trial 361
     for management of gastric cancer, in a combination regimen 350
     for palliation in oesophageal cancer 162
   cocetaxel, in a multiple drug regimen for treating oesophagogastric cancer 351
   epirubicin, cisplatin, 5-fluorouracil regimen for treating oesophagogastric cancer 351
     for gastric cancer, in a combination regimen for chemotherapy 350
   ethambutol, for treating tuberculous enteritis 109
   etoposide, for management of gastric cancer, in a combination regimen 350
   5-fluorouracil, in a definitive chemoradiotherapy trial 365
     in management of adenocarcinoma of the jejunum and ileum 202
     in management of gastric cancer 350
     for palliation in oesophageal cancer 162
   imatinib mesylate, for treating gastrointestinal stromal tumours 215
   iminodiacetic acid (IDA) derivatives 303
   infliximab, contraindications to therapy with 106
     for treating Crohn's disease 106
   irinotecan, for chemoradiotherapy in oesophageal cancer 364
     in a multiple drug regimen for treating oesophagogastric cancer 351
   isoniazid, for treating tuberculous enteritis 109
   lansoprazole, for treating peptic ulcer disease 93
   leucovorin, in adenocarcinoma management 202
     in gastric cancer management 350
   lidocaine throat spray, using in endoscopy 281
   methotrexate, for management of gastric cancer 350
   metronidazole, for perianal disease 106
   mitomycin-C, for management of gastric cancer, in a combination regimen 350

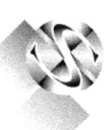

Drugs (*cont.*)
    montelukast, for treating eosinophilic oesophagitis 78
    nifedipine, for treating diffuse oesophageal spasm 81
    octreotide, for radiopharmaceutical imaging 304
    oxaliplatin, for chemoradiotherapy in oesophageal cancer 364
        in a multiple drug regimen for treating oesophagogastric cancer 351
    paclitaxel, for chemoradiotherapy in oesophageal cancer 364
    penicillin, after splenectomy 150-151, 228
    pentostatin, for treating hairy cell leukemia 63
    ranitidine, effects on acid secretion 34
        for treating peptic ulcer disease 93
    rifampicin, for treating tuberculous enteritis 109
    sulfasalazine, for treating Crohn's disease 105-106
    taxanes, in a multiple drug regimen for treating oesophagogastric cancer 351
Drugs, benzodiazepines, for sedation in endoscopy 281-282
Dumping syndrome
    avoiding with partial proximal gastrectomy 345-346
    as a complication of gastrectomy 177
    after gastric surgery 96
Duodenal ampulla, role in digestion 41
Duodenal diverticula 111
Duodenal mucosa, production of the cholecystokinin in 42
Duodenogastric reflux, after gastric surgery 97
Duodenopancreatectomy, partial, for treating gastrointestinal stromal tumours 215. *See also* Pancreaticoduodenectomy
Duodenotomy, for managing bleeding duodenal ulcers 94
Duodenum
    adenocarcinomas of 201-202
    adenomas of 201
    benign lesions arising in, limited resection in 193
    blood supply to 23
    carcinomas of, association with adenomatous polyposis coli 197
    defined 39
    defining, for upper gastrointestinal endoscopy 280
    embryonic development of 19
    gastrointestinal stromal tumours of, treating 215
    nerves of 26
    physiology of 40-41
    therapeutic endoscopy for cancer of 285
    vasoactive intestinal peptide of 32
Duplications
    accessory spleens 132-134
    of the embryological oesophagus 86
    of the stomach, complete and incomplete 19
Dyes, as diagnostic adjuncts in upper gastrointestinal endoscopy 280-281
Dysphagia, after antireflux surgery 76
Dysplasia
    defined 274
    and gastric cancer 97, 274
    glandular, in the oesophagus and stomach 251-253
    high grade, and risk of adenocarcinoma 263
    natural history of 263

## E

Eastern Cooperative Oncology Group (ECOG), randomised trial of chemoradiotherrapy versus radiotherapy, for squamous carcinoma 361
E-cadherin
    role in Barrett's oesophagus 262
    role in diffuse gastric cancer 169, 275
ECF (epirubicin, cisplatin, 5-fluorouracil) regimen, for treating oesophagogastric cancer 351
Efficacy, of lymph node dissection in stomach cancer 338-339
Elastic properties, of the diaphragm 50
Elastin fibres, of the body of the oesophagus 6
Electrical activity, resting, within the stomach 35
Embolisation
    of the spleen, risks and utility of 151-153
    splenic infarct resulting from 146-147
Embryology
    of the diaphragm 46-48
    of the oesophagus 1-2
        anomalies arising during development 241
    of the small intestine 43-44
    of the spleen 59, 127-128
    of the stomach 17-19
En bloc resection, defined 340
Encephalin, of the gastrointestinal tract 33
Endopeptidases, in the stomach 30
Endoscopic anatomy, of the oesophagus 5
Endoscopic mucosa resection (EMR)
    for gastric cancer 174
    for oesophageal dysplasia and cancer, outcomes 266
    for tumours of the distal oesophagus 332-333
Endoscopic treatment, of oesophageal cancer 162-163
Endoscopic ultrasound (EUS)
    for assessing mucosal associated lymphoid tissue lymphoma 235-236
    for diagnosing gastrointestinal cancer 211
    for diagnosing oesophageal cancer 159-161
    gastrointestinal evaluation using 297
Endoscopy
    appearance of gastric lymphoma on 231
    oesophageal, for diagnosing cancer 157
    small bowel, for diagnosing tumours 200-201
    upper gastrointestinal 279-286

# INDEX

Enteric neurones, secretion of acetylcholine by 35
Enterochromaffin cells, of the pyloric zone of the stomach 30
Enteroclysis, for diagnosing small bowel tumours 200, 301–302
Enterocrinin, secretion of, from the duodenal mucosa 42
Enteroendocrine cells, location and function of 40
Enterogastric reflex 35
Enteroglucagon, as a factor in adaptation of the small bowel after resection 113
Enterokinase, secretion of, in the small intestine 40
Enteropathy-associated T-cell lymphoma (EATL) 203
Enteroscopy, techniques of 285
Environmental factors, in development of gastric atrophy 271–272
Eosinophilic oesophagitis 77
Epidemiology
   of Barrett's oesophagus 259–264
   of Crohn's disease 101
   of gastric cancer 170–171
   of gastrointestinal stromal tumours 210
   of oesophageal squamous papilloma 267
   of small bowel neoplasms 194
   of squamous epithelial dysplasia 264–265
Epidermal growth factor (EGF)
   duodenal juice as a source of 113
   R2 receptor for, overexpression in gastric cancer 274
   receptor for, potential for drugs targeting 351
Epidermolysis bullosa, association with pyloric atresia 19
Epigastric arteries, path between the sternal and costal margins of the diaphragm 48
Epiphrenic diverticula 84
Epirubicin, for gastric cancer, in a combination regimen for chemotherapy 350
Epithelial dysplasia, squamous oesophageal, as a premalignant lesion 259
Epithelial neoplasms, of the stomach 167–180
Epithelial tumours, of the small bowel
   benign 201
   malignant 201–202
Epithelium
   lining the stomach 28
   squamous, of the oesophageal mucosa 6
Eradication therapy
   for *Helicobacter pylori* infection, in mucosal associated lymphoid tissue 235
   for peptic ulcer disease caused by *Helicobacter pylori* 93
*Escherichia coli*, infection by, after splenectomy 66
Ethambutol, for treating tuberculous enteritis 109
Ethyl alcohol, absorption from the stomach 33
Etoposide, for management of gastric cancer, in a combination regimen 350
Eventration of the diaphragm 122–123
Exocrine secretions, suppression of release in the pancreas, by somatostatin 32
Extended lymph node dissection (D2 dissection), indications for 339–340
Extracorporeal membrane oxygenation (ECMO), for managing infants with congenital diaphragmatic hernia 121
Extraintestinal features, of Crohn's disease 104
Extramural system, of zones of lymphatic drainage of the stomach 24–25
Extraperitoneal lymph vessels, path across the diaphragm 48

## F

Familial adenomatous polyposis (FAP)
   association with small bowel neoplasms 196–197
   duodenal polyps in 201
Familial oesophageal and upper gastrointestinal leiomyomatosis 209
Fas gene, effect of mucosal inflammation on expression of 262–263
Fasting state, physiology of the oesophagus in 8–9
Fiberoptic direct visualisation endoscopy, for diagnosing gastrointestinal disease 279
Finney type stricturoplasty, in Crohn's disease 108
Fistulas
   of the small bowel 112–113
   splenic, as a complication of splenic abscess 137–138
   tracheo-oesophageal 2
Fitness, assessment of, in treating gastric cancer 173
Flow cytometry, for evaluating biopsy specimen, oesophageal 264
Fluid retention, after D2 dissection 340
5-Fluorouracil
   in a definitive chemoradiotherapy trial 365
   in management of adenocarcinoma of the jejunum and ileum 202
   in management of gastric cancer 350
   for palliation in oesophageal cancer 162
Focal disease, of the spleen 136–137
Follicular lymphoma, splenic, relationship with hepatic schistosomiasis 143
Follow-up, in achalasia management 313–314
Foramen
   of Morgagni 117
   of Winslow, anatomy of 21
      formation of 19
Foramen, diaphragmatic 118–119
Foramen ovale, failure to close in neonates with congenital diaphragmatic hernia 120–121
Foreign bodies, ingested
   removal from the stomach 283
   small bowel damage from 114
Free radicals, in ulcerated gastro-oesophageal mucosa, effects of 262

French University Association for Surgical Research, randomised trial, radiotherapy or no further treatment after oesophagectomy 360
Fryns syndrome, diaphragmatic hernia in 119
Functional foregut disorder (FFD), association with upper gastrointestinal dysfunction 78–79
Fundic glands (principal glands), of the oxyntic zone of the stomach 29
Fundoplication, in treating gastro-oesophageal reflux disease 75

## G

Galactose, absorption by the stomach 33
Galanin 33
Gallstones, as a complication of congenital spherocytosis 141
Ganglionated sympathetic trunks, transmission through the diaphragm 48
Gastrectomy
  Billroth II, for treating bleeding gastric ulcers 94
  total versus subtotal 335–336
Gastric acid
  formation and secretion of, in parietal cells of the stomach 31
  secretion of, control mechanisms 33–35
  suppression of release in the stomach, by somatostatin 32
Gastric artery
  left, oesophageal branches of 4–5
    supply of blood to the stomach by 21–22
  right, anatomy of 22
Gastric atrophy, defined 271
Gastric cancer
  adjuvant therapy for 352
  association with gastric surgery 97
  direct spread to the spleen 225
  distal, pandemic 170
  lymph node dissection in 337–339
  neoadjuvant chemotherapy for 353
  therapeutic endoscopy for 284–285
Gastric dilatation, acute, as a complication of surgery 98
Gastric emptying
  delayed, after truncal vagotomy 97
  radiopharmaceuticals for studying 304–305
Gastric epithelium, characteristics of, versus intestinal epithelium 243
Gastric glands, cells of the epithelial lining of the stomach continuing into 28
Gastric hormones 31–33
Gastric ileus, after splenectomy 227
Gastric lymphoma 231
  large cell 237
Gastric motility
  control of 17, 36
  and hunger contraction 35–36
Gastric mucosa, zones of 28–30
Gastric nodes, drainage from the stomach into 24–25
Gastric outlet obstruction, barium meal to indicate the nature of 172
Gastric phase, of stimulated secretion 35
Gastric pits, glands of the stomach opening into 28–29
Gastric polyps 275–276
Gastric secretions 30–31
  effect of vasoactive intestinal peptide on 32
  regulation of 33–36
Gastric Surgical Adjuvant Radiotherapy Consensus Report, on planning postoperative chemoradiotherapy 367
Gastric therapy
  endoscopic 283
  types of resection 335–337
Gastric tone, effects of abnormalities in 35–36
Gastric ulcer, differentiating from gastric cancer 172
Gastric varices, management of, endoscopically 283
Gastric veins, anatomy of 23
Gastric volvulus, association of, with para-oesophageal hiatus hernia 98
Gastrin
  secretion of, increase in *Helicobacter pylori* infection 92
    in the stomach 30
  sources and characterisation of 31–32
  suppression of release in the stomach, by somatostatin 32
Gastrin peptide vaccine G17dt, for treating gastric cancer 180
Gastritis
  acute, gastrointestinal haemorrhage from 97
  chronic, risk of gastric cancer associated with 98
  of the oesophagus 244–246
  reactive 244
Gastroduodenal artery, anatomy of 22
Gastroduodenal Crohn's disease, surgery for 108
Gastroduodenal junction, anatomy of 20
Gastroenteric reflex 41–42
Gastroenterostomy, outcomes of 178–179
Gastroepiploic arteries 22
  left, branch of the splenic artery 60
Gastroepiploic nodes
  left, drainage from the stomach into 25
  right, drainage from the stomach into 24
Gastroepiploic veins, anatomy of 23–24
Gastro-esophageal junction, cancer at 187–191
Gastroileal reflex 41–42
Gastrointestinal autonomic nerve tumours (GANT), c-KIT positive 209
Gastrointestinal features, of Crohn's disease 103–104

# INDEX

Gastrointestinal stromal tumours (GIST) 155, 254–255
  defined 204
  differentiating from other mesenchymal tumours 208–209
Gastrojejunostomy
  for managing Crohn's disease 108
  for managing duodenal ulcer 95
Gastro-oesophageal junction
  anatomy of 20
  cancer at 181–192
  defined 5
Gastro-oesophageal reflux
  evaluating with contrast radiography 292–293
  investigation of 13–14
Gastro-oesophageal reflux disease (GORD) 69–76
  aetiology of 260–261
  chronic, associated with congenital diaphragmatic hernia 122
  defined 69
  detecting with oesophageal transit scintigraphy 307
  and incidence of squamous oesophageal cancer 156
  oesophageal adenocarcinoma risk associated with 182
  oesophageal rings associated with 85
  oesophageal spasm associated with 81
  in overweight individuals 187–188
  physiology of 14
Gastroschisis 44
Gastrosplenic ligament, embryonic formation of 59
Gastrosplenic omentum, anatomy of 21
Gaucher's disease (GD) 145
  splenomegaly due to 61
G cells, of the stomach and duodenum 31–32
Genes
  Bcl10, translocations associated with MALT lymphoma 234
  c-KIT, role in gastrointestinal stromal tumour development 208–209
  *c-kit* proto-oncogene, role in tumourigenesis 204
  for DNA mismatch repair, mutation in hereditary non-polyposis colorectal cancer 197
  homeobox HOXDII, embryological control of splenogenesis by 134–135
  NOD2, mutations associated with Crohn's disease 102
  p16, inactivation of, in Barrett's oesophagus, non-dysplastic premalignant 261–262
  p53, role in Barrett's oesophagus progression to adenocarcinoma 261–262
    role in intestinal metaplasia 275
    role in squamous cell carcinoma 265–266
  for serine threonine kinase, mutation in Peutz-Jeghers syndrome 197

Genetic disorders
  familial adenomatous polyposis, duodenal polyps in 201
  familial oesophageal and upper gastrointestinal leiomyomatosis 209
  gastric cancer as 169
  predisposition to gastro-oesophageal reflux disease 70
  *See also* Chromosomes; Congenital abnormalities
Genetics, of Crohn's disease 101
German Lymphoma study group, data on resection in large cell gastric lymphoma 237
Glands of Brunner, of the duodenum 27
Glucagon, suppression of release in the pancreas, by somatostatin 32
ß-Glucocerebrosidase, deficiency of, in Gaucher's disease 145
Glucose-dependent insulinotropic peptide (GIP), effect on insulin release from pancreatic islet cells 42
Glycoproteins, secretion of, by parietal cells of the stomach 31
Grading
  of gastritis 246
  of gastrointestinal stromal tumours of the stomach 215–216
  of oesophagitis 70
  of splenic injury and bleeding 65–66
  of squamous cell carcinomas of the oesophagus 247
  *See also* Staging
Growth factor receptor, c-KIT, expression in gastrointestinal stromal tumours 208
Growth hormone (GH), inhibition of, by somatostatin 32

## H

Haemangioendotheliomas, splenic 223
Haemangioma, of the spleen 138, 222
Haematological disorders
  involvement of the spleen in 139–142
  malignancy involving the spleen 223–224
  rupture of the spleen due to 149
  splenectomy for managing 61
Haematological functions, of the spleen 128–131
Haematological studies, to identify causes of splenomegaly 148
Haematopoietic cells
  embryonic formation of, in the spleen 59
  formation of, in the spleen 60
Haemocytopoiesis, by the spleen 128
Haemolytic anaemia
  hereditary 63
  in spherocytosis 141
  splenectomy for treating 150
*Haemophilus* B, immunisation against, after splenectomy 228

*Haemophilus influenzae*, infection by, after splenectomy 66
Haemorrhage
  from peptic ulcers, arresting 94
  after splenectomy 227
  subcapsular, splenic rupture due to 149
  from typhoid enteritis 110
  *See also* Bleeding
Hairy cell leukaemia (HCL), splenomegaly in 63, 223
Halstedian cancer model, of metastasis 337–339
Hamartomas, splenic 138
Hamman's mediastinal crunch, as a clinical sign of oesophageal perforation 87
Heineke-Mikulicz pyloroplasty, for closure in duodenotomy for bleeding peptic ulcers 94
Heineke-Mikulicz stricturoplasty, in Crohn's disease 108
Heinz bodies, removal from erythrocytes in the spleen 129
*Helicobacter pylori*
  association of, with atrophic gastritis 271
    with gastric adenocarcinoma 250–251
    with gastritis 244
  as a cause, of gastric cancer 169–170, 254, 272
    of stomach cancer 184
  discovery of, and surgery for peptic ulcer disease 91–92
  eradication of, in treating MALT lymphoma 235
  infection with, correlation with gastric lymphoma 234–235
    correlation with stomach cancer 181
Heller's myotomy, for treating achalasia 80–81
Hemi-azygos vein, passage through the diaphragm 48
Hepatic artery, supply of blood to the stomach by 22
Hepatisation, of the spleen 154
Hepato-gastric ligament (lesser omentum), anatomy of 20
Hereditary non-polyposis colorectal cancer (HNPCC), risk of small bowel cancer associated with 197
Hernia, diaphragmatic 242
Herpes simplex virus (HSV), oesophagitis due to 77, 243
Hiatus hernia 242
  correction of, in antireflux surgery 75
  para-oesophageal, gastric volvulus associated with 98
  rolling, evaluating in a gastro-oesophageal reflux disease patient 72
  sliding, evaluating in a gastro-oesophageal reflux disease patient 72
    from a weakened phreno-oesophageal ligament 5

High frequency oscillatory ventilation (HFOV), for managing infants with congenital diaphragmatic hernia 121
Histology
  of adenocarcinomas of the oesophagus and stomach 250–251
  of the columnar lined oesophagus 243
  of gastrointestinal stromal tumours 212–214
  of the intestinal wall 40
Histopathology, in primary lymphomas of the gut 233
Hodgkin's disease 62–63
  splenomegaly in 224
Homeobox gene HOXDII, embryological control of splenogenesis by 134–135
Hormones
  effects of, on gastric motility 17
  intestinal 42
  secretion of, in the stomach 30
Howell-Jolly bodies
  as indicators of accessory spleens 134
  removal from erythrocytes in the spleen 129
Human immunodeficiency virus (HIV) infection, spleen involvement in 144
Human papilloma virus (HPV) infection, association with oesophageal squamous papilloma 267–268
Hunger contractions 36
Hydramnios, association with pyloric atresia 19
Hyoid muscles, action in swallowing 9–10
Hypersplenism 136
  splenomegaly due to 61
Hypertensive lower oesophageal sphincter 82
Hypertrophic gastropathy (Ménétrier's disease) 246
Hypervolaemia, and splenic pooling 129–130
Hypogammaglobulinemia, association with lymphoma of the small intestine 196
Hypoglycaemia, secondary to hyperinsulaemia, after gastric surgery 96
Hypokalaemic metabolic alkalosis, association with pyloric stenosis 95
Hypothalamus, role in hunger sensations 36
Hypovolaemia, correcting, in splenic sequestration from sickle cell disease 140
Hypoxaemia, in neonates with congenital diaphragmatic hernia 121

I

Iatrogenic disorders
  oesophageal perforation 87–88
  splenic embolisation 146–147
Idiopathic thrombocytopenic purpura (ITP)
  in patients with human immunodeficiency virus infection 145
  splenectomy to manage 140–141
    laparoscopic 153–154
Ileocaecal resection, in Crohn's disease 108
Ileogram, retrograde 296

# INDEX

Ileum
  adenocarcinoma of, management of 202
  defined 39
  tumours of, similarity to adenocarcinoma of the colon 193
Imaging
  in gastrointestinal surgery 287–305
  of the small bowel 193
Imatinib mesylate (tyrosine kinase inhibitor), for treating gastrointestinal stromal tumours 215
Iminodiacetic acid (IDA) derivatives, for biliary imaging 303
Immune responses
  generation of, in the spleen 60
  splenomegaly due to disorders of 61
  uninhibited, in Crohn's disease 102
  *See also* Autoimmune disorders
Immune status, compromised, and effects of splenectomy 144–145
Immune thrombocytopenic purpura (ITP), splenectomy for treating 61–62
Immunisation
  before splenectomy 226
  after splenectomy 228
Immunocompromise, and infective oesophagitis 77, 243
Immunoglobulins. *See* Antibodies
Immunohistochemistry, for diagnosing gastrointestinal stromal tumours 212–214
Immunological functions, of the spleen 131–132
  results of loss of 135
Immunosuppression
  after allogeneic hepatocyte transplantation 154
  risk of visceral tumours associated with 196
  for treating Crohn's disease 106
Incidence
  of diaphragmatic rupture 123–124
  of stomach cancer 182–185
Incisions, diaphragmatic 118
Incisura angularis, anatomy of 20
Indications
  for antireflux surgery 73–74
  for pancreaticosplenectomy with total gastrectomy 344
  for splenectomy 61, 149–150, 226
    laparoscopic 154
    in sickle cell disease 140
  for splenorrhaphy 153
  for surgery, in Crohn's disease 107–108
    in tuberculous enteritis 109
Indigo-carmine dye, to aid recognition of mucosal patterns in the stomach 280
Indium-111, for white cell scanning 302–303
Infections
  and incidence of Crohn's disease 101
  after splenectomy 66
  splenomegaly due to 61

Inflammation
  after ingestion of caustic substances 243
  of the stomach 97–98
Inflammatory bowel disease, association with oesophagitis 78
Inflammatory cell, infiltrate of, as a cause of gastritis 244–245
Inflammatory myofibroblastic tumour, in children 210
Infliximab (Remicade), for treating Crohn's disease 106
Injection therapy, palliative, for oesophageal cancer 162
Insulin, suppression of release in the pancreas, by somatostatin 32
Intensity modulated radiotherapy (IMRT) 364
Intercostal nerves, sensory fibres to the diaphragm from 49
Interferon, for treating hairy cell leukemia 63
Interleukin 1ß (IL-1ß), implication in neoplastic progression of Barrett's oesophagus 262
Interleukin 1 genotype, and development of benign ulcer or cancer in *Helicobacter pylori* infection 169
Intermediary system
  of lymphatic drainage of the stomach 24
Intermuscular network, of lymphatic drainage of the stomach 24
International Extra Nodal Lymphoma Study Group (IELSG), comparison of chemotherapy in large cell gastric lymphoma 237
International Society for Diseases of the Esophagus (ISDE), definition of the extent of lymphadenectomy for oesophageal cancer 323
Interprandial gastric acid secretion, stimulated gastric acid secretion 33
Interstitial cells of Cajal (ICC), c-KIT expression in 208
Intestinal crypts 40
Intestinal epithelium, characteristics of, versus gastric epithelium 243
Intestinal metaplasia
  in Barrett's oesophagus 260
  in *Helicobacter pylori* infection 244, 273–274
Intestinal phase, of stimulated secretion in the stomach 35
Intra-abdominal pressure, diaphragmatic recruitment to relieve 57–58
Intragastric pressure, and hunger contraction 35
Intraluminal tumours, oesophageal benign 86
Intramural plexuses, of the oesophagus 8
Intramural pseudodiverticulosis 82
Intramural tumours, oesophageal benign 86
Intrinsic factor, secretion of, by parietal cells of the stomach 31
Intubation, for palliation in oesophageal cancer 163

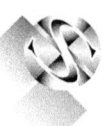

Intussusception, small bowel tumours presenting with 198
Investigations
  of Crohn's disease 104–105
  of gastric cancer 172
  of gastro-oesophageal reflux 13–14
  of lymphoma 232
  of oesophageal neoplasms 157–162
  of peristalsis 10–11
  of splenomegaly 148
In vivo observations, relaxation of the diaphragm 55–56
Ionising radiation, justification of the use of 287
Iran, incidence of oesophageal cancer in 182
Irinotecan
  for chemoradiotherapy in oesophageal cancer 364
  in a multiple drug regimen for treating oesophagogastric cancer 351
Iron, reabsorption of, in the stomach 97
Irritable bowel syndrome (IBS) 78–79
Isometric relaxation of muscles, defined 54–55
Isoniazid, for treating tuberculous enteritis 109
Isotonic relaxation of muscles, defined 54–55
Isotope scanning, to diagnose splenic neoplasms 225
Ivemark's syndrome, as bilateral right-sidedness 135
Ivor Lewis approach, in junctional tumour surgery 176

**J**

Japan, screening programme for stomach cancer in 181
Japanese Clinical Oncology Group (JCOG)
  prospective trial of D2 total gastrectomy with and without splenectomy 341
  trial of para-aortic nodal dissection for gastric cancer 346
Japanese Research Society for Esophageal Cancer, classification of lymph node groups 324–325
Japanese Research Society for Gastric Cancer (IRSGC)
  on degrees of differentiation of epithelial neoplasms 167–168
  histological classification of adenocarcinoma by 250–251
  staging system for oesophageal and gastric carcinomas 255–256
Jejunal ileal region, involvement in small bowel Crohn's disease 108
Jejunal interposition, for reconstruction after total gastrectomy 344
Jejunum
  adenocarcinoma of, management of 202
  defined 39
  physiology of 41
  tumours of, similarity to adenocarcinoma of the colon 193
Junctional cancer 170–171
Junctional tumours, surgery for oesophagogastric junction tumours 175–176

**K**

Kala-azar (visceral leishmaniasis), spleen involvement in 142
Kaposi's sarcoma, of the gastrointestinal tract 196
Kidney, left, radiation dose to, in treating gastric lymphoma 238
Killian's triangle, origin of a pharyngeal pouch in 5

**L**

Lacteals, intestinal transport of materials by 40
Lamina propria
  of the small intestine 40
  of the stomach 28
Lansoprazole (proton pump inhibitor), for treating peptic ulcer disease 93
Laparoscopic splenectomy 64–65, 153–154
  risks of 226–227
Laparoscopic ultrasound, for staging in gastric cancer 173
Laparoscopy, for diagnosing oesophageal cancer 158–159
Laryngotracheal diverticulum, development of 2
Lateral soft tissue neck, imaging with plain radiology 287
Lauren classification, for gastric tumours 167–169, 250
Law of Laplace, constancy of intragastric pressure 35
Lectin, binding of, changes in squamous epithelial dysplasia 266
Leiomyomas
  bleeding due to 94
  gastrointestinal 209
  of the oesophagus, management of 214–215
  of the small bowel 204–205
    computed tomography for diagnosing 199–200
Leiomyosarcoma
  gastrointestinal 209
  metastasis to the lung 216
  of the small bowel 205
    computed tomography for diagnosing 199–200
  obstruction in 198
*Leishmania donovani*, effect on the spleen 142
Leucovorin
  in adenocarcinoma management 202
  in gastric cancer management, in a combination regimen 350
Leukaemia
  chronic and hairy cell, splenic involvement in 63
  splenic involvement in 223–224
  splenomegaly due to 61

# INDEX

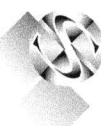

Lewis-Tanner operation, for oesophageal cancer 164
Lidocaine, throat spray using, in endoscopy 281
Lifestyle, modifying, in peptic ulcer disease 92–93
Linitis plastica 250
   differentiating from gastric cancer 172
   lymph node dissection in 340
Lipase, acid-resistant, secretion of, in the stomach 30–31
Lipomas of the small bowel 205
Littoral cell angiomas 222–223
Liver, impaired function of, and risk in D2 dissection to manage gastric cancer 340
Los Angeles system, for grading oesophagitis 70–71
Lower oesophageal sphincter (LOS) 6–7
   role of, in swallowing 11–12
Lugano modification, Ann Arbor staging system, for gastrointestinal lymphoma 233
Lugol iodine solution, for diagnosing squamous epithelial dysplasia 266
Lumbar elements of the diaphragm 117
Lung hypoplasia, association with congenital diaphragmatic hernia 119–120
Lung volume, effect of, on the action of the diaphragm on the rib cage during breathing 53
Lupus erythematosus, oesophageal motility affected by 83
Lymphadenectomy
   D2, for squamous cell oesophageal cancer 330
   extended, in surgery for oesophageal cancer 317–334
   limited, in surgery for gastric gastrointestinal stroma tumours 214–215
   for oesophageal cancer 321–329
Lymphangioma, splenic 138, 223
Lymphatic drainage
   of the diaphragm 49
   of the oesophagus 7–8
   of the spleen 128
   of the stomach 24–25
Lymph nodes
   dissection of, in resection of the stomach 335
   en bloc dissection of, in resection of gastric cancer 174
   status of, and prognosis in oesophageal carcinoma 8
   TNM system for staging 256
Lymphocytes. *See* B lymphocytes; T lymphocytes
Lymphocytic gastritis 244
Lymphoid hyperplasia, of the small bowel 202–203
Lymphoid tissue, spleen as 128–132
Lymphomas 231–240
   B cell, association with coeliac disease 196
   gastric high grade and low grade, radiotherapy for treating 238
   malignant, of the small bowel 203
   mucosal associated lymphoid tissue, low grade 234–235
   oesophageal 254
   risk of, associated with acquired immunodeficiency syndrome 196
   small bowel obstruction as a presenting factor 198
   splenic 138
   splenomegaly associated with 61, 223–224
   of the stomach 254
   T cell
      association with coeliac disease 196
      enteropathy-associated 203
Lymphoproliferative disorders, of the small bowel 202–204
Lymph plexus, at each surface of the diaphragm 49–50
Lymph vessels, of the diaphragm 49–50
Lysosomal sphingolipid storage disorders, Gaucher's disease 145

## M

McKeown oesophagectomy 164
Mackler's triad, as a clinical sign of oesophageal perforation 87
Macroscopic features, of Crohn's disease 102–103
Magnetic resonance cholangio-pancreatography (MRCP) 299–302
Magnetic resonance imaging (MRI)
   for confirming traumatic diaphragmatic rupture 125
   cross-sectional, for gastrointestinal evaluation 299–302
   for defining gastrointestinal stromal tumours 211–212
   for diagnosis, of oesophageal cancer 159
   of splenic neoplasms 225–226
   enteroclysis with, for diagnosing small bowel tumours 200
Malaria
   acute, non-traumatic splenic rupture caused by 149
   hypersplenism in 136
   risk of, in blood transfusion in the tropics 143
   tropical splenomegaly syndrome from 142
Malignancy, secondary, involving the spleen 224–225
Malignant change, in benign duodenal ulcers 96
Malignant melanoma
   metastasis to the small bowel 205
   of the oesophagus 255
Management
   of atrophic gastritis 273
   of eosinophilic oesophagitis 77–78
   of gastric polyps 276
   of gastrointestinal bleeding 93
   of gastrointestinal stromal tumours 214–215
   of gastro-oesophageal reflux disease 70–72
   of intestinal metaplasia 274–275
   long-term, after splenectomy 227–228
   of lymphomas, small bowel 203
   of small bowel fistulas 112–113

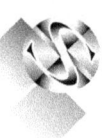

of small bowel neoplasms 201–202
Management (*cont.*)
  of splenic trauma 149
  surgical, in eventration of the diaphragm and phrenic nerve palsies 123
    of gastric cancer 174–179
    of segmental splenectomy 152
    in splenic infarction 147
    for splenorrhaphy 153
    in traumatic diaphragmatic rupture 125
  *See also* Surgery; Treatment
Manometry
  correlation with oesophageal transit scintigraphy data 309–311
  oesophageal, for diagnosing achalasia 79–80
  with pH monitoring, for evaluating oesophageal motility disorders 307
Mantle cell lymphoma 254
Marimastat (matrix metalloproteinase inhibitor), for gastric cancer 180, 351
Markers
  of intestinal dysplasia 275
  molecular, for predicting tumour response 357
Maximum relaxation rate (MRR), of the diaphragm, measurement from pressure decay curves 55
Meckel's diverticulum
  appearance on scan of 303–304
  development of, with vitello-intestinal duct abnormalities 44
  source and management of 111
Medical Research Council, study comparing surgery with neoadjuvant chemotherapy for oesophagogastric cancers 353–355
Medical treatment, of Crohn's disease 105–107
Medication, long-term, versus surgery for gastro-oesophageal reflux disease 74
Meissner's plexus, in achalasia of the cardia 8
Melanoma, malignant, metastasis to the small bowel 205
Memorial Sloan Kettering Cancer Center
  study of gastrointestinal stromal tumour survival after resection 216
  study of mesenchymal gastrointestinal neoplasms 209
Ménétrier's disease, infection by, after splenectomy 66
Merendino's operation, for reconstruction after proximal gastrectomy 336
Mesenchymal neoplasms, differentiating from gastrointestinal stromal tumours 208–209
Mesenteric artery
  branches of 40
  superior, blood supply to the midgut through 43–44
Mesenteric vein, superior, draining the small intestine 40

Mesentery
  dorsal, of the oesophagus, fusing of the pleuroperitoneal membranes with, during gestation 47
  of the small intestine 39
    embryological development of 43
Mesocolon, transverse, anatomy of 21
Metaplasia
  in Barrett's oesophagus, development of 261
  natural history of 263
Metastasis
  distant, of oesophageal cancers 256
    of oesophageal cancers as a prognostic factor 318–320
  of gastric cancer 168
    modes of 337–339
  lymphatic spread of oesophageal cancer, patterns in 321–323
  lymph node, in oesophageal cancer for determining prognosis 319
  to the oesophagus and stomach 255
  to the spleen 224–225
Methotrexate, for management of gastric cancer, in a combination regimen 350
Methylene blue, to stain mucosal abnormalities 280
Metronidazole, for perianal disease, in Crohn's disease 106
Microorganisms, clearance of, by the spleen 60
Microscopic anatomy, of the stomach 27–28
Microscopic features, of Crohn's disease 103
Mid-oesophageal diverticula 84
Minimum dataset information, from an oesophageal or gastric resection specimen 257
Mitomycin-C (MMC), for management of gastric cancer, in a combination regimen 350
Molecular biology
  of Barrett's oesophagus 261–263
  of squamous epithelial dysplasia 265–266
Molecular markers predicting tumour response 357
Molybdenum, soil levels of, and incidence of squamous epithelial dysplasia and carcinoma 265
Montelukast, for treating eosinophilic oesophagitis 78
Morbid obesity, gastric surgery for managing 98–99
Morphology, of gastrointestinal stromal tumours 204
Mortality
  in adenocarcinoma of the small bowel 202
  association with morbid obesity 98–99
  in congenital diaphragmatic hernia 122
  after D2 distal gastrectomy with splenectomy 345
  in diagnostic endoscopy 281
  in diaphragmatic rupture 124
  in enteropathy-associated T-cell lymphoma (EATL) 203
  in gastric cancer after D2 lymph node dissection 338–340

# INDEX

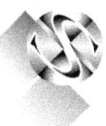

in mucosal associated lymphoid tissue lymphoma 234–235
in non-operative management of splenic injury 65
in oesophageal cancer 155
in oesophageal perforation 88
after oesophagectomy 1, 155–156
in post-splenectomy sepsis 66
from small bowel fistulas 112
in splenectomy 151
following splenectomy for hyper-reactive malarial splenomegaly 142
in stomach cancer, change in rate with percentage of nodal metastases 337
    change in rate with sex and age 182–183
in surgery for peptic ulcer disease 92–93
in surgical management of small bowel fistulas 113
in total gastrectomy for managing gastrointestinal haemorrhage 97
Motilin, suppression of release in the intestine, by somatostatin 32
Motility disorders, oesophageal 79–83
    evaluating with contrast radiography 293–294
    non-specific 82–83
Mucoepidermoid carcinoma 253
Mucosa, of the stomach 27–28
Mucosa associated lymphatic follicles, conditions associated with 234–235
Mucosa associated lymphoid tissue (MALT)
    of the gut, involvement in gastric lymphoma 231
    lymphoma of 203, 254
        response to antibiotic therapy 367
    of stomach tumours, *Helicobacter pylori* eradication for treating 273
Mucosal inflammation, role in Barrett's oesophagus 262–263
Mucosal resection, endoscopic 282–283, 284
Mucosal zones, of the stomach 28–30
Mucous cells, of the oxyntic zone 29
Mucus secretions, from epithelial cells of the stomach 30
Muscles
    diaphragm, mechanical aspects of relaxation in 54–55
    slow- and fast-twitch fibres of, sarcoplasmic reticulum calcium ion uptake in 54
Muscularis externa, of the stomach 27
Muscularis mucosae
    of the small intestine 40
    of the stomach 27
Musculophrenic artery, aperture across the diaphragm for 48
*Mycobacterium bovis*, milk contaminated with, as a cause of tuberculous enteritis 109
Myelofibrosis, involvement of the spleen in 145–146
Myenteric plexus 8

Myositis, oesophageal motility affected by 83
Myotomy
    to treat achalasia 80–81
    to treat oesophageal diverticula 83

## N

National Cancer Database, analysis of information about adenocarcinoma of the small bowel 202
Natural history
    of atrophic gastritis 272–273
    of intestinal metaplasia 273–275
Nausea, excitation of the medulla oblongata in 37
Neoadjuvant therapy
    chemoradiotherapy, for oesophageal cancer 355–356, 360–361
        safety of resection following 330
    for oesophageal cancer 164–165
    in oesophagogastric cancer 352–353
    radiotherapy, for oesophageal cancer 359
Neoplasms
    primary, causing splenic enlargement 222–223
    of the small bowel 193–206
        secondary 205
    of the stomach and oesophagus 247–257
Nerve supply
    of the diaphragm 49, 118
    of the oesophagus 8
    of the stomach 25–27
Neuroendocrine cells
    defined 27
    of the oxyntic zone of the stomach 29
    of the pyloric zone of the stomach 30
Neurofibromas of the small bowel 205
Neurofibromatosis (von Recklinghausen's disease), risk for small bowel neoplasms associated with 197–198
Neurotensin, in the pyloric zone of the stomach 33
Niemann-Pick disease 145
Nifedipine, for treating diffuse oesophageal spasm 81
Nissen fundoplication 75
Nissen Rosetti modification, of the Nissen fundoplication 75
Nitrate, dietary, role in development of cancers at the gastro-esophageal junction 188
Nitrous oxide (NO), role in swallowing 11
N-nitrosamines, role in squamous epithelial dysplasia and carcinoma development 265
Non-Hodgkin's lymphoma (NHL)
    gastric, study of resection with post-operative radiation to treat 237
    management of involvement of the spleen in 63
    primary oesophageal T-cell, treatment of 365
    of the small bowel 203
    splenomegaly in 224

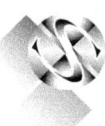

Non-steroidal anti-inflammatory drugs (NSAIDs)
    absorption from the stomach 33
    aspirin, damage to the stomach by 30
        reduction of oesophageal COX-2 by 262–263
    association of atrophic gastritis type B with 272
    as a cause of peptic ulcer disease 91–92
    reactive gastritis due to use of 244
Non-surgical treatment, of oesophageal neoplasms 163–164
North American Intergroup trial, evaluation of chemoradiotherapy for gastric cancer after surgery 352
Nuclear medicine, for managing high risk lesions in the oesophagus 307–315
Nutcracker oesophagus (NCE) 81–82
    oesophageal transit scintigraphy for identifying 309
Nutrition
    deficiencies in, after gastrectomy 177
        after gastric surgery 96–97
    and reduction in incidence of stomach cancer 182
    and risk of squamous cell carcinogenesis 265
    See also Diet
Nutritional therapy
    in Crohn's disease 106–107
    in managing small bowel fistula 112
    after resection for surgery in small bowel syndrome 114

# O

Obesity
    morbid, gastric surgery for managing 98–99
    as a risk factor in D2 dissection to manage gastric cancer 340
Obstruction
    from gastrointestinal stromal tumours 211
    from small bowel tumours 198
Octreotide, for radiopharmaceutical imaging 304
Oesophageal cancer
    adjuvant therapy for 352
    classification of, by location and histologic type 317–318
    demographics of 181–182
    neoadjuvant chemoradiotherapy for managing 355–356
    neoadjuvant chemotherapy for managing 353–355
    radiotherapy for managing 359–366
    survival of 186–187
    therapeutic endoscopy for 283–284
    variation in incidence of, with deprivation 185–186
Oesophageal foramen (aperture), in the diaphragm 48, 118
Oesophageal lymphomas 231
Oesophageal perforation 87–88
Oesophageal phase, of swallowing 9
Oesophageal rests, defined 86
Oesophageal squamous papilloma 267–268
Oesophageal transit scintigraphy (ETS) 307–309
Oesophagectomy
    as part of a treatment plan in oesophageal cancer 164
    risks of 155–156
Oesophagitis 243–244
    infective 77
    non-reflux 76–79
    progression to Barrett's metaplasia 263
    progression to Barrett's oesophagus 260–261
Oesophagogastric cancer, advanced, chemotherapy for management of 349–350
Oesophagogastric junction, physiology of the antireflux mechanism involving 13
Oesophagojejunostomy, for reconstruction after gastrectomy 96
Oesophagotomy, to remove intra luminal polyps or tumours 87
Oesophagus
    anatomy and physiology of 1–15
    benign disease of 69–89
    cervical, anatomy of 3
    columnar lined 243
    epithelial neoplasms of the 155–166
    high risk lesions in, and nuclear medicine 307–315
    iodine solution to visualise mucosal abnormalities in 280
    pathology of 241–257
    premalignant lesions of 259–269
    transit studies using technetium labelling 304
Omenta, anatomy of 21
Omentectomy, with resection of the anterior sheet of the mesocolon 341
Omphalocele (exomphalos), mortality associated with 43
Openings, of the stomach 20
Open splenectomy, description of 64, 226–227
Oral feeding, reintroduction of, after resection in small bowel syndrome 114
Organ Injury Scaling, for grading spleen trauma 65
Oropharyngeal phase of swallowing 9
Outcomes
    of antireflux surgery 76
    of Crohn's disease 108
    of eradication therapy for mucosal associated lymphoid tissue lymphoma 236–237
    of lymphadenectomy, for adenocarcinoma of the distal oesophagus 328–329
        for squamous cell oesophageal cancer 327–328
    of surgery, for eventration of the diaphragm 123
        for gastric cancer 177
    of untreated traumatic diaphragmatic rupture 125–126
Overwhelming post-splenectomy infections (OPSI) 150–151, 227

# INDEX

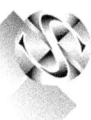

Oxaliplatin
  for chemoradiotherapy in oesophageal cancer 364
  in a multiple drug regimen for treating oesophagogastric cancer 351
Oxyntic zone, of the stomach 29
  somatostatin in 32
  substance P of 33
  vasoactive intestinal peptide of 32

## P

p16 gene, inactivation of, in Barrett's oesophagus, non-dysplastic premalignant 261–262
p53 gene
  role in Barrett's oesophagus progression to adenocarcinoma 261–262
  role in intestinal metaplasia 275
  role in squamous cell carcinoma 265–266
Paclitaxel, for chemoradiotherapy in oesophageal cancer 364
Pain
  abdominal, in Crohn's disease 103
  presentation of angiosarcoma with 222
  presentation of oesophageal perforation with 87
  presentation of small bowel tumours with 198
Palliation
  in gastric cancer management 178
  in oesophageal cancer management 162–163
    endoscopic 284–285
    radiotherapy for 365
Pancreas
  embryonic development of 19
  heterotropic 242–243
  somatostatin from the islet D cells of 32
  suppression of release of glucagon in 32
  tail of, managing in laparoscopic splenectomy 153
    managing in open splenectomy 64
Pancreatic artery, dorsal, relationship to the splenic artery 23, 128
Pancreatic cancer, therapeutic endoscopy for 285
Pancreatic lymphomas, primary 231
Pancreaticoduodenectomy (Whipple's procedure) 193
  for adenocarcinoma of the duodenum, studies 201–202
  for adenomatous polyp management 201
Pancreaticosplenectomy, with total gastrectomy, D2 344
Pancreatic tissue, ectopic 19
Papilloma, squamous oesophageal 250, 267–268
  as a premalignant lesion 259
Para-aortic nodal dissection, for advanced gastric cancer 346
Parasympathetic nerve supply
  of the oesophagus 8
  of the stomach 25–26

Parietal cells
  effects of, on gastric secretions 34
  of the pyloric zone of the stomach 29
Parkinson's disease, achalasia caused by 79
Partial proximal gastrectomy (PPG) 345–346
Parvalbumin, muscle relaxation rate and concentration of 54
Pathogenesis, of Crohn's disease 102
Pathology
  assessing, with upper gastrointestinal endoscopy 280
  of atrophic gastritis 272
  of Crohn's disease 102–103
  of gastric cancer 167–169
  of the oesophagus and stomach 241–257
Pathophysiology, in achalasia 79–80
Patient factors
  desire for antireflux surgery 73–74
  effect on outcomes of D2 dissection in gastric cancer 340
  fitness and antireflux surgery 74
Patient identification, after splenectomy, bracelets or cards for 228
Pelvic floor muscles, correlation with intra-abdominal pressure in postural tasks 56–57
Pentostatin, for treating hairy cell leukemia 63
Pepsin
  precursors of, from the zymogenic cells of the oxyntic zone 29
  suppression of release in the stomach, by somatostatin 32
Pepsinogen
  relative secretions of 1 and 2 forms, as a marker for atrophic gastritis 272
  secretion of, increase in *Helicobacter pylori* infection 92
    in the stomach 30
  serum measures of, as a test for gastric cancer 171
Peptic ulcer disease 91–95, 246
Peptidergic nervous system
  anatomy and embryology of 27
  defined 25
Peptides
  of amine precursor uptake and decarboxylation cells of the gut 27
  terminal, of gastrin forms 32
Perforation
  oesophageal, causes of 87–88
  due to peptic ulcer 94–95
Pericardiacophrenic arteries, of the diaphragm 118
Pericardium, defined 50
Perinatal management, of congenital diaphragmatic hernias 121
Peristalsis
  control of, in swallowing 11
  evaluating with contrast radiography 294
  investigation of 10–11

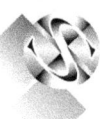

Peristalsis (cont.)
  primary, in swallowing 9–10
  response to oesophageal reflux 14
  secondary, in swallowing 10
  in the small intestine, effect on absorptive capacity 41
Peritoneum, relationships with the diaphragm 50
Pernicious anaemia
  association with autoimmune atrophic gastritis 271
  risk of gastric cancer in 98
Peutz-Jeghers syndrome
  gastric polyps in 246–247
  risk for small bowel malignancies in 197
Peyer's patches, in the ileum 41
pH
  of duodenal contents, change in with location 41
  effect on gastrin release 35
  response of pepsin to 30
Phagocytosis
  promotion of, by opsonic proteins of the spleen 60
  by the spleen, outcomes of loss of 134–135
Photodynamic therapy (PDT), for treating oesophageal dysplasia or cancer 266–267
Phrenic nerves
  palsy of, differentiating from eventration of the diaphragm 122
  paralysis of, breathing with bending or lifting in 57
  passage through the diaphragm 48
  supply to the diaphragm 49
Phreno-oesophageal ligament, attachment of the oesophagus to 5, 48
Physical signs, of Crohn's disease 104
Physiology
  of the diaphragm 50–58
  of the oesophagus 8–14
  of the small intestine 40–43
  of the spleen 60, 128–132, 221
  of the stomach 30–31
Pitting, removal of intra-erythrocyte inclusions by the spleen through 129, 135
Plasmapheresis, for treating thrombotic thrombocytopenic purpura 62
Platelets
  sensitisation of, by antiplatelet IgG autoantibodies 140–141
  transfusion of, before splenectomy 226
Pleura, separation of the diaphragm from the lung by 50
Pleural cavities, expansion of, during gestation 47
Pleural pressure, during relaxation, relationship with diaphragm muscle relaxation 55–56
Pleuroperitoneal membranes, embryologic development of 47
Plummer-Vinson/Patterson-Kelly syndrome 84

Plummer-Vinson syndrome, surveillance of patients with, for squamous cell carcinoma 266
Pneumatosis cystoides intestinalis 110–111
Polar artery, superior, branch of the splenic artery 60
Polypectomy, for gastric adenoma removal 283
Polyps, gastric 246–247
Polysplenia, association with congenital anomalies 135
Portal hypertension
  oesophageal varices as a complication of 242
  in patients with splenic arteriovenous fistula 147–148
Positron emission tomography (PET)
  with 18-fluorodeoxyglucose, to detect distant metastases before surgery 366
  for staging oesophageal cancer 320, 356
Posterior nerve of Latarjet, regulation of, by the spleen 26
Posterior vagus nerve, of the stomach 26
Postero-inferior surface, of the stomach 20–21
Postoperative care, after D2 dissection 346
Postural control, effect of the diaphragm on 56–57
Posture, effects of, on the diaphragm during breathing 52–53
Prednisone, for treating immune thrombocytopenic purpura 62
Preoperative evaluation, for splenorrhaphy 153
Preoperative preparation
  for splenectomy 226
  for surgery, in Crohn's disease 107
Presentation. See Clinical presentation
Pressure difference, across the diaphragm 50–51
Prevention, of gastrointestinal haemorrhage from acute gastritis 97
Primary care, for gastro-oesophageal reflux disease 70–72
Prognosis
  in Barrett's adenocarcinoma associated with aneuploidy 262
  in gastrointestinal stromal tumours 215–216
  in oesophageal adenocarcinoma 263
  in squamous cell and adenocarcinoma of the oesophagus 318–320
Prophylaxis, anti-thrombus, after surgery for Crohn's disease 107
Proton pump, gastric, production of hydrochloric acid by 29
Proton pump inhibitors
  in managing small bowel syndrome 114
  for treating Barrett's oesophagus 264
  for treating gastro-esophageal reflux 188
Proto-oncogene, bcl-2, role in oesophageal dysplasia to carcinoma sequence 262
Proximal gastrectomy (PG), indications for 336
Public Health Laboratory Service (PHLS), data on pneumococci-resistant penicillin 228
Pyloric atresia 19

# INDEX

Pyloric dilatation, balloons for 283
Pyloric sphincter, role of, in gastric motility 36
Pyloric stenosis 95, 242
Pyloric zone, of the stomach 29–32
Pylorus
    anatomy of 20
    congenital double 19
Pylorus preserving gastrectomy (PPG) 336–337
Pyruvate kinase, reticulocytes deficient in, in spherocytosis 141

## Q

Quality of life, and choice of treatment
    for gastro-oesophageal reflux disease 74
    for oesophageal cancer 350–351

## R

Radiation Therapy Oncology Group, randomised trial of chemoradiotherapy for oesophageal squamous carcinoma 361
Radical radiotherapy, for oesophageal cancer patients not suitable for resection 359–360
Radiochemotherapy, for stomach cancer, comparison with surgery alone 338
Radiology
    for detecting small bowel Crohn's disease 104–105
    to diagnose splenic neoplasms 225
    for diagnosis of traumatic diaphragmatic rupture 124–125
    in gastrointestinal surgery 287–292
Radionuclide imaging 302–305
    of lymphatic flow from the oesophagus 8
Radiotherapy
    after antibiotic therapy for mucosal associated lymphoid tissue lymphoma 237
    for gastric cancer 179–180
        lymphomas 237–239
    for oesophageal cancer management 359–366
    for palliation in oesophageal cancer 162
    to the stomach, limitations on 366
    technique of 364
        for treating gastric lymphoma 238–239
    in upper gastrointestinal tract neoplasms 359–368
Randomised trials
    comparing chemotherapy regimens in oesophagogastric cancer 351
    comparing chemotherapy with best supportive care, for gastric cancer chemotherapy 349–350
    of neoadjuvant chemotherapy with radiotherapy and surgery, list 165, 179
    of neoadjuvant radiochemotherapy versus surgery alone in oesophageal cancer 360–361
    of surgery with and without radiotherapy, for stomach cancer 366

Ranitidine
    effects of, on acid secretion 34
    for treating peptic ulcer disease 93
Rapid-eye-movement sleep, paradoxical movement of the rib cage with inspiration during 53–56
Recent Ionising Radiation Medical Exposure Regulations (IRMER) 287
Reconstruction, after transthoracic oesophagectomy 330
Recurrence rate, of peptic ulcer disease after surgery 92
Red blood cells
    abnormal, removal from circulation in the spleen 60
        splenomegaly due to 61
    transfusion to manage splenic sequestration in sickle cell disease 140
Red pulp, of the spleen 60
    involution of 128
Reed-Sternberg cells
    for characterisation of Hodgkin's disease 62
    in Hodgkin's disease, splenomegaly associated with 224
Reflux
    and development of gastric cancer 170
    oesophageal response to 14
Reflux oesophagitis 243
Regional enteritis/ileitis (Crohn's disease) 101–109
    as a predisposing factor for small bowel neoplasms 195
Region of interest (ROI), analysis over, in an oesophageal transit study 308–309
Relationships, anatomical, of the oesophagus 3–5
Relaxation, of the diaphragm 53–56
Renal failure, chronic, effect on fasting levels of gastrin 32
Replacement, oesophageal, evaluating 314
Resection
    combined organ, for lymphadenectomy 340–341
    D2, for oesophageal cancer 325
    endoscopic mucosal 284
    laparoscopic, in gastric cancer 174
    for leiomyosarcoma management 214
    for malignant oesophageal gastrointestinal stromal tumours 214
    for oesophageal cancer, role of extended lymphadenectomy 317–334
    open curative, in gastric cancer 174–178
    segmental, for benign lesions of the small bowel 193
    surgical, in managing oesophageal cancer, aims of 320–321
    of the stomach, with lymph node dissection 335
Resolution, of endoscopic ultrasound 160
Respiration, the role of diaphragm relaxation in 56
Retching, description of 37

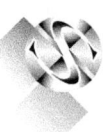

Reticulocytes, pyruvate kinase deficient, haemolysis in 141
Reticuloendothelial system, development of, from sinusoids of the splenic artery 59
Revised European-American Lymphoma (REAL) classification 203
Rheumatoid arthritis, oesophageal motility in 83
Rib cage
  effect of diaphragmatic contraction on 51-52
  stabilization of, by intercostal muscles 56
Rifampicin, for treating tuberculous enteritis 109
Rings, oesophageal 85
Risk analysis, for selecting patients for oesophagectomy and reconstruction 320
Risk factors
  for Barrett's adenocarcinoma 263
  for small bowel neoplasms 195-198
  in splenectomy, laparoscopic 226-227
  for stomach cancer 181
Roux-en-Y, for reconstruction after gastrectomy 96, 344
Royal Marsden Hospital, United Kingdom, on combination regimen for chemotherapy
  in gastric cancer 350
  in oesophagogastric cancer, randomised trials 351
Rupture
  oesophageal, site of 5
  splenic 148-149
    as a complication of splenic abscess 137-138

## S

Safety margin, of lymphadenectomy 327
*Salmonella Typhi*, typhoid fever caused by 109-110
Sarco(endo)-plasmic reticulum $Ca^{2+}$-ATPase (SERCA), in the human diaphragm 54
Sarcomas, defined 207
Sarcomeres, auxotonic relaxation of 55
Sarcoplasmic reticulum (SR), calcium ion pumping by 53-54
Savary-Miller system, for grading oesophagitis 70-71
Scavenging, by the spleen 135
Schatzki ring 85
Schilling's test, for diagnosing blind loop syndrome 112
*Schistosoma mansoni* infection, effect of, on the spleen 143
Schwannomas, gastrointestinal 209
Scleroderma, oesophageal 82-83
  transit scintigraphy for identifying 309
Screening
  for Barrett's oesophagus 263-264
  for squamous cell carcinoma, regional variations in 266
Secondary care, for gastro-oesophageal reflux disease 70-72

Second look operation, in small bowel syndrome 114
Secretin
  production of, in enteroendocrine cells of intestinal crypts 40
    in response to acid 42
  release in the small intestine, effect on gastric activity 35
  suppression of release in the intestine, by somatostatin 32
Secretions, in the small intestine 42
Sedation, techniques in endoscopy 281-282
Selective tyrosine kinase inhibitor (STI-571), for treating gastrointestinal stromal tumours 204
Self-expanding metal stents (SEMS), for malignant disease management 284
Sensation, oesophageal 14
Sentinel lymphadenectomy, for early Barrett's cancer 333
Sepsis
  control of, in small bowel fistula management 112
  in overwhelming post-splenectomy infection 150-151
Septum transversum, development of the diaphragm from 46-47
Sequestration, splenic, in sickle cell anaemia 139-140
Serine threonine kinase, gene for, mutation in Peutz-Jeghers syndrome 197
Serotonin, synthesis by neuroendocrine cells of the oxyntic zone of the stomach 29
Serous coat (adventitia), of the stomach 27
Serous membranes, association of the diaphragm with 50
Sex
  and incidence of adenocarcinoma of the oesophagus 188-189
  and incidence of Barrett's oesophagus 259
  and incidence of stomach cancer 182
  and mortality from gastric gastrointestinal stromal tumours 216
  and survival of stomach cancer 186-187
Short bowel syndrome 113-114
Sickle cell disease (SCD)
  hereditary, splenectomy for treating 63
  involvement of the spleen in 139-140
  splenic infarction in 146-147
Sinogram, gastrointestinal 296
Skin-stoma care, for small bowel fistula management 112-113
Small bowel
  anatomy and physiology of 39-44
  benign disease of 101-115
  diverticular disease of 111
  emptying of, radionuclide study 305
  enema for gastrointestinal evaluation 296

# INDEX

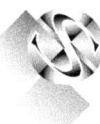

fistulas of 112–113
   massive resection of, effect on fasting levels of gastrin 32
   for gastrointestinal stromal tumour management 215
   neoplasms of 193–206
   radiotherapy for managing neoplasms of 367
Small bowel adenocarcinoma (SBA), predisposing factors for 195
Small cell carcinoma, of the oesophagus 365
Smoking
   and recurrence of ileocolic involvement in Crohn's disease 108
   as a risk factor, for atrophic gastritis 272
      for gastric cancer 170
      for squamous cell carcinoma of the oesophagus 182, 247
Somatostatin
   distribution of 32
   for small bowel fistula management 112
Spasm, diffuse oesophageal 81
Spherocytosis, hereditary, splenectomy for treating 63, 141
Sphincters
   oesophageal 2–3
      functions of 1
      gastro-oesophageal reflux disease from failure of 70
   vasoactive intestinal peptide nerves of 32
Sphingomyelin, accumulation of, in Niemann-Pick disease 145
Spindle cell carcinoma, of the oesophagus 247
Splanchnic nerves, transmission through the diaphragm 48
Spleen 59–67
   benign diseases of 127–154
   embryonic development of, attachment to the stomach 19
   neoplasms of 221–230
Splenectomy 149–151
   alternatives to 151–153
   in D2 total gastrectomy, randomized control trial for evaluating 341
   elective, principles of 64–65
   indications for 226
   laparoscopic 64–65, 153–154, 226–227
   partial, advantages of 151–152
      in Gaucher's disease 145
   segmental 152
      for treating schistosomiasis 143
   in sickle cell disease, indications for 140
   after trauma 65–66
   for treatment, of hematologic disorders 61–64
      of hyper-reactive malarial splenomegaly 142
      of hypersplenism 136
      of splenic abscess 147
      of thalassemia 142
Splenic arteriovenous fistula 147–148

Splenic artery
   aneurysm of 146
   blood supply to the spleen by 128
   blood supply to the stomach by 22–23
Splenic contraction, in haematemesis 130–131
Splenic enlargement, causes of 222–225
Splenic index 148
   for determining suitability of laparoscopic splenectomy 64
Splenic infarct 146–147
Splenic torsion (ectopic spleen) 135
Splenic vein, thrombosis of 146
Splenogonadal fusion 135
Splenomegaly 61
   in bilharzia 143
   causes of 148, 223–225
   in diffuse splenic disease 139
   due to thalassaemia major 142
Splenorenal ligament, embryonic formation of 59
Splenorrhaphy 153
Splenosis, defined 147–148
Spontaneous oesophageal perforation 87
Squamocolumnar junction, endoscopic visualisation of 5
Squamous carcinoma
   association with achalasia 81
   association with oesophageal diverticula 83
Squamous cell carcinoma (SCC)
   epidemiology of 264–265
   oesophageal 156
      radiotherapy for 163
      results of lymphadenectomy for 327–328
      surgical approach to 329–330
Squamous epithelial dysplasia 250
   oesophageal, as a premalignant lesion 259, 264–267
Squamous papilloma, oesophageal, as a premalignant lesion 259
Stage migration
   in evaluating gastric cancer 168–169, 175
   in evaluating nodal dissection for gastric cancer 338
   in evaluating oesophageal cancer 327
Staging
   with 18-fluorodeoxyglucose positron emission tomography 366
   of adenocarcinoma of the small bowel, TNM system for 202–203
   of gastric cancer 168–169, 172–174
   of gastric carcinomas 255–256
   of Hodgkin's disease 62
   of non-Hodgkin's lymphoma, gastric 233
   of oesophageal cancer 255–256
      investigations for 157–162
      before surgery 320
      and survival rates 186–187
   of oesophageal carcinoma 255–256

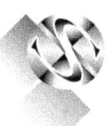

Staging (cont.)
    of small bowel tumours, computed tomography for 200
    of splenic trauma 149
    of stomach cancer, and survival rates 186–187
    See also Grading
Standard distal gastrectomy 344–345
Standard mediastinal lymphadenectomy, defined 275, 324
*Staphylococcus*, infection by, after splenectomy 66
Stem cells, Barrett's oesophagus and dysplasia arising from 261
Stenosing tumours, endoscopic dilatation in 284
Stenosis, rectal and anal, in Crohn's disease 104
Stents, for managing oesophageal cancer 163, 284
Sternal elements of the diaphragm 117
Steroids, for treating Crohn's disease 106–107
Stomach
    anatomy and physiology of 17–37
    benign diseases of 91–99
    carcinoma of 182–187, 366–367
    epithelial neoplasms of 167–180
    high risk lesions in 271–277
    pathology of 241–257
    See also Gastric *entries*
Stoma site, preoperative marking of 107
Stout's bizarre smooth muscle tumours, defined 207
*Streptococcus pneumoniae*, infection by, after splenectomy 66
Stricturoplasty, in Crohn's disease surgery 107–108
Stromal tumours
    gastrointestinal 204
    of the oesophagus and stomach 255
    upper gastrointestinal 207–219
Stromal tumours of uncertain malignant potential (STUMP), defined 207
Structure of the oesophagus 5–7
Subcardial gastric carcinoma 318
Submucosal network of lymphatic drainage of the stomach 24
Submucous coat of the stomach 27
Subpyloric glands, drainage from the stomach through 24–25
Subserosal network, of lymphatic drainage of the stomach 24
Substance P
    of the duodenum 32
    in the gastrointestinal tract 33
Succus entericus, flow of secretions across the small bowel mucosa 42
Sugars, absorption by the stomach 33
Sulfasalazine, for treating Crohn's disease 105–106
Suprapyloric nodes, drainage from the stomach into 24
Surfaces, of the stomach 20–21

Surgery
    for adenocarcinoma of the small bowel 193–194
    approach to oesophageal cancer 329–333
    approach to the oesophagus, by segment 4–5
    for congenital diaphragmatic hernia 122
    for Crohn's disease 107–108
    gastrointestinal, imaging in 287–305
    for gastrointestinal stromal tumours 214–215
    oesophageal perforation during 88
    risks of, in large cell gastric lymphoma 237
    role in bleeding peptic ulcer management 94
    for small bowel syndrome 114
    See also Management; Resection; Treatment
Surveillance, in Barrett's oesophagus 263–264
Surveillance, Epidemiology, and End-Results (SEER) Program, reported incidence of small bowel tumours 194
Swallowing, physiology of the oesophagus in 9–10
Swallowing centre, of the brainstem 8
Sydney classification, of gastritis 246
Sympathetic nerve supply
    of the oesophagus 8
    of the stomach 26–27
Symptoms, of eventration of the diaphragm 122–123

T

Taxanes, in a multiple drug regimen for treating oesophagogastric cancer 351
T cell lymphoma, enteropathy-associated 203
$^{99m}$Technetium, for white cell scanning 302–303
$^{99m}$Technetium-sulphur colloid scintigraphy, of splenic cysts 137
Telomerase, activity of, in Barrett's oesophagus 262
Temporal trends
    in oesophageal cancer incidence and mortality 183
    in stomach cancer incidence and mortality 182–183
Thalassaemia
    hereditary, splenectomy for treating 63
    uptake of damaged cells by the spleen 141–142
Therapeutic endoscopy
    for benign disease 282–283
    for malignant disease 283–285
Thermal ablation, for palliative treatment of oesophageal cancer 162–163
Thoracic duct
    lymphatic drainage by 4
    passage through the diaphragm 48
Thoracic oesophagus, anatomy of 3–4
Thoracic outlet, effect of, on the diaphragm 45–46
Thoracic plexus, of the diaphragm 49
Three-dimensional conformal radiotherapy (3D-CRT), for planning radiotherapy 238

# INDEX

Thrombocytopenic purpura
    idiopathic 140–141
    immune, splenectomy for treating 61–62
    splenectomy for treating 150
    thrombotic, mortality in 62
Thrombocytosis, after splenectomy 66, 227
Thrombotic thrombocytopenic purpura (TTP), mortality in 62
Thymidylate synthase (TS), elevated levels of, and resistance to 5-fluorouracil 357
Thyroid-stimulating hormone (THS), suppression of release of, by somatostatin 32
Tight junctions, of the epithelial lining of the stomach 28, 30
Time activity curves (TACs), for evaluating oesophageal transit 308–309
T lymphocytes
    effector, development of, in the spleen 131–132
    mucosal, activation in Crohn's disease 102
    periarteriolar, in the white pulp of the spleen 60
    the spleen as a reservoir of 134–135
Toluidine, to stain mucosal abnormalities 280
Topoisomerase I inhibitor, in a multiple drug regimen for treating oesophagogastric cancer 351
Total gastrectomy (TG), pancreas preserving 341–344
Total parenteral nutrition (TPN), after surgery for small bowel syndrome 114
Toupet operation 75–76
Toxicity, of radiotherapy and chemoradiotherapy 364–365
TP 53 mutations, and development of squamous cell carcinoma 265–266
Tracheal bifurcation, types of tumours above and below 318
Tracheobronchial tree bronchoscopy, for staging oesophageal carcinoma 320
Tracheo-oesophageal fistulas (TOF) 85–86
Tracheo-oesophageal septum, development of 2
Transcutaneous ultrasound, for diagnosing oesophageal cancer 158
Transdiaphragmatic pressure (Pdi)
    elevation of, during lifting 57
    variation of maximum relaxation rate with 55
Transforming growth factor-ß (TGF-ß) receptor, role in gastric carcinogenesis 274
Transient lower oesophageal sphincter (tLOS), relaxation of 12
Transit studies, with radiopharaceuticals 304–305
Translocations, chromosomal, in low grade mucosal associated lymphoid tissue 234
Transmediastinal oesophagectomy, comparison with transthoracic oesophagectomy 329
Transthoracic oesophagectomy
    comparison with transmediastinal oesophagectomy 329
    reconstruction after 330

Trauma
    diaphragmatic rupture due to 123–126
    oesophageal perforation from 88
    responses of the spleen to 65
    rupture 148–149
    splenectomy for managing injuries from 61, 149–150
    splenic arteriovenous fistula leading to 147–148
    to the stomach and duodenum 98
Treatment
    of achalasia 80–81
    of Barrett's oesophagus 264
    choice of, after staging 173
    of intraluminal polyps of tumours 87
    of lymphoma 233–234
    of oesophageal cancer 162–165
        with curative intent 163–165
    of oesophageal perforation 88
    of oesophageal squamous papilloma 268
    of oesophagitis due to caustic injury 76–77
    of peptic ulcer disease 92–93
    of perforation in gastric ulcers 95
    of small bowel syndrome 113–114
    of splenic abscesses 138
    of squamous epithelial dysplasia 266
    of tuberculous enteritis 109
    See also Adjuvant therapy; Eradication therapy; Gastric therapy; Management; Neoadjuvant entries; Nutritional therapy; Surgery
Trisomy 3, in mucosal associated lymphatic disorders 234
Tropical diseases, involving the spleen 142
Tropical splenomegaly syndrome (hyper-reactive malarial splenomegaly) 142
Troponin C (TnC), removal of calcium ion from, in muscle relaxation and contraction 54
Truncal vagotomy, effects of, on gastric motility 36
Trunk, stability of, effect of the diaphragm on 56–57
*Trypanosoma cruzi*, achalasia caused by 79
Tuberculosis
    extrapulmonary, association with infliximab administration 106
    intestinal, as a risk factor for lymphoma 196
Tuberculous enteritis 109
Tuberculous splenomegaly 144
Tuftsin, production in the spleen 132
Tumour, Node, Metastasis (TNM) classification. See Classification
Tumour factors, in D2 dissection in gastric cancer 339–340
Tumour necrosis factor-ß (TNF-ß), role in neoplastic progression of Barrett's oesophagus 262
Tumour necrosis factor-ß, inhibition of, to treat Crohn's disease 106

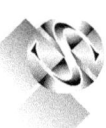

Tumours, oesophageal
  differentiating benign from malignant with contrast radiography 293
  spread of 156–157
Tylosis, association of oesophageal squamous papilloma with 267
Typhoid enteritis 109–110
Tyrosine kinase receptor, roles of 208

## U

Ulceration, non-specific, of the small bowel 111–112
Ultrasonography
  for gastrointestinal evaluation 296–297
  of splenic abscess 137–138
  for splenic cyst identification 137
  for splenic neoplasm diagnosis 225
  for traumatic diaphragmatic rupture confirmation 124–125
  for tuberculous splenomegaly identification 144
Umbilical herniation, physiological, during embryologic development of the small intestine 43
Umbilicus, fistula connecting the small intestine with 44
Union Internacional Contra la Cancrum (UICC), TNM classification of, for gastric cancer 338
Union Internacional Contra la Cancrum/American Joint Committee on Cancer, guidelines for resection in oesophageal cancer 318
University of Hong Kong, randomised trial, radiotherapy or no treatment after oesophagectomy 360
Upper gastrointestinal endoscopy 279–286
Upper oesophageal diverticula 83
Upper oesophageal sphincter (UOS)
  physiology of, during swallowing 9
  structure of 5

## V

Vaccines, prophylactic, before splenectomy 150
Vaculolating cytotoxin (Vac A), effect on development of gastric carcinoma 272
Valvulae conniventes, association with absorption from the small intestine 41
Varices
  endoscopy for management of 282
  oesophageal, clinical importance of 7
  in portal hypertension 242
Vascular diseases, of the spleen 146–148
Vascular ring (dysphagia lusoria) 85
Vascular supply, to the diaphragm 118. *See also* Arteries
Vasoactive intestinal peptide (VIP)
  nerves utilizing 32
  production of, response to chyme entering the duodenum 42–43

Vasodilatation, by vasoactive intestinal peptide 32
Veins, splenic, anatomy of 60
Vena caval aperture of the diaphragm 48
Venous drainage
  of the diaphragm 49
  of the oesophagus 7
  of the stomach 23–24
Ventilation, correction of hypoxaemia with, in congenital diaphragmatic hernia 121
Ventral mesogastrium, embryonic formation of 17–18
Verrucous carcinoma, defined 250
Video clips, to evaluate motility disorders, with contrast radiography 293–294
Vimentin, as a marker for mesenchymal tissue 212–214
Viral replication, in the spleen 144–145
Vitamins
  $B_{12}$, dependence of intestinal absorption of on intrinsic factor 31
    malabsorption of, after resection of the small bowel 113
    replacement therapy after total gastrectomy 97
  C, inhibition of conversion of nitrates to nitroso-mutagens by 273
  E, reversal of intestinal metaplasia by 273
Vitello-intestinal duct, abnormalities of 44
Vocal cord palsy, from surgical trauma to the laryngeal nerves 3
Vomiting, description of 36–37
Von Recklinghausen's disease, risk for small bowel neoplasms associated with 197–198

## W

Water, absorption from the stomach 33
Water-soluble contrast swallow, in contrast radiography 294
Webs, oesophageal 84
Whipple's procedure (pancreaticoduodenectomy) 193
  for adenomatous polyp management 201
White cell scanning, with radiopharmaceuticals 302–303
White pulp, of the spleen
  B lymphocytes of 60
  involution of 128
  involvement in lymphoma 138
Widal test, for typhoid 110
World Congress of Gastroenterology, guidelines for classifying and grading gastritis 246, 251–253
World Health Organisation (WHO)
  classification of adenocarcinoma, oesophageal 250
  TNM staging system of 157

# INDEX

**X**

X-rays, plain abdominal, for diagnosing small bowel tumours 199. *See also* Radiology

**Z**

Zenker's diverticulum 83
Zinc, deficiency of, and oesophageal cancer 182
Z-line, squamocolumnar junction visibility as 5
Zollinger-Ellison syndrome (gastrinoma)
    effect of, on fasting levels of gastrin 32
    excluding in treating peptic ulcer disease 93
    gastrin-secreting tumours in 246
Zymogenic cells, pepsin precursors in 29

Lightning Source UK Ltd.
Milton Keynes UK
UKHW050048061218
333496UK00021B/698/P